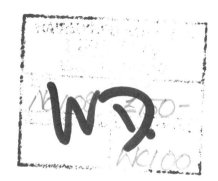

Infectious Diseases
in Critical Care
Medicine

INFECTIOUS DISEASE AND THERAPY

Series Editor

Burke A. Cunha

Winthrop-University Hospital
Mineola, and
State University of New York School of Medicine
Stony Brook, New York

1. Parasitic Infections in the Compromised Host, *edited by Peter D. Walzer and Robert M. Genta*
2. Nucleic Acid and Monoclonal Antibody Probes: Applications in Diagnostic Methodology, *edited by Bala Swaminathan and Gyan Prakash*
3. Opportunistic Infections in Patients with the Acquired Immunodeficiency Syndrome, *edited by Gifford Leoung and John Mills*
4. Acyclovir Therapy for Herpesvirus Infections, *edited by David A. Baker*
5. The New Generation of Quinolones, *edited by Clifford Siporin, Carl L. Heifetz, and John M. Domagala*
6. Methicillin-Resistant *Staphylococcus aureus*: Clinical Management and Laboratory Aspects, *edited by Mary T. Cafferkey*
7. Hepatitis B Vaccines in Clinical Practice, *edited by Ronald W. Ellis*
8. The New Macrolides, Azalides, and Streptogramins: Pharmacology and Clinical Applications, *edited by Harold C. Neu, Lowell S. Young, and Stephen H. Zinner*
9. Antimicrobial Therapy in the Elderly Patient, *edited by Thomas T. Yoshikawa and Dean C. Norman*
10. Viral Infections of the Gastrointestinal Tract: Second Edition, Revised and Expanded, *edited by Albert Z. Kapikian*
11. Development and Clinical Uses of *Haemophilus b* Conjugate Vaccines, *edited by Ronald W. Ellis and Dan M. Granoff*
12. *Pseudomonas aeruginosa* Infections and Treatment, *edited by Aldona L. Baltch and Raymond P. Smith*
13. Herpesvirus Infections, *edited by Ronald Glaser and James F. Jones*
14. Chronic Fatigue Syndrome, *edited by Stephen E. Straus*
15. Immunotherapy of Infections, *edited by K. Noel Masihi*
16. Diagnosis and Management of Bone Infections, *edited by Luis E. Jauregui*
17. Drug Transport in Antimicrobial and Anticancer Chemotherapy, *edited by Nafsika H. Georgopapadakou*
18. New Macrolides, Azalides, and Streptogramins in Clinical Practice, *edited by Harold C. Neu, Lowell S. Young, Stephen H. Zinner, and Jacques F. Acar*

Infectious Diseases in Critical Care Medicine

Second Edition

edited by

Burke A. Cunha

Winthrop-University Hospital
Mineola
and
State University of New York School of Medicine
Stony Brook, New York, U.S.A.

Informa Healthcare USA, Inc.
270 Madison Avenue
New York, NY 10016

© 2007 by Informa Healthcare USA, Inc.
Informa Healthcare is an Informa business

No claim to original U.S. Government works
Printed in the United States of America on acid-free paper
10 9 8 7 6 5 4 3 2 1

International Standard Book Number-10: 0-8493-3617-1 (Hardcover)
International Standard Book Number-13: 978-0-8493-3617-1 (Hardcover)

Library of Congress Cataloging-in-Publication Data

Infectious diseases in critical care medicine / edited by Burke A. Cunha. --2nd ed.
    p. ; cm. -- (Infectious disease and therapy ; 40)
  Includes bibliographical references and index.
  ISBN-13: 978-0-8493-3617-1 (hardcover : alk. paper)
  ISBN-10: 0-8493-3617-1 (hardcover : alk. paper)
  1. Nosocomial infections. 2. Critical care medicine. 3. Intensive care units. I. Cunha, Burke A. II. Series.
  [DNLM: 1. Communicable Diseases--diagnosis. 2. Critical Care. 3. Diagnosis, Differential. 4. Intensive Care Units. W1 IN406HMN v.40 2006 / WC 100 I4165 2006]

RC112.I4595 2006
616.9'0475--dc22   2006046567

Visit the Informa Web site at
www.informa.com

and the Informa Healthcare Web site at
www.informahealthcare.com

For
Marie

Peerless wife and mother,
Provider of domestic peace and harmony,
Paragon of truth and beauty,
Paradigm of earthly perfection . . .

With gratitude for love and constant support.

Foreword

In the United States, there are over 4000 intensive care units containing 87,000 beds. While the number of hospitals has been more than decreasing in the United States over the past decade, the number of intensive care unit beds has increased. From 1985 to 2000, while the total number of U.S. hospitals decreased by 8.9% and total beds decreased by 26.4%, the number of intensive care unit beds increased by 26.2% (1–3).

Intensive care unit beds have a high occupancy rate (over 65% nationally). The acuity of patients in those beds is rising. The costs associated with intensive care unit care have risen at a faster rate from 1985 to 2000 (190%) than the cost of hospital care in general (150%) and the gross domestic product (133%). Analyses have estimated that intensive care unit care cost the United States $33 billion to $55 billion in 1995 (3–5). Thus, these numbers give a numerical background to the trend obvious to all health care providers: a larger and larger fraction of hospitalized patients have high acuity and require extensive resources if the patients needing such care are to benefit from the impressive advances medical science has made over the past several decades.

Intensive care units have become such an integral part of the health care complex over the past 40 years because medical science has developed the technical and cognitive skills to reverse life-threatening processes with an increasingly higher success rate than was conceivable even one or two decades ago. Victims of trauma, cancer, acute infections, myocardial damage, hemorrhagic diatheses, renal failure, hepatic failure, or neurologic catastrophes are examples of patients who have a far better prognosis in 2005 if they can have prompt access to modern critical care facilities.

In terms of the infections that bring patients to intensive care units, patient outcome has improved substantially. These improvements include a more sophisticated understanding of pathophysiology, more accurate and less invasive diagnostic approaches, and a dramatic expansion of therapeutic options. These improvements have permitted patients to survive despite sepsis, human immunodeficiency virus infection, fungal disease, or viral processes to a degree not imagined two decades ago.

Many other patients, however, are admitted to intensive care units with noninfectious catastrophes, only to have their courses complicated or their lives terminated by infections they acquired in the intensive care unit. Thus, ventilator-associated pneumonia, intravascular catheter-associated sepsis, urosepsis due to a urethral catheter or fungal superinfection, and candidemia are examples of processes that can be prevented to a substantial degree by improved strategies to prevent such complications. When infections do occur, they are more likely to be due to antibiotic-resistant pathogens because of heavy antibiotic exposure in the intensive care unit and the contamination of patients with pathogens transmitted from other sick patients by aerosols, droplets, fomites, or health care staff. As many as 45% of nosocomial infections occur in intensive care unit patients, although intensive care unit beds account for only 13% of all hospital beds.

In this book edited by Burke A. Cunha, 32 chapters summarize the current knowledge concerning infectious diseases occurring in the field of critical care medicine. The material described in this book is written by an impressive team of experienced clinicians who deal regularly with patients in intensive care units. The material covered in these chapters is a compilation of information on general concepts, specific syndromes, and current management strategies that combines material that is derived from disparate sources. For intensivists, and for hospitalists, house officers, and consultants who spend much of their time caring for patients in intensive care units, this focused book will be most useful.

Critical care medicine is an expanding aspect of health care in the developed world. Proper management of infectious complications is an important priority, given the magnitude and impact of the infections on patient outcome. Regular updates of this book will be most useful.

Henry Masur
Department of Critical Care
National Institutes for Health
Bethesda, Maryland, U.S.A.

REFERENCES

1. Angus DC, Kelley MA, Schmitz RJ, White A, Popovich J Jr., Committee von Manpower for Pulmonary and Critical Care Societies (COMPACCS). Caring for the critically ill patient. Current and projected workforce requirements for care of the critically ill and patients with pulmonary disease: can we meet the requirements of an aging population? JAMA 2000; 284(21):2762–2770.
2. Cooper RA. The COMPACCS Study: questions left unanswered. The Committee on Manpower for Pulmonary and Critical Care Societies. Am J Respir Crit Care Med 2001; 163(1):10–11.
3. Halpern NA, Pastores SM, Greenstein RJ. Critical care medicine in the United States 1985–2000: an analysis of bed numbers, use, and costs. Crit Care Med 2004; 32:1254–1259.
4. Jacobs P, Noseworthy TW. National estimates of intensive care utilization and costs: Canada and the United States. Crit Care Med 1990; 18:1282–1286.
5. Halpern N, Bettes I, Greenstein R. Federal and nationwide intensive care units and health care costs: 1986–1992. Crit Care Med 1994; 4:2366–2373.

Preface

Infectious diseases continue to represent a major diagnostic and therapeutic challenge in the critical care unit. Infectious diseases maintain their preeminence in the critical care unit setting because of their frequency and importance in the critical care unit patient population. Since the first edition of *Infectious Disease in Critical Care Medicine*, there have been newly described infectious diseases to be considered in differential diagnosis, and new antimicrobial agents have been added to the therapeutic armamentarium. The second edition of *Infectious Diseases in Critical Care Medicine* continues the clinical orientation of the first edition. Differential diagnostic considerations in infectious diseases continue to be the central focus of the second edition.

Clinicians caring for acutely ill patients in the critical care unit are confronted with the common problem of differentiating noninfectious disease mimics from their infectious disease counterparts. For this reason, the differential diagnosis of noninfectious diseases remains an important component of infectious diseases in the second edition. The second edition of *Infectious Diseases in Critical Care Medicine* emphasizes differential clinical features that enable clinicians to sort out complicated diagnostic problems.

Because critical care unit patients often have complicated/interrelated multisystem disorders, subspecialty expertise is essential for optimal patient care. Early utilization of infectious disease consultation is important to assure proper application/interpretation of appropriate laboratory tests and for the selection/optimization of antimicrobial therapy. Selecting the optimal antimicrobial for use in the critical care unit is vital. As important is the optimization of antimicrobial dosing to take into account the pharmacokinetic and pharmacodynamic attributes of the antibiotic. The infectious disease clinician, in addition to optimizing dosing considerations, is also able to evaluate potential antimicrobial side effects as well as drug–drug interactions, which may affect therapy. Infectious disease consultations can be helpful in differentiating colonization ordinarily not treated from infection that should be treated. Physicians who are not infectious disease clinicians lack the necessary sophistication in clinical infectious disease training, medical microbiology, pharmacokinetics/pharmacodynamics, and diagnostic experience. Physicians in critical care units should rely on infectious disease clinicians as well as other consultants to optimize care for these acutely ill patients.

The second edition of *Infectious Diseases in Critical Care Medicine* has been streamlined while maintaining its clinical focus. Again, the authors have been selected for their expertise and experience. The contributors are world-class teachers/ clinicians who have, in their writings, imparted their clinical experience for the benefit of the critical care unit physicians and their patients. The second edition of *Infectious Diseases in Critical Care Medicine* remains the only book dealing with infections in critical care.

Burke A. Cunha

Contents

PART II: CLINICAL SYNDROMES

PART IV: THERAPEUTIC CONSIDERATIONS

Contributors

John G. Bartlett   Department of Medicine, School of Medicine, Johns Hopkins University, Baltimore, Maryland, U.S.A.

Emilio Bouza   Clinical Microbiology and Infectious Diseases Department, Hospital General Universitario "Gregorio Marañón," Universidad Complutense, Madrid, Spain

Richard B. Brown   Division of Infectious Disease, Baystate Medical Center and Tufts University School of Medicine, Springfield, Massachusetts, U.S.A.

John L. Brusch   Department of Medicine, Harvard Medical School, Cambridge, Massachusetts, U.S.A.

Almudena Burillo   Department of Clinical Microbiology, Hospital Madrid-Montepríncipe, Madrid, Spain

Brian W. Cooper   Division of Infectious Disease, Hartford Hospital, Hartford, and University of Connecticut School of Medicine, Farmington, Connecticut, U.S.A.

April Correll   Winthrop-University Hospital, Mineola, New York, U.S.A.

Giampaolo Corti   Infectious Disease Unit, University of Florence School of Medicine, Florence, Italy

Burke A. Cunha   Infectious Disease Division, Winthrop-University Hospital, Mineola, and State University of New York School of Medicine, Stony Brook, New York, U.S.A.

Marci Drees   Department of Geographic Medicine and Infectious Diseases, Tufts-New England Medical Center, Boston, Massachusetts, U.S.A.

Lee S. Engel   Department of Medicine, Louisiana State University Health Science Center, New Orleans, Louisiana, U.S.A.

Donald E. Fry   Department of Surgery, University of New Mexico School of Medicine, Albuquerque, New Mexico, U.S.A.

Sherwood L. Gorbach Nutrition/Infection Unit, Department of Public Health and Family Medicine, Tufts University School of Medicine, Boston, Massachusetts, U.S.A.

Eric V. Granowitz Division of Infectious Disease, Baystate Medical Center and Tufts University School of Medicine, Springfield, Massachusetts, U.S.A.

Diane H. Johnson Infectious Disease Division, Winthrop-University Hospital, Mineola, and State University of New York School of Medicine, Stony Brook, New York, U.S.A.

Meghann L. Kaiser Department of Surgery, University of California, Irvine School of Medicine, Orange, California, U.S.A.

Seung H. Kim Burn Center, United States Army Institute of Surgical Research, San Antonio, Texas, U.S.A.

Jason M. Lazar Department of Cardiology, State University of New York Downstate Medical Center, Brooklyn, New York, U.S.A.

Fred A. Lopez Department of Medicine, Louisiana State University Health Science Center, New Orleans, Louisiana, U.S.A.

Larry I. Lutwick Department of Infectious Diseases, VA New York Harbor Health Care System, and State University of New York Downstate Medical School, Brooklyn, New York, U.S.A.

C. Glen Mayhall Division of Infectious Diseases and Department of Healthcare Epidemiology, University of Texas Medical Branch at Galveston, Galveston, Texas, U.S.A.

Patricia Muñoz Clinical Microbiology and Infectious Diseases Department, Hospital General Universitario "Gregorio Marañón," Universidad Complutense, Madrid, Spain

Franco Paradisi Infectious Disease Unit, University of Florence School of Medicine, Florence, Italy

Laurel C. Preheim Departments of Medicine, Medical Microbiology and Immunology, Creighton University School of Medicine, University of Nebraska College of Medicine, and VA Medical Center, Omaha, Nebraska, U.S.A.

Basil A. Pruitt Division of Trauma and Emergency Surgery, Department of Surgery, University of Texas Health Science Center, and Burn Center, United States Army Institute of Surgical Research, San Antonio, Texas, U.S.A.

Charles V. Sanders Department of Medicine, Louisiana State University Health Science Center, New Orleans, Louisiana, U.S.A.

Louis D. Saravolatz Division of Infectious Disease, Department of Medicine, St. John Hospital and Medical Center, and Wayne State University School of Medicine, Detroit, Michigan, U.S.A.

David Schlossberg Infectious Disease Section, Department of Medicine, Temple University School of Medicine, Philadelphia, Pennsylvania, U.S.A.

Mamta Sharma Division of Infectious Disease, Department of Medicine, St. John Hospital and Medical Center, and Wayne State University School of Medicine, Detroit, Michigan, U.S.A.

John N. Sheagren Department of Internal Medicine, Advocate Illinois Masonic Medical Center, Chicago, Illinois, U.S.A.

Jihad Slim Infectious Disease Division, Department of Medicine, Seton Hall P.G. School of Medicine, and St. Michael's Medical Center, Newark, New Jersey, U.S.A.

Leon G. Smith Infectious Disease Division, Department of Medicine, Seton Hall P.G. School of Medicine, and St. Michael's Medical Center, Newark, New Jersey, U.S.A.

Donna Sym College of Pharmacy and Allied Health Professions, St. John's University, and North Shore University Hospital, Jamaica, New York, U.S.A.

Damary C. Torres College of Pharmacy and Allied Health Professions, St. John's University, Jamaica, and Winthrop-University Hospital, Mineola, New York, U.S.A.

María V. Torres Clinical Microbiology and Infectious Diseases Department, Hospital General Universitario "Gregorio Marañón," Universidad Complutense, Madrid, Spain

David R. Tribble Department of Enteric Diseases, Infectious Diseases Directorate, Naval Medical Research Institute, Silver Spring, Maryland, U.S.A.

Kenneth F. Wagner Independent Consultant, Infectious Diseases and Tropical Medicine, Islamorada, Florida, U.S.A.

Samuel E. Wilson Department of Surgery, University of California, Irvine School of Medicine, Orange, California, U.S.A.

Steven E. Wolf Division of Trauma and Emergency Surgery, Department of Surgery, University of Texas Health Science Center, and Burn Center, United States Army Institute of Surgical Research, San Antonio, Texas, U.S.A.

1

Methicillin-Resistant *Staphylococcus aureus*/Vancomycin-Resistant Enterococci Colonization and Infection in the Critical Care Unit

C. Glen Mayhall
Division of Infectious Diseases and Department of Healthcare Epidemiology, University of Texas Medical Branch at Galveston, Galveston, Texas, U.S.A.

INTRODUCTION

Methicillin-resistant *Staphylococcus aureus* (MRSA) and vancomycin-resistant enterococci (VRE) are among the most common antibiotic-resistant nosocomial pathogens in health care in general and in critical care units (CCUs) in particular. Although discovered shortly after its introduction, resistance to methicillin was first reported in the United States in 1968 (1,2). Since then, MRSA have spread throughout the world and have continued to spread in the United States. In many healthcare facilities, ≥50% of *S. aureus* isolates are MRSA. In intensive care units (ICUs), MRSA now make up 60% of *S. aureus* isolates (3).

As hospital-acquired methicillin-resistant *S. aureus* (HA-MRSA) continues to spread within healthcare facilities, sites where healthcare is delivered face a new threat from community-acquired methicillin-resistant *S. aureus* (CA-MRSA). These latter strains from the community first appeared in the 1990s and now have been detected throughout the United States and in many other countries throughout the world (4–12). Infections due to CA-MRSA occur in patients with no risk factors or recent contact with healthcare facilities. They commonly occur in healthy children and most commonly manifest as skin and soft-tissue infections (13–15). Most patients require treatment, and 23% to 29% have required hospitalization (14,15).

The appearance of CA-MRSA raises concerns about an additional reservoir for MRSA for healthcare facilities. Indeed, reports have begun to appear of the introduction and spread of CA-MRSA in hospitals (16,17). Thus hospital epidemiologists and infection-control professionals will have to protect ICU patients from both HA-MRSA and CA-MRSA.

VRE are resistant gram-positive cocci that have appeared more recently in hospitals and ICUs. VRE were first noted in November 1986 and reported in January 1988 (18). In July 1988, VRE colonization of hematology patients was reported from

Paris (19). In 1989, 0.3% of enterococci (0.1% in ICUs) isolated from patients in hospitals participating in the National Nosocomial Infection Surveillance (NNIS) system at the Centers for Disease Control and Prevention (CDC) were resistant to vancomycin (20). In 1993, 7.9% of enterococci isolated in NNIS system hospitals (13.6% in ICUs) were resistant to vancomycin. By 2003, 28.5% of enterococci isolated in NNIS system hospital ICUs were resistant to vancomycin (21).

As normal flora, enterococci are not nearly as invasive as are *S. aureus*. Approximately 1 in 10 patients colonized with VRE develop infection (22), although this may vary with the degree of immunosuppression of the patients (23,24). The most serious infections with VRE are bacteremia, endocarditis, and meningitis. Urinary tract infections are less serious and easier to treat. Infections at other body sites are difficult to document, because VRE isolated from other sites frequently represent colonization and not infection (25,26).

METHICILLIN-RESISTANT *S. AUREUS*

Types of MRSA

Nosocomial Methicillin-Resistant S. aureus

Nosocomial methicillin-resistant *S. aureus* (NA-MRSA) first appeared in the United States in 1968 (2). It has spread across the United States over the last three-and-a-half decades by lateral transfer among hospital patients and by transfer of patients between hospitals and between hospitals and long-term care facilities. Most circulating strains of NA-MRSA appear to have originated from two or three clones of MRSA (27,28).

Methicillin resistance and resistance to all betalactam antibiotics are conferred by the staphylococcal cassette chromosome *mec* (SCC*mec*), which carries the *mecA* gene that encodes a protein designated "penicillin-binding protein 2a" or "penicillin-binding protein 2′." These altered penicillin-binding proteins bind betalactam antibiotics poorly, permitting cell wall synthesis to continue in the presence of these antimicrobial agents.

There are three types of SCC*mec* in HA-MRSA, types I, II, and III (4,29). Type I contains no additional resistance determinants, but types II and III contain resistance determinants in addition to *mecA*; these additional genetic elements account for the antimicrobial resistance to many antibiotics in addition to the beta-lactam agents. The three SCC*mec* types contained in NA-MRSA have an identical chromosomal integration site and the cassette chromosome recombinase genes, which are responsible for horizontal transfer of SCC*mec* (4). Thus, NA-MRSA are resistant to many antibiotics and have a selective advantage as they are spread among patients by the hands of personnel and other contaminated surfaces. The presence of underlying diseases and multiple types of instrumentation and procedures predisposes patients to colonization and infection by the multiply resistant strains of NA-MRSA.

Community-Acquired MRSA. CA-MRSA have appeared gradually over about the last 15 years. Early on there was uncertainty about the origin of CA-MRSA, and it was unclear whether CA-MRSA were different from NA-MRSA. Some investigators believed that most of the CA-MRSA infections could be traced back to some previous contact with the healthcare system. More recently, it has become clear that these infections occur in young healthy persons with no recent healthcare contacts and no risk factors for NA-MRSA. It has also become clear that CA-MRSA have evolved in the community through an evolutionary pathway entirely separate from NA-MRSA.

It appears that all four of the SCC*mec* types have risen from *Staphylococcus sciuri*, the most ubiquitous and ancient species of *Staphylococcus* (30). Due to their large size, SCC*mec* types I, II, and III have rarely been transferred to the cells of methicillin-susceptible *S. aureus* (MSSA). On the contrary, CA-MRSA has an SCC*mec* type IV that is small enough to be transferred between cells by transduction or phage-mediated transformation (30,31). There is some evidence that transfer of type IV SCC*mec* from CA-MRSA to MSSA can occur (29).

Given that many infections caused by CA-MRSA are treated in hospitals and other healthcare facilities, there must be some concern that CA-MRSA may become another type of MRSA in hospitals. In addition to infections, it is likely that patients admitted to hospitals for a variety of indications will be colonized with CA-MRSA.

In addition to adding to the burden of MRSA in the hospital, CA-MRSA appear to be more virulent than NA-MRSA. The MW2 strain of CA-MRSA, a common strain in the United States, has 18 toxins which were not found in five comparative *S. aureus* genomes (32). The majority of CA-MRSA contain the genetic element for the Panton-Valentine leukocidin. This toxin has been associated with necrotizing pneumonia in healthy children (6). The MW2 strain of CA-MRSA contains genes for 11 exotoxins and four enterotoxins. All of these toxins are super-antigens (32). CA-MRSA may also contain genes for exfoliative toxins and for hemolysins (33).

CA-MRSA most commonly cause skin and soft tissue infections in persons with no risk factors for NA-MRSA. However, they may cause severe disease, and hospital patients may be at particularly high risk for serious disease. It is very important that infection control programs be on guard for ingress of CA-MRSA into hospitals, and this is particularly true for ICUs.

Types of Infections Caused by MRSA

Infections Caused by NA-MRSA

Adult ICUs. Bacteremia and pneumonia are the most common NA-MRSA infections encountered when all types of ICUs are considered (34–39). Other NA-MRSA infections reported include urinary tract infections (34,35), empyema (35), and bacteremia associated with hemofiltration (38). Surgical site infections due to NA-MRSA are reported from ICUs that care for surgical patients, although most all of these infections were acquired in the operating room and not in the ICU (35,36).

Neonatal ICUs. NA-MRSA are recovered from many more sites of infection in patients in neonatal intensive care units (NICUs) compared with patients in adult ICUs. As is the case in adult ICUs, reports on sites of infection due to NA-MRSA in neonates are from publications of outbreak investigations. Table 1 shows the sites of infection due to NA-MRSA reported from outbreaks in NICUs.

Infections Caused by CA-MRSA

Adult ICUs. To date, all cases of CA-MRSA acquired in the hospital by adults have been reported from Australia (45–47). There were no reports of

Table 1   Sites of Infection Due to Nosocomial Methicillin-Resistant
Staphylococcus aureus in Patients in Neonatal Intensive Care Units

Sites of infection
Bacteremia, primary
Pneumonia
Skin and soft tissue abscess
Peritonitis or necrotizing enterocolitis
Ventriculitis or meningitis
Osteomyelitis or septic arthritis
Urinary tract infection
Eye infection
Wound infection
Endocarditis
Thrombophlebitis
Ear, nose and throat infection
Omphalitis

Source: From Refs. 40–44.

outbreaks in the ICUs of these hospitals. None of the isolates were tested for type of SCC*mec* or for Panton-Valentine leukocidin or other toxins often found in CA-MRSA. The strains of CA-MRSA were isolated from 24% to 42% of inhabitants in two communities remote from the urban area where patients from these communities were hospitalized. Only one of these reports provided limited information on the sites of infections (46). In the latter report, there were 19 episodes of bacteremia in 16 patients.

Neonatal ICUs.   Two outbreaks due to CA-MRSA have been reported from NICUs (17,48). In one outbreak, the isolates were identified as CA-MRSA by detection of a type IV SCC*mec* (17). However, virulence factors frequently found in CA-MRSA, including the element coding for Panton-Valentine leukocidin, were not detected in the outbreak strain. The second outbreak in an NICU was stated to be due to CA-MRSA, but no testing for the type of SCC*mec* or virulence factors was done (48). The mother of the index case had had contact with the healthcare system, and the antibiogram of the isolates suggested that they were likely NA-MRSA.

An outbreak has also been reported in a newborn nursery and associated maternity units (49). The isolates from this outbreak were shown to have the type IV SCC*mec* and genes for Panton-Valentine leukocidin and staphylococcal enterotoxin K.

Epidemiology of NA-MRSA Infections in Critical Care

Epidemiology of NA-MRSA

Adult ICUs.   The risk for adult patients who are culture-negative for NA-MRSA on admission to an ICU, where NA-MRSA is endemic, for acquiring NA-MRSA ranges between 4.5% and 11.7% for cumulative incidence (36,50) and between 7.9 and 9.9 per 1000 patient days for incidence density (51,52). In one study, it was observed that NA-MRSA was acquired at about 1% per day in the first week after admission and then at 3% per day thereafter (38).

Sources of NA-MRSA. The sources of NA-MRSA include colonized or infected patients, colonized or infected healthcare workers (HCWs), and contaminated environmental surfaces. One of the best indications of the importance of colonized and infected patients as an important source of NA-MRSA is the significant relationship between colonization pressure and acquisition of NA-MRSA colonization or infection by patients who have no colonization or infection due to NA-MRSA at the time of admission to an ICU (50). Colonization pressure is defined as the number of patient days for patients with cultures positive for NA-MRSA divided by the number of total patient days (53). Colonization pressure can be calculated for any day or for a given period of time. The most common site of MRSA colonization is the external nares (35,54,55). The second most common site of colonization is skin and soft tissue other than surgical sites (34%) (54). Other sites of colonization include rectal (11–28.9%), respiratory tract (11%), and urinary tract (6%) (35,54,55).

Another source of NA-MRSA is colonized or infected healthcare personnel. Acquisition of NA-MRSA in an ICU from a respiratory therapist with chronic sinusitis due to NA-MRSA has been reported, as well as surgical site infections due to colonization of the external nares and an area of dermatitis on the hand of a surgeon (56,57). The surgical site infections caused by the colonized surgeon were initiated at the time of surgery but became manifest postoperatively in the ICU. HCWs often become colonized with NA-MRSA from patient contacts when providing healthcare but are not often implicated in transmission to patients. To implicate a colonized HCW as a source for colonization or infection of patients, it is first necessary to epidemiologically establish an association between contact with the colonized or infected HCW and acquisition of NA-MRSA by patients. Then it is necessary to prove that the strain from the HCW and the patient is the same using molecular techniques such as pulsed-field gel electrophoresis (PGFE) after restriction endonuclease digestion of genomic DNA.

Contaminated surfaces of equipment and environmental surfaces appear to make up another source of NA-MRSA for transmission to patients (58,59). NA-MRSA has been recovered from cultures of computer terminals, the floor next to the patient's bed, bed linens, patient gowns, over-bed tables, blood pressure cuffs, bedside rails, infusion pump buttons, door handles, bedside commodes, stethoscopes, and window sills. In the latter study, 27% of 350 environmental surface cultures yielded NA-MRSA (59). It has also been shown in in vitro studies that outbreak isolates of NA-MRSA survive at significantly higher concentrations and for longer periods of time on an inanimate surface than do sporadic NA-MRSA isolates (60). Thus, environmental contamination is likely another important source for transmission of NA-MRSA to patients.

Mode of Transmission of NA-MRSA. The most common mode of transmission of NA-MRSA to patients is by indirect contact. Several studies have shown that NA-MRSA is frequently transmitted to the hands and clothing of HCWs from colonized or infected patients. Two studies have shown that NA-MRSA can be recovered from 14% to 17% of HCWs' hands after patient contact (61,62).

Another study showed that 7 out of 12 (58%) nurses who cared for patients with NA-MRSA in a wound or urine had NA-MRSA on their gloves, recoverable by direct plating to solid media (59). Culture of 13 of 20 (65%) nurses' uniforms or gowns who cared for these same patients yielded NA-MRSA. When cultures were taken from gloves of 12 personnel who touched only environmental surfaces in the rooms of these patients, five (42%) had NA-MRSA recovered on culture. Arbitrary-primed polymerase chain reaction (PCR) typing demonstrated that isolates recovered from patients and environment had very similar banding patterns (59). Although additional studies are needed, data continue to accumulate in support of indirect transfer of NA-MRSA to patients from contaminated hands and clothing of HCWs.

NA-MRSA also appear to have an advantage over MSSA in colonizing patients after transmission (63). During an epidemic of NA-MRSA colonizations and infections in a surgical ICU, 23 patients were exposed to six patients admitted to the ICU with NA-MRSA colonization. PFGE of isolates showed that all secondary cases had NA-MRSA PFGE patterns identical to the PFGE patterns of the strain recovered from the patients to whom they were exposed. None of the PFGE patterns of the isolates of MSSA cultured from patients and HCWs were the same. The authors concluded that NA-MRSA may have spread more easily between patients due to selection through antibiotic pressure.

Airborne transmission of NA-MRSA may occur, but the importance of this route of transmission has not been established. The CDC has not recommended airborne precautions for patients with NA-MRSA colonization or infection (64). Theoretically, NA-MRSA could be transferred by the airborne route after aerosolization from contaminated environmental surfaces or by aerosolization from nasal carriers. One study has shown that NA-MRSA can be aerosolized from environmental surfaces, i.e., changing bed sheets (65). Molecular typing showed that environmental isolates and patient isolates were identical. However, the authors did not investigate other possible routes of transmission of NA-MRSA to the patients.

Several studies have been published on the dissemination of *S. aureus* from the upper respiratory tracts of HCWs. To the author's knowledge, no such studies have been published on dissemination of NA-MRSA from HCWs. One study has epidemiologically implicated a HCW with chronic sinusitis and nasal colonization with *S. aureus* in spread of *S. aureus* to patients. The relationship was confirmed by molecular typing (56). There appears to be a strong relationship between shedding of *S. aureus* by HCWs and having a viral upper respiratory tract infection (66,67). In one study, nasal carriers of *S. aureus* who volunteered were experimentally infected with rhinovirus (67). Investigators were able to quantify the *S. aureus* colony-forming units (CFU) released into the air under varying conditions including type of clothes worn and whether or not a mask was worn. They documented that the *S. aureus* released into the air was from the experimentally infected volunteers by molecular typing. Studies on airborne dissemination of NA-MRSA using these techniques are needed.

Risk Factors for Acquisition of NA-MRSA.   Risk factors for acquisition of NA-MRSA in ICUs vary depending on the type of ICU. Risk for NA-MRSA colonization/ infection identified in recent well-designed studies making use of multivariable analysis is shown in Table 2.

Neonatal ICUs.   The epidemiology of NA-MRSA colonization and infection has been less well studied in NICUs than in adult ICUs. Few, if any, reports on outbreaks of NA-MRSA in NICUs published in the 1990s and up to the present have included data on the risk of acquisition of NA-MRSA during outbreaks or analytic epidemiologic studies to identify risk factors for acquisition. One study provided time-and-intensity-of-care-adjusted incidence density for infections. In the intensive care section of the unit this incidence density was 0.73 infections/1000 patient-care hours (40). In the intermediate-care area the incidence density was 0.62 infections/1000 patient-care hours. There are no data on the rate of acquisition of NA-MRSA colonization.

Table 2 Risk Factors for Acquisition of Nosocomial Methicillin-Resistant *Staphylococcus aureus* in Adults

Publications	Type of ICU	Risk factors	Adjusted odds ratio (95% CI)	p Value
Marshall et al. (36)	Medical surgical	Previous admission to the ICU	3.3 (1.7–6.6)	
		Previous admission to trauma/ orthopedics ward	2.9 (1.2–7.2)	
		Previous admission to the neurology/endocrinology/ rheumatology/renal ward	2.6 (1.0–6.9)	
		LOS more than three days prior to admission to the ICU	8.6 (4.4–16.9)	
		Being a trauma patient	3.9 (1.8–8.7)	
		LOS 2–7 days in the ICU	11.1 (1.4–86)	
		LOS more than 7 days in the ICU	109.8 (14.5–833)	
Merrer et al. (50)	Medical	Weekly colonization pressure >40%	5.8 (1.7–20.1)	<0.0001
Grundmann et al. (52)	Interdisciplinary	Clustered cases		
		Days of staff deficit	1.05 (1.020–1.084)	0.001
		Sporadic cases		
		Urgent/emergency admission	3.50 (1.328–9.209)	0.011
		APACHE II score at 24 hr	1.07 (1.002–1.147)	0.044
		Bronchoscopy	3.68 (1.38–9.84)	0.009
Marshall et al. (68)	Trauma	Laparotomy	6.3 (1.4–28.9)	
		Motor vehicle accident	10.4 (1.2–93.7)	
		Ticarcillin–clavulanic acid	4.5 (1.3–15.0)	
		Glycopeptide	5.9 (1.7–21.0)	

Abbreviations: ICU, intensive care unit; LOS, length of stay; APACHE, acute physiology and chronic health evaluation.

There are few data on the source of NA-MRSA in NICUs. In one recent study, patients would have to be presumed to be the source of NA-MRSA, as personnel or the environment could not be implicated (42). In another study based on molecular typing, environmental cultures were all negative and a HCW was thought to have transferred the NA-MRSA outbreak strain from an adult hospital (44). However, the HCW was not epidemiologically implicated as the source. In all of the latter studies, transmission between patients by the hands of HCWs is suggested (40,42,44).

No case–control studies to identify risk factors for colonization or infection with NA-MRSA in NICUs have been published to the author's knowledge. Using a different approach, one study implicated overcrowding and understaffing as risk factors for acquisition of NA-MRSA colonization or infection (40).

Epidemiology of CA-MRSA

Adult ICUs. Although outbreaks of CA-MRSA infections have been described in hospitals in Australia, there were no reports of such outbreaks in ICUs (45–47). There have been no reports of infections due to CA-MRSA in adult ICUs in the United States.

Neonatal ICUs. There are three published reports of transmission of CA-MRSA in NICUs (17,48,69). In one report, the strain was identified as CA-MRSA by recovery from both the mother and neonate within the first 48 hours after admission (48). However, the isolate was susceptible only to gentamicin, rifampin, and vancomycin, and the mother had had contact with the healthcare system for prenatal care. The isolate was not tested for either the SCC*mec* type or the gene that encodes for Panton-Valentine leukocidin. Strains from the other two studies were both tested for the SCC*mec* type and Panton-Valentine leukocidin (17,69). Isolates from these two investigations had SCC*mec* type IV identified, but one did not carry the gene for Panton-Vanentine leukocidin (17) and the other was not tested for the latter virulence factor (69).

One study provided an incidence rate of 18.5 cases per 1000 hospitalized neonates (17). There are no published data on modes of transmission or risk factors for acquisition of CA-MRSA in NICUs. Although there are few published epidemiologic data on the spread of CA-MRSA in NICUs, it is clear that CA-MRSA may enter NICUs and cause outbreaks with resultant colonization and infection of neonates. It is likely that CA-MRSA will continue to enter many areas of hospitals, and more definitive studies will be needed to better understand how to prevent entry of CA-MRSA and to control it once present in healthcare facilities.

Prevention and Control of MRSA in ICUs

Prevention of MRSA transmission and control of ongoing dissemination among patients receiving healthcare require a number of preventive and control measures. The approach to control is similar for adult and neonatal patients and for NA-MRSA and CA-MRSA. Differences for adults versus neonates and for NA-MRSA versus CA-MRSA will be noted.

Screening Patients on Admission and During Hospitalization

The most important measures for control of MRSA in ICUs are active surveillance for patients infected or colonized with MRSA at the time of admission followed by prompt isolation of those patients identified as colonized or infected and weekly cultures for patients remaining in the ICU to detect acquisition of MRSA from patients who may have escaped detection on admission, from colonized or infected HCWs, or from contaminated environmental surfaces (34,44,63,70–84). It is important to identify every colonized patient so that all colonized as well as all infected patients can be placed on contact precautions. Surveillance cultures for MRSA should always include samples from the anterior nares (70).

Screening patients for colonization with MRSA has been done by taking swab samples from the anterior nares and other sites of possible MRSA colonization, such as the oropharynx, axilla, inguinal area, perirectal areas, and from open wounds and skin eruptions. Samples were then inoculated to broth or solid media containing antibiotics or other agents to select out MRSA. Although effective, results are not immediately available due to the delay for incubation and identification of isolates. More rapid techniques for detection of MRSA based on the PCR have been developed and published (85). Such techniques permit detection of MRSA from swab specimens within two hours.

Screening for MRSA colonization and infection on admission is particularly important for patients admitted from other hospitals, from long-term care facilities, or who have been hospitalized in the past year. Although it is not yet clear as to the impact of CA-MRSA on the influx of MRSA into hospitals, this potential reservoir for MRSA must be kept in mind. It may be necessary to screen everyone entering the hospital from the community regardless of whether they have one of the above-mentioned risk factors for MRSA colonization or infection.

Barrier Precautions

Gloves should be worn before entry of HCWs into rooms of patients isolated for MRSA (70). There is good evidence that HCWs acquire MRSA on gloved and ungloved hands when in contact with patients colonized or infected with MRSA (61,62). Hands should be washed before and after glove use.

Gowns should be worn on entry into the room except when there will be no contact between the HCW and the patient or between the HCW and environmental surfaces (70). Studies have shown that the clothing of HCWs becomes contaminated after contact with patients and patient-care surfaces (59,86).

Whether or not masks are needed for contact precautions for MRSA is controversial. The CDC has not recommended that masks be used for isolation of patients colonized or infected by MRSA (64). Masks are recommended by the Society for Healthcare Epidemiology of America (SHEA) Guidelines for preventing nosocomial transmission of multidrug-resistant strains of *S. aureus* and *Enterococcus* (70). However, the recommendation is categorized as a type II. Definitive studies are needed to determine whether or not masks are needed for isolation of patients with MRSA colonization or infection.

Decontamination of the Environment

There is growing evidence that the environment may be an important source for MRSA for patient colonization and infection (59,87,88). One study has shown that strains of MRSA survive for about 7 to 10 months on glass surfaces (60). It was also shown that outbreak strains of MRSA survived longer than sporadic strains. There is evidence that enhanced disinfection is an important measure for controlling epidemic MRSA (89,90). Thus, attention should be paid to thorough cleaning and disinfection of environmental surfaces in patient rooms and other areas where patients receive care.

Hand Hygiene

Hand hygiene is very important in conjunction with barrier precautions in preventing the spread of MRSA between patients and from patients to HCWs (70). Hand hygiene practices have been suboptimal for many years, and efforts to improve them have had little impact on compliance rates, which average about 40%. Risk factors for poor compliance include being a physician or a nursing assistant, working in an ICU, working during weekdays performing activities with a high risk for transmission, and having many opportunities for hand hygiene per hour of patient care (70). Most of these risk factors for poor hand hygiene are commonly present in ICUs.

HCWs must be taught to decontaminate their hands with an antiseptic-containing agent (an alcohol-based hand rub or a hand washing preparation containing an antiseptic agent). If hands are visibly soiled with urine, feces, blood, or other body fluids, they must be washed with soap and water followed by application of an alcohol-based hand rub or washed with soap containing an antiseptic.

Hands must be decontaminated before and after contact with each patient. This includes decontamination by washing with an antimicrobial soap or application of an alcohol-based hand rub after removal of gloves (91). HCWs should be strongly encouraged to apply moisturizing hand lotions, but it is important to establish that such preparations are compatible with the cleansing products and glove materials used by the HCWs. HCWs must be thoroughly educated about microbial contamination of their hands and why hand hygiene is important. Hand hygiene should be monitored and feedback should be given to HCWs about their performance on a continuous basis. It is unlikely that occasional feedback will change hand-hygiene practice.

Decolonization of Patients Who Are Carriers of MRSA

Decolonization of patients as a way to prevent and control outbreaks of colonization and infections due to both MRSA and MSSA has been studied for decades. In spite of the introduction of mupirocin as one of the most potent topical antistaphylococcal antibiotics discovered to date, decolonization of patients colonized with MRSA remains a challenge (92). In a number of studies, patients often become recolonized with the same or a different strain of MRSA. Few randomized controlled clinical trials with long-term follow-up (≥12 weeks after intranasal application of mupirocin) have been conducted. Decolonization is often attempted using a combination of mupirocin applied to the nares and showers with an antiseptic agent such as chlorhexidine. Very little published data suggest that chlorhexidine baths may add to the efficacy of mupirocin (93). One of the major problems in the use of mupirocin for decolonization of patients, in addition to failure to maintain long-term decolonization, is development of resistance (94). Resistance is particularly likely to develop with extensive use such as application to wounds. Resistance to mupirocin after use for treatment of both colonization and infection can be effectively controlled by limiting its use to the treatment of colonization (94).

Use of mupirocin for decolonization of patients in ICUs must be very judicious. Several of the risk factors for failure are present in many ICU patients (92). These include (i) colonization of multiple body sites; (ii) chronic nonhealing wounds; and (iii) the presence of colonized foreign bodies such as tracheostomy tubes or gastrostomy tubes. Treatment for colonization should be limited to the nares. Attempts at decolonization of patients with colonization at multiple body sites, with chronic nonhealing wounds, and the presence of foreign bodies should be avoided. If mupirocin is used on multiple patients over long periods of time (months), MRSA isolates from patients should be tested for susceptibility to mupirocin.

Another approach to decolonization of MRSA carriers has been instillation of vancomycin into the gastrointestinal tract by way of a nasogastric tube. In a recent study, the ICU patients had surveillance cultures of throat and rectum for MRSA over an eight-month period (95). The patients were part of a study of prevention of infection in mechanically ventilated patients. The patients were receiving oral antimicrobial agents for selective decontamination of the digestive tract. The authors designed a study to determine whether oral administration of vancomycin could eliminate MRSA from the intestinal tract. The study was not randomized and did not have concurrent controls. The authors noted a significant decrease in MRSA infections in the treated group compared with the historical group. They were able to show elimination of MRSA from the gastrointestinal tract based on rectal swab cultures. The weaknesses of the study included nonrandomization, the use of historic controls, and the simultaneous administration of other oral antimicrobial agents. The strengths included eradication of gastrointestinal carriage of MRSA and the careful monitoring of vancomycin resistance in MRSA and enterococci. No resistance was detected in many isolates of MRSA and enterococci tested for vancomycin susceptibility during the study. The authors also noted that by eradicating rectal carriage with vancomycin and preventing infection, they administered only 25% as much vancomycin to the group given oral vancomycin prophylaxis as was needed to treat the infections in the control group. Additional studies are required to better define the role of oral vancomycin for decolonization of the gastrointestinal tract, but this modality of decolonization appears to be of potential benefit and is worthy of further investigation.

Decolonization of patients in NICUs is similar to that in adult ICUs but has not been as well studied. In one report of a MRSA outbreak, four patients were treated with nasal mupirocin three times a day for five days and bathed with diluted (1:10); 4% chlorhexidine gluconate once daily for three days (17). Two of the four neonates were successfully decolonized and two remained colonized with MRSA. The latter two were decolonized after the regimen was repeated. In a report of a second outbreak, colonized neonates were treated with mupirocin twice daily to the anterior nares and the umbilical area for seven days (96). The authors did not report the results of their decolonization regimen.

In an account of a MRSA outbreak in an NICU, one control measure was application of triple dye to the umbilical area of the patients (40). This was one of several control measures implemented. Other control measures instituted included reducing overcrowding and understaffing and placing an infection control nurse in the NICU. Because all of these control measures were implemented at the same time, it was not possible to determine what effect the triple dye had in controlling the outbreak.

Decolonization of Healthcare Workers Who Are MRSA Carriers

Decolonization of HCWs is necessary when they have been epidemiologically implicated in the transmission of MRSA to patients from a colonized body site, which is most often the nose. Eradication of MRSA carriage from HCWs has been shown to help control outbreaks (56). For MRSA, mupirocin will decolonize the external nares effectively 91% of the time, although recolonization may occur in about one quarter of individuals so treated within four weeks (97). It has also been shown that decolonization of HCWs with nasal carriage of MSSA results in a substantial decrease in hand carriage (98). Temporary decolonization of most of the colonized HCWs in an ICU for a few weeks may help control an outbreak. Although there are few data on decolonization of HCWs carrying MRSA, it is likely that mupirocin will eradicate MRSA from the nares and hands of HCWs.

A second area where HCWs may be colonized with MRSA is at the site of dermatitis on their hands or forearms. It is important that hands and forearms of HCWs be examined and areas of dermatitis be cultured during an outbreak investigation. Other sites of colonization or infection are less common but may have to be sought if epidemiologically indicated. Table 3 lists the control measures for MRSA in ICUs.

Cost Effectiveness of MRSA Control

One study of the cost-effectiveness of MRSA control in an medical intensive care unit (MICU) has concluded that identification of patients who are carriers of MRSA on admission and during hospitalization and isolating of these carriers is cost effective (34). In spite of an ongoing MRSA carriage prevalence in admitted patients of 4%, the authors were able to reduce the incidence of ICU-acquired MRSA infection and colonization by fourfold. They observed that costs for single-room isolation of patients were $1480 and that the extra cost of an MRSA infection was $9275. They estimated that control was cost effective when MRSA carriage on admission is between 1% and 7% and when the MRSA transmission rate from colonized to isolated patients is at least fivefold less than to patients not isolated. Additional studies are needed on the cost effectiveness of MRSA control.

VANCOMYCIN-RESISTANT ENTEROCOCCI

Mechanism of Resistance

Although there are many species of *Enterococcus*, relatively few species make up the VRE that cause endemic and epidemic nosocomial colonization and infection in healthcare facilities. The most important species are *E. faecium* and *E. faecalis.* Two other species, *E. gallinarum* and *E. casseliflavus*, are motile and display intrinsic vancomycin resistance (99).

Vancomycin resistance in enterococci is mediated by the production of D-Alanine:D-Alanine ligases of altered substrate specificity (100). The most common ligases with altered substrate specificity are *vanA* and *vanB*. Both of these ligases condense D-Ala with D-Lac (lactate). Vancomycin does not bind to D-Lac, thus permitting cell wall synthesis to continue. The *vanA* trait is carried on a transposon, Tn*1546*. This transposon is most often carried on a plasmid and can be transferred to other gram-positive cocci. The genes that code for both *vanA* and *vanB* are similar. The *vanB* genes are carried on a large mobile element found on the chromosome. The *vanB* trait can be transferred to other enterococci (99). VRE containing the *vanA* ligase are resistant to vancomycin and another glycopeptide, teicoplanin, whereas *vanB* isolates are resistant to vancomycin but are susceptible to teicoplanin. Enterococci carrying *vanA* have minimal inhibitory concentrations (MICs) to vancomycin of >64 µg/mL, whereas isolates with *vanB* have MICs to vancomycin of 16 to >1000 µg/mL (99).

Other types of ligases with altered substrate specificities are *vanC* [D-Ala-D-Ser (serine)], *vanD* (D-Ala-D-Lac), and *vanE* (D-Ala-D-Ser). The *vanE* genes are found on

Table 3 Control Measures for Methicillin-resistant *Staphylococcus aureus* in
Intensive Care Units

Measure	Comments
Culture all patients on admission and weekly while in the ICU until they become positive for MRSA or they are discharged	Use selective culture media Always take cultures from the external nares Culture wounds and skin eruptions Consider perirectal cultures if other sites are negative Flag patients' charts or flag patients in the hospital computer system who are MRSA positive
Place patients with MRSA infection and colonization on contact precautions	Place patients flagged for MRSA on contact precautions on admission Wear gloves to enter the room Wear a gown for contact with the patient or environment Use of a mask is optional Remove gloves and gown prior to leaving the room
Practice hand hygiene after leaving room	Wash hands with soap containing an antiseptic or apply an alcohol hand rub If hands are visibly soiled, wash with a soap containing an antiseptic or wash with plain soap followed by application of an alcohol hand rub
Culture environmental surfaces to assess extent of contamination with MRSA	Obtain specimens with sterile swabs moistened with sterile saline without bacteriostatic agents Use selective culture media to maximize efficiency of laboratory identification of MRSA
Decontaminate environmental surfaces often enough to keep them free of MRSA	Thoroughly clean surfaces followed by application of a hospital-grade disinfectant Culture environmental surfaces to determine effectiveness of cleaning and disinfection methods Do not use phenolic disinfectants in NICUs for environmental decontamination
Determine what sites to clean and the frequency of cleaning based on environmental culture data	
Attempts at decolonization of patients with MRSA should be done only under the supervision of infection control staff	Mupirocin is the agent of choice Follow the manufacturer's instructions for use Decolonization should be attempted for nasal colonization only Attempts at nasal decolonization should not be done for patients with the following conditions: Colonization of multiple body sites Chronic nonhealing wounds

(*Continued*)

Table 3 Control Measures for Methicillin-resistant *Staphylococcus aureus* in Intensive Care Units (*Continued*)

Measure	Comments
	Presence of colonized foreign bodies such as tracheostomy tubes or gastrostomy tubes
	Take cultures after treatment for decolonization and 12 wks later
Healthcare workers who have nasal colonization with MRSA and who have been epidemiologically implicated in transmission to patients should be furloughed from patient care and treated with mupirocin for decolonization	Nasal decolonization is the same in NICUs
	Mupirocin should be applied to the external nares according to manufacturer's instructions
	Follow up cultures of the external nares should be taken after therapy and again at 2, 6, and 12 wks to detect relapse or recolonization
	When decolonization is unsuccessful on the first attempt, retreatment may be successful
When healthcare workers are infected with MRSA or have colonization of dermatitis, they should be furloughed from patient care and treated for infection or dermatitis until the condition clears	Sites of infection or colonization should be culture negative before the healthcare worker returns to patient care

Abbreviations: MRSA, methicillin-resistant *Staphylococcus aureus*; ICU, intensive care unit; NICUs, neonatal intensive care units.

the chromosomes of *E. gallinarum* and *E. casseliflavus*. These latter species have intrinsic low-level resistance to vancomycin (8–16 µg/mL).

More recently, it has been discovered that *E. faecium* strains of VRE have acquired genes that appear to code for two virulence factors (101,102). The *esp* gene was found only in outbreak strains of *E. faecium* on three continents and not in nonepidemic isolates and isolates from healthy individuals or farm animals (101). Isolates carrying the *esp* gene seem to be associated with in-hospital spread and possibly with increased virulence. The hyl_{Efm} gene is found primarily in vancomycin-resistant *E. faecium* in nonstool cultures obtained from patients hospitalized in the United States (102). This observation suggests that specific *E. faecium* strains may contain determinants that are associated with clinical infections. The appearance of virulence determinants in microorganisms that were considered nonvirulent normal flora in the past makes control of VRE even more urgent than when the only concern was resistance to glycopeptides.

Types of Infections Caused by VRE

Adult ICUs

The most important type of infection caused by VRE is bacteremia. Such infections are usually related to intravascular catheters (103–109). Mortality due to VRE bacteremia has not been studied extensively. One study concluded that VRE bacteremia had a negative impact on survival (107). The best study was a historical cohort study that found an attributable mortality of 37% (95% CI 10–64%) (106). Nosocomial meningitis has been reported rarely (110,111). VRE is frequently cultured from urine, but only about 13% of patients with positive urine cultures have a urinary tract infection. Bacteremia from the infected urinary tract occurs but is uncommon (112). A univariate analysis of patients with and without a urinary tract infection revealed a significant relationship between having a malignancy and a urinary tract infection (112).

Neonatal ICUs

As in adults, neonates may also develop serious infections caused by VRE (113–115). The most common infection is bacteremia. Meningitis due to VRE has been reported in neonates, and two cases of VRE meningitis developed in patients after ventriculoperitoneal shunt placement (114). Urinary tract infection and lower respiratory tract infection with VRE has also been reported (114). Similar to adult patients, only about 1 in 10 colonized patients develop infection.

Epidemiology of VRE in ICUs

Sources of VRE

The main source/reservoir for VRE in hospitalized patients is the gastrointestinal tract (116–119). The first sites from which VRE are recovered on culture in newly colonized patients 86% of the time are the rectum or groin (116). Rectal cultures for VRE remain positive 100% of the time while patients are hospitalized. Gastrointestinal colonization may be very prevalent in ICU patients even in the absence of an outbreak (118). Patients with gastrointestinal colonization with VRE have very high concentrations of VRE in stool (median 10^8 CFU/g) (117). VRE are the predominant aerobic microorganisms in the gastrointestinal tracts of colonized patients, outnumbering gram-negative bacilli and vancomycin-susceptible enterococci. Given the high concentrations of VRE in stool, it is not surprising that many body sites in the patient carrying VRE become colonized (116).

Transmission of VRE in the ICU

Transmission of VRE to patients is by indirect contact with the hands of HCWs and fomites. There is no evidence that VRE are spread by the airborne route. Four studies show that gloved hands in contact with colonized patients and their environments become culture positive for VRE (120–123). When patients have diarrhea, the likelihood of HCWs picking up VRE on their gloves when in contact with these patients is greater than when in contact with patients who do not have diarrhea (121). It has also been shown that VRE isolates in the environment surrounding a colonized patient are easily transferred on to the gloved hands of HCWs after contact with environmental surfaces (122). Isolates from patients, environmental surfaces, and gloved hands of HCWs were the same strains by PFGE. Isolates from patients' intact skin or environmental surfaces may also be transferred to clean sites on patients by HCWs hands or gloves (123).

Two studies have shown that environmental surfaces have a lower density of VRE than do perirectal swabs (123,124). Both studies showed that broth amplification was often necessary to recover VRE from environmental surface samples. However, low density of VRE on environmental surfaces did not prevent transfer. Sixty-nine percent of surfaces from which VRE were transferred were positive by broth amplification culture only (123).

Another concern about transfer of VRE from environmental surfaces is that the microorganism can survive on inanimate surfaces from seven days to two months (125,126). Further evidence that VRE may survive for a prolonged period on an inanimate surface and then be transferred to a patient is provided by a report on a VRE outbreak in a burn unit (119). After initial control of the outbreak for five weeks, the outbreak recurred from an electrocardiogram (EKG) lead that had not been cleaned since use on the last patient. In the five-week period, during which the outbreak had been cleared, all weekly patient surveillance cultures and 317 environmental cultures were negative for VRE. The VRE cultured from the EKG lead, the prior patient on which the lead had been used and the patient who acquired the VRE from the EKG lead, were shown to be the same strain by PFGE. The time from use of the EKG lead on the first patient to use on the second patient was 38 days. VRE have also been transmitted between patients by electronic thermometers during an outbreak (127). Restriction endonuclease analysis of plasmid DNA indicated that all clinical isolates and isolates from handles of the electronic thermometers were identical.

Risk Factors for Acquisition of VRE in ICUs

Adult ICUs. Although many published studies have examined risk factors for nosocomial acquisition of VRE, most have not been well designed. When trying to ascertain risk factors for acquisition, it is important to determine the exact time of colonization or infection by VRE, to use controls that are negative for VRE [as opposed to controls positive for vancomycin-susceptible enterococci (VSE)], and to use multivariable statistics to identify independent risk factors. Some studies of risk factors have included ICUs in addition to other areas of the hospital (Table 4), and others have been limited to ICUs (Table 5).

Several of the studies included in Tables 4 and 5 have identified a significant relationship between prior administration of an antimicrobial agent and acquisition of VRE. Drugs listed included cephalosporins, metronidazole, vancomycin, carbapenems, ticarcillin–clavulanate, and quinolones. The antibiotic most often identified as a risk factor was vancomycin. In an extensive study of the effects of antimicrobial agents on fecal flora, it was found that antianaerobic antibiotics promoted high-density

Table 4 Risk Factors for Acquisition of Vancomycin-Resistant Enterococci from Studies of Mixed Patient Populations

Publications	Risk factors	Adjusted odds ratio (95% CI)	p Value
Loeb et al. (128)	Cephalosporin use	13.8 (2.5–76.3)	0.01
Byers et al. (129)	Proximity to an unisolated patient	2.04 (1.32–3.14)	0.0014
	History of major trauma	9.27 (1.43–60.3)	0.020
	Therapy with metronidazole	3.04 (1.05–8.77)	0.040
Cetinkaya et al. (130)	Vancomycin use	3.2 (1.7–6.0)	0.0003
	Gastrointestinal bleeding[a]	0.26 (0.08–0.79)	0.02
	Presence of central venous lines	2.2 (1.04–4.6)	0.04
	Antacid use	2.9 (1.5–5.6)	0.002
	Mean daily dose of Vicodin[R;a]		0.0003

[a]Protective factors.

Table 5 Risk Factors for Acquisition of Vancomycin-Resistant Enterococci from Studies in Intensive Care Units

Publications	Type of ICU	Risk factors	Adjusted odds ratio (95% CI)	p Value
Karanfil et al. (131)	Cardiothoracic surgery	Vancomycin use	Sole predictor in the logistic regression model	
Slaughter et al. (132)	Medical	Length of stay in ICU ≤5 day	0.08 (0.02–0.39)[a]	
		Enteral feeding	6.09 (1.56–23.7)	
		Sucralfate	3.26 (1.09–9.72)	
Bonten et al. (53)	Medical	Colonization pressure	1.032 (1.012–1.052)[b]	0.002
		Proportion of days with enteral feeding	1.009 (1.000–1.017)[b]	0.05
		Proportion of patient days with cephalosporin use	1.007 (0.999–1.015)[b]	0.11
Falk et al. (119)	Burn	Presence of diarrhea	43.9 (5.5–infinity)	0.0001
		Administration of an antacid	24.2 (2.9–infinity)	0.002
Gardiner et al. (133)	Medical	Enteral feedings	19 (2.02–177.9)	< 0.05
Padiglione et al. (134)	Multicenter study—mixed ICUs and transplant units	Renal unit patients	4.62 (1.22–17)[b]	0.02
		Carbapenems	2.84 (1.02–7.96)[b]	0.048
		Ticarcillin–clavulanate	3.64 (1.13–11.64)[b]	0.03
Martinez et al. (135)	Medical	Hospitalization for more than one week before MICU admission	18.5 (1.1–301.0)	0.04
		Administration of vancomycin before or during an ICU admission	6.3 (1.2–34.0)	0.03
		Administration of quinolones before or during MICU admission	14.8 (1.2–180.0)	0.04
		Location in a high risk MICU room[c]	81.7 (2.2–3092.0)	0.02
Warren et al. (136)	Medical	Increasing age	1.02 (1.01–1.03)	
		Hospitalization in the 6 mo prior to current admission	2.74 (2.21–3.40)	
		Admission from a long-term care facility	1.30 (1.14–1.47)	

[a]Protective factor.
[b]Hazard ratios.
[c]A room that proved to be contaminated after postpatient discharge cleaning.
Abbreviations: ICU, intensive care unit; MICU, medical intensive care unit.

colonization of stool with VRE (136). Administration of vancomycin had no effect on the concentration of VRE in stool. Although antianaerobic agents increased the concentration of VRE in stool, it is unclear whether these agents or vancomycin predispose to acquisition of VRE.

Several case–control studies have shown that vancomycin is a risk factor for acquisition of VRE. In an assessment of studies showing a relationship between vancomycin and acquisition of VRE by meta-analysis, the authors concluded that the apparent relationship between administration of vancomycin and colonization with VRE is due to selection of VSE as the reference group, confounding by duration of hospitalization and publication bias (137). However, several studies have been published in which the reference group was appropriately selected (VRE-negative patients and not VSE-culture positive) and duration of hospitalization was included to control for confounding due to longer exposure time (130,131,138,139). Thus, the issue of whether vancomycin is a risk factor for acquisition of VRE is unsettled.

Risk factors from Tables 4 and 5 that appear greater than or equal to two times are use of antacids and enteral feedings. One study noted that a length of stay of less than or equal to five days in an MICU was protective against VRE acquisition, whereas another study observed that hospitalization for more than one week prior to MICU admission was a risk factor for acquisition of VRE. In summary the most frequently identified risk factors for acquiring VRE from these studies are administration of antibiotics and antacids, enteral feedings, and longer length of stay.

Neonatal ICUs. There are six reports of outbreaks of VRE in NICUs (113–115,140–142). Analytical epidemiology was used in only one of the studies to identify risk factors for acquisition of VRE (113). This study examined a large number of variables by univariate analysis and found many variables apparently related to VRE colonization. However, multivariable analysis by logistic regression identified days of antimicrobial therapy (OR 1.21, 95% CI 1.045–1.400, $p = 0.01$) and birth weight (OR 0.92, 95% CI 0.862–0.979, $p = 0.009$) as the only independent associations with acquisition of VRE. Additional studies are needed to further define the variables associated with acquisition of VRE in this population.

Prevention and Control of VRE in ICUs

Although less data were available 10 years ago on the epidemiology and control of VRE, recommendations of the CDC's Hospital Infection Control Practices Advisory Committee (HICPAC) have stood the test of time (143). Virtually all of HICPAC's recommendations to prevent and control the spread of VRE have been supported by the studies published in the last 10 years. Thus, the focus for control and prevention is on the following: (i) detection of colonized patients by surveillance cultures; (ii) barrier isolation; (iii) hand hygiene; (iv) environmental decontamination; (v) decolonization of HCWs; and (vi) control of antimicrobial (particularly vancomycin) use. The HICPAC guideline also emphasized that prevention and control should start in ICUs and other areas where the VRE transmission rate is the highest.

Culture Surveillance

Because only about 10% of patients colonized with VRE develop infection, most patients who make up the reservoir of VRE in the hospital are colonized and not infected. Colonization can be detected only by surveillance cultures. Colonized patients have been detected by screening stool specimens submitted to the clinical microbiology laboratory for *Clostridium difficile* toxin assay (144). Stool may be collected and sent from the ICU to the clinical microbiology laboratory, but in most cases perirectal swab specimens are cultured in broth or streaked to solid agar. One group of authors found that a rectal swab sample had a sensitivity of 58% in detecting VRE compared to culture of stool (145). These authors also noted that the concentration of VRE in stool increased with the number of antibiotics administered and duration of their administration. It is likely that perirectal swab cultures will have a higher sensitivity for detection of VRE in ICUs where many patients are on antibiotics.

In another study in a burn unit, the authors observed that perirectal swabs had the same sensitivity for detecting VRE whether inoculated to broth or to solid media (124). This suggests that small numbers of VRE detected by broth amplification can also be detected by growth on solid media. This may have been due to the extensive use of antimicrobial agents in the burn unit where the study was performed. The HICPAC guideline also recommends culturing urine and wounds for VRE (143). This will likely increase the sensitivity of surveillance cultures.

Surveillance cultures can be made more efficient by using a selective culture media to suppress growth of other microorganisms that will likely contaminate the specimens (124,143). It is likely that most patients who are colonized with VRE in an ICU will be detected by perirectal swabs and swabs of open wounds and other skin sites inoculated to selective media. This recommendation is further supported by a study that found that rectal and perirectal swabs had approximately the same sensitivity (79%) (146).

Surveillance cultures and isolation of colonized and infected patients has been shown in many studies to control VRE in both acute care and long-term care facilities (117,119,120,129,147–150). One publication describes the effective control of VRE in four acute-care hospitals and in 26 long-term care facilities in the Siouxland region of Iowa, Nebraska, and South Dakota (147).

Barrier Precautions

Patients with VRE infections and VRE colonization detected by surveillance cultures should be immediately placed on barrier or isolation precautions. The HICPAC guideline recommends placement of patients in a single room or in the same room as other patients with VRE (143). The guideline also recommends donning clean nonsterile gloves prior to entering the room. Use of a gown is recommended only for substantial contact with the patient or environment. Many health care facilities now require that a gown be worn as well as gloves to enter the room of a patient with VRE. This is based on several studies. The first report noted that an outbreak in an ICU was not contained until personnel began to wear gowns in addition to gloves (151). In a prospective, controlled nonrandomized study in an MICU in a hospital in which VRE were endemic, half the patients were isolated with glove use alone and the other half were cared for by HCWs wearing both gloves and gowns (132). The authors observed that there was no difference in transmission from patients isolated with glove use only and those isolated with HCWs wearing gowns and gloves.

Two prospective nonrandomized studies using historical controls and multivariable analysis carried out in MICUs both observed a significantly lower rate of transmission of VRE when gowns and gloves rather than gloves alone were used for isolation (152,153). In the former study, the addition of gowns was protective only for those patients exposed to VRE for more than 15 days.

Use of gowns in addition to gloves is further supported by the findings from a study that evaluated the proportion of gloves, gowns, and stethoscopes that were contaminated after a structured physical examination of patients colonized or infected with VRE (154). Gloves were contaminated in 63%, gowns in 37%, and stethoscopes in 31% of the examinations. Available published data support a recommendation that both gloves and gowns be worn when entering a room where a patient is isolated for VRE colonization or infection.

There are few data on when patients colonized or infected with VRE may be taken off of isolation. The CDC's HICPAC recommendation was that isolation be discontinued when three sets of cultures taken from stool or by rectal swab and all previous positive body sites were culture negative for VRE on three occasions at least one week apart (143). One study has been published that supports the recommendation made by HICPAC that patients may be taken off of isolation after three consecutive negative cultures (155).

Decontamination of the Environment

That VRE can remain viable on inanimate surfaces from seven days to two months has already been established (119,125,126). In addition to hard surfaces, upholstered surfaces in hospitals can be contaminated with VRE (156). VRE were recovered at 72 hours and one week after inoculation to an upholstered surface. VRE were also recovered from 3 of 10 seat cushions that were cultured in the room of a VRE patient. The authors state that an easily cleanable nonporous material is the preferred upholstery in hospitals.

Extensive cultures of environmental surfaces in rooms of patients colonized with VRE in an MICU and a burn ICU identified contaminated surfaces in 12% and 13.5%, respectively (116,119). It has also been shown that at least one environmental surface was positive in the rooms of 63% to 92% of patients colonized with VRE (116,122). Three studies have demonstrated that VRE are easily transferred to gloves or hands of HCWs after contact with the environment (121–123). In one of the latter studies, VRE were transferred from a culture-positive site to a culture-negative site in 10.6% of the opportunities (123). VRE were transferred from patient to environment and from environment to patient. VRE were transferred from sites with low-density contamination or colonization (cultured from broth only) 69% of the time. Environmental contamination has also been shown to be more widely distributed in the areas around the bed of a colonized patient with diarrhea (151).

Further evidence for the importance of environmental contamination in the acquisition of VRE in an MICU was the finding in a case–control study that environmental contamination was a risk factor for patients acquiring VRE (135).

The effectiveness of decontamination of the environment depends on the method used. In one study, the investigators observed that cleaning environmental surfaces with a cleaning rag sprayed with a quaternary ammonium disinfectant was significantly less effective than dipping the cleaning rag into a bucket of the same disinfectant, drenching all surfaces, allowing the surfaces to remain wet for 10 minutes, and then wiping the surfaces dry with a clean towel (157). The authors referred to the latter method as the bucket method. Using the method in which the disinfectant was sprayed on the cleaning rag took 2.8 applications to eradicate VRE from environmental surfaces compared with one application using the bucket method. In addition to a greater efficiency at removing VRE from surfaces, the bucket method also cost less than the method of spraying disinfectant on a cleaning rag. Based on this study, the bucket method is the preferred method for decontaminating environment surfaces.

Hand Hygiene

Excellent hand hygiene must always be practiced for the prevention of nosocomial infections, but it is particularly important in providing effective isolation of patients with VRE. Given the frequent contamination of gloved and ungloved hands of HCWs in contact with VRE-colonized patients and environmental surfaces, excellent hand hygiene must be an integral part of barrier precautions for VRE (121–123,154). After patient contact, hands should be washed with an antiseptic-containing soap or an alcohol hand rub should be applied.

Colonization of Healthcare Workers

Colonization of HCWs with VRE has not been reported in the literature during outbreaks of VRE infection and colonization. A study of 55 stool specimens from HCWs in a hospital where 15% of enterococci were VRE found that all cultures of stool specimens were negative for VRE (158). The authors concluded that colonization resistance was sufficient to prevent colonization of HCW's gastrointestinal tracts in the absence of acute illness or severe underlying comorbidities.

Antimicrobial Agents

Antimicrobial agents have been identified as risk factors for acquisition of VRE as shown in Tables 4 and 5. Vancomycin has been considered as a risk factor for acquisition of VRE, but several studies have failed to identify vancomycin as a risk factor (128,129,132,134). The HICPAC recommendations included a list of indications for use of vancomycin and a list of contraindications for use of this antibiotic (143). A more recent publication from the CDC reports on a study performed in cooperation with 20 hospitals in the NNIS system that joined the Intensive Care Antimicrobial Resistance Epidemiology (ICARE) Project. These hospitals contributed data from 50 ICUs on grams of selected antibiotics used each month and on susceptibility tests for selected microorganisms recovered from patients in these units each month (159). The data submitted to Project ICARE was used to create benchmarks for vancomycin use. Those ICUs that instituted changes in practice observed significant decreases in vancomycin use and in VRE prevalence. Although some controversy remains about whether vancomycin use is a risk factor for acquisition of VRE, the bulk of the data to date is in favor of limiting vancomycin use in ICUs as part of the control programs for VRE.

Other antibiotics that have been identified as risk factors for acquisition of VRE include cephalosporins, metronidazole, carbapenems, ticarcillin–clavulanate, and quinolones (128,129,134,135). A study of the effect of antimicrobial therapy on the concentration of VRE in patients' stools observed that concentrations of VRE increased significantly in stools of those patients who received antianaerobic antibiotics. The authors made the point that vancomycin has antianaerobic activity and showed that VRE increased in concentration in stools of patients who were treated with vancomycin (137). The authors also showed that patients with high concentrations of VRE in stools caused greater environmental contamination and observed that eight patients with VRE cultured from blood, urine, and a sacral wound had ≥6 logs of VRE per gram of stool. Therefore, avoiding the use of antianaerobic antimicrobial therapy in patients when possible may aid in control of VRE by reducing environmental contamination. Limiting the concentration of VRE in stool may also reduce the risk of invasive disease due to VRE. Limiting the use of antianaerobic agents and vancomycin appears important in the control of VRE.

Table 6 Control Measures for Vancomycin-Resistant Enterococci in Intensive Care Units

Measure	Comments
Culture patients on admission who are transferred from other healthcare facilities or long-term care facilities and those hospitalized in the last year and weekly while in the ICU until they become positive for VRE or they are discharged	Use selective culture media Take specimens for culture from perirectal area and wounds Flag patients' charts or flag patients in the hospital computer system who are VRE-positive
Place patients with VRE infection and colonization on contact precautions	Place patients flagged for VRE on contact precautions on admission Healthcare workers should wear both gown and gloves Masks are not needed Remove gown and gloves prior to leaving the room
Practice hand hygiene after leaving the room	Wash hands with a soap containing an antiseptic or apply an alcohol hand rub If hands are visibly soiled, wash with a soap containing an antiseptic or wash with plain soap followed by application of an alcohol hand rub
Culture environmental surfaces to assess extent of contamination with VRE	Obtain specimens with sterile swabs moistened with sterile saline without bacteriostatic agents Use selective culture media to maximize efficiency of laboratory identification of VRE Use bucket method to clean and disinfect environmental surfaces Culture environmental surfaces to determine the effectiveness of the cleaning and disinfection methods Do not use phenolic disinfectants in NICUs for environmental decontamination
When possible, limit use of those antimicrobial agents that have been identified as risk factors for VRE acquisition or that increase the concentration of VRE in stool	Antimicrobial agents that have been identified as risk factors for the acquisition of VRE include cephalosporins (particularly third generation cephalosporins), vancomycin, metronidazole, carbapenems, and ticarcillin–clavulanate Antimicrobial agents that have been shown to increase the concentration of VRE in stools include clindamycin, metronidazole, cefoxitin, and ceftriaxone Piperacillin-tazobactam may protect against acquisition of VRE
Patients may be taken off of contact precautions when they have had three consecutive sets of negative cultures for VRE, each taken ≥1 wk apart	Cultures should be taken from the perirectal area and all previously positive sites

Abbreviations: VRE, vancomycin-resistant enterococci; ICU, intensive care unit; NICUs, neonatal intensive care units.

Another approach to controlling VRE through changes in the use of anti-microbial agents is to replace the use of antimicrobials to which VRE are resistant with antimicrobials to which VRE are more susceptible. Piperacillin/tazobactam has been considered to be a good candidate for suppressing the growth of VRE, because it has good antimicrobial activity against *E. faecium*, which is the most common VRE species, and because it is concentrated in bile. Five studies on the use of piperacillin–tazobactam in place of third-generation cephalosporins and ticarcillin–clavulanate have been published (160–164). Only one of the latter studies was adequately designed to provide definitive results (164). There was a significant reduction in the acquisition of VRE after ticarcillin–clavulanate was replaced by piperacillin–tazobactam. As the authors pointed out, additional studies are needed for this control strategy as the study was carried out in a single institution and the reduction in acquisition of VRE was associated with the formulary change, but causality could not be established. When other measures have failed to control the spread of VRE, this approach could be tried.

In summary when measures are being instituted in an attempt to control VRE, it would appear prudent to limit the use of vancomycin, cephalosporins, metronidazole, clindamycin, and ticarcillin–clavulanate. Initiating the use of piperacillin–tazobactam might add to the effectiveness of manipulating antimicrobials as part of the control measures for VRE.

Other risk factors that should be addressed are the use of enteric feedings, the use of antacids, and effectively removing VRE from environmental surfaces. Table 6 lists the control measures for VRE in ICUs.

Cost Effectiveness of VRE Control

The high cost of VRE control is often mentioned in the literature, and many infection control programs have decided to apply very limited control measures to prevent and control the spread of VRE. However, several recent studies on the cost effectiveness of VRE control have all concluded that effective VRE control with a reduction in infections caused by VRE is cost effective (165–168). In three of the studies, control of VRE was cost effective with savings to the hospitals of between $100,000 and $500,000 per year (165,166,168). The other study estimated the costs of VRE infections in a hospital using a retrospective matched cohort study (167). The authors estimated that the effects of VRE infections on patients would include 15 cases of in-hospital deaths, 22 major operations, 26 ICU admissions, and 1445 additional hospitalization days with excess costs of $2,974,478 during the study period. It is reasonable to conclude from the available data that control of VRE is cost effective.

REFERENCES

1. Jevons MP. "Celbenin"– resistant staphylococci. Br Med J 1961; 1:124–125.
2. Barrett FF, McGehee RF, Finland M. Methicillin-resistant *Staphylococcus aureus* at Boston City Hospital. N Engl J Med 1968; 279:441–448.
3. http://www.cdc.gov/ncidod/hip/Aresist/ICU-RES Trend 1995–2004.pdf (accessed June2005).
4. Daum RS, Ito T, Hiramatsu K, et al. A novel methicillin-resistance cassette in community-acquired methicillin-resistant *Staphylococcus aureus* isolates of diverse genetic backgrounds. J Infect Dis 2002; 186(9):1344–1347.

5. Salmenlinna S, Lyytikäinen O, Vuopio-Varkila J. Community-acquired methicillin-resistant *Staphylococcus aureus,* Finland. Emerg Infect Dis 2002; 8(6):602–607.

6. Österlund A, Kahlmeter G, Bieber L, et al. Intrafamilial spread of highly virulent *Staphylococcus aureus* strains carrying the gene for Panton-Valentine leukocidin. Scand J Infect Dis 2002; 34:763–764.

7. Liassine N, Auckenthaler R, Descombes M-C, et al. Community-acquired methicillin-resistant *Staphylococcus aureus* isolated in Switzerland contains the Panton-Valentine leukocidin or exfoliative toxin genes. J Clin Microbiol 2004; 42(2):825–828.

8. Stemper ME, Shukla SK, Reed KD. Emergence and spread of community-associated methicillin-resistant *Staphylococcus aureus* in rural Wisconsin, 1989 to 1999. J Clin Microbiol 2004; 42(12):5673–5680.

9. Diep BA, Sensabaugh GF, Somboona NS, et al. Widespread skin and soft-tissue infections due to two methicillin-resistant *Staphylococcus aureus* strains harboring the genes for Panton-Valentine Leucocidin. J Clin Microbiol 2004; 42(5):2080–2084.

10. Cooms GW, Nimmo GR, Bell JM, et al. Genetic diversity among community methicillin-resistant *Staphylococcus aureus* strains causing outpatient infections in Australia. J Clin Microbiol 2004; 42(10):4735–4743.

11. Witte W, Braulke C, Cuny C, et al. Emergence of methicillin-resistant *Staphylococcus aureus* with Panton-Valentine leukocidin genes in central Europe. Eur J Clin Microbiol Infect Dis 2005; 24:1–5.

12. Lu P-L, Chin L-C, Peng C-F, et al. Risk factors and molecular analysis of community methicillin-resistant *Staphylococcus aureus* carriage. J Clin Microbiol 2005; 43(1):132–139.

13. Hussain FM, Boyle-Vavra S, Daum RS. Community-acquired methicillin-resistant *Staphylococcus aureus* colonization in healthy children attending an outpatient pediatric clinic. Pediatr Infect Dis J 2001; 20(8):763–767.

14. Naimi TS, LeDell KH, Boxrud DJ, et al. Epidemiology and clonality of community-acquired methicillin-resistant *Staphylococcus aureus* in Minnesota 1996–1998. Clin Infect Dis 2001; 33(7):990–996.

15. Fridkin SK, Hageman JC, Morrison M, et al. Methicillin-resistant *Staphylococcus aureus* disease in three communities. N Engl J Med 2005; 352(14):1436–1444.

16. Morel A-S, Wu F, Della-Latta P, et al. Nosocomial transmission of methicillin-resistant *Staphylococcus aureus* from a mother to her preterm quadruplet infants. Am J Infect Control 2002; 30(3):170–173.

17. Regev-Yochay G, Rubinstein E, Barzilai A, et al. Methicillin-resistant *Staphylococcus aureus* in neonatal intensive care unit. Emerg Infect Dis 2005; 11(3):453–456.

18. Uttley AH, Collins CH, Naidoo J, et al. Vancomycin-resistant enterococci. Lancet 1988; 1(1):57–58.

19. Leclercq R, Derlot E, Duval J, et al. Plasmid-mediated resistance to vancomycin and teicoplanin in *Enterococcus faecium*. N Engl J Med 1998; 319(3):157–161.

20. Nosocomial enterococci resistant to vancomycin-United States, 1989–1993. Morbid Mortal Wkly Rep 1993; 42(30):597–600.

21. Centers for Disease Control and Prevention. National Nosocomial Infections Surveillance (NNIS) system report, data summary from January 1992 through June 2004, issued October 2004. Am J Infect Control 2004; 32(12):470–485.

22. Montecalvo MA, de Lencastre H, Carraher M, et al. Natural history of colonization with vancomycin-resistant *Enterococcus faecium*. Infect Control Hosp Epidemiol 1995; 16(12):680–685.

23. Henning KJ, de Lencastre H, Eagan, J, et al. Vancomycin-resistant *Enterococcus faecium* on a pediatric oncology ward: duration of stool shedding and incidence of clinical infection. Pediatr Infect Dis J 1996; 15(10):848–854.

24. Patel R. Clinical impact of vancomycin-resistant enterococci. J Antimicrob Chemother 2003; 51(suppl 3):iii13–iii21.

25. McGeer AJ, Low DE. Vancomycin-resistant enterococci. Semin Respir Infect 2000; 15(4):314–326.

26. Murray BE. Drug therapy: vancomycin-resistant enterococcal infections. N Engl J Med 2000; 342(10):710–721.

27. Kreiswirth B, Kornblum J, Arbeit RD, et al. Evidence for a clonal origin of methicillin resistance in *Staphylococcus aureus*. Science 1993; 259(1):227–230.

28. Musser JM, Kapur V. Clonal anaylsis of methicillin-resistant *Staphylococcus aureus* strains from intercontinental sources: association of the *mec* gene with divergent phylogenetic lineages implies dissemination by horizontal transfer and recombination. J Clin Microbiol 1992; 30:2058–2063.

29. Mongkolrattanothai K, Boyle S, Kahana MD, et al. Severe *Staphylococcus aureus* infections caused by clonally related community-acquired methicillin-susceptible and methicillin-resistant isolates. Clin Infect Dis 2003; 37(8):1050–1058.

30. Eady EA, Cove JH. Staphylococcal resistance revisited: community-acquired methicillin resistant *Staphylococcus aureus* – an emerging problem for the management of skin and soft tissue infections. Curr Opin Infect Dis 2003; 16:103–124.

31. Charlebois ED, Perdreau-Remington F, Kreiswirth B, et al. Origins of community strains of methicillin-resistant *Staphylococcus aureus*. Clin Infect Dis 2004; 39(1):47–54.

32. Baba T, Takenchi F, Kuroda M, et al. Genome and virulence determinants of high virulence community-acquired MRSA. Lancet 2002; 359:1819–1827.

33. Eguia JM, Chambers HF. Community-acquired methicillin-resistant *Staphylococcus aureus*: epidemiology and potential virulence factors. Curr Infect Dis Rep 2003; 5: 459–466.

34. Chaix C, Durand-Zaleski I, Alberti C, et al. Control of endemic methicillin-resistant *Staphylococcus aureus*: a cost-benefit analysis in an intensive care unit. JAMA 1999; 282(18):1745–1751.

35. Squier C, Rihs JD, Risa J, et al. *Staphylococcus aureus* rectal carriage and its association with infections in patients in a surgical intensive care unit and a liver transplant unit. Infect Control Hosp Epidemiol 2002; 23(9):495–501.

36. Marshall C, Harrington G, Wolfe R, et al. Acquisition of methicillin-resistant *Staphylococcus aureus* in a large intensive care unit. Infect Control Hosp Epidemiol 2003; 24(5):322–326.

37. Cassone M, Campanile F, Pantosti A, et al. Identification of a variant "Rome clone" of methicillin-resistant *Staphylococcus aureus* with decreased susceptibility to vancomycin, responsible for an outbreak in an intensive care unit. Microb Drug Resist 2004; 10:43–49.

38. Thompson DS. Methicillin-resistant *Staphylococcus aureus* in a general intensive care unit. JR Soc Med 2004; 97:521–526.

39. Gastmeier P, Sohr D, Geffers C, et al. Mortality risk factors with noscomial *Staphylococcus aureus* infections in intensive care units: results from the German Nosocomial Infection Surveillance System (KISS). Infection 2005; 33(2):50–55.

40. Haley RW, Cushion NB, Tenover FC, et al. Eradication of endemic methicillin-resistant *Staphylococcus aureus* infections from a neonatal intensive care unit. J Infect Dis 1995; 171(3):614–624.

41. Andersen BM, Lindermann R, Bergh K, et al. Spread of methicillin-resistant *Staphylococcus aureus* in a neonatal intensive unit associated with understaffing, overcrowding and mixing of patients. J Hosp Infect 2002; 50(1):18–24.

42. Nambiar S, Herwaldt LA, Singh N. Outbreak of invasive disease caused by methicillin-resistant *Staphylococcus aureus* in neonates and prevalence in the neonatal intensive care unit. Pediatr Crit Care Med 2003; 4(2):220–226.

43. Isaacs D, Fraser S, Hogg G, et al. *Staphylococcus aureus* infections in Australasian neonatal nurseries. Arch Dis Child Fetal Neonatal Ed 2004; 89:F331–F335.

44. Saiman L, Cronquist A, Wu F, et al. An outbreak of methicillin-resistant *Staphylococcus aureus* in a neonatal intensive care unit. Infect Control Hosp Epidemiol 2003; 24(5): 317–321.

45. Udo EE, Pearman JW, Grubb WB. Genetic analysis of community isolates of methicillin-resistant *Staphylococcus aureus* in Western Australia. J Hosp Infect 1993; 25:97–108.

46. Maguire GP, Arthur AD, Boustead PJ, et al. Clinical experience and outcomes of community-acquired and nosocomial methicillin-resistant *Staphylococcus aureus* in a northern Australian hospital. J Hosp Infect 1998; 38:273–281.
47. O'Brien FG, Pearman JW, Gracy M, et al. Community strain of methicillin-resistant *Staphylococcus aureus* involved in a hospital outbreak. J Clin Microbiol 1999; 37(9): 2858–2862.
48. Eckhardt C, Halvosa JS, Ray SM, et al. Transmission of methicillin-resistant *Staphylococcus aureus* in the neonatal intensive care unit from a patient with community-acquired disease. Infect Control Hospital Epidemiol 2003; 24(6):460–461.
49. Bratu S, Eramo A, Kopec R, et al. Community-associated methicillin-resistant *Staphylococcus aureus* in hospital nursery and maternity units. Emerg Infect Dis 2005; 11(6): 808–813.
50. Merrer J, Santoli F, Appéré-De Vecchi C, et al. "Colonization pressure" and risk of acquisition of methicillin-resistant *Staphylococcus aureus* in a medical intensive care unit. Infect Control Hosp Epidemiol 2000; 21(11):718–723.
51. Troché G, Joly L-M, Guibert M, et al. Detection and treatment of antibiotic-resistant bacterial carriage in a surgical intensive care unit: a 6-year prospective survey. Infect Control Hosp Epidemiol 2005; 26(2):161–165.
52. Grundmann H, Hori S, Winter B, et al. Risk factors for the transmission of methicillin-resistant *Staphylococcus aureus* in an adult intensive care unit: fitting a model to the data. J Infect Dis 2002; 185(4):481–488.
53. Bonten MJM, Slaughter S, Ambergen AW, et al. The role of "colonization pressure" in the spread of vancomycin-resistant enterococi. An important infection control variable. Arch Intern Med 1998; 158:1127–1132.
54. Simor AE, Ofner-Agostini M, Bryce E, et al. The evolution of methicillin-resistant *Staphylococcus aureus* in Canadian hospitals: 5 years of national surveillance. CMAJ 2001; 165(1):21–26.
55. Dupeyron C, Campillo B, Bordes M, et al. A clinical trial of mupirocin in the eradication of methicillin-resistant *Staphylococcus aureus* nasal carriage in a digestive disease unit. J Hosp Infect 2000; 52(4):281–287.
56. Boyce JM, Opal SM, Potter-Bynoe G, et al. Spread of methicillin-resistant *Staphylococcus aureus* in a hospital after exposure to a healthcare worker with chronic sinusitis. Clin Infect Dis 1993; 17(3):496–504.
57. Wang J-T, Chang S-C, Ko W-J, et al. A hospital-acquired outbreak of methicillin-resistant *Staphylococcus aureus* infection initiated by a surgeon carrier. J Hosp Infect 2001; 47(2):104–109.
58. Devine J, Cooke RPD, Wright EP. Is methicillin-resistant *Staphylococcus aureus* (MRSA) contamination of ward-based computer terminals a surrogate marker for nosocomial MRSA transmission and handwashing compliance? J Hosp Infect 2001; 48(1):72–75.
59. Boyce JM, Potter-Bynoe G, Chenevert C, et al. Environmental contamination due to methicillin-resistant *Staphylococcus aureus*: possible infection control implications. Infect Control Hosp Epidemiol 1997; 18(9):622–627.
60. Wagenvoort JHT, Sluijsmans W, Penders RJR. Better environmental survival of outbreak versus sporadic MRSA isolates. J Hosp Infect 2000; 45(3):231–234.
61. Bhalla A, Pultz NJ, Gries DM, et al. Acquisition of nosocomial pathogens on hands after contact with environmental surfaces near hospitalized patients. Infect Control Hosp Epidemiol 2004; 25(2):164–167.
62. McBryde ES, Bradley LC, Whitby M, et al. An investigation of contact transmission of methicillin-resistant *Staphylococcus aureus.* J Hosp Infect 2004; 58(2):104–108.
63. Vriens MR, Fluit AC, Troelstra A, et al. Is methicillin-resistant *Staphylococcus aureus* more contagious than methicillin-susceptible *S. aureus* in a surgical intensive care unit? Infect Control Hosp Epidemiol 2002; 23(9):491–494.
64. http://www.cdc.gov/ncidod/hip/ARESIST/mrsahcw.htm (accessed July, 2005).

65. Shiomori T, Miyamoto H, Makishima K. Significance of airborne transmission of methicillin-resistant *Staphylococcus aureus* in an otolaryngology-head and neck surgery unit. Arch Otolaryngol Head Neck Surg 2001; 127(6):644–648.

66. Sherertz RJ, Bassetti S, Bassetti-Wyss B. "Cloud" health-care workers. Emerg Infect Dis 2001; 7(2):241–244.

67. Bassetti S, Bischoff WE, Walter M, et al. Dispersal of *Staphylococcus aureus* into the air associated with a rhinovirus infection. Infect Control Hosp Epidemiol 2005; 26(2):196–203.

68. Marshall C, Wolfe R, Kossmann T, et al. Risk factors for acquisition of methicillin-resistant *Staphlococcus aureus* (MRSA) by trauma patients in the intensive care unit. J Hosp Infect 2004; 57(3):245–252.

69. Healy CM, Hulten KG, Palazzi DL, et al. Emergence of new strains of methicillin-resistant *Staphylococcus aureus* in a neonatal intensive care unit. Clin Infect Dis 2004; 39:1460–1466.

70. Muto CA, Jernigan JA, Ostrowsky BE, et al. SHEA Guideline for preventing nosocomial transmission of multidrug-resistant strains of *Staphylococcus aureus* and *Enterococcus*. Infect Control Hosp Epidemiol 2003; 24(5):362–386.

71. Boyce JM, Havill NL, Kohan C, et al. Do infection control measures work for methicillin-resistant *Staphylococcus aureus*? Infect Control Hosp Epidemiol 2004; 25(5):395–401.

72. Jernigan JA, Titus MG, Groschel DHM, et al. Effectiveness of contact isolation during a hospital outbreak of methicillin-resistant *Staphylococcus aureus*. Am J Epidemiol 1996; 143:496–504.

73. Salmenlinna S. Lyytikäinen O, Kotilainen P, et al. Molecular epidemiology of methicillin-resistant *Staphylococcus aureus* in Finland. Eur J Clin Microbiol Infect Dis 2000; 19:101–107.

74. Thompson RL, Cabezudo I, Wenzel RP. Epidemiology of nosocomial infections caused by methicillin-resistant *Staphylococcus aureus*. Ann Intern Med 1982; 97:309–317.

75. Jernigan JA, Clemence MA, Stott GA, et al. Control of methicillin-resistant *Staphylococcus aureus* at a university hospital: one decade later. Infect Control Hosp Epidemiol 1995; 16(12):686–696.

76. Jans B, Suentens C, Struelens M. Decreasing MRSA rates in Belgian hospitals: results from the national surveillance network after introduction of national guidelines. Infect Control Hosp Epidemiol 2000; 21(6):419.

77. Harbarth S, Martin Y, Rohner P, et al. Effect of delayed infection control measures on a hospital outbreak of methicillin-resistant *Staphylococcus aureus*. J Hosp Infect 2000; 46(1):42–49.

78. Back NA, Linnemann CC Jr., Staneck JL, et al. Control of methicillin-resistant *Staphylococcus aureus* in a neonatal intensive-care unit: use of intensive microbiologic surveillance and mupirocin. Infect Control Hosp Epidemiol 1996; 17(4):227–231.

79. Nicolle LE, Dyck B, Thompson G, et al. Regional dissemination and control of epidemic methicillin-resistant *Staphylococcus aureus*. Infect Control Hosp Epidemiol 1999; 20(3):202–205.

80. Law MR, Gillon. Hospital-acquired infection with methicillin-resistant and methicillin-sensitive staphylococci. Epidemiol Infect 1988; 101:623–629.

81. Murray-Leisure KA, Gei S, et al. Control of epidemic methicillin-resistant *Staphylococcus aureus*. Infect Control Hosp Epidemiol 1990; 11:343–350.

82. Kotilainen P, Routamaa M, Peltonen R, et al. Eradication of methicillin-resistant *Staphylococcus aureus* from a health center ward and associated nursing home. Arch Intern Med 2001; 161:859–863.

83. Lucet J-C, Chevret S, Durand-Zaleski I, et al. Prevalence and risk factors for carriage of methicillin-resistant *Staphylococcus aureus* at admission to the intensive care unit. Arch Intern Med 2003; 163:181–188.

84. Girou E, Pujade G, Legrand P, et al. Selective screening of carriers for control of methicillin-resistant *Staphylococcus aureus* (MRSA) in high-risk hospital areas with a high level of endemic MRSA. Clin Infect Dis 1998; 27(3):543–550.

85. Francois P, Pittet D, Bento M, et al. Rapid detection of methicillin-resistant *Staphylococcus aureus* directly from sterile or nonsterile clinical samples by a new molecular assay. J Clin Microbiol 2003; 41:254–260.

86. Boyce JM, Chenevert C. Abstracts of Papers, Eighth Annual Meeting of the Society for Healthcare Epidemiology of America, Orlando, FL, Apr 5–7, 1998.

87. Dietze B, Rath A, Wendt C, et al. Survival of MRSA on sterile goods packaging. J Hosp Infect 2001; 49(4):255–261.

88. Embil J, McLeod J, Al-Barrak AM, et al. An outbreak of the methicillin-resistant *Staphylococcus aureus* on a burn unit: potential role of contaminated hydrotherapy equipment. Burn 2001; 27:681–688.

89. Rampling A, Wiseman S, Davis L, et al. Evidence that hospital hygiene is important in the control of methicillin resistant *Staphylococcus aureus*. J Hosp Infect 2001; 49: 109–116.

90. Farr BM. Prevention and control of methicillin-resistant *Staphylococcus aureus* infections. Curr Opin Infect Dis 2004; 17:317–322.

91. Arnold MS, Dempsey JM, Fishman M, et al. The best hospital practices for controlling methicillin-resistant *Staphylococcus aureus*: on the cutting edge. Infect Control Hosp Epidemiol 2002; 23(2):69–76.

92. Boyce JM. MRSA patients: proven methods to treat colonization and infection. J Hosp Infect 2001; 48(suppl A):S9–S14.

93. Watanakunakorn C, Axelson C, Bota B, et al. Mupirocin ointment with and without chlorhexidine baths in the eradication of *Staphylococcus aureus* nasal carriage in nursing home residents. Am J Infect Control 1995; 23:306–309.

94. Vivoni AM, Santos KRN, de-Oliveira MP, et al. Mupirocin for controlling methicillin-resistant *Staphylococcus aureus*: lessons from a decade of use at a university hospital. Infect Control Hosp Epidemiol 2005; 26(7):662–667.

95. Silvestri L, Milanese M, Oblach L, et al. Enteral vancomycin to control methicillin-resistant *Staphylococcus aureus* outbreak in mechanically ventilated patients. Am J Infect Control 2002; 30(7):391–399.

96. Khoury J, Jones M, Grim A, et al. Eradication of methicillin-resistant *Staphylococcus aureus* from a neonatal intensive care unit by active surveillance and aggressive infection control measures. Infect Control Hosp Epidemiol 2005; 26(7):616–621.

97. Doebbeling BN, Breneman DL, Neu HC, et al. Elimination of *Staphylococcus aureus* nasal carriage in healthcare workers: analysis of six clinical trials with calcium mupirocin ointment. Clin Infect Dis 1993; 17(9):466–474.

98. Reagan DR, Doebbeling BN, Pfaller MA, et al. Elimination of coincident *Staphylococcus aureus* nasal and hand carriage with intranasal application of mupirocin calcium ointment. Ann Intern Med 1991; 114(2):101–106.

99. Chenoweth CE. *Enterococcus* species. In: Mayhall CG, ed. Hospital Epidemiology and Infection Control. 3rd ed. Philadelphia: Lippincott Williams and Wilkins, 2004:529–544.

100. Bugg TDH, Dutka-Malen S, Arthur M, et al. Identification of vancomycin resistance protein VanA as a D-Alanine: D-Alanine ligase of altered substrate specificity. Biochemistry 1991; 30(8):2017–2021.

101. Willems RJL, Homan W, Top J, et al. Variant *esp* gene as a marker of a distinct genetic lineage of vancomycin-resistant *Enterococcus faecium* spreading in hospitals. Lancet 2001; 357:853–855.

102. Rice LB, Carias L, Rudin S, et al. A potential virulence gene, hyl_{Efm}, predominates in *Enterococcus faecium* of clinical origin. J Infect Dis 2003; 187(3):508–512.

103. Shay DK, Maloney SA, Monetcalvo M, et al. Epidemiology and mortality risk of vancomycin-resistant enterococcal bloodstream infections. J Infect Dis 1995; 172(10): 993–1000.

104. Montecalvo MA, Shay DK, Patel P, et al. Bloodstream infections with vancomycin-resistant enterococci. Arch Intern Med 1996; 156:1458–1462.

105. Stroud L, Edwards J, Danzig L, et al. Risk factors for mortality associated with enter-ococcal bloodstream infections. Infect Control Hosp Epidemiol 1996; 17(9):576–580.
106. Edmond MB, Ober JF, Dawson JD, et al. Vancomycin-resistant enterococcal bactere-mia: natural history and attributable mortality. Clin Infect Dis 1996; 23(12):1234–1239.
107. Stosor V, Peterson LR, Postelnick M, et al. *Enterococcus faecium* bacteremia. Does van-comycin resistance make a difference? Arch Intern Med 1998; 158:522–527.
108. Zaas AK, Song X, Tucker P, et al. Risk factors for development of vancomycin-resistant enterococcal bloodstream infection in patients with cancer who are colonized with vancomycin-resistant enterococci. Clin Infect Dis 2002; 35(10):1139–1146.
109. Raad II, Hanna HA, Boktour M, et al. Catheter-related vancomycin-resistant *Entero-coccus faecium* bacteremia: clinical and molecular epidemiology. Infect Control Hosp Epidemiol 2005; 26(7):658–661.
110. Hussain Z, Shaikh A, Peloquin CA, et al. Successful treatment of vancomycin-resistant *Enterococcus faecium* meningitis with linezolid: case report and literature review. Scan J Infect Dis 2001; 33:375–379.
111. Steinmetz MP, Vogelbaum MA, DeGeorgia MA, et al. Successful treatment of vancomy-cin-resistant enterococcus meningitis with linezolid: case report and review of the literature. Crit Care Med 2001; 29(12):2383–2385.
112. Wong AHM, Wenzel RP, Edmond MB. Epidemiology of bacteriuria caused by vancomycin-resistant enterococci: a retrospective study. Am J Infect Control 2000; 28(4):277–281.
113. Malik RK, Montecalvo MA, Reale MR, et al. Epidemiology and control of vancomycin-resistant enterococci in a regional neonatal intensive care unit. Pediatr Infect Dis J 1999; 18(4):352–356.
114. Singh N, Leger M-M, Campbell J, et al. Control of vancomycin-resistant enterococci in the neonatal intensive care unit. Infect Control Hosp Epidemiol 2005; 26(7):646–649.
115. Sherer CR, Sprague BM, Campos JM, et al. Characterizing vancomycin-resistant enter-ococci in neonatal intensive care. Emerg Infect Dis 2005; 11(9):1470–1472.
116. Bonten MJM, Hayden MK, Nathan C, et al. Epidemiology of colonization of patients and environmental with vancomycin-resistant enterococci. Lancet 1996; 348:1615–1619.
117. Montecalvo MA, Shay DK, Gedris C, et al. A semiquantitative analysis of the fecal flora of patients with vancomycin-resistant enterococci: colonized patients pose an infection control risk. Clin Infect Dis 1997; 25(10):929–930.
118. Ostrowsky BE, Venkataraman L, D'Agata EMC, et al. Vancomycin-resistant entero-cocci in intensive care units: high frequency of stool carriage during a non-outbreak period. Arch Intern Med 1999; 159(13):1467–1472.
119. Falk PS, Winnike J, Woodmansee C, et al. Outbreak of vancomycin-resistant enterococci in a burn unit. Infect Control Hosp Epidemiol 2000; 21(9):575–582.
120. Boyce JM, Mermel LA, Zervos MJ, et al. Controlling vancomycin-resistant enterococci. Infect Control Hosp Epidemiol 1995; 16(11):634–637.
121. Tenorio AR, Badri SM, Sahgal NB, et al. Effectiveness of gloves in the prevention of hand carriage of vancomycin-resistant *Enterococcus* species by health care workers after patient care. Clin Infect Dis 2001; 32(5):826–829.
122. Ray AJ, Taub TF. Nosocomial transmission of vancomycin-resistant enterococci from surfaces. JAMA 2002; 287(11):1400–1401.
123. Duckro AN, Blom DW, Lyle EA, et al. Transfer of vancomycin-resistant enterococci via health care worker hands. Arch Intern Med 2005; 165:302–307.
124. Reisner BS, Shaw S, Huber ME, et al. Comparison of three methods to recover vanco-mycin-resistant enterococci (VRE) from perianal and environmental samples collected during a hospital outbreak of VRE. Infect Control Hosp Epidemiol 2000; 21(12):775–779.
125. Noskin GA, Stosor V, Cooper I, et al. Recovery of vancomycin-resistant enterococci on fingertips and environmental surfaces. Infect Control Hosp Epidemiol 1995; 16(10):577–581.

126. Bonilla HF, Zervos MJ, Kauffman CA. Long-term survival of vancomycin-resistant *Enterococcus faecium* on a contaminated surface. Infect Control Hosp Epidemiol 1996; 17(12):770–771.

127. Livornese LL Jr., Dias S, Samel C, et al. Hospital-acquired infection with vancomycin-resistant *Enterococcus faecium* transmitted by electronic thermometers. Ann Intern Med 1992; 117(2):112–116.

128. Loeb M, Salama S, Armstrong-Evans M, et al. A case-control study to detect modifiable risk factors for colonization with vancomycin-resistant enterococci. Infect Control Hosp Epidemiol 1999; 20(11):760–763.

129. Byers KE, Anglim AM, Anneski CJ, et al. A hospital epidemic of vancomycin-resistant *Enterococcus*: risk factors and control. Infect Control Hosp Epidemiol 2001; 22(3): 140–147.

130. Cetinkaya Y, Falk PS, Mayhall CG. Effect of gastrointestinal bleeding and oral medications on acquisition of vancomycin-resistant *Enterococcus faecium* in hospitalized patients. Clin Infect Dis 2002; 35(8):935–942.

131. Karanfil LV, Murphy M, Josephson A, et al. A cluster of vancomycin-resistant *Enterococcus faecium* in an intensive care unit. Infect Control Hosp Epidemiol 1992; 13(4):195–200.

132. Slaughter S, Hayden MK, Nathan C, et al. A comparison of the effect of universal use of gloves and gowns with that of glove use alone on acquisition of vancomycin-resistant enterococci in a medical intensive care unit. Ann Intern Med 1996; 125(6):448–456.

133. Gardiner D, Murphey S, Ossman E, et al. Prevalence and acquisition of vancomycin-resistant enterococci in a medical intensive care unit. Infect Control Hosp Epidemiol 2002; 23(8):466–468.

134. Padiglione AA, Wolfe R, Grabsch EA, et al. Risk factors for new detection of vancomycin-resistant enterococci in acute-care hospitals that employ strict infection control procedures. Antimicrob Agents Chemother 2003; 47(8):2492–2498.

135. Martinez JA, Ruthazer R, Hansjosten K, et al. Role of environmental contamination as a risk factor for acquisition of vancomycin-resistant enterococci in patients treated in a medical intensive care unit. Arch Intern Med 2003; 163:1905–1912.

136. Warren DK, Nitin A, Hill C, et al. Occurrence of co-colonization or co-infection with vancomycin-resistant enterococci and methicillin-resistant *Staphylococcus aureus* in a medical intensive care unit. Infect Control Hosp Epidemiol 2004; 25(2):99–104.

137. Donskey CJ, Chowdhry TK, Hecker MT, et al. Effect of antibiotic therapy on the density of vancomycin-resistant enterococci in the stool of colonized patients. N Engl J Med 2000; 343(26):1925–1932.

138. Carmeli Y, Samore MH, Huskins WC. The association between antecedent vancomycin treatment and hospital-acquired vancomycin-resistant enterococci. A meta-analysis. Arch Intern Med 1999; 159:2461–2468.

139. D'Agata EMC, Green WK, Schulman G, et al. Vancomycin-resistant enterococci among chronic hemodialysis patients: a prospective study of acquisition. Clin Infect Dis 2001; 32(1):23–29.

140. Lee HK, Lee WG, Cho SR. Clinical and molecular biological analysis of a nosocomial outbreak of vancomycin-resistant enterococci in a neonatal intensive care unit. Acta Pediatr 1999; 88:651–654.

141. Yüce A, Karaman M, Gülay Z, et al. Vancomycin-resistant enterococci in neonates. Scand J Infect Dis 2001; 33:803–805.

142. Rupp ME, Marion N, Fey PD, et al. Outbreak of vancomycin-resistant *Enterococcus faecium* in a neonatal intensive care unit. Infect Control Hosp Epidemiol 2001; 22(5):301–303.

143. Recommendations for preventing the spread of vancomycin resistance. Hospital Infection Control Practices Advisory Committee (HICPAC). Infect Control Hosp Epidemiol 1995; 16(2):105–113.

144. Leber AL, Hindler JF, Kato EO, et al. Laboratory-based surveillance for vancomycin-resistant enterococci: utility of screening stool specimens submitted for *Clostridium difficile* toxin assay. Infect Control Hosp Epidemiol 2001; 22(3):160–164.

145. D'Agata EMC, Gautam S, Green WK, et al. High rate of false-negative results of the rectal swab culture method in detection of gastrointestinal colonization with vancomycin-resistant enterococci. Clin Infect Dis 2002; 34(2):167–172.

146. Weinstein JW, Tallapragada S, Farrel P, et al. Comparison of rectal and perirectal swabs for detection of colonization with vancomycin-resistant enterococci. J Clin Microbiol 1996; 34(1):210–212.

147. Ostrowsky BE, Trick WE, Sohn AH, et al. Control of vancomycin-resistant enterococcus in health care facilities in a region. N Engl J Med 2001; 344(19):1427–1433.

148. Siddiqui AH, Harris AD, Hebden J, et al. The effect of active surveillance for vancomycin-resistant enterococci in high-risk units on vancomycin-resistant enterococci incidence hospital-wide. Am J Infect Control 2002; 30(1):40–43.

149. Calfee DP, Giannetta ET, Durbin LJ, et al. Control of endemic vancomycin-resistant *Enterococcus* among inpatients at a university hospital. Clin Infect Dis 2003; 37(3): 326–332.

150. Price CS, Paule S, Noskin GA, et al. Active surveillance reduces the incidence of vancomycin-resistant enterococcal bacteremia. Clin Infect Dis 2003; 37(7):921–928.

151. Boyce JM, Opal SM, Chow JW, et al. Outbreak of multidrug-resistant *Enterococcus faecium* with transferable *vanB* class vancomycin resistance. J Clin Microbiol 1994; 32(5):1148–1153.

152. Puzniak LA, Leet T, Mayfield J, et al. To gown or not to gown: the effect on acquisition of vancomycin-resistant enterococci. Clin Infect Dis 2002; 35(1):18–25.

153. Srinivasan A, Song X, Ross T, et al. A prospective study to determine whether cover gowns in addition to gloves decrease nosocomial transmission of vancomycin-resistant enterococci in an intensive care unit. Infect Control Hosp Epidemiol 2002; 23(8):424–428.

154. Zachary KC, Bayne PS, Morrison VJ, et al. Contamination of gowns, gloves and stethoscopes with vancomycin-resistant enterococci. Infect Control Hosp Epidemiol 2001; 22(9):560–564.

155. Byers KE, Anglim AM, Anneski CJ, et al. Duration of colonization with vancomycin-resistant *Enterococcus*. Infect Control Hosp Epidemiol 2002; 23(4):207–211.

156. Noskin GA, Bednarz P, Suriano T, et al. Persistent contamination of fabric covered furniture by vancomycin-resistant enterococci: implications for upholstery selection in hospitals. Am J Infect Control 2000; 28(4):311–313.

157. Byers KE, Durbin LJ, Simonton BM, et al. Disinfection of hospital rooms contaminated with vancomycin-resistant *Enterococcu faecium*. Infect Control Hsop Epidemiol 1998; 19(4):261–264.

158. Carmeli Y, Venkataraman L, DeGirolami PC, et al. Stool colonization of healthcare workers with selected resistant bacteria. Infect Control Hosp Epidemiol 1998; 19(1):38–40.

159. Fridkin SK, Lawton R, Edwards JR, et al. Monitoring antimicrobial use and resistance: comparison with a national benchmark on reducing vancomycin use and vancomycin-resistant enterococci. Emerg Infect Dis 2002; 8(7):702–707.

160. Quale J, Landman D, Saurina G, et al. Manipulation of a hospital antimicrobial formulary to control an outbreak of vancomycin-resistant enterococci. Clin Infect Dis 1996; 23(11):1020–1025.

161. May AK, Melton SM, McGwin G, et al. Reduction of vancomycin-resistant enterococcal infections by limitation of broad-spectrum cephalosporin use in a trauma and burn intensive care unit. Shock 2000; 14(3):259–264.

162. Chavers LS, Moser SA, Funkhouser E, et al. Association between antecedent intravenous antimicrobial exposure and isolation of vancomycin-resistant enterococci. Microb Drug Resist 2003; 9(suppl 1):S69–S77.

163. Stiefel U, Paterson DL, Pultz NJ, et al. Effect of the increasing use of piperacillin/ tazobactam on the incidence of vancomycin-resistant enterococci in four academic medical centers. Infect Control Hosp Epidemiol 2004; 25(5):380–383.
164. Winston LG, Charlebois ED, Pang S, et al. Impact of a formulary switch from ticarcillin-clavulanate to piperacillin-tazobactam on colonization with vancomycin-resistant enterococci. Am J Infect Control 2004; 32(8):462–469.
165. Montecalvo MA, Jarvis WR, Uman J, et al. Costs and savings associated with infection control measures that reduced transmission of vancomycin-resistant enterococci in an endemic setting. Infect Control Hosp Epidemiol 2001; 22(7):437–442.
166. Muto CA, Giannetta ET, Durbin LJ, et al. Cost-effectiveness of perirectal surveillance cultures for controlling vancomycin-resistant *Enterococcus*. Infect Control Hosp Epidemiol 2002; 23(8):429–435.
167. Carmeli Y, Eliopoulos G, Mozaffari E, et al. Health and economic outcomes of vancomycin-resistant enterococci. Arch Intern Med 2002; 162:2223–2228.
168. Puzniak LA, Gillespie KN, Leet T, et al. A cost-benefit analysis of gown use in controlling vancomycin-resistant *Enterococcus* transmission: is it worth the price? Infect Control Hosp Epidemiol 2004; 25(5):418–424.

2

Outbreak Investigation in the Critical Care Unit

Brian W. Cooper

Division of Infectious Disease, Hartford Hospital, Hartford, and University of Connecticut School of Medicine, Farmington, Connecticut, U.S.A.

INTRODUCTION

The term "outbreak" is a loaded word that tends to precipitate severe anxiety in hospital staff. Outbreaks of nosocomial infection, however, are quite common and often occur in critical care settings. An estimated 4% of all patients acquiring a nosocomial infection develop the infection as part of an outbreak (1). Outbreaks occur periodically in all institutions, and all clinicians should be aware of the potential dangers of outbreaks and the need for systematic surveillance and analysis of data in order to interdict clusters of infection as early as possible.

Outbreaks are defined as an increase in the rate of occurrence of an event compared with past experience. The past experience is the baseline or endemic rate of event occurrence. Sometimes outbreaks are identified by large explosive increases in rates of infection. Such outbreaks are often easily identified. A three-fold increase in bacteremias due to *Enterobacter cloacae* during one month in an intensive care unit (ICU) would be a good example. Other outbreaks are more subtle and require careful analysis of surveillance data to recognize. For example, Kool et al. describe an outbreak of unrecognized hospital transmission of Legionnaires disease in transplant patients which ran over a two-year period before being recognized (2).

Commonly, outbreaks may involve a single organism producing infections at a single site, as noted above. Other outbreaks involve clusters of particular types of infection caused by several different organisms. An example would be an increase in urinary tract infections arising due to poor technique in handling the catheters on a particular unit. Such an outbreak may involve infections due to several organisms. Sometimes outbreaks involve infections at several sites, as might happen with cutaneous infections, conjunctivitis, and bacteremia after introduction of *Staphylococcus aureus* into a neonatal ICU. Still other outbreaks may be quite difficult to detect. In particular, outbreaks of infections with long incubation periods are not easily discerned. Examples include nosocomial outbreaks of tuberculosis or hepatitis B viral infection. Outbreaks may also involve unusual sources of infection. For example,

Gaillot et al. describe the spread of an extended spectrum beta lactamase (ESBL) producing Klebsiella strain, which was transmitted in ultrasonography gel (3).

SURVEILLANCE

Surveillance of nosocomial infections provides the foundation for investigation of out-break control efforts. It is the means by which a baseline or endemic rate is established. Surveillance of nosocomial infections involves systematic collection and analysis of data on the occurrence of infection. Care needs to be taken to make sure that well accepted definitions of nosocomial infection are followed by those conducting surveillance to ensure database validity. In addition, changes in surveillance methodology or case-finding methods will affect the comparability of data from one time period to another. When surveillance methods are significantly changed, data collected by the new surveillance activity can no longer be compared to data collected in prior time periods.

Surveillance of nosocomial infections in hospitals is commonly carried out by infection control and hospital epidemiology personnel. Some critical care units may wish to supplement this surveillance activity with surveillance data of their own col-lected as part of a unit quality-improvement program. Such efforts need to be closely coordinated with infection-control personnel. Other sources of data in outbreaks include reports from clinicians or nursing units who may have noticed an unusual increase in particular infections.

Mere collection of surveillance data is not sufficient in itself to detect clusters. The data must be analyzed periodically and compared with past experience. The most common means for this involves calculating a rate; one divides the crude number of infections by an appropriate denominator. Appropriate denominators are often derived from the patient census on a unit. The sensitivity of data analysis can be increased by using incidence density-adjusted denominators. For example, the rate of primary bacter-emias in a given month or quarter may be expressed as a ratio of the number of infections to patients admitted to the unit. If, during a given quarter, six primary bacter-emias are identified and 240 patients were admitted to the unit, the rate of infection may be expressed as $6/240 = 3.3\%$. However, because some patients may be admitted to the unit only briefly while others have long-term stays, a more efficient denominator may be patient-days. When patient-days are used as a denominator, the rate is often multiplied by some constant such as 1000 to make the decimal point more manageable. In our example, if the 240 patients admitted to the unit accrued 1200 patient-days, the rate might be expressed as $6/1200 \times 1000 = 5$ infections per 1000 patient-days.

An even better way of calculating this rate would be to adjust for exposure to central intravenous catheters and use catheter-days as the denominator. Such rates more accurately reflect the exposure of patients to risk factors such as central intra-venous catheters.

Rates of infection collected in surveillance data should be compared with base-line rates using valid statistical methods to determine if a statistically significant increase in rate has occurred.

INVESTIGATION OF CLUSTERS OF INFECTION

Outbreak investigation is a time- and resource-consuming process. Although there is no set script for all investigations, it is usually wise to proceed in a systematic fashion. Epidemiologists have derived a series of steps which comprise essential

Table 1 Systemic Steps in Outbreak Investigations

Confirm the outbreak
Establish a case definition and define the pre-epidemic and epidemic periods
Notify appropriate hospital personnel
Construct an epidemic curve to describe events in time, place, and person
Review the literature
Develop a line listing, chart review, and summary analysis of data
Develop hypotheses and institute preliminary control measures
Evaluate the effectiveness of control measures
If necessary, proceed to further studies, such as case-control studies

milestones in the workup of an outbreak (Table 1). The order of these steps does not need to be followed precisely, but the first few steps listed are best completed initially.

Confirming the Outbreak

Because outbreak investigation is so resource-intensive, it is a waste of time to investigate small clusters that are not epidemics. When rates of infection are significantly elevated above baseline rates, an outbreak may be occurring. The investigator should next consider the possibility of a pseudo-outbreak. Pseudo-outbreaks usually occur when noninfecting organisms contaminate patient culture material. A good example has been described in the literature (4). Occasionally, pseudo-outbreaks occur when bias is introduced into case-finding methods, such as a change in definitions or surveillance methodology in the epidemic and pre-epidemic periods. Sometimes, changes in laboratory techniques during the pre-epidemic and epidemic periods may lead to pseudo-outbreaks.

Establish a Case Definition

In order to minimize bias in data collection, a precise written definition of cases needs to be developed. The definition should be broad enough that all potential cases are included yet not so broad as to bias the investigator with noncases. At times, the case definition may need to be redefined as the investigation proceeds. The definition should include the chief characteristics of the case diagnoses as well as appropriate factors indicating time, place, and person. An example of case definition for our fictitious outbreak of bacteremias may resemble the following: "A case was defined as any patient in the surgical ICU with *Enterobacter cloacae* isolated from blood cultures in the period after December 1, 1995."

All potential cases must fit the proposed definition or be rejected from the analysis. This allows uniformity in further data collection.

The development of the case definition should also establish the pre-epidemic and epidemic periods. The epidemic period is usually the time from the first identified case to the present. The time period for the pre-epidemic period varies. In general, it is unwise to use a pre-epidemic period of less than six months. If the epidemic period is long or cases are few, then the pre-epidemic period should be lengthened. A one-year pre-epidemic period is commonly used in investigations of nosocomial outbreaks.

NOTIFICATION OF APPROPRIATE INDIVIDUALS

Good communication is essential in unraveling an outbreak investigation. Early in the investigation, the microbiology lab should be notified and the means developed to save outbreak organisms for possible epidemiologic typing later.

Sometimes acute and convalescent serum needs to be collected and preserved. Numerous other details often need to be discussed with the laboratory director, and good lines of communication are essential. Affected chiefs of service, department heads, ICU directors, head nurses, and other clinical staff should be notified of the investigation. Often important information and direction can be gleaned by talking to these sources early on in the investigation.

Outbreaks have political and sometimes public relations aspects as well. The hospital public relations director should be kept apprised of the investigation, but unsolicited press releases are usually not wise. When the press involves itself in an outbreak investigation and the investigators must talk to members of the media, it is best to be forthright and honest with information. All information released to the media should be channeled through a single hospital source to minimize confusion.

Legal implications often flow from an outbreak investigation as well. At the outset, a new file should be opened and all decisions and meetings documented thoroughly.

Outbreaks involving reportable diseases should, of course, be promptly reported to the state public health authorities. In some states, all outbreaks are required to be reported to the state. The list of reportable diseases also varies from state to state.

CONSTRUCT AN EPIDEMIC CURVE

Epidemic curves are simple graphic tools which can convey surprising amounts of information concisely characterizing the outbreak. In an epidemic curve, individual cases are graphed over time. Additional data, such as mortality, location, or comorbid factors may be coded and superimposed on this curve. An additional graphic tool such as a spot map of a unit or wing may be useful in characterizing the epidemic's geographic factors. Bed or room locations of cases can be easily displayed on the spot map.

REVIEW THE LITERATURE

It is useful early in the investigation to gather information about the infection. The biology of the infecting organism, its reservoirs, and it mode of transmission should be carefully reviewed. Past outbreaks reported in the literature are important sources of information. Other investigations may have already dealt with similar situations, and solutions to your problems may have been suggested.

Sources of information to search are myriad but should include computerized Medline searches, textbook sources, and Index Medicus searches. The medical librarian can be an invaluable resource to the investigator. We have found that a combination of computerized Medline searches and manual searches in textbooks and Index Medicus yields the best results.

DEVELOP A LINE LISTING

A line listing is merely a questionnaire consisting of data from case records which the investigator deems potentially useful. Included are demographic data such as age, sex, and race, as well as patient diagnosis and location. Major diagnostic and therapeutic procedures that the patient has undergone are also helpful. Underlying illnesses and medications administered are important to indicate. Listing the health care personnel taking care of the patient is often important, especially if a cluster of infections may be related to a health-care worker colonized with a pathogenic organism. Richman et al. (5) described an outbreak of Group A streptococcal surgical wound infections linked to exposure to an operating room staff member who was a rectal carrier of the organism. In addition, the line listing should consider all other potential risk factors for the illness noted by the investigator, including health-care or hygienic practices that may lead to illness in unusual ways. Claesson et al. (6) described an outbreak of Group A streptococcal endometritis on a maternity ward linked to use of a shower head.

Data for the line listing are usually collected by chart review and stored in a computer database for ease of analysis. Preliminary analysis of the case is conducted by examining simple frequency rates and descriptions of the collected data. Clues to the outbreak may be apparent in the initial pattern of data collected. Risk factors that most cases have in common may be clues to solving an outbreak; however, in many cases the initial review of data is insufficient to establish the cause, and one must proceed to a case-control study as noted below.

DEVELOP HYPOTHESES AND INSTITUTE PRELIMINARY CONTROLS

Even when initial data analysis is not sufficient to establish cause for the epidemic, the investigator commonly has developed early in the investigation several potential hypotheses regarding the underlying cause. Further analysis or data gathering may be necessary to prove out the likely hypothesis, but often at this stage some preliminary controls can be instituted. At times in an outbreak investigation, the preliminary control measures must be instituted early and empirically in the investigation due to the urgency of the situation. For example, in our institution, a case of nosocomial *Salmonella gastroenteritis* was noted in the newborn ICU (7). A quick review of the situation indicated that several staff members in the newborn ICU had been ill with mild gastrointestinal disturbance the week prior to the index case. While further investigation proceeded, preliminary controls were focused quickly on controlling exposure of newborns to potentially infected or colonized hospital staff. Ultimately, the investigation showed that no hospital staff were infected or colonized with *S. gastroenteritis* and that the infant was infected by her chronically colonized but asymptomatic mother.

Control measures instituted early in the investigation should be based on hypotheses drawn from certain clues from the data gathered, which may suggest a source for the outbreak. For example, an outbreak of *Serratia marcescens* urinary tract infections among catheterized patients in an ICU might suggest problems in aseptic technique during catheter care. Control measures might include an education program stressing reinforcement of proper aseptic techniques in catheter care as well as redoubled efforts to encourage hand washing on the unit.

EVALUATE THE EFFECTIVENESS OF CONTROL MEASURES

While control measures are being implemented, it is important to continue intensive surveillance for any new cases that continue to accrue. If new cases accumulate, one should question the effectiveness of the control measures. The investigator needs to be careful to take into account the incubation period of the infection during this period, however. Illnesses with relatively long incubation period such as a varicella may continue to accumulate after preliminary control measures were put into effect.

FURTHER STUDIES

If cases continue to accumulate beyond the institution of empiric controls, the investigator must question the accuracy of the hypothesis. Further hypotheses can be developed by evaluating multiple risk factors in a case-control study. In this type of study, case patients and appropriately chosen control patients are compared with regard to exposure to various risk factors. The investigator is looking for statistically significant association of certain risk factors with cases as opposed to controls. In an investigation of fever and hypotension on a surgical ICU, Trilla et al. (8) conducted a case-control study and found that volume of plasma expanders used was significantly associated with symptoms in case versus controls ($p = .0029$).

Proper selection of control patients can be critical to the success of a case-control study. The art of selecting proper controls can be complicated, and the reader is referred to literature specifically dealing with this subject (9–11). Most importantly, care should be taken to ensure that cases and controls have an equal likelihood of being exposed to a set of risk factors. As a rule of thumb, three control patients should be chosen for each case patient.

At the conclusion of the case-control study, a new understanding about relationships between risk factors and cases may suggest a need for a new set of control measures for the outbreak.

SUMMARY

Investigations of clusters or epidemics of nosocomial infection are often difficult, time- and resource-consuming activities. They tax the abilities and skills of infection-control personnel severely. However, outbreak investigations are among the most satisfying of infection control activities because of their far-reaching preventive effects. The proper response to a cluster of infections may mean the difference between a few cluster cases and a large-scale epidemic with significant morbidity and possible mortality. The reader is referred to the following references as examples of modern outbreak investigation. (12–18)

REFERENCES

1. Wenzel RP, Thompson RL, Landry SM, et al. Hospital acquired infections in intensive care unit patients: an overview with emphasis on epidemics. Infect Control 1983; 4:371–375.
2. Kool JL, Fiore AE, Kioski CM, et al. More than 10 years of unrecognized nosocomial transmission of Legionnaires disease among transplant patients. Infect Control Hosp Epidemiol 1998; 19:905–910.
3. Gaillot O, Maruejouls C, Abachin E, et al. Nosocomial outbreak of Klebsiella pneumoniae producing SHV5 extended spectrum beta lactamase originating from a contaminated ultrasonography coupling gel. J Clin Microbiology 1998; 36:1357–1360.
4. Auerbach SB, McNeil MM, Brown JM, Lasker BA, Jarvis WR. Outbreak of pseudoinfections with *Tsukamurella paurometabolum* traced to laboratory contamination: efficacy of joint epidemiological and laboratory investigation. Clin Infect Dis 1992; 14:1015–1022.

5. Richman DD, Bretton SJ, Goldman DA. Scarlet fever and group A streptococcal surgical wound infection traced to an anal carrier. J Pediatr 1977; 90:387–390.
6. Claesson BE, Claesson UL. An outbreak of endometritis in a maternity ward caused by spread of group A streptococci from a shower head. J Hosp Infect 1985; 6:304–311.
7. Cooper, B. Unpublished observation.
8. Trilla A, Codina C, Salles M, et al. A cluster of fever and hypotension on a surgical intensive care unit related to the contamination of plasma expanders by cell wall products of Bacillus stearothermophilus. Infect Control Hosp Epidemiol 1995; 16:335–339.
9. Cole P. The evolving case control study. J Chron Dis 1979; 32:15–27.
10. Feinstein AR. Experimental requirements and scientific principles in case control studies. J Chron Dis 1985; 38:127–133.
11. Hayden GF, Kramer MS, Horwitz RI. The case control study: a practical review for the clinician. JAMA 1982; 247:326–331.
12. Pimental JD, Low J, Styles K, et al. Control of an outbreak of multi-drug-resistance Acinetobacter baumannii in an intensive care unit and a surgical ward. J Hosp Infect 2005; 59(3):249–253.
13. Jeong SH, Bae IK, Kwon SB, et al. Investigation of a nosocomial outbreak of Acinetobacter baumannii producing PER-1 extended spectrum beta lactamase in an intensive care unit. J Hosp Infect 2005; 59(3):242–248.
14. Qavi A, Segal-Maurer S, Mariano N, et al. Increased mortality associated with a clonal outbreak of ceftazidime-resistant Klebsiella pneumoniae: a case-control study. Infect Control Hosp Epidemiol 2005; 26(1):63–68.
15. Zawacki A, O'Rourke E, Potter-Bynoe G, et al. An outbreak of Pseudomonas aeruginosa pneumonia and bloodstream infection associated with intermittent otitis externa in a healthcare worker. Infect Control Hosp Epidemiol 2004; 25(12):1083–1089.
16. Behari P, Englund J, Alcasid G, et al. Transmission of methicillin-resistant Staphylococcus aureus to preterm infants through breast milk. Infect Control Hosp Epidemiol 2004; 25(9):778–780.
17. Bukholm G, Tannaes T, Kjelsberg AB, et al. An outbreak of multidrug-resistant Pseudomonas aeruginosa associated with increased risk of patient death in an intensive care unit. Infect Control Hosp Epidemiol 2002; 23(8):441–446.
18. Lehours P, Rogues AM, Occhialini A, et al. Investigation of an outbreak due to Alcaligenes xylosoxidans subspecies xylosoxydans by random amplified polymorphic DNA analysis. Eur J Clin Microbiol Infect Dis 2002; 21(2):108–113.

3

Clinical Approach to Fever in the Critical Care Unit

Burke A. Cunha
Infectious Disease Division, Winthrop-University Hospital, Mineola, and State University of New York School of Medicine, Stony Brook, New York, U.S.A.

INTRODUCTION

Overview

Fever is a cardinal sign of disease. Fever may be caused by a wide variety of infectious and noninfectious disorders. The number of disorders that occur in seriously ill patients in critical care unit (CCU) is more limited than in the non-CCU population. The main clinical problems in the CCU are to differentiate between noninfectious and infectious causes of fever rather than to try and determine the specific cause of the patient's fever.

The clinical approach to fever in the CCU is based on a careful analysis of the acuteness/chronicity of the fever, the characteristics of the fever pattern, the relationship of the pulse to the fever, the duration of the fever, and the defervescence pattern of the fever. It is the task of the infectious disease consultant to relate aspects of the patient's history and physical, laboratory, and radiological tests with the characteristics of the patient's fever, which together determine differential diagnostic possibilities. After the differential diagnosis has been narrowed by analysis of the fever's characteristics and the patient-related factors mentioned, it is usually relatively straightforward to order tests to arrive at a specific diagnosis.

Most patients in the CCU have some degree of temperature elevation. Trying to determine the cause of fever in CCU patients is the daily task of the physicians concerned. Fever in the CCU can be a perplexing problem, because the clinician must determine whether the patient's underlying disorder is responsible for the fever or fever is a superimposed phenomenon on the patient's underlying problem responsible for admission to the CCU. The infectious disease consultant's clinical skills are best demonstrated by the rapidity and excellence of arriving at a cause for the patient's fever (1–10).

DIAGNOSTIC CONSIDERATIONS

The clinician's initial assessment of the febrile patient is based on the temperature elevation/patterns, underlying disorders, assessment of medications, and clinical appearance. CCU patients may be grouped into three categories. The first group of patients is the one that has been admitted to the hospital and directly put in the CCU. Such patients need immediate/appropriate diagnostic tests, and if an infectious etiology is likely, empiric antibiotic therapy based on organ system involvement is needed. Some patients with lymphoma, vasculitis, or systemic lupus erythematosus (SLE) may be febrile/critically ill and in the CCU, but these disorders usually have a less fulminant clinical presentation.

The second group of CCU patients is those transferred to the CCU after hospitalization. This group of patients has been hospitalized for a variety of reasons, and some catastrophic event during hospitalization requires transfer to the CCU for intensive evaluation/organ support. The usual infectious diseases in this group include nosocomial pneumonia, intravenous (IV)-line infections, *Clostridium difficile* colitis, postoperative rupture of a viscus, or leakage of a partially drained/undrained abscess. Equally important are noninfectious diseases occurring in hospitalized patients who require transfer to the CCU. Commonly, these include acute myocardial infarction, pulmonary emboli/infarcts, acute pancreatitis, acute adrenal insufficiency and internal/gastrointestinal hemorrhage. Unless urologically instrumented during hospitalization, urosepsis is rare; but if there is renal disease, SLE, or diabetes, it may occur.

The third group of patients has underlying infectious/noninfectious disorders that may flare and be superimposed on the patient's underlying medical disorders. Most disorders in this group are noninfectious diseases and present in the stabilized hospital patient with a new fever. Such disorders include an acute attack of gout, thrombophlebitis, phlebitis, *C. difficile* diarrhea, or connective tissue diseases (usually SLE or rheumatoid arthritis), atelectasis/dehydration, pleural effusions, and drug fever (1,5,6,10).

CAUSES OF FEVER IN THE CCU

Noninfectious Causes of Fever in the CCU

A wide variety of disorders are associated with a febrile response. Both infectious and noninfectious disorders may cause acute/chronic fevers that may be low, i.e., $\geq 102°F$, or high grade, i.e., $\leq 102°F$. Of the multiplicity of conditions that may be encountered in the CCU with a few notable exceptions, most noninfectious disorders are associated with fevers of $\leq 102°F$. Exceptions to the 102°F fever rule include malignant hyperthermia, adrenal insufficiency, massive intracranial hemorrhage, central fever, drug fever, collagen vascular disease flare, particularly SLE flare, heat stroke, vasculitis, and certain malignancies, particularly lymphomas.

The most common noninfectious disorders encountered in the CCU either have no fever or have low-grade fevers $\leq 102°F$, and include acute myocardial infarction, pulmonary embolism/infarct, phlebitis, catheter-associated bacteriuria, acute pancreatitis, viral hepatitis, acute hepatic necrosis, dry gangrene, uncomplicated wound infections, subacute bacterial endocarditis, cerebrovascular accidents, small-moderate intracerebral bleeds, pulmonary hemorrhage, acute respiratory distress syndrome (ARDS), bronchiolitis obliterans with organizing pneumonia (BOOP), pleural effusions, atelectasis, cholecystitis, noninfectious diarrheas, *C. difficile* diarrhea, ischemic colitis, splenic infarcts, renal infarcts, pericardial effusion, dry gangrene, gas gangrene, surgical toxic shock syndrome, acute gout, small bowel obstruction, and cellulitis.

The clinical approach to the noninfectious disorders with fever is usually relatively straightforward, because they are readily diagnosable by history, physical, or routine laboratory or radiology tests. Having known that noninfectious disorders are not associated with fevers >102°F in patients, the clinician can look for an alternate explanation in these patients. The difficulty usually arises when the patient has a multiplicity of conditions and sorting out the infectious from the noninfectious causes can be a daunting task. For example, if a patient in the CCU following cancer resection of the large bowel postoperatively develops extremity gangrene, phlebitis, pulmonary infiltrates, leukocytosis, myocardial infarction, hematomas/ seromas, atelectasis, dehydration, and catheter-associated bacteriuria, has a stroke, is on multiple medications, and has just had a blood transfusion, the clinical analysis of the fever in this patient would go as follows. The patient spiked to 102.8°F on the seventh postoperative day and 24 hours after receiving the blood transfusion. Postoperatively, if there was no peritonitis, the temperatures due to hematoma/healing should be <102°F. The patient's condition of phlebitis, peripheral gangrene, stroke, and myocardial infarction all do not explain the fever more than 102°F. The problem is to evaluate the fever, leukocytosis, and infiltrates on chest X ray in the proper clinical context. The fever, leukocytosis, and pulmonary infiltrates, if due to a nosocomial pneumonia, could certainly have a fever ≥102°F. Temporal relationships are also important in detecting different causes of fever. The patient's fever, leukocytosis, and pulmonary infiltrates could easily be explained on the basis of heart failure secondary to the patient's recent postoperative myocardial infarction. However, because the fever spike was temporally related to the blood transfusion, the cause of the 102.8°F fever was best explained by the recent blood transfusion (1,5–10).

Infectious Causes of Fever in the CCU

Most infections that are not toxin-mediated elicit a febrile response. Although all infections do not manifest temperatures >102°F, they have the potential to do so, e.g., nosocomial pneumonia may be associated with temperatures <102°F or >102°F. Although all infectious diseases will not present with temperatures ≥102°F, they are the disorders most frequently associated with temperatures in the ≤102°F range.

Infectious diseases encountered in the CCU usually associated with temperatures ≥102°F include postoperative abscesses, acute meningitis, acute encephalitis, brain abscess, septic thrombophlebitis, jugular septic vein thrombophlebitis, septic pelvic thrombophlebitis, septic pulmonary emboli, pericarditis, acute bacterial endocarditis, perivalvular/myocardial abscess, community-acquired pneumonia (CAP), pleural empyema, lung abscess, cholangitis, intrarenal/perinephric abscess, prostatic abscess, urosepsis, central-line infections, contaminated infusates, pylephlebitis, liver abscess, *C. difficile* colitis, complicated skin and soft tissue infections/abscesses, AV graft infections, foreign body–related infections (infected pacemakers/automatic implantable cardioveter defibrillator (AICD)s, central IV catheters, Hickman/ Broviac catheters), and septic arthritis. Infectious diseases likely to be present in the CCU setting with temperatures <102°F include osteomyelitis, sacral decubitus ulcers, uncomplicated wound infections, cellulitis, etc. (Table 1) (1–4,10).

Table 1 Causes of Fever in the Critical Care Unit

System	Infectious Etiology	Noninfectious Etiology
Central nervous	Meningitis	Cerebral infarction
	Encephalitis	Cerebral hemorrhage
	Brain abscess	Posterior Fossa syndrome
		Seizures
		CNS tumors
Cardiovascular	Endocarditis	Myocardial infarction
	IV line sepsis	Dressler's syndrome
	Septic thrombophlebitis	Postpericardiotomy syndrome
	Thrombophlebitis	Cholesterol emboli syndrome
	Postperfusion syndrome (CMV)	Deep vein thrombosis
	Pericarditis	Atrial myomas
	Pacemaker/defibrillator infection	
Pulmonary	Pneumonia	Atelectasis
	Empyema	SLE pneumonitis
	Tracheobronchitis	Pleural effusion
	Lung abscess	Pulmonary emboli/infarction
	Empyema	ARDS
		Pulmonary drug reactions
		BOOP
		Fat emboli
Gastrointestinal	Liver abscess	Gastrointestinal hemorrhage
	Splenic abscess	Acalculous cholecystitis
	Intra-abdominal abscess	Nonviral hepatitis
	Cholecystitis/cholangitis	Pancreatitis
	Viral hepatitis	Inflammatory bowel disease
	Peritonitis	Non–*C. difficile* diarrhea
	Appendicitis	Ischemic/non–*C. difficile* colitis
	Diverticulitis	Splenic infarct
	C. difficile diarrhea/colitis	
Renal	Urinary tract infection	Renal infarct
	Pyelonephritis	
	Renal abscess	
Rheumatologic	Osteomyelitis	Acute gout/pseudogout
	Septic arthritis	SLE/RA flare
		Vasculitis
Skin/soft tissue	Cellulitis	Hematoma
	Wound infection	Intramuscular injections
	Decubitus ulcer	Burns
Endocrine/metabolic		Acute adrenal insufficiency
		Hyperthyroidism/thyroiditis
		Alcohol withdrawal/DTs
GU	Prostatic abscess	Hemorrhage into ovarian cyst
	PID	
	Tubo-ovarian abscess	
Other	Transient bacteremias	Drug fever
	Septicemia	Blood/blood products transfusion
	Parotitis	
	Pharyngitis	
	Transient bacteremia	

Abbreviations: PIDS, pelvic infectious disease syndrome; DTs, delirium tremens; SLE, systemic lupus erythematus; RA, rheumatoid arthritis; ARDS, acute respiratory distress syndrome, BOOP, bronchiolitis obliterans with organizing pneumonia; CNS, central nervous system; IV, intravenous; CMV, cytomegalovirus; GU, genitourinary; *C. difficile*, *Clostridium difficile*.
Source: From Refs. 1, 3, 5.

Cunha's "102°F Rule" is useful clinically in differentiating most common causes of fever in the CCU. The clinician should analyze the fever relationships in the clinical context and correlate these findings with other aspects of the patient's clinical condition to arrive at a likely cause for the patient's temperature elevation. The clinical approach utilizes not only the height of the fever but also the abruptness of onset, the characteristics of the fever curve, the duration of the fever, and the defervescence pattern which all have diagnostic importance (Table 2) (1,6,10).

CLINICAL SIGNIFICANCE OF FEVER PATTERNS

Extreme Hyperpyrexia (≥106°F)

Infectious diseases usually present with some degree of fever. Most infectious diseases encountered in the CCU setting have temperatures in the 102°F to 106°F range. Causes of extreme hyperpyrexia (>106°F) include heat stroke, malignant hyperthermia, central fevers, malignant neoplastic syndrome, and drug fever. These hyperpyrexia disorders are usually readily diagnosed because of associated features, i.e., fever immediately following surgery/general anesthesia (malignant hyperthermia), prolonged high temperatures/dehydration (prolonged heat exposure), central nervous system (CNS) disorders with hypothalamic involvement (tumors, neurosurgical procedures, and trauma), or sensitivity medications (drug fever). Temperatures in excess of 106°F should suggest a noninfectious etiology (Table 3) (1,10,11).

Single Fever Spikes >102°F

Patients in the CCU who have been afebrile or had low-grade fevers, i.e., ≤102°F, may suddenly develop a single fever spike >102°F. Single fever spikes are never infectious in origin. The causes of single fever spikes include insertion/removal of a urinary catheter or a venous catheter, suctioning/manipulation of an endotracheal tube, wound packing/lavage, wound irrigation, etc. Any procedure that involves a manipulation of a colonized/infected surface can induce a transient bacteremia. Because of their short duration, i.e., less than five minutes, such bacteremias do not result in sustaining infection or spread infection to other organs, and for this reason may not be treated. Single fever spikes of the transient bacteremias are a diagnostic not a therapeutic problem.

The other common cause of single fever spikes in the CCU is blood-product transfusions. Fever secondary to blood products/blood transfusions are a frequent occurrence, and are most commonly manifested by fever following the infusion. The distribution of fever is bimodal, following a blood transfusion. Most reactions occur within the first 72 hours after the blood/blood product transfusion, and most reactions within the 72-hour period occur in the first 24 to 48 hours. There are very few reactions after 72 hours, but a smaller peak five to seven days after the blood transfusion, which although is very uncommon, may occur. Temperature elevations associated with late blood transfusion reactions are lower than those with reactions occurring soon after blood transfusion.

The fever subsequent to the transient bacteremia results from cytokine release and is not indicative of a prolonged exposure to the infecting agent, but rather represents the postbacteremia chemokine-induced febrile response. The temperature elevations from manipulation of a colonized or infected mucosal surface persist long after the bacteremia has ceased.

Table 2 Clinical Applications of the 102°F Rule in the Critical Care Unit

Common causes of temperature	Comments
	≤102°F
Acute myocardial infarction	H/O chest pain/CAP
	EKG/cardiac enzymes
Pulmonary embolism	H/O PE underlying reasons predisposing to pulmonary emboli
	VQ scan positive (pulmonary angiography for large emboli)
	↑ FSPs with multiple small pulmonary emboli
GI bleed	Hyperactive BS, BRB per rectum/melena
	↑ BUN (except in alcoholic liver disease)
	Endoscopy/abdominal CT scan → bleeding source
Acute pancreatitis	Severe abdominal pain: may be associated with ARDS
	↑ amylase and ↑ lipase or pancreatitis on abdominal CT scan
Hematomas	H/O recent surgery/bleeding diathesis
	Visible on skin, e.g., Grey-Turner's/Cullen's sign, or on CT scan
Phlebitis	Local erythema without suppuration/vein tenderness
Catheter-associated bacteriuria	Urine with bacteria and WBCs nearly always represent colonization, not infection
	Bacteremia (urosepsis) does not result from bacteriuria unless pre-existing renal disease, urinary tract obstruction, or patient has SLE, DM, steroids, etc.
Pleural effusions	Bilateral effusions are never due to infection: look for a noninfectious etiology
	Except for gas gangrene and streptococcal cellulitis, temperatures are usually low grade
Uncomplicated wound infections	"Wounds" with temperatures ≥102°F should prompt a search for an underlying abscess
Atelectasis/dehydration	Temperatures usually ≤101°F
	May be confused with pulmonary emboli/early pneumonia
Tracheobronchitis	Purulent endotracheal secretions with negative chest X ray for pneumonia
	Tracheobronchitis does not → temperatures ≥102°F
Thrombophlebitis	Warm, tender calf/foot veins ± palpable cord
	Thrombophlebitis does not → pulmonary emboli
	Phlebothrombosis → pulmonary emboli
Clostridium difficile	Stools positive for *C. difficile* toxin
	Fecal WBC positive ~50%. Stools are watery, green, foul smelling
	If temperatures ≥102°F with blood/mucous diarrhea, diagnosis is probable
	>102°F
Nosocomial pneumonia/ventilator-associated pneumonia	May have temperatures ≤102°F also
	Pulmonary infiltrate consistent with a bacterial pneumonia occurring ≥1 wk after hospitalization
	Must be differentiated from ARDS, LVF, etc.
	Definitive diagnosis by quantitative protected catheter-tip culture (PBB/BAL)
	Endotracheal secretions represent upper airway colonization and are not reflective of lower respiratory tract organisms causing vent-associated pneumonia

(Continued)

Table 2 Clinical Applications of the 102°F Rule in the Critical Care Unit (*Continued*)

Common causes of temperature	Comments
	Endotracheal respiratory secretion cultures should not be cultured or covered
IV-line infections	Overdue central lines usual cause
	Organisms from blood cultures taken from noninvolved extremity same as positive semiquantitative catheter culture (≥15 colonies)
	If all other sources of fever are ruled out, consider IV-line infection, especially with overdue lines (even if site not infected visually)
C. difficile	Stools positive for *C. difficile* toxin
	Bloody diarrhea, temperature ≥102°F
	Abdominal CT scan shows thumbprinting/colitis/toxic megacolon
Drug fever	In patients with otherwise unexplained temperatures, consider drug fever
	Blood cultures are negative (excluding contaminants)
	Patients with drug fever usually have ≥102°F accompanied by relative bradycardia
	↑ WBC with left shift is common as is ↑ ESR
	Mild-moderate serum transaminases common
	Eosinophils nearly always present but eosinophils less common
	Patient with infection may also have a drug fever
	Commonest causes of drug fever are diuretics, pain/sleep medications, sulfa-containing stool softeners as well as sulfa drugs, and β-lactam antibiotics
Blood/blood product transfusion	Single fever spike (1–3 or 5–7 days posttransfusion)
Transient bacteremia due to manipulation of a colonized/infected mucosal surface	Single temperature spike 1–3 days, postmanipulative, that spontaneously resolves without treatment
September invasive infectious diseases	Blood culture variably positive as a function of time
	Usually associated with temperatures ≤102°F in normal hosts

Abbreviations: GI, gastrointestinal; CT, computed tomography; ARDS, acute respiratory distress syndrome; SLE, systemic lupus erythematosus; IV, intravenous; WBC, white blood cells; DM, diabetes mellitus; PBB, protected bronchial brushings; BAL, bronchoalveolar lavage; ESR, erythrocyte sedimentation rate; CAP, community-acquired pneumonia; PE, pulmonary emboli; FSPs, fibrin split products.
Source: Adapted from Refs. 3, 5.

Table 3 Causes of Extreme Hyperpyrexia (>106°F)

Hypothalamic dysfunction
Malignant neuroleptic syndrome
Central fevers (hemorrhagic, trauma, malignancy)
Heat stroke
Malignant hyperthermia
Drug fever

In patients with fever spikes due to transient bacteremias following manipulation of a colonized or infected mucosal surface, or secondary to a blood product/blood transfusion, may be inferred by the temporal relationship of the event and the appearance of the fever. In addition to the temporal relationship between the fever and the transient bacteremia or transfusion-related febrile response, the characteristic fever curve, i.e., a single isolated temperature spike resolves spontaneously without treatment (1,6,10,11).

Multiple Fever Spikes >102°F

Multiple fever spikes >102°F may be infectious or noninfectious in origin, because a hectic, septic fever pattern does not in itself suggest a particular etiology. Because this fever pattern is common but not specific, the clinician must rely upon associated findings in the history and physical, or among laboratory or radiology tests, to determine the cause of the fever. Pulse temperature relationships are also of help in differentiating the causes of fever in patients with multiple temperature spikes over a period of days. Assuming that there is no characteristic fever pattern, the presence or absence of a pulse temperature deficit is useful.

Patients with a pulse temperature deficit, i.e., relative bradycardia, are limited to relatively few infectious and noninfectious disorders. In the CCU setting, patients with multiple spiking fevers and a pulse temperature deficit should suggest Rocky Mountain spotted fever (RMSF), typhus, arboviral hemorrhagic fevers, central fevers, lymphoma-related fevers, legionnaires' disease, Q fever, psittacosis, or drug fever. The diagnostic significance of relative bradycardia can only be applied in patients who have normal pulse temperature relationships, i.e., those who do not have pacemaker-induced rhythms, have third-degree heart block, those with arrhythmias, and those on β-blocker therapy. Any patient on β-blocker medications who develops a fever will develop relative bradycardia, thus eliminating the usefulness of this important diagnostic sign in patients with relative bradycardia. If these conditions are eliminated, narrowing diagnostic possibilities is relatively straightforward.

If the patient has pneumonia and relative bradycardia, then *Legionella*, psittacosis, or Q fever is suggested. Patients with relative bradycardia may accompany lymphoma or central fever, and in those conditions should not suggest an alternative diagnosis. Typhus or RMSF will be suggested by the pattern/nature of their rash as well as other findings, and relative bradycardia is an ancillary finding in those situations. Similarly, the arboviral hemorrhagic fevers do not require the presence of a pulse temperature deficit for diagnosis. In those situations, epidemiology/recent travel history, systemic toxemia, and hemorrhagic nature of the rash are the primary diagnostic determinants (1,5,10,11).

Drug fever, i.e., a hypersensitivity reaction to medications without rash, occurs in approximately 10% of hospitalized patients. In the CCU where multiple medications are being used, drug fever is a common cause of obscure fever. Drug fever is a diagnosis of exclusion, and its presence is suggested by the presence of relative bradycardia in the absence of another explanation for the fever. Drug fever with relative bradycardia may also be a problem that is related to the therapy of the underlying disorder that prompted CCU admission. Aside from being a diagnosis of elimination, drug fever is suggested by negative blood cultures excluding contaminants, increase in the erythrocyte sedimentation rate (ESR), and an early mild/transient increase in the serum transaminases serum glutamate oxaloacetate transaminase/serum glutamate pyruvate transaminase (SGOT/SGPT). Drug fevers <102°F may occur, but most occur in the 102°F to 104°F range, and some drug fevers may exceed 106°F. High spiking fevers due to medications often confuse the clinician who has not thought of the diagnosis. Drug fevers also mimic infection in that they are usually accompanied by an increase in the white count with a left shift. Fever with rash is a hypersensitivity reaction to a drug with cutaneous manifestations. Because of the rash, the clinician is alerted to the differential diagnostic possibilities. Without a rash, the drug fever as the manifestation of a hypersensitivity reaction often goes unnoticed (1,12–16).

Low-Grade Fevers of Short Duration (Three to Five Days) in the CCU

Most of the acute, noninfectious disorders that occur in the CCU are accompanied by low-grade fevers, i.e., ≤102°F for a short period of time. Fever secondary to acute myocardial infarction, pulmonary embolus, and acute pancreatitis are associated with fevers of relatively short duration. In such patients with these diagnoses, fever >102°F for more than three days should suggest a complication or alternate diagnosis. Other disorders with prolonged low-grade fevers include dehydration, atelectasis, wound healing, hematoma, seromas, ARDS, BOOP, deep vein thromboses, pleural effusions, tracheobronchitis, decubitus ulcers, cellulites, and phlebitis. Prolonged low-grade fevers (≤102°F) are usually noninfectious. Clinicians should try to identify the noninfectious disorder causing the fever so that undue resources will not be expended looking for an infectious explanation for the fever (1,10,17–24).

Low-Grade Prolonged Fevers (more than five days) in the CCU: Nosocomial FUOs

There are relatively few causes of prolonged fevers in the CCU that last for over a week. Such low-grade prolonged fevers lasting over a week have been termed nosocomial fevers of unknown origin (FUO). There are relatively few causes of nosocomial FUO in contrast to its community-acquired counterpart. Low-grade infections or inflammatory states account for most of the causes of nosocomial FUO. Nosocomial FUOs are usually due to central fevers, drug fevers, postperfusion syndrome, atelectasis, dehydration, undrained seromas, tracheobronchitis, and catheter-associated bacteriuria.

Prolonged fevers that become high spiking fevers should suggest the possibility of nosocomial endocarditis related to a central line or invasive cardiac procedure. Prolonged high spiking fevers can also be due to septic thrombophlebitis or an undrained abscess. Nosocomial sinusitis due to prolonged nasotracheal intubation is a rare cause of nosocomial FUO (1,10,25).

Special Fever Patterns

Camel Back/Domedary Fevers

Fever patterns are often considered as nonspecific in nature therefore having limited diagnostic specificity. It is true that fevers in patients being intermittently given antipyretics and being instrumented in a variety of anatomical locations, do have complex fever patterns. However, these are usually easily sorted out on the basis of clinical findings. Fever patterns that remain useful to diagnose certain entities in the hospital include a "domedary" or "camel back" fever pattern, i.e., increase in fever over two to three days followed by a decrease followed a few days later by two to three more days of fever. Such a fever pattern should suggest the possibility of Colorado tick fever, dengue, leptospirosis, brucellosis, lymphocytic choriomeningitis, yellow fever, the African hemorrhagic fevers, rat bite fever, and smallpox.

Sustained/Remittent Fevers

Continuous fevers are those that rise slowly over days to peak levels and then plateau until defervescence. The causes of continuous/sustained fevers include typhoid fever, drug fever, scarlet fever, RMSF, psittacosis, Kawasaki's disease, brucellosis, human herpes virus six (HHV-6) infections, and central fevers. Remittent fevers are characteristic of viral respiratory tract infection, malaria, acute rheumatic fever, legionnaires' disease, *Legionella/mycoplasma* CAP, tuberculosis (TB), and viridans streptococcal subacute bacterial endocarditis (SBE).

Hectic/Septic Fevers

Hectic/septic fevers are repetitive fever spikes over days that may or may not decrease to normal between fever spikes. Hectic/septic fevers may be due to gram-negative or gram-positive sepsis, renal, abdominal, or pelvic abscesses, acute bacterial endocarditis, Kawasaki's disease, malaria, miliary TB, peritonitis, or toxic shock syndrome. Noninfectious causes include lymphomas or overzealous administration of antipyretics.

Double Quotidian Fevers

Double quotidian fevers, i.e., two fever spikes in 24 hours, not artificially induced by antipyretics, should suggest right-sided gonococcal endocarditis, mixed malarial infections, miliary TB, visceral leishmaniasis, or adult Still's disease. Double quotidian fevers are helpful, when present, in narrowing diagnostic possibilities enabling the clinician to order specific diagnostic testing for likely diagnostic possibilities (Table 4) (1,3,10,11).

Relapsing Fevers

Relapsing fevers are those that are separated by afebrile intervals. Causes of noninfectious relapsing fevers include Crohn's disease, Behçet's disease, relapsing funiculitis, leukoclastic angiitis, Sweet's syndrome, familial Mediterranean fever, fever aphthous ulcer pharyngitis adenopathy (FAPA) syndrome, hyper IgG syndrome, and SLE. The infectious causes of relapsing fevers include viral infections, i.e., cytomegalovirus (CMV), Epstein–Barr virus, lymphatic choriomeningiti virus (LCM), dengue, yellow fever, and Colorado tick fever. Zoonotic bacterial infections include leptospirosis, bartonellosis, brucellosis, rat bite fever (*S. minus*), visceral leishmaniasis, malaria, babesiosis, ehrlichiosis, Q fever, typhoid fever, trench fever, and relapsing fever. Fungal infections tend to relapse, as do melioidosis and TB. Chronic meningococcemia by definition is prone to relapse (Table 5) (1,3,10,11).

PULSE–TEMPERATURE RELATIONSHIPS

Diagnostic Importance of Relative Bradycardia

Relative bradycardia is a pulse temperature deficit inappropriate for the degree of fever. A temperature increase of normally 1°F is accompanied by an appropriate

Table 4 Diagnostic Significance of Fever Patterns

Fever pattern	Usual causes
Single fever spike	Manipulation of a colonized/infected mucosal surface (not systemic infectious disease)
	Blood/blood products transfusion
	Infusion-related sepsis (contaminated infusate)
	Temperature error
Intermittent (hectic/septic) fevers	Gram-negative/positive sepsis
	Abscesses (renal, abdominal, pelvic)
	Acute bacterial endocarditis
	Kawasaki disease
	Malaria
	Miliary TB
	Peritonitis
	Toxic shock syndrome
	Antipyretics
Remittent fevers	Viral upper respiratory tract infections
	Plasmodium falciparum malaria
	ARF
	Legionella
	Mycoplasma
	TB
	SBE (*viridans streptococci*)
Continuous/sustained fevers	Central fevers
	Roseola infantum (human herpesvirus-6)
	Brucellosis
	Kawasaki disease
	Psittacosis
	RMSF
	Scarlet fever
	Enterococcal SBE (tularemia)
	Typhoid fever
	Drug fever
Double quotidian fevers	Adult Still's disease (adult–juvenile rheumatoid arthritis)
	Visceral leishmaniasis
	Miliary TB
	Mixed malarial infections
	Right-sided gonococcal endocarditis
Biphasic (Camelback) fevers	Colorado tick fever
	Dengue fever
	Leptospirosis
	Brucellosis
	Lymphocytic choriomeningitis
	Yellow fever
	Poliomyelitis
	Smallpox
	Rat-bite fever (*Spirillum minus*)
	Chikungunya fever
	Rift Valley fever

(*Continued*)

Table 4 Fevers Prone to Relapse (*Continued*)

Fever pattern	Usual causes
Relapsing fevers	African hemorrhagic fevers (Marburg, Ebola, Lassa, etc.)
	Echovirus (Echo 9)
	Relapsing fever (*B. recurrentis*)
	Yellow fever
	Smallpox
	Ascending (intermittent) cholangitis
	Brucellosis
	Dengue
	Chronic meningococcemia
	Malaria
	Rat-bite fever (*S. moniliformis*)

Abbreviations: RMSF, Rocky Mountain spotted fever; SBE, subacute bacterial endocarditis; TB, tuberculosis; ARF, acute rheumatic fever.
Source: From Ref. 11.

pulse increase of 10 beats/min. If the pulse response is less than it should be for any degree of temperature increase (>102°F), then the term relative bradycardia may be applied. Relative bradycardia combined in a patient with an obscure fever is an extremely useful diagnostic sign. Fever plus relative bradycardia immediately limits

Table 5 Fevers Prone to Relapse

Infectious causes	
Relapsing fever (*Borrelia recurrentis*)	Colorado tick fever
Trench fever (*Rochalimaea quintana*)	Dengue fever
Q fever	Leptospirosis
Typhoid fever	Brucellosis
Vibrio fetus	Bartonellosis (Oroyo fever)
Syphilus	Acute rheumatic fever
TB	Rate-bite fever (*Spirillum minus*)
Histoplasmosis	Visceral leishmaniasis
Coccidioidomycosis	Lyme disease
Blastomycosis	Malaria
Pseudomonas pseudomallei (meliodosis)	Noninfluenzal respiratory viruses
LCM	Babesiosis
Dengue fever	EBV
Yellow fever	CMV
Chronic meningococcemia	
Noninfectious causes	
Behcet's disease	Familial Mediterranean fever
Crohn's disease	Fever, adenitis, pharyngitis, aphthous ulcer
Weber-Christian disease (panniculitis)	syndrome
Leukoclastic angitis	SLE
Sweet's syndrome	Hyper IgD syndrome

Abbreviations: EBV, Epstein–Barr virus, CMV, cytomegalovirus; SLE, systemic lupus erythematosus; TB, tuberculosis; LCM, lymphatic choriomeningitis virus.
Source: From Ref. 11.

diagnostic possibilities to central fevers, drug fevers, lymphomas, and the noninfectious disorders commonly causing fever in the CCU. Among the infectious causes of fever in the CCU, relative bradycardia in patients with pneumonia narrows diagnostic possibilities to *Legionella*, psittacosis, or Q fever pneumonia. Patients without pneumonias with fevers in the CCU, limit diagnostic possibilities to a variety of arthropod-borne infections, i.e., RMSF, typhus, typhoid fever, and arthropod-borne hemorrhagic fevers, i.e., yellow fever, Ebola, and dengue fever. Relative bradycardia like other signs should be used in concert with other clinical findings to prompt further diagnostic testing for the infectious diseases and to eliminate from further consideration the noninfectious disorders associated with relative bradycardia (Table 6; Fig. 1) (1,10,26,28–31).

Table 6 Causes of Relative Bradycardia

Infectious	Noninfectious
Legionella	Beta blockers
Psittacosis	Verapamil, or diltiazem
Q fever	CNS lesions
Typhoid fever	Lymphomas
Typhus	Factitious fever
Babesiosis	Drug fever
Malaria	
Leptospirosis	
Yellow fever	
Dengue fever	
Viral hemorrhagic fevers	
RMSF	

Determination of relative bradycardia
Inclusive criteria
    Patient must be an adult, i.e., >13 yr
    Temperature >102°F
    Pulse must be taken simultaneously with the temperature elevation
Exclusive criteria
    Patient has NSR without arrhythmia, second-or third-degree heart block or
        pacemaker-induced rhythm
    Patient must not be on β-blocker medications
Appropriate Temperature-Pulse Relationships

Pulse (beats/min)	Temperature
150	41.1°C (106°F)
140	40.6°C (105°F)
130	40.7°C (104°F)
120	39.4°C (103°F)
110	38.9°C (102°F)

Relative bradycardia refers to heart rates that are inappropriately slow relative to body temperature (pulse must be taken simultaneously with temperature elevation). Applies to adult patients with temperature ≥102°F; does not apply to patients with second/third-degree heart block, pacemaker-induced rhythms, or those taking beta-blockers.

Abbreviations: CNS, central neurous system; RMSF, Rocky Mountain spotted fever; NSR, normal sinus rhythm.

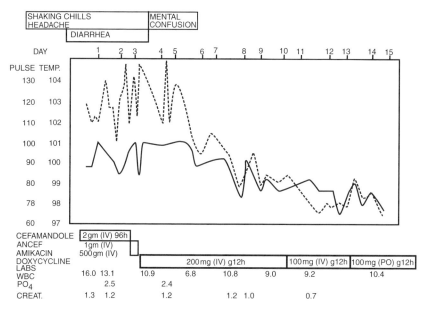

Figure 1 Temperature chart showing relative bradycardia in a patient with legionnaires' disease prior to initiation of doxycycline treatment on day 5. Solid line represents temperature; dotted line represents pulse. *Source*: From Ref. 27.

DIAGNOSTIC SIGNIFICANCE OF FEVER DEFERVESCENCE PATTERNS

Overview

Most of this chapter has been concerned with the diagnosis of fever in the CCU by analyzing the rapidity of onset of the fever, the height of the fever, the relationship of the fever to the pulse, the fever patterns, and the duration of the fever. Particularly in perplexing cases of fever, the characteristics of fever resolution also have diagnostic significance. Fever defervescence patterns may be interpreted in two ways. The rapidity and completeness of the fever pattern resolution attests to the effective treatment or resolution of the noninfectious or infectious process. Fever defervescence patterns are as predictable and useful as fever patterns in predicting complications secondary to the disorder or therapy (5,10,11).

Meningitis in the CCU

With bacterial meningitis, temperature resolution with appropriate therapy is related to the pathogen causing the meningitis. Meningococcal meningitis defervesces quickly over one to three days, whereas *Haemophilus influenzae* meningitis resolves over three to five days, and severe pneumococcal meningitis may take a week or longer for the fever to decrease/become afebrile. Viral causes of meningitis or encephalitis defervesce very slowly over a seven-day period, and by fever defervescence pattern easily differentiate viral meningitis/encephalitis from bacterial meningitis. Because fever defervescence patterns may also point to complications, the astute clinician will monitor the fever pattern post-therapy, looking for an unexpected temperature spike after the patient has defervesced.

H. influenzae meningitis, for example, defervesces after three to five days but if the patient spikes a temperature after five days, this would suggest either a complication of the infection, i.e., subdural empyema, or a complication of therapy, i.e., drug fever secondary to antimicrobial therapy (1,5,10).

Endocarditis in the CCU

In patients with endocarditis, the fever defervescence pattern is also pathogen related. Patients with SBE have fevers <102°F, and defervesce after a few days of effective antimicrobial therapy. A subsequent temperature spike after the fever with *Streptococcus viridans* SBE has resolved should suggest either a complication of SBE, i.e., septic emboli/infarcts, or a complication of SBE therapy, i.e., drug fever. With *S. aureus* acute bacterial endocarditis (ABE), patients have temperatures ≥102°F (excluding IVDAs). Patients with *S. aureus* endocarditis defervesce within three to five days after initiation of effective anti–*S. aureus* therapy. The persistence of fever in a patient being treated appropriately for *S. aureus* ABE should suggest the possibility of a paravalvular/mild myocardial abscess. With *S. aureus* ABE, the reappearance of fever after initial defervescence should suggest a septic complication, i.e., septic emboli/infarcts, paravalvular/myocardial abscess, or complication of antimicrobial therapy, e.g., drug fever (5,10,11).

Patients with enterococcal endocarditis have a fever defervescence pattern intermediate between *S. viridans* SBE and *S. aureus* ABE. Patients with enterococcal endocarditis usually defervesce slowly over five days, and recrudescence of fever in patients with enterococcal endocarditis should suggest a septic complication or drug fever.

CAP in the CCU

Fever defervescence patterns are also important in patients with CAP as well as nosocomial pneumonias (NP). In normal hosts with CAP due to typical bacterial pathogens, i.e., *S. pneumoniae, H. influenzae,* or *Moraxella catarrhalis*, fever resolves rapidly over the first few days with effective treatment. *S. pneumoniae* CAP has three possible fever defervescence patterns, the first and most common is a rapid decrease in temperature similar to that found in *H. influenzae* or *M. catarrhalis* CAP in normal hosts. The second fever defervescence pattern with pneumococcal pneumonia is that of initial defervescence followed in three to five days by a secondary rise in fever. A secondary fever rise is a normal variant and does not indicate an infectious complication. The third defervescence pattern with *S. pneumoniae* is found in patients with impaired humoral immunity, i.e., patients with alcoholic cirrhosis, multiple myeloma, chronic lymphatic leukemia (CLL) etc. In patients with impaired B-lymphocyte function, the fever slowly remits during the first week of therapy.

Patients with overwhelming pneumococcal sepsis, with no humoral immunity, i.e., asplenia, remain febrile and critically ill until the infection resolves or there is a fatal outcome.

NP in the CCU

Patients with NP often have temperature elevations >102°F, but fever is not helpful in ruling in or out the diagnosis of nosocomial pneumonia. The NP is an imprecise diagnosis and is routinely given to most patients in the CCU who have fever, leukocytosis, and pulmonary infiltrates. Therefore, most patients who have a working diagnosis of NP in fact do not have NP but have infiltrates, fever, and leukocytosis due to other causes. Patients being treated appropriately with monotherapy or combination therapy for NP defervesce rapidly if the infiltrates do in fact represent NP. Monotherapy or combination therapy for NP should be with at least one agent that has a high degree of anti–*P. aeruginosa* activity. Patients with bona fide NP defervesce within a week (32–37).

The persistence of fever, i.e., lack of a fever in patients with possible NP, suggests two possibilities; firstly, the patient has a noninfectious disorder that is mimicking NP and for this reason is not responding to antimicrobial therapy. Secondly, the patient could have an infectious disease, a process that is unresponsive to antipseudomonal antimicrobial therapy, i.e., herpes simplex virus 1 (HSV-1) pneumonia.

HSV-1 pneumonia is common in the CCU setting and presents as persistent fever and infiltrates unresponsive to antibiotics, or as "failure to wean" in ventilated patients. Patients who present as "failure to wean" have persistent fevers and did not have antecedent severe lung disease that would compromise their ability to come off the respirator. NP with empiric treatment should see an improvement/resolution of infiltrates and a defervescence of fever within two weeks. Persistence of fever with or without infiltrates after two weeks, in the absence of another cause for the fever, should suggest HSV-1 pneumonia until proven otherwise.

HSV-1 pneumonia is diagnosed by bronchoscopy, demonstrating cytopathic effects from cytology specimens, or direct fluorescent antibody (DFA)/monoclonal tests of respiratory secretions will be positive for HSV. Importantly, no vesicles are present in the bronchi in bronchoscoped patients with HSV-1 pneumonitis (38,39).

OBSCURE FEVERS IN THE CCUs

Drug Fever

Drug fevers are so important in the CCU setting because of the multiplicity of medications. Physicians should always be suspicious of the possibility of drug fever when other diagnostic possibilities have been exhausted. Drug fever may occur in individuals who have just recently been started on the sensitizing medication, or more commonly who have been on a sensitizing medication for a long period of time without previous problems. Patients with drug fever do not necessarily have multiple allergies to medications, and are not usually atopic. However, the likelihood of drug fever is enhanced in patients who are atopic with multiple drug allergies. Patients with drug fever, i.e., hypersensitivity reaction without rash may present with any degree of fever, but most commonly drug fevers are in the 102°F to 104°F range. Other conditions aside, patients look "inappropriately well" for the degree of fever that is different than the toxemic patient with a serious bacterial systemic infection. Relative bradycardia is invariably present excluding patients on β-blocker therapy, those with arrhythmias, heart block, or pacemaker-induced rhythms. Laboratory tests include an increase in WBC count with a shift to the left. Eosinophils are often present early in the differential count, but less commonly is their actual eosinophilia. The ESR is increased with drug fever but this may be marked by other causes of increased ESR by one/more acute disorders in CCU patients. The sedimentation rate also is increased after surgical procedures, negating the usefulness of this test in the postoperative fever patient. Serum transaminases, i.e., SGOT/SGPT are also mildly/transiently elevated early in cases of drug fever. Such mild increases in the serum transaminases are often overlooked by clinicians as acute phase reactants or not being very elevated.

However, in a patient with an obscure otherwise unexplained fever the constellation of nonspecific findings including relative bradycardia, slightly increased serum transaminases, and eosinophils in the differential count, are sufficient to make a presumptive diagnosis of drug fever. It is a popular misconception that antibiotics are the most common cause of drug fever. Among the antibiotics, β-lactams and sulfonamides are the most common causes of drug fever in the CCU setting. More common causes of fever in the CCU setting are anti-arrhythmics, anti-seizure medications, sulfa-containing loop diuretics (furosemide) or stool softeners (Colace) or tranquilizers, sedatives/sleep medications, antihypertensive medications, and β-blockers. As patients are usually receiving multiple medications, it is not always possible to discontinue an agent likely to be the cause of the drug fever. Often two or three agents have to be discontinued simultaneously. The clinician should discontinue the most likely agent that is not life supporting or essential first, in order properly interpret the decrease in temperature if indeed that was the sensitizing agent responsible for the drug fever.

If the agent that is likely to cause the drug fever cannot be discontinued, every attempt should be made to find an equivalent nonallergic substitute, i.e., ethacrinic acid in place of furosemide as a loop diuretic for congestive heart failure and a carbapenem in place of a β-lactam. If the agent responsible for the drug fever is discontinued, temperatures will decrease to near normal/normal within 72 hours. If the temperature does not decrease within 72 hours, then the clinician should discontinue sequentially one drug at a time, those that are likely to be the causes of drug fever. Resolution of drug fever means that not only the temperature returns to normal, but also the leukocytosis decreases and the eosinophils disappear in the differential WBC count (Tables 7 and 8) (1,3,5,10,12–24).

IV-Line Infections

Any invasive intravascular device may be associated with infection, but central IV lines are the ones most likely to result in IV-line sepsis. Other causes of IV-line sepsis

Table 7 Clinical Features of Drug Fever

History
  Many individuals are atopic
  "sensitizing medication" taken for days or years
Physical examination
  Look "inappropriately well" for degree of fever
  Low to high-grade fevers ($102°F \geq 106°F$)
  Relative bradycardia (with temperature $\geq 102°F$ if not on β-blockers, etc.)
  No rash[a]
Laboratory tests
  ↑ WBC count (often with left shift)
  Eosinophils usually present in peripheral smear (often missed with autonated counters)
  Eosinophilia is uncommon
  ↑ ESR in most (may reach ≥ 100 mm/hr)
  Mild/transient ↑of serum transaminases (early)

Abbreviations: WBC, white blood cells; ESR, erythrocyte sedimentation rate.
[a]If present, diagnosis is drug rash with fever.
Source: From Refs. 11–15.

Table 8 Drug Fever (2° Sensitizing Medications)

Common causes	Rare causes
Antibiotics	Digoxin
β-lactams	Steroids
Sleep medications	Diphenhydramine (Benadryl)
Antiseizure medications	Aspirin
Sulfa-containing drugs	Vitamins
Stool softeners (Colace)	Tetracyclines
Diuretics (Lasix)	Erythromycins
Antimicrobials (TMP-SMX, pentamidine)	Ketolides
Antidepressants/tranquilizers	Clindamycin
Antiarrhythmics	Aminoglycosides
β-blockers	Chloramphenicol
Ace inhibitors	Vancomycin
	Teichoplanin
	Aztreonam
	Carbapenems
	Quinolones
	Quinipristin/dalfopristin
	Daptomycin
	Tigecycline

Abbreviation: TMP-SMX, trimethoprim–sulfamethoxazole.
Source: From Ref. 12.

that may be encountered in the CCU are an infected Hickman/Broviac, Pik line, or pacemaker lead/generator infection, Quinton catheter. Patients with AV-graft infections resemble, in clinical presentation, those with central IV-line sepsis. The diagnosis of IV-line infection may be obvious or less straightforward. The likelihood that a patient in the CCU has IV-line infection is related to the duration that the central IV line is in place. Central IV-line infections are rare in less than or equal to seven days after line placement. There is progressive increase in the incidence of central IV-line infection following seven days of catheter insertion, i.e., the longer the central IV line is in the more likely that IV sepsis will ensue. Central IV-line infections often present as otherwise unexplained obscure fevers. Half of the patients will have obvious signs of infection at the catheter entry site. This is all that is required for a presumptive diagnosis of IV-line infection, and the catheter should be removed and semiquantitative catheter-tip cultures and blood cultures should be obtained to confirm the diagnosis.

The more common problem is in the other half of patients who have no local signs of infection at the site of IV catheter insertion. IV-line infection should be suspected after other diagnostic possibilities have been eliminated in patients who have had a central IV line in place for days/weeks. Blood cultures should be obtained and the catheter removed for semiquantitative culture of the catheter tip. The finding of a positive catheter-tip culture is one with ≥15 colonies plated in the method of Maki/Cleary. Positive catheter-tip culture without bacteremia indicates only a colonized catheter. Bacteremia without positive catheter-tip culture with the same organism indicates bacteremia but not secondary to the IV line. IV-line infection is diagnosed by demonstrating the same organism in the blood and the catheter tip.

The treatment for central IV-line infection is to remove the central IV line. If no further central venous access is necessary, the line may be discontinued, but if continued central IV line access is required, the catheter may be changed over a guide wire. Changing the catheter over a guide wire does not subject the patient to the possibility of a pneumothorax from a subclavian insertion. Alternately, after the catheter is removed, another catheter may be placed in a different anatomical location. Femoral catheters are the ones most likely to be infected, followed by IJ-inserted catheters. The subclavian inserted central IV lines are those least likely to be infected over time. Central IV-line infections are treated by catheter removal and antibiotics are usually given, even though the source of the bacteremia has been removed.

The organisms from the skin, i.e., *S. aureus*, *S. epidermidis*/coagulase-negative staphylococci (CoNS), are the most frequent cause, but aerobic gram-negative bacilli and to a lesser extent enterococci are also important causes of IV-line sepsis in the CCU. Many times catheters are often needlessly changed when patients, particularly postoperative patients, spike a fever in the first two to three days postoperatively. Catheter change so early is unnecessary because IV-line infections are rare before being in place at least seven days.

If antibiotics are used to treat IV-line infections after the central line is removed, treatment is ordinarily for seven days for gram-negative organisms and for two weeks for gram-positive organisms (excluding CoNS). CoNS are not ordinarily treated because they are low virulence pathogens and are incapable of infection in the absence of prosthetic metal or plastic materials. Even if prosthetic materials are in place in a patient with a CoNS bacteremia, patients have endothelialized their appliances and the likelihood of infection from a transient bacteremia associated with a central line diminishes. It cannot be emphasized too strongly that the clinician should have a high index of suspicion for central IV-line infection the longer the catheter has been in place in patients without an alternate explanation for their prolonged fevers. Catheter lines should not be changed/removed prophylactically if they are in place for less than seven days unless there are obvious signs of infection at the catheter site entry point (1,5,10,40–42).

Persistence of Fever

The clinical approach to the delayed resolution of fever, persistence of fever, or new appearance of fever related to a complication of therapy, i.e., drug fever after initial improvements in temperature/fever, a recrudescence of fever manifested by new fever/fever spikes may be related to the infectious process, or may be related to a noninfectious complication unrelated to therapy, i.e., myocardial infarction, gastrointestinal hemorrhage, acute pancreatitis, acute gout, deep vein thrombosis, phlebitis, and pulmonary emboli/infarcts. The time that the fever spike occurs in relation to the initial defervescence, pulse temperature relationships, and other associated findings are the key determinants diagnostically in sorting out possible explanations for the reappearance of fever in CCU patients. The recrudescence of fever is virtually never due to resistant organisms. Recrudescence of fever may be due to other infectious processes, i.e., candidemia, invasive aspergillosis, in patients with central lines, or on prolonged/high dose steroid or immunosuppressive therapy. Lack of response to antimicrobial therapy suggests inadequate spectrum or insufficient activity against the pathogen in the antibiotic regimen that is selected (Table 9) (42–44).

Table 9 Persistent Fever in the Critical Care Unit

Antibiotic related problems
Inadequate coverage/spectrum
Inadequate antibiotic blood levels
Inadequate antibiotic tissue levels
   Undrained abscess
   Foreign body–related infection
   Protected focus
     Abscess
     Foreign body
     Chronic osteomyelitis, etc.
   Organ hypoperfusion/diminished local blood supply
In vitro susceptibility but inactive in vivo
Antibiotic tolerance (gram-positive cocci)
Drug-induced interactions
   Antibiotic inactivation
   Antibiotic antagonism
Nonantibiotic related problems
Treating colonization
Noninfectious diseases mimics
   SLE
   Drug reactions
   Drug fever
   Atelectasis
   Pleural effusions
   Seroma
   Dehydration
   Acute pancreatitis
   Pulmonary emboli
   Acute myocardial infarction
   CNS hemorrhage/cerebrovascular accident
Antibiotic-unresponsive infectious diseases
   Viral infection

Abbreviations: SLE, systemic lupus erythematosus; CNS, central nervous system.
Source: From Refs. 1, 3, 5.

CLINICAL DIAGNOSTIC APPROACH TO FEVER IN THE CCU

Patients in the CCU with fever are admitted for a primary problem but also arrive with a variety of pre-existing disorders that may interact or complicate the primary reason for admission to the CCU. Problems that occur in the CCU related to new problems, complications of the original/new problems, plus the effect of multiple medications make diagnostic possibilities to explain fever in the CCU complex. The cause of fever may be suggested by epidemiologic factors as well as the history, physical, laboratory, and radiology tests. If the main thrust of the diagnostic approach is to identify reversible/curable causes of fever, analysis of the fever characteristics is the best way to sort out differential diagnostic possibilities in the CCU. Careful attention should be given to whether the fever spike is isolated or sustained, whether the fever is > or <102°F, the duration of the fever, and the relationship of the temperature to the pulse. Careful review of all the medications is essential not only to recognize drug side effects/interactions, but also to entertain the possibility

Table 10 Clinical Syndromic Approach to Fever in the Critical Care Unit

System	Community Acquired	Nosocomial	Either	Usual maximum temp. at presentation	
				≥102°F	≤102°F
CNS	Meningitis			+	+
	Encephalitis			+	+
	Brain abscess	Neurosurgical shunt infection		+	+
		Posterior fossa syndrome			+
			Central fevers	+	+
			Cerebrovascular accident	+	
			Massive intraventricular hemorrhage		+
			Seizures		+
Cardiovascular	SBE		Acute bacterial endocarditis	+	+
			Myocardial infarction		+
	Permanent IV/central line/infected pacemaker	Temporary IV/central line/ infected pacemaker		+	
		Postpericardiotomy syndrome			
	Viral pericarditis		Myocardial/perivalvular abscess	+	+
	Postperfusion syndrome	Balloon pump fever		+	+
		Sternal osteomyelitis			+

(Continued)

Table 10 Clinical Syndromic Approach to Fever in the Critical Care Unit (*Continued*)

System	Community Acquired	Nosocomial	Either	Usual maximum temp. at presentation	
				≥102°F	≤102°F
Pulmonary	CAP			+	
	Lung abscess			+	
		VAP		+	
			Pulmonary emboli/infarction		−
			ARDS		−
	Empyema			+	
			Pleural effusion		−
			Atelectasis/dehydration		+
	SLE pneumonitis			+	
			Tracheobronchitis		+ +
	BOOP				+ +
	Broncogenic carcinomas (without postobstructive pneumonia)				+
	Pulmonary cytotoxic drug reactions				
			Mediastinitis	+	
GI					
	Cholecystitis		Intra-abdominal abscess	+	
			Cholangitis	+	
			Viral hepatitis		+
			Acalculous cholecystitis	+	
			Peritonitis	+	
			Pancreatitis		
	Ischemic colitis	GI			+ + +
			Hemorrhage		
			Antibiotic-associated diarrhea (*Clostridium difficile*)	+	

Urinary tract	Pyelonephritis	+
	Cystitis	+
	Urosepsis	+
Skin/soft tissue	Cellulitis	+
	Catheter-associated bacteremia	+
	Uncomplicated wound Infection	+
	Gas gangrene	+
	Mixed soft tissue infection with gas	+
Bone/joint	Decubitus ulcer	+
	Chronic osteomyelitis	+
	Acute osteomyelitis	+
	Septic arthritis	+
	Acute gout	+
	RA joint flare	+
Other	Fat emboli	+
	Transient bacteremias	+
	Blood/blood product transfusion	+
	Sinusitis	+
	Adrenal insufficiency hematomas	+
	Antibiotic-associated colitis (*C. difficile*)	+
	Alcohol withdrawal syndrome	+
	Delirium tremens	+
	SLE flare	+

Abbreviations: CNS, central nervous system; GI, gastrointestinal; SBE, subacute bacterial endocarditis; IV, intravenous; CAP, community-acquited pneumonia; ARDS, acute respiratory distress syndrome; SLE, systemic lupus erythematosus; RA, rheumatoid arthritis; BOOP, bronchiolitis obliterans with organizing pneumonia; VAP, ventilation associated pneumonia.

Source: From Refs. 1, 5.

of drug fever if other diagnoses are unlikely. Clinicians should also be familiar with the fever defervescence patterns of infectious and noninfectious disorders (Table 10) (1,5,10,45–49).

Most situations are fairly straightforward, e.g., a steroid-dependent patient with SLE and flare who is in the CCU for the management of renal insufficiency and develops fevers >102°F without relative bradycardia, which are sustained. Although there are many possibilities to explain these fevers, i.e., superimposed CMV or bacterial infections, the most important correctable factor to identify as the cause of the fever is inadequate steroid dosage. Patients on chronic corticosteroids when admitted to the CCU should require stress doses of corticosteroids. Without increasing the corticosteroid daily dose, patients develop either a fever from a flare of their SLE/relative bradycardia or adrenal insufficiency, which presents as otherwise unexplained fever in such patients (Table 11) (1,10,47–49).

CLINICAL THERAPEUTIC APPROACH

General therapeutic interventions should be done as soon as possible. Gastrointestinal hemorrhage may require blood transfusion, collagen vascular diseases/vasculitis may require high dose corticosteroid therapy, pulmonary emboli may require anticoagulation, myocardial infarction may require balloon pump support or cardiac interventional procedures/surgery, IV lines should be removed and sent for semi-quantitative catheter-tip cultures and peripheral blood cultures. Patients with

Table 11 Clinical Diagnostic Approach to Fever in Critical Care Unit

Early infectious disease consultation	
All febrile CCU patients should have an infectious disease consultation	
Infectious disease consultation to evaluate mimics of infections (pseudosepsis) and microbiologic data	
Persistent low grade fevers (≤102°F)	
Noninfectious medical diseases most likely	
Infectious disease causes also important	
Acute high, spiking fevers (≥102°F)	
Infectious disease etiology most likely	
Medical disorders excluded by fevers ≥102°F:	
MI/LVF	Thrombophlebitis
PE	*C. difficile*
	diarrhea
Acute pancreatitis	GI hemorrhage
ARDS	Cholecystitis
Atelectasis/dehydration	Uncomplicated
Hematomas	wound infection
Only noninfectious diseases with temperatures ≥102°F in CCU	
Drug fevers	
Malignant neuroleptic syndrome	
Central fevers	
Fevers 2° to blood/blood product transfusion	
Transient bacteremias 2° to manipulation of a colonized/infected mucosa	

Abbreviations: CCU, critical care unit; ARDS, acute respiratory distress syndrome; GI, gastrointestinal, MI, myocardial infarction; LVF, left ventricular failure; PE, pulmonary emboli.
Source: From Refs. 1, 3.

ARDS should be on PEEP with high oxygen concentrations. Abscesses should be drained as soon as possible. Abdominal computed tomography (CT) scanning is invaluable in accessing abdominal pain in a febrile patient in the CCU. Plain films of the abdomen are helpful, and ultrasound is (except for biliary tract obstruction) insufficiently accurate compared to a CT scan. Because CCU problems are time critical, the abdominal CT scan should be obtained on an urgent basis and serially if necessary (Table 12) (50–53).

Infectious diseases should be treated with appropriate empiric antimicrobial therapy. Coverage should be directed against the usual pathogen(s) associated with the infected organ system involved. Once again, infectious disease consultation is invaluable in determining adequate and appropriate antibiotic therapy without being excessive. Infectious disease consultants can also streamline the antibiotic regimen and make adjustments for drug allergies as well as hepatic and/or renal insufficiency, and take into account significant drug interactions/side effects to tailor the antimicrobial therapy to the patient's condition. The antibiotic selected should have a spectrum appropriate for the site of infection, be started as soon as possible, have a low resistance potential, have excellent safety profile, and be inexpensive. Coverage should be adequate for likely pathogens, but colonization should not be treated. The infectious disease consultant is in the best position to analyze complex/

Table 12 Therapeutic Approach to Fever in the Critical Care Unit

Microbiologic data evaluation
Critical to differentiate colonization from infection:
    Respiratory secretion isolates
    Urinary isolates
    Analysis of origin of blood culture isolates
Rule out pseudo-infections
Common causes of fevers
Nosocomial pneumonia/VAP
    Chest X ray
      If negative, no nosocomial pneumonia/VAP
      If positive, rule out LVF, ARDS, etc.
    Perform semiquantitative BAL to confirm diagnosis
Check central IV lines
    Duration of insertion
      The longer the IV line is overdue, the more likely the fever is due to IV-line infection
      Otherwise unexplained fevers in a patient with overdue IV lines should be regarded
        as IV line infection until proven otherwise
    Evidence of infections at local site
      If IV shows sign of infection, remove IV line immediately, send tip for
        semiquantitative culture, and obtain blood cultures from peripheral vein
      If IV site non-erythematous, IV line infection not ruled out, remove/replace IV line
        and send removed catheter tip for semiquantitative culture
If nosocomial pneumonia and IV-line infection eliminated from diagnostic consideration,
  consider drug fever
Early empiric therapy
Coverage based on site/organism correlations: colonization should not be treated
Infectious disease consultant recommendations should be followed.

Abbreviations: IV, intravenous; ARDS, acute respiratory distress syndrome; BAL, bronchoalveolar lavage; VAP, ventilation associated pneumonia; LVF, left ventricular failure.
Source: From Refs. 1, 3, 5.

Table 13 Enzyme Antibiotic Therapy in Sepsis/Septic Shock

Subset	Usual pathogens	Preferred IV therapy	Alternate IV therapy	IV-to-PO switch
Unknown source	Enterobacteriaceae B. fragilis	Meropenem 1 g (IV) q8h × 2 wk or piperacillin/tazobactam 4.5 g (IV) q8h × 2 wk or imipenem 500 mg (IV) q6h × 2 wk or ertapenem 1 g (IV) q24h × 2 wk or combination therapy with ceftriaxone 1 g (IV) q24h × 2 wk plus metronidazole 1 g (IV) q24h × 2 wk	Quinolone[a] (IV) × 2 wk plus either metronidazole 1 g (IV) q24h × 2 wk or clindamycin 600 mg (IV) q8h × 2 wk	Moxifloxacin 400 mg (PO) q24h × 2 wk or combination therapy with clindamycin 300 mg (PO) q8h × 2 wk plus either ciprofloxacin 500 mg (PO) q12h × 2 wk or gatifloxacin 400 mg (PO) q24h × 2 wk or levofloxacin 500 mg (PO) q24h × 2 wk
	Group D streptococci[b] E. faecalis E. faecium (VRE)	Meropenem 1 g (IV) q8h × 2 wk or piperacillin/tazobactam 4.5 g (IV) q8h × 2 wk Linezolid 600 mg (IV) q12h × 2 wk or quinupristin/dalfopristin 7.5 mg/ kg (IV) q8h × 2 wk	Ampicillin/sulbactam 3 g (IV) q6h × 2 wk or Quinolone[c] (IV) × 2 wk Chloramphenicol 500 mg (IV) q6h × 2 wk or Doxycycline 200 mg (IV) q12h × 3 days, then 100 mg (IV) q12h × 11 days	Quinolone[c] (PO) × 2 wk Linezolid 600 mg (PO) q12h × 2 wk or doxycycline 100 mg (PO) q12h × 2 wk
Lung source	S. pneumoniae, H. influenzae, K. pneumoniae	Ceftriaxone 1 g (IV) q24h × 2 wk or cefepime 2 g (IV) q12h × 2 wk	Quinolone[c] (IV) q24h × 2 wk or any second generation cephalosporin (IV) × 2 wk	Quinolone[c] (PO) q24h × 2 wk or doxycycline 200 mg (PO) q12h × 3 days, then 100 mg (PO) q12h × 11 days
IV-line sepsis Bacterial (Treat initially for MSSA; if later identified as MRSA, treat accordingly)	S. epidermidis, S. aureus (MSSA), Klebsiella, Enterobacter, Serratia	Meropenem 1 g (IV) q8h × 2 wk or cefepime 2 g (IV) q12h × 2 wk	Ceftriaxone 1 g (IV) q24h × 2 wk or quinolone[d] (IV) q24h × 2 wk	Quinolone[d] (PO) q24h × 2 wk or cephalexin 500 mg (PO) q6h × 2 wk

S. aureus (MRSA)	Daptomycin 6 g/kg (IV) 24 h or linezolid 600 mg (IV) q12h × 2 wk	Vancomycin 1 g (IV) q12h × 2 wk or linezolid 600 mg (IV) q12h × 2 wk or quinupristin/dalfopristin 7.5 mg/kg (IV) q8h × 2 wk	Linezolid 600 mg (PO) q12h × 2 wk or minocycline 100 mg (PO) q12h × 2 wk
Fungal (Treat initially for non-albicans Candida; if later identified as *C. albicans*, treat accordingly) *Candida albicans*	Preferred IV therapy: fluconazole 800 mg (IV) × 1, then 400 mg (IV) q24h × 2 wk Alternate IV therapy: or Caspofungin 70 mg (IV) × 1 dose, then 50 mg (IV) q24h × 2 wk or lipid-associated formulation of amphotericin B (p. 369) (IV) q24h × 2 wk or amphotericin B deoxycholate 0.7 mg/kg (IV) q24h × 2 wk or voriconazole (see "usual dose," p. 480) or itraconazole 200 mg (IV) q12h × 2 days, then 200 mg (IV) q24h × 2 wk	Preferred IV therapy: fluconazole 800 mg (IV) × 1, then 400 mg (IV) q24h × 2 wk Alternate IV therapy: or caspofungin 70 mg (IV) × 1 dose, then 50 mg (IV) q24h × 2 wk or lipid-associated formulation of amphotericin B (p. 369) (IV) q24h × 2 wk or amphotericin B deoxycholate 0.7 mg/kg (IV) q24h × 2 wk or voriconazole (see "usual dose," p. 480) or itraconazole 200 mg (IV) q12h × 2 days, then 200 mg (IV) q24h × 2 wk	Fluconazole 400 mg (PO) q24h × 2 wk or voriconazole (see "usual dose," p. 480) Itraconazole 200 mg (PO) solution q12h × 2 wk
Non-albicans Candida[e]	Caspofungin or lipid amphotericin B or amphotericin B deoxycholate (see *C. albicans*, above) × 2 wk	Caspofungin or itraconazole (see *C. albicans*, above) or voriconazole (see "usual dose," p. 480) × 2 wk	Fluconazole (see *C. albicans*, above) or itraconazole 200 mg (PO) solution q24h or voriconazole (see "usual dose," p. 480) × 2 wk[e]
Aspergillus	Voriconazole (see "usual dose", p. 480) × 2 wk or caspofungin 70 mg (IV) × 1 dose, then 50 mg (IV) q24h × 2 wk or itraconazole 200 mg (IV) q12h × 2 days, then 200 mg (IV) q24h × 2 wk	Lipid-associated formulation of amphotericin B (p. 369) (IV) q24h × 2 wk or amphotericin B deoxycholate 1–1.5 mg/kg (IV) q24h × 2 wk	Voriconazole (see "usual dose," p. 480) × 2 wk or itraconazole 200 mg (PO) solution q12h × 2 days, then 200 mg (PO) solution q24h × 2 wk

(Continued)

Table 13 Enzyme Antibiotic Therapy in Sepsis/Septic Shock (*Continued*)

Subset	Usual pathogens	Preferred IV therapy	Alternate IV therapy	IV-to-PO switch
Intra-abdominal/pelvic source	Enterobacteriaceae *B. fragilis*	Meropenem 1 g (IV) q8h × 2 wk or piperacillin/tazobactam 4.5 g therapy with (IV) q8h × 2 wk or tigacycline 100 mg (IV) × 1 dose then 50 mg (IV) of 12 h×2 wk or combination therapy with ceftriaxone 1 g (IV) of 24h × 2 wk plus metronidazole 1 g (IV) q24h × 2 wk	Quinolone[a] (IV) × 2 wk plus either metronidazole 1 g (IV) q24h × 2 wk or clindamycin 600 mg (IV) q8h × 2 wk	Moxifloxacin 400 mg (PO) q24h × 2 wk or combination therapy with clindamycin 300 mg (PO) q8h × 2 wk plus either ciprofloxacin 500 mg (PO) q12h × 2 wk or gatifloxacin 400 mg (PO) q24h × 2 wk or levofloxacin 500 mg (PO) q24h × 2 wk
Urosepsis Gram (−) bacilli	Enterobacteriaceae	Ceftriaxone 1 g (IV) q24h × 1–2 wk	Aztreonam 2 g (IV) q8h × 1–2 wk or Any aminoglycoside (IV) × 1–2 wk	Quinolone (PO)[a] × 1–2 wk
Gram + streptococci (treat initially for *E. faecalis*; if later identified as VRE, treat accordingly)	Group B streptococci *E. faecalis*	Quinolone (IV)[a] × 1–2 wk	Ampicillin 1–2 g (IV) q4h × 1–2 wk or vancomycin 1 g (IV) q12h × 1–2 wk	Amoxicillin 1 g (PO) q8h × 1–2 wk or quinolone (PO)[a] × 1–2 wk
Treat initially for *E. faecium*; if later identified as VRE, treat accordingly)	*E. faecium* (VRE)	Linezolid 600 mg (IV) q12h × 1–2 wk or quinupristin/dalfopristin 7.5 mg/kg (IV) q8h × 1–2 wk	Linezolid 600 mg (IV) q12h × 1–2 wk or quinupristin/dalfopristin 7.5 mg/kg (IV) q8h × 1–2 wk	Linezolid 600 mg (PO) q12h × 1–2 wk or doxycycline 200 mg (PO) q12h
Organism not known	Enterobacteriaceae Group B, D streptococci	Quinolone (IV)[a] × 2 wk	Piperacillin/tazobactam 4.5 g (IV) q8h × 1–2 wk	Quinolone (PO[a]) × 2 wk
Asplenia or hyposplenia	*S. pneumoniae, H. influenzae, N. meningitidis*	Ceftriaxone 2 g (IV) q24h × 2 wk or Quinolone[f] (IV) q24h × 2 wk	Cefepime 2 g (IV) q12h × 2 wk or Cefotaxime 2 g (IV) q6h × 2 wk	Quinolone[f] (PO) q24h × 2 wk

Steroids (high chronic dose)	Candida, Aspergillus	Treat the same as for fungal infection (pp. 118–119)	Treat the same as for fungal infection (pp. 118–119)	Treat the same as for fungal infection (pp. 118–119)
Miliary TB	M. tuberculosis	Treat the same as pulmonary TB (p. 47) plus steroids × 1–2 wk	Treat the same as pulmonary TB (p. 47) plus steroids × 1–2 wk	Treat the same as pulmonary TB (p. 47) plus steroids × 1–2 wk
Miliary BCG (disseminated)	BCG	Treat with 4 anti-TB drugs (NIH, rifampin, ethambutol, cycloserine) q24h × 6–12 months plus steroids (e.g., prednisone 40 mg q24h) × 1–2 wk	Treat with 4 anti-TB drugs (NIH, rifampin, ethambutol, cycloserine) q24h × 6–12 months plus steroids (e.g., prednisone 40 mg q24h) × 1–2 wk	Treat with 4 anti-TB drugs (NIH, rifampin, ethambutol, cycloserine) q24h × 6–12 months plus steroids (e.g., prednisone 40 mg q24h) × 1–2 wk
Severe sepsis	Gram-negative or gram-positive bacteria	Appropriate antimicrobial therapy plus surgical decompression/drainage if needed ±	±drotrecogin alpha (Xigris) 24 µg/kg/hr	Appropriate antimicrobial therapy plus surgical decompression/drainage if needed plus drotrecogin alpha (Xigris) 24 µg/kg/hr

Note: Duration of therapy represents total time IV or IV + PO.

Loading dose not needed PO if given IV with the same drug.

Most patients on IV therapy able to take PO meds should be switched to PO therapy after clinical improvement.

a Ciprofloxacin 400 mg (IV) or 500 mg (PO) q12h or gatifloxacin 400 mg (IV or PO) q24h or levofloxacin 500 mg (IV or PO) q24h.

b Treat initially for *E. faecalis*; if later identified as *E. faecium* (VRE), treat accordingly.

c Ciprofloxacin 400 mg (IV) or 500 mg (PO) q12h or gatifloxacin 400 mg (IV or PO) q24h or levofloxacin 500 mg (IV or PO) q24h or moxifloxacin 400 mg (IV or PO) q24h.

d Gatifloxacin 400 mg or levofloxacin 500 mg or moxifloxacin 400 mg.

e Best agent depends on infecting species. Fluconazole-susceptibility varies predictably by species. *C. glabrata* (usually) and *C. krusei* (almost always) are resistant to fluconazole. *C. lusitaniae* is often resistant to amphotericin B (deoxycholate and lipid-associated formulations). Others are generally susceptible to all agents.

f Gatifloxacin 400 mg or levofloxacin 500 mg or moxifloxacin 400 mg.

Abbreviations: IV, intravenous; BCG, bacillus Calmette–Guerin; MSSA/MRSA, methicillin-sensitive/resistant *S. aureus*; TB, tuberculosis; VRE, vancomycin resistant enterococci; INH, isoniazid.

Source: From Ref. 53.

Table 14 Treatment of Fever in the Critical Care Unit

Obligatory Reduction in Temperatures >106°F
Heat stroke
Malignant hyperthermia
Malignant neoplastic syndrome
Central fevers
Drug fever
Obligatory reduction in temperatures >102°F[a]
Acute myocardial infarction
Borderline pulmonary function
CNS trauma
Optional Reduction of Temperatures >102°F[a]
Blood/blood product transfusion reactions
Postdiagnosis of infectious/noninfectious diseases febrile disorders

[a]Temperatures should be lowered to <102°F.
Abbreviation: CNS, central nervous system.
Source: From Refs. 1, 56.

conflicting culture data and select the optimal antibiotic regimen in the proper clinical context (1,10).

Antibiotic therapy alone eliminates infection due to undrained abscesses, IV-lines, infections associated with prosthetic material/foreign bodies, obstructed biliary, gastrointestinal, or urinary tracts. Antibiotics will not eliminate fever due to noninfectious diseases, e.g., hemorrhage, hematoma, atelectasis, drug fever, vasculitis, and fever due to malignancies. Drug fever is a common problem in CCU patients because of the variety of nonantibiotic medications associated with drug fever. The most common causes of drug fever in the CCU are anti-seizure medications, β-blockers, angiotensin converting enzyme inhibitors, sleep medications, or sulfa-containing medications, i.e., diuretics/pentamidine, stool softeners (Colace), and sensitizing medication, but it is a common error to add/change antibiotics instead (Table 13) (52,53).

Unless fever could be detrimental to the patient, fever should be treated per se. In those with good cardiopulmonary function, fever >106°F should be treated to reduce the temperature to 102°F to 104°F range. Patients with CNS trauma, recent myocardial infarction, or borderline cardiopulmonary function should have temperatures maintained at ~102°F. Temperatures >102°F in sick patients could worsen neurologic daze in those with CNS trauma or precipitate an acute myocardial infarction, chronic heart failure, or pulmonary decompensation in those with advanced cardiopulmonary disease (Table 14) (54–56).

REFERENCES

1. Cunha BA. Clinical approach to fever in the Critical Care Unit. Crit Care Clin 1998; 8: 1–14.
2. Clarke DE, Kimelman J, Raffin TA. The evaluation of fever in the intensive care unit. Chest 1991; 100:213–220.
3. Cunha BA. Fever in the intensive care unit. Intensive Care 1999; 25:648–651.
4. Marik PE. Fever in the ICU. Chest 2000; 117:855–869.
5. Cunha BA, Shea KW. Fever in the intensive care unit. Infect Dis Clin North Am 1996; 10:185–209.

6. McGowan JE, Rose RC, Jacobs NF, et al. Fever in hospitalized patients. Am J Med 1987; 82:580–586.
7. O'Grady NP, Barie PS, Bartlett J, et al. Practice parameters for evaluating new fever in critically ill patients. Task Force of the American College of Critical Care Medicine of the Society of Critical Care Medicine in collaboration with the Infectious Disease Society of America. Crit Care Med 1998; 26:392–408.
8. Stumacher RJ. Fever in the ICU. Infect Dis Pract 1996; 20:89–92.
9. Ryan M, Levy MM. Clinical review: fever in intensive care unit patients. Crit Care 2003; 7:221–225.
10. Cunha BA. Approach to fever. In: Gorbach SL, Bartlett JB, Blacklow NR, eds. Infectious Diseases in Medicine Surgery. 4th ed. Baltimore: Lippincott Williams & Wilkins, 2005: 54–63.
11. Cunha BA. The diagnostic significance of fever curves. Infect Dis Clin North Am 1996; 10:33–44.
12. Johnson DH, Cunha BA. Drug fever. Infect Dis Clin North Am 1996; 10:85–91.
13. Mackowiak PA, LeMaistre CF. Drug fever: a critical appraisal of conventional concepts. Ann Intern Med 1987; 106:728–733.
14. Mackowiak PA. Drug fever: mechanisms, maxims and misconceptions. Am J Med Sci 1987; 294:275–286.
15. Cunha BA. The diagnostic approach to rash and fever in the critical care unit. Crit Care Clin 1998; 8:35–54.
16. Cunha BA. Rash and fever in the intensive care unit. In: Abraham E, Vincent JL, Kochanek P, eds. Textbook of Critical Care Medicine. 5th ed. Philadelphia: Elsevier, 2005:113–119.
17. Cunha BA. Fever in malignant disorders. Infect Dis Pract 2004; 28:335–336.
18. Ginsberg MD, Busto R. Combating hyperthermia in acute stroke: a significant clinical concern. Stroke 1998; 29:529–534.
19. Wood AJJ. Adverse drug reactions. In. Fauci AS, Braunwald E, Isselbacher KJ, et al., eds. Harrison's Principles of Internal Medicine. New York: McGraw–Hill, 1998:422–430.
20. Ferrara JL. The febrile platelet transfusion reaction: a cytokine shower. Transfusion 1995; 35:89–90.
21. Fenwick JC, Cameron M, Naiman SC, et al. Blood transfusion as a cause of leucocytosis in critically ill patients. Lancet 1994; 344:855–856.
22. Marx N, Neumann FJ, Ott I, et al. Induction of cytokine expression in leukocytes in acute myocardial infarction. J Am Coll Cardiol 1997; 30:165–170.
23. Murray HW, Ellis GC, Blumenthal DS, et al. Fever and pulmonary thromboembolism. Am J Med 1979; 67:232–235.
24. Engoren M. Lack of association between atelectasis and fever. Chest 1995; 107:81–84.
25. Cunha BA. FUO in the ICU. In Bouza E, Picazo JJ, eds. Infeccion. Madrid, Spain, 2004.
26. Cunha BA. The diagnostic significance of relative bradycardia in infectious disease. Clin Microbiol Infect 2000; 6:633–634.
27. Cotton LM, Strampfer MJ, Cunha BA. Legionella and mycoplasma pneumonia: a community hospital experience. Clin Chest Med 1987; 8:441–453.
28. Ostergaard L, Huniche B, Andersen PL. Relative bradycardia in infectious diseases. J Infect 1996; 33:185–191.
29. Cunha BA. Diagnostic significance of relative bradycardia. Infect Dis Pract 1997; 21: 38–40.
30. Cunha BA. Relative bradycardia as a diagnostic clue. Intern Med 1999; 20:42–46.
31. Wittesjo B, Bjornham A, Eitrem R. Relative bradycardia in infectious diseases. J Infect 2000; 38:246–247.
32. Meduri GU, Mauldin GI, Wunderink RG, et al. Causes of fever and pulmonary densities in patients with clinical manifestations of ventilator-associated pneumonia. Chest 1994; 106:221–235.

33. Meduri GU. Diagnosis and differential diagnosis of ventilator-associated pneumonia. Clin Chest Med 1995; 16:61–93.
34. Santos E, Talusan, Brandstetter RD. Roentgenographic mimics of pneumonia in the critical care unit. Crit Care Clin 1998; 14:91–104.
35. Cunha BA. Severe community-acquired pneumonia. Crit Care Clin 1998; 14:105–117.
36. Cunha BA. Nosocomial pneumonia: diagnostic and therapeutic considerations. Med Clin North Am 2001; 85:79–114.
37. Cunha BA. Pneumonia Essentials. Michigan: Physicians Press, 2006.
38. Eisenstein L, Cunha BA. Herpes simples virus type I (HSV-I) pneumonia presenting as failure to wean. Heart Lung 2003; 32:65–66.
39. Cunha BA. Herpes simplex-1 (HSV-1) pneumonia. Infect Dis Pract 2005; 29:375–378.
40. Maki DG. Pathogenesis, prevention, and management of infections due to intravascular devices used for infusion therapy. In: Bisno A, Waldvogel F, eds. Infections Associated with Indwelling Medical Devices. Washington, D.C.: American Society for Microbiology, 1989:161–177.
41. Cunha BA. Intravenous line infections. Crit Care Clin 1998; 8:339–346.
42. Garibaldi RA, Brodine S, Matsumiya S, et al. Evidence for the noninfectious etiology of early postoperative fever. Infect Control 1985; 6:273–277.
43. Kitaichi M. Differential diagnosis of bronchilitis obliterans organizing pneumonia. Chest 1992; 102:44–49.
44. Fry DE. Postoperative fever. In: Mackowiak PA, ed. Fever: Basic Mechanisms and Management. New York: Raven Press, 1991:243–254.
45. Warren JW. Catheter-associated urinary tract infections. Infect Dis Clin North Am 1997; 11:609–619.
46. Paradisi F, Corti G, Mangani V. Urosepsis in the critical care unit. Crit Care Clin 1998; 114:165–180.
47. Tu RP, Cunha BA. Significance of fever in the neurosurgical intensive care unit. Heart Lung 1988; 17:608–611.
48. Bouza E, Munoz P, Alonso R. Clinical manifestations, treatment and control of infections caused by *Clostridium difficile*. Clin Microbiol Infect 2005; 4:57–64.
49. Caines C, Gill MV, Cunha BA. Non-*Clostridium difficile* nosocomial diarrhea in the intensive care unit. Heart Lung 1997; 26:83–84.
50. Mieszczanska H, Lazar J, Cunha BA. Cardiovascular manifestations of sepsis. Infect Dis Pract 2003; 27:183–186.
51. Brun–Buisson C, Doyon F, Carlet J, et al. Incidence, risk factors, and outcome of severe sepsis and septic shock in adults: a multicenter prospective study in intensive care units. French ICU Group for Severe Sepsis. JAMA 1995; 274:968–974.
52. Cunha BA. Antibiotic treatment of sepsis. Med Clin North Am 1995; 79:551–558.
53. Cunha BA. Antibiotic Essentials. (5th Ed) Michigan: Physicians Press, 2006.
54. Plaisance KI, Mackowiak PA. Antipyretic therapy: physiologic rationale, diagnostic implications, and clinical consequences. Arch Intern Med 2000; 160:449–456.
55. Mackowiak PA. Physiological rationale for suppression of fever. Clin Infect Dis 2000; 31(suppl 5):S185–S189.
56. Cunha BA. Should fever be treated in sepsis. In: Vincent JL, Carlet J, Opal S, eds. Sepsis. 21st Symposium on Intensive Care and Emergency Medicine. New York: Kluwer Academic Publishers, 2001:705–717.

4

Sepsis and Its Mimics in the Critical Care Unit

Burke A. Cunha

Infectious Disease Division, Winthrop-University Hospital, Mineola, and
State University of New York School of Medicine, Stony Brook, New York, U.S.A.

INTRODUCTION

Sepsis refers to bacteremia or fungemia with hypotension and organ dysfunction. The main clinical problem with the "septic" patient is to determine if the patient is septic or has a noninfectious condition that mimics sepsis by hemodynamic or laboratory parameters. In the intensive care setting it is of critical importance to differentiate between sepsis and its mimics (1–6).

Diagnostic Approach

Many patients with fever and hypotension are not septic. Several clinical disorders resemble sepsis. Patients do not become septic without a major breach in host defenses. The most important clinical consideration in determining whether a patient is septic is to identify the source of infection. Sepsis is a complication with only relatively few infections. Infections limited to specific infections in a few organ systems are the only ones with septic potential. Most sepsis is derived from perforated obstructions or abscesses of the gastrointestinal (GI) tract/pelvis, hepatobiliary tract, and genitourinary (GU) tract, or may be related to central intravenous (IV) lines. Even though the GI tract is the most frequent focus of infection leading to sepsis, not all GI disorders including infections have a septic potential. Lower GI tract perforations, intra-abdominal/pelvic abscesses, and pylephlebitis commonly result clinically in sepsis. In contrast, gastritis and nonperforating gastric ulcer are rarely associated with sepsis. Cholangitis in the hepatobiliary tract results in sepsis, but rarely, if ever, complicates acute/chronic cholecystitis (6–13). IV line sepsis represents the ultimate breach in host defenses, as the pathogenic organisms from central catheters are introduced directly into the bloodstream in high concentrations (14,15).

The primary task is to search for GI, GU, or an IV source of sepsis. It is almost always possible to identify the septic source by physical exam, laboratory, or radiology tests. Without local signs of entry site infection, IV-line sepsis should not be entertained if the central IV line has been in place less than seven days.

If intraabdominal and GU sources have been eliminated as diagnostic possibilities, central IV lines, either temporary or long term, should be considered as a cause of sepsis. The longer a central IV line is in place, the more likely the central IV line may be the cause of fever/hypotension. Signs of infection at entry sites of central IV lines indicate likely IV-line sepsis, but no superficial erythema/swelling does not rule out IV-line sepsis (14–16).

Disorders that mimic sepsis should be recognized to treat the condition and not to avoid inappropriate treatment with antibiotics. Disorders that mimic sepsis (pseudosepsis) include GI hemorrhage, pulmonary embolism, myocardial infarction, acute pancreatitis, diabetic ketoacidosis, systemic lupus erythematosus (SLE) flare, and relative adrenal insufficiency, inadequate (maintenance, not stress dosed), or too rapidly typed steroid therapy, ventricular pseudo-aneurysm, massive aspiration or atelectasis, systemic vasculitis, and diuretic-induced hypovolemia (Table 1) (6,17–21).

Clinical Signs of Sepsis

Excluding the elderly, compromised hosts, and uremic patients, fever is a cardinal sign of inflammation or infection. Fever should not be equated with infection as the chemical mediators of inflammation and infection, i.e., cytokines, induce a febrile response mediated via the preoptic nucleus of the anterior hypothalamus. All that is febrile is not infectious, and most, but not all diseases causing sepsis are accompanied by temperatures $\geq 102°F$. With the exceptions of drug fever and adrenal insufficiency, the disorders that mimic sepsis and pseudosepsis have temperatures $\leq 102°F$. The temperature relationships are critical when considered together with organ involvement, i.e., GI, GU, etc. are key factors in determining if the patient is septic or has a noninfectious disorder resembling sepsis. Hyperthermia $\geq 106°F$ is only caused by noninfectious disorders. Hypothermia is an important clinical clue to bacteremia, particularly in renal insufficiency. In normal hosts with fever, sepsis should not be a diagnostic consideration if temperatures are $<102°F$ or $>106°F$ (Table 2) (22–25).

LABORATORY ABNORMALITIES IN SEPSIS

The usual hemodynamic parameters associated with sepsis include decreased peripheral resistance (PR) with increased cardiac output (CO) accompanied by tachycardia/respiratory alkalosis. Patients with fever are often diagnosed as septic. Although sepsis is associated with hemodynamic abnormalities, i.e., ↓ PR/↑ CO, many disorders mimicking sepsis also have similar findings, i.e., acute pancreatitis, GI bleed, etc. If hemodynamic abnormalities are present but are not accompanied by GI, GU, or IV clinical disorders associated with sepsis, then it should be assumed that the patient has a noninfectious mimic of sepsis.

As with hemodynamic parameters, laboratory data may mislead the unwary in incorrectly ascribing laboratory abnormalities to an infectious rather than a noninfectious process. An increase in white peripheral blood cell count with a shift to the left is a nonspecific reaction to stress, and is not specific for infection. Leukocytosis does not differentiate bacterial from viral infections. An increase in white count with a shift to the left is a measure of the intensity of the systemic response to stress of infectious or noninfectious disorders.

Similarly, an increase in fibrin split products and lactic acid, decrease in serum albumin, α-2 globulins, and fibrinogen, or an increase in prothrombin time/partial thromboplastin time are compatible but not characteristic of infection.

Table 1 Clinical Conditions Associated with Sepsis Disorders

Associated with sepsis (fevers $\geq 102°F$)	Not associated with sepsis (fevers $\leq 102°F$)
GI source	*GI source*
Liver	Esophagitis
Abscess	Gastritis
Gallbladder	Pancreatitis
Gallbladder "wall abscess"	GI bleed
Cholangitis	*Genitourinary source*
Colon	Urethritis
Colitis	Cystitis (normal hosts)
Diverticulitis	Cervicitis
Toxic megacolon	Vaginitis
Perforation	PID
Obstruction	Catheter-associated bacteriuria (normal hosts)
Abscess	*Upper respiratory source*
Genitourinary source	Pharyngitis
Renal	Sinusitis
Pyelonephritis	Mastoiditis
Intra/perinephric abscess	Bronchitis
Calculi	Otitis
Urinary tract obstruction	*Lower respiratory source*
Partial	CAP (normal host)
Total	*Skin/soft tissue source*
Prostate	Osteomyelitis
Abscess	Uncomplicated wound infections
Pelvic source	*Cardiovascular source*
Pelvic peritonitis	Subacute bacterial endocarditis
Tubo-ovarian abscess	*Central nervous system source*
Pelvic septic thrombophlebitis	Bacterial meningitis (excluding meningococcal meningitis with meningococcemia)
Lower respiratory source	Intravascular source
CAP	A-lines
Asplenia/hyposplenism	Peripheral IV lines
Empyema	
Lung abscess	
Nosocomial pneumonia	
Intravascular source	
IV line infection	
Central IV lines	
PICC lines	
Hickman/Broviac catheters	
Infected prosthetic devices	
AV grafts	
Jugular vein septic thrombophlebitis	
Cardiovascular source	
Acute bacterial endocarditis	
Myocardial abscess	
Paravalvular abscess	
Other	
Toxic shock syndrome	

Abbreviations: GI, gastrointestinal; IV, intravenous; PID, pelvic inflammatory disease; CAP, community acquired pneumonia; BPH, benign prostatic hyperpertrophy PICC, peripherally inserted central catheter; AV, arteriovenous.
Source: From Refs. 9, 22.

Table 2 Clinical Mimics of Sepsis

Acute gastrointestinal hemorrhage
Acute pulmonary embolism
Acute myocardial infarction
Acute pancreatitis
Diabetic ketoacidosis
SLE flare
Relative adrenal insufficiency
Diuretic-induced hypovolemia
Rectus sheath hematoma

Source: From Refs. 9, 22.

Laboratory parameters that are more indicative of infection include leukopenia or thrombocytopenia. The only laboratory abnormalities that are specific for sepsis are organisms in the blood, i.e., gram/acridine orange stains of buffy-coat smears/high grade positivity in blood cultures (excluding contaminants). Increased cytokine/endotoxin levels are also suggestive. Highly elevated C-reactive protein (CRP) levels have also been described as a marker for sepsis. Positive buffy-coat smears are not present in all patients with bacteremia, but when positive are diagnostic and rapid. The bacteria/fungi present in buffy-coat smears are helpful in determining the origin of the septic process by their association with particular organ system involvement, i.e., poorly stained pleomorphic gram-negative bacilli (*Bacteroides fragilis*)

Table 3 Sepsis vs. Mimics of Sepsis

Parameters	Disorders mimicking sepsis	Sepsis (bacteremia from GI/pelvic GU, IV source)
Microbiologic	Negative blood cultures (excluding skin contaminants)	Positive buffy-coat smear
		Bacteremia (excluding skin contaminants)
Hemodynamic	↓ PVR	↓ PVR
	↑ CO	↑ CO
Laboratory	↑ WBC (with left shift)	↑ WBC (with left shift)
	Normal platelet count	↓ Platelet count
	↓ Albumin	↓ Albumin
	↑ FSP	↑ FSP
	↑ Lactate	↑ Lactate
	↑ D-dimers	↑ D-dimers
	↑ PT/PTT	↑ PT/PTT
	↓ Fibrinogen	
	↓ α_2 globulins	
Clinical	≤102°F	≥102°F
	Hypotension	Hypotension
	Tachycardia	Tachycardia
	Respiratory alkalosis	Respiratory alkalosis

Abbreviations: PVR, peripheral vascular resistance; CO, cardiac output; FSP, fibrin split products; WBC, white blood cell; PT/PTT, prothrombin time/partial thromboplastin time; GI, gastrointestinal; GU, genitourinary; IV, intravenous.
Source: From Refs. 9, 22.

point to a GI, but not GU/IV source. The morphology/arrangement of the bacteria in buffy-coat smears is also useful in selecting appropriate empiric antibiotic coverage (Table 3) (26–30).

EMPIRIC ANTIMICROBIAL THERAPY

The selection of appropriate antibiotic therapy for sepsis depends on accurate localization of the infectious process to the abdomen/pelvis, GU tract, or IV line. Because each organ has its normal resident flora that become the pathogenic flora when the organ function is disrupted, empiric coverage is directed against the normal resident flora (Table 4). Factors in antibiotic selection include hepatic/renal insufficiency, allergic status of the patient, tissue penetration of the antibiotic, safety profile of the antibiotic, resistance potential of the antibiotic, and cost.

If the spectrum is appropriate for the source of sepsis, no regimen is superior to others in terms of clinical outcome. However, clinicians should utilize the most

Table 4 Empiric Therapy of Sepsis Based on Organ System Involved

Source/usual organisms	Empiric therapy usual organisms	
	Monotherapy	Combination therapy
Lower GI tract/pelvis (common coliforms plus *Bacteroides fragilis*)	Meropenem tigacycline Ertapenem Piperacillin/tazobactam	Aztreonam or aminoglycoside plus either clindamycin or metronidazole
GU tract/kidneys/prostate (aerobic gram-negative bacilli)	Quinolone Third-generation cephalosporin Aztreonam	
(Enterococci non-VRE)	Ampicillin Piperacillin Meropenem	
(Enterococci VRE)	Linezolid Daptomycin Quinupristin-dalfopristin	
Organism unknown	Meropenem Piperacillin/tazobactam tigacycline	
Bloodstream IV line (aerobic gram-negative bacilli, *Staphylococcus aureus*, Enterococci)	Meropenem[a]	Cefepime plus vancomycin
Lung nosocomial pneumonia/ vent-associated pneumonia (aerobic gram-negative bacilli)	Meropenem Cefepime Cefoperazone Levofloxacin	Meropenem or cefepime plus either levofloxacin or aztreonam or amikacin

[a]Vancomycin, daptomycin, or linezolid if most intravenous-line infections in institution due to methicillin-resistant *Staphylococcus aureus* (MRSA).
Abbreviations: IV, intravenous; GI, gastrointestinal; GU, genitourinary; VRE, vancomycin-resistant enterococci.
Source: From Ref. 32.

clinically/cost-effective regimens with a low resistance potential and begin therapy as soon as the diagnosis of sepsis is made. The basis of empiric therapy for sepsis depends on eliminating the source of sepsis and covering the patient with antibiotic therapy appropriate for the septic source. The use of steroids and anti-cytokine therapies remains controversial and is of unproven benefit (31–44).

SUMMARY

The immediate task of the clinician is to determine whether the patient has sepsis or a mimic of sepsis. The diagnostic process may be approached from the negative perspective, i.e., if the patient does not have a GI, GU, and IV process usually associated with sepsis, then the patient in all probability does not have sepsis, and the workup should be directed to diagnosed disorders that mimic sepsis.

The temperature of the patient is of key importance in determining if the patient has sepsis or a noninfectious mimic. In temperatures $\geq 106°F$ and $\leq 102°F$, a noninfectious disease process is likely and argues against a diagnosis of sepsis. Antibiotic therapy should be instituted as soon as there is a basis for the diagnosis of sepsis, i.e., characteristic (perforation, obstruction, or abscess) organ system of infection, GI, GU, and IV site. Coverage should be based on the usual pathogens associated with the involved organ system. Antibiotics with appropriate spectrum, good safety profile, low resistance potential, and anti-endotoxin qualities are preferred. In sepsis related to perforation, obstruction, or abscess, surgical intervention is paramount and should be done as soon as the diagnosis is confirmed.

REFERENCES

1. Annane D, Bellisant E, Cavaillon JM. Septic shock. Lancet 2005; 365:63–78.
2. Hardaway RM. A review of septic shock. Am Surg 2000; 66:22–29.
3. Murray MJ, Kumar M. Sepsis and septic shock. Postgrad Med 1991; 90:199–202.
4. Sibbald WJ, Marshall J, Christou N, et al. "Sepsis"—clarity of existing terminology or more confusion? Crit Care Med 1991; 19:996–998.
5. Sharma S, Kumar A. Septic shock, multiple organ failure, and acute respiratory distress syndrome. Curr Opin Pulm Med 2003; 9:199–209.
6. Cunha BA. Sepsis and its mimics. Intern Med 1992; 13:48–55.
7. Lazaron V, Barke RA. Gram-negative bacterial sepsis and the sepsis syndrome. Urol Clin North Am 1999; 26:687–699.
8. Cunha BA. Urosepsis. J Crit Illness 1997; 12:616–625.
9. Marshall JC. Intra-abdominal infections. Microbes Infect 2004; 6:1015–1025.
10. Sacks-Berg A, Calubiran OV, Cunha BA. Sepsis associated with transhepatic cholangiography. J Hosp Infect 1992; 20:43–50.
11. Carpenter HA. Bacterial and parasitic cholangitis. Mayo Clin Proc 1998; 73:473–478.
12. Alberti C, Brun-Buisson C. The sources of sepsis. In: Vincent JL, Carlet J, Opal SM, eds. The Sepsis Text. Boston: Kluwer Academic Publishers, 2002:491–503.
13. Cruz K, Dellinger RP. Diagnosis and source of sepsis: the utility of clinical findings. In: Vincent JL, Carlet J, Opal SM, eds. The Sepsis Text. Boston: Kluwer Academic Publishers, 2002:11–28.
14. Bouza E, Burillo A, Munoz P. Catheter-related infections: diagnosis and intravascular treatment. Clin Microbiol Infect 2002; 8:265–274.

15. Gill MV, Cunha BA. IV line sepsis. In: Cunha BA, ed. Infectious Diseases in Critical Care Medicine. New York: Marcel Dekker, 1998:57–65.
16. Cunha BA. Intravenous line infections. Crit Care Clin 1998:339–346.
17. Hamid N, Spadafora P, Khalife ME, Cunha BA: Pseudosepsis: rectus sheath hematoma mimicking septic shock. Heart & Lung 2006; 35:528–530..
18. McCriskin JW, Baisden CE, Spaccevento LJ, et al. Pseudosepsis after myocardial infarction. Am J Med 1987; 83:577–580.
19. Melby MJ, Bergman K, Ramos T, et al. Acute adrenal insufficiency mimicking septic shock: a case report. Pharmacotherapy 1988; 8:69–71.
20. Gabbay DS, Cunha BA. Pseudosepsis secondary to bilateral adrenal hemorrhage. Heart Lung 1998; 27:348–351.
21. Wilson PG, Manji M, Neoptolemos JP. Acute pancreatitis as a model of sepsis. J Antimicrob Chemother 1998; 41(suppl A):51–63.
22. Cunha BA. Fever in the critical care unit. Crit Care Clin 1998; 14:1–14.
23. Opal SM, Cohen J. Clinical gram-positive sepsis: does it fundamentally differ from gram-negative bacterial sepsis. Crit Care Med 1999; 27:1608–1616.
24. Levy B, Bollaert PE. Clinical manifestations and complications of septic shock. In: Dhainaut JG, Thijs LG, Park G, eds. Septic Shock. Philadelphia: WB Saunders, 2000: 339–352.
25. Court O, Kumar A, Parrillo JE, et al. Clinical review: myocardial depression in sepsis and septic shock. Crit Care 2002; 6:500–508.
26. Ristuccia PA, Hoeffner RA, Digamon-Beltran M, et al. Detection of bacteremia by buffy coat smears. Scand J Infect Dis 1987; 19:215–217.
27. Llewelyn M, Cohen J. Intern Sepsis Forum. Diagnosis of infection in sepsis. Intensive Care Med 2001; 27(suppl 1):S10–S32.
28. Mieszczanska H, Lazar J, Cunha BA. Cardiovascular manifestations of sepsis. Infect Dis Prac 2003; 27:183–186.
29. Takala A, Nupponen I, Kylanpaa-Back ML, et al. Markers of inflammation in sepsis. Ann Med 2002; 34:614–623.
30. Povoa P. C-reactive protein: a valuable marker of sepsis. Intensive Care Med 2002; 28:235–243.
31. Cunha BA. Antibiotic treatment of sepsis. Med Clin North Am 1995; 79:551–558.
32. Cunha BA. Antibiotic Essentials. (5th Ed) Royal Oak Physicians Press, 2006.
33. Kollef MH. Inadequate antimicrobial treatment: an important determinant of outcome for hospitalized patients. Clin Infect Dis 2000; 31(suppl 4):S131–S138.
34. Finch RG. Empirical choice of antibiotic therapy in sepsis. JR Coll Physicians Lond 2000; 34:528–532.
35. Bochud PY, Glauser MP, Calandra T, et al. Antibiotics in sepsis. Intensive Care Med 2001; 27(suppl 1):S33–S48.
36. Lepper PM, Held TK, Schneider EM, et al. Clinical implications of antibiotic-induced endotoxin release in septic shock. Intensive Care Med 2002; 28:824–833.
37. Danner RL, Elin RJ, Hosseini JM, et al. Endotoxemia in human septic shock. Chest 1991; 99:169–175.
38. Dellinger RP. Current therapy for sepsis. Infect Dis Clin North Am 1999; 13:495–509.
39. Vincent JL. International Sepsis Forum. Hemodynamic support in septic shock. Intensive Care Med 2001; 27(suppl 1):S80–S92.
40. Carlet J. Antibiotic management of severe infections in critically ill patients. In: Dhainaut JG, Thijs LG, Park G, eds. Septic Shock. Philadelphia: WB Saunders, 2000:445–460.
41. Marshall JC. Control of the source of sepsis. In: Vincent JL, Carlet J, Opal SM, eds. The Sepsis Text. Boston: Kluwer Academic Publishers, 2002:525–538.
42. Callister ME, Evans TW. Haemodynamic and ventilatory support in severe sepsis. JR Coll Physicians Lond 2000; 34:522–528.
43. Annane D. Corticosteroids for septic shock. Crit Care Med 2001; 29(suppl):S117–S120.
44. Healy DP. New and emerging therapies for sepsis. Ann Pharmacother 2002; 36:648–654.

5
Meningitis and Its Mimics in the Critical Care Unit

Burke A. Cunha

Infectious Disease Division, Winthrop-University Hospital, Mineola, and State University of New York School of Medicine, Stony Brook, New York, U.S.A.

OVERVIEW

There are several diagnostic difficulties in patients presenting with the possibility of acute bacterial meningitis. Critically ill patients with meningitis are usually transferred to the critical care unit (CCU) for intensive supportive care. Meningitis may be mimicked by a variety of infectious and noninfectious disorders. The mimics of meningitis are readily ruled out on the basis of the history/physical exam and, if any doubt remains, then a lumbar puncture with cerebrospinal fluid (CSF) analysis will include or exclude the diagnosis of acute bacterial meningitis. Early and appropriate empiric antimicrobial therapy of acute bacterial meningitis in the CCU may be lifesaving. In contrast to the differential diagnostic problem of encephalitis in the CCU, acute bacterial meningitis in the CCU is not usually a diagnostic problem but is primarily a therapeutic problem.

Acute bacterial meningitis is, in the main, caused by bacterial neuropathogens. Acute bacterial meningitis occurs in normal and compromised hosts and may be acquired naturally or as a complication of open head trauma or neurosurgical procedures. Regardless of the pathogen or mode of acquisition, the definitive diagnosis of acute bacterial meningitis rests on analysis of the CSF profile and gram stain/culture of the CSF. Acute bacterial meningitis in normal and compromised hosts presents clinically with meningeal irritation, i.e., nuchal rigidity. Nuchal rigidity must be differentiated from other causes of neck stiffness, i.e., meningismus associated with the mimics of meningitis. There are relatively few nonbacterial causes of meningitis, and it is important to differentiate aseptic or viral meningitis from bacterial meningitis. In general, patients with aseptic or viral meningitis are less critically ill than are those with acute bacterial meningitis. Patients ill enough to be admitted to the CCU usually are more likely to have bacterial versus viral meningitis. Aseptic viral meningitis may be diagnosed by analysis of the CSF profile, as well as specific viral culture/polymerase chain reaction (PCR) determinations. Patients with acute meningitis, either bacterial or viral, will have various degrees of nuchal rigidity with intact mental status. Patients with mental confusion, i.e., encephalopathy, have encephalitis, and these patients do not have nuchal rigidity. Central nervous system (CNS) infection caused by a few organisms, i.e., Herpes simplex virus (HSV)-1, *Mycoplasma pneumoniae*, and *Listeria monocytogenes*, may present with a combination of stiff neck and mental confusion, i.e., meningoencephalitis. Any patient with fever and otherwise unexplained neck stiffness should have a lumbar puncture performed to confirm the diagnosis of acute bacterial meningitis. If acute bacterial meningitis is suspected, lumbar puncture should be performed prior to head computed tomography (CT)/magnetic resonance imaging (MRI) (1–6).

Therefore, the challenge of meningitis in the CCU setting is to arrive at a correct diagnosis by ruling out the noninfectious mimics of meningitis, and then differentiating viral meningitis from bacterial meningitis. Patients with signs of meningeal irritation and mental confusion, i.e., meningoencephalitis, are diagnosed on the basis of the CSF profile and extra-CNS signs, symptoms, and/or laboratory abnormalities. The objective of arriving at a presumptive diagnosis of acute bacterial meningitis is to begin appropriate empiric therapy as soon as possible. Appropriate empiric therapy for acute bacterial meningitis is determined by predicting the likely range of pathogens. In acute bacterial meningitis, the most likely pathogen is determined by the age of the patient, mode of onset, epidemiological history/predisposing factors, physical signs, e.g., rash, rhinorrhea, cranial nerve abnormalities, etc., specific host defense defects and associated underlying disorders, and the morphology/arrangement of organisms seen on the gram stain of the CSF (1,2,4).

CLINICAL DIAGNOSIS OF ACUTE BACTERIAL MENINGITIS

Overview

Excluding open CNS trauma or neurosurgical procedures, bacteria causing acute meningitis reach the CSF hematogenously. Many bacteria have a bacteremic potential, i.e., bacteremias are part of their infection process, but relatively few are able to cross the blood–brain barrier and cause meningitis. Acute bacterial meningitis usually involves the leptomeninges or the covering of the brain. Leptomeningeal irritation is responsible for the nuchal rigidity, Kernig's and Brudzinski's signs associated with acute bacterial meningitis (7,8). Because the leptomeninges cover the brain parenchyma, meningitis is not associated with changes in mental status that require parenchymal invasion. The majority of pathogens causing acute bacterial meningitis are respiratory tract organisms. Acute bacterial meningitis may also result from contiguous spread from a local source in close proximity to the brain. Infections that cause meningitis by contiguous spread include sinusitis or mastoiditis. Cracks in the cribriform plate are another example of a mode of entry via a contiguous bacterial source. Meningitis may also occur by hematogenous spread of nonrespiratory pathogens, e.g., *Listeria, Escherichia coli*, and *Staphylococcus aureus*, as part of secondary bacteremia with CNS seeding. Acute bacterial endocarditis due to *S. aureus* is not infrequently complicated by acute purulent bacterial meningitis as a suppurative complication (9). The insertion of CNS shunts for hydrocephalus/increased intracranial pressure, if complicated by meningitis, reflects either the flora of the skin introduced during the insertion process, or the flora at the distal end of the shunt, i.e., a ventricular peritoneal shunt. Open head trauma introduces the bacteria into the CSF/brain parenchyma (Table 1) (1–5,10–13).

Meningoencephalitis due to *L. monocytogenes* is recognizable by clues from the CSF profile and is common in the elderly/immunosuppressed. *M. pneumoniae*

Table 1 Symptoms and Signs of Acute Bacterial Meningitis

Symptoms	Signs
Headache	Fever
Photophobia	Meningismus
Nausea and vomiting	Kernig's sign
	Brudzinski's sign
	Acute deafness
	Cranial nerve palsies
	Seizures

meningoencephalitis is being recognized as part of the clinical presentation of *M. pneumoniae* atypical pneumonia. *M. pneumoniae* meningoencephalitis occurs in patients with *Mycoplasma* community–acquired pneumonia with very high cold agglutinin levels ($>$1:512).

The viruses, e.g., enteroviruses, that cause meningitis are relatively few compared to their bacterial counterparts. Some viruses, i.e., HSV-1 cause a spectrum of CNS infections in normal hosts from aseptic meningitis to encephalitis. Partially treated meningitis is bacterial meningitis following initial treatment for meningitis. Partially treated bacterial meningitis is diagnosed by history, and findings in the CSF, i.e., pleocytosis with a variably decreased glucose and a moderately elevated CSF lactic acid (4–6 mmol/L). Partially treated meningitis requires retreatment with antimicrobials with the same spectrum and dosage as to treat acute bacterial meningitis (1–3,14,15).

THE MIMICS OF MENINGITIS

Overview

Because a stiff neck or nuchal rigidity is the hallmark of acute bacterial meningitis, any condition that is associated with neck stiffness may mimic meningitis. Patients with acute torticollis, muscle spasm of the head/neck, cervical arthritis, or meningismus due to a variety of head and neck disorders can all mimic bacterial meningitis. Fortunately, most of these causes of neck stiffness or meningismus are not associated with fever. Fever plus nuchal rigidity is the distinguishing hallmark of acute bacterial meningitis. It may be difficult in elderly patients to rule out meningitis on the basis of fever and nuchal rigidity alone because many elderly individuals have fever due to a variety of non-CNS infections, and may have a stiff neck due to cervical arthritis. In such situations, analysis of the CSF profile will readily distinguish the mimics of meningitis from actual infection (1–5).

Noninfectious Mimics of Acute Bacterial Meningitis

Disorders that commonly may be mistaken for meningitis include drug-induced meningitis, meningeal carcinomatosis, serum sickness, collagen vascular diseases, granulomatous angiitis of the CNS, Behçet's disease, systemic lupus erythematosus (SLE), and neurosarcoidosis. The diagnostic approach to the mimics of meningitis is related to the clinical context in which they occur. For example, lupus cerebritis would rarely present as the sole manifestation of SLE. Similarly, with Behçet's disease, patients developing neuro-Behçet's disease have established Behçet's, and have multiple manifestations, which should lead the clinician to suspect the diagnosis in such a patient. Similarly, with neurosarcoid, the presentation is usually subacute or chronic rather than acute, and occurs in patients with a known history of sarcoidosis (Table 2) (16–21).

Drug-Induced Meningitis

Drug-induced meningitis may present with a stiff neck and fever. The time of meningeal symptoms after consumption of the medication is highly variable. The most

Table 2 Mimics of Acute Bacterial Meningitis

Drug-induced aseptic meningitis
Toxic/metabolic abnormalities
NSAIDs
OKT®3
ATG
TMP-SMX
Azathioprine
CNS vasculitis
SLE cerebritis
Sarcoid meningitis
Bland emboli from SBE or marantic endocarditis
(nonbacterial thrombocytic endocarditis)
Tumor emboli
Primary or metastatic CNS malignancies
(meningeal carcinomatosis)
AML
ALL
Hodgkin's lymphoma
Non-Hodgkin's lymphoma
Melanoma
Breast carcinomas
Bronchogenic carcinomas
Hypernephromas (renal cell carcinomas)
Germ cell tumors
Legionnaires' disease
Posteria fossa syndrome
Subarachnoid hemorrhage
Intracerebral hemorrhage
CNS leukostasis
Thrombocytopenia
DIC
Abnormal platelet function
Coagulopathy
CNS metastases
Embolic and thrombotic strokes
Partially treated bacterial meningitis
Meningoencephalitis

Abbreviations: AML, acute myelogenous leukemia; ALL, acute lymphoblastic leukemia; DIC, disseminated intravascular coagulation; CNS, central nervous system; SLE, systemic lupus erythematosus; NSAIDs, nonsteroidal inflammatory drugs; ATG, antithymoglobulin; SBE, subacute endocarditis; TMP-SMX, trimethoprim-sulfamethoxazole.
Source: From Refs. 1–6.

common drugs associated with drug-induced meningitis include use of nonsteroidal inflammatory drugs. In addition, trimethoprim alone (TMP-SMX), and to a lesser extent, azathioprine may present as a drug-induced aseptic meningitis. Leukocytosis in the CSF with a polymorphonuclear predominance is typical with drug-induced meningitis, and the clinical clue to the presence of drug-induced meningitis is the presence of eosinophils in the CSF. In drug-induced meningitis, the CSF also contains increased protein, but the CSF glucose is rarely decreased. RBCs or an increased CSF lactic acid level are not features of drug-induced meningitis. Treatment is discontinuation of the offending agent (1,16,17).

Serum Sickness

Serum sickness is a systemic reaction to the injection of serum-derived antitoxin derivatives. Because such toxins are not used much anymore, serum sickness is now most commonly associated with the use of certain medications, including β-lactam antibiotics, sulfonamides, and streptomycin among the antimicrobials. Nonantimicrobials associated with serum sickness include hydralazine, alpha methyldopa, propanolol, procainamide, quinidine, phenylbutazone, naproxen, catapril, and diphenyl hydantoin. Symptoms typically begin about two weeks after the initiation of drug therapy, and are characterized by fever, arthralgias/arthritis, and immune complex–mediated renal insufficiency. Urticaria, abdominal pain, or lymphadenopathy may or may not be present. Neurologic abnormalities are part of the systemic picture and include a mild meningoencephalitis, which occurs early in the first few days with serum sickness. Ten percent of patients may have papilledema, seizures, circulatory ataxia, transverse myelitis, or cranial nerve palsies. The clues to serum sickness systemically are an increased sedimentation rate, a decreased serum complement, microscopic hematuria/RBC casts, and hypergammaglobulinemia. The CSF typically shows a mild lymphocytic pleocytosis, and protein is usually normal but may be slightly elevated as is the CSF glucose. The cause of the patient's fever and meningeal symptoms may be related to serum sickness if the clinician appreciates the association of the CNS findings and extra-CNS manifestations of serum sickness. Treatment is with corticosteroids (1–4).

Collagen Vascular Diseases

SLE often presents with CNS manifestations ranging from meningitis to cerebritis, and encephalitis. The most frequent CNS manifestation of SLE is aseptic meningitis, which needs to be differentiated from acute bacterial meningitis. CNS manifestations of SLE usually occur in patients who have established multisystem manifestations of SLE. CNS SLE is usually present as part of a flare of SLE. SLE flare may be manifested by fever, an increase in the signs/symptoms of SLE manifested in previous flares. Laboratory tests suggesting flare include new or more severe leukopenia, thrombocytopenia, increased erythrocyte sedimentation rate (ESR), polyclonal gammopathy, and proteinuria/microscopic hematuria. The CSF in patients with SLE includes a lymphocytic predominance (usually $<100\,WBCs/mm^3$). Polymorphonuclear neutrophils (PMNs) may predominate early in SLE and aseptic meningitis. The RBCs are not present in the CSF with SLE and aseptic meningitis, and the CSF lactic acid level is also normal. The definitive test for diagnosing CNS SLE is to demonstrate a decreased C_4 level in the CSF. Unfortunately, patients with a flare of CNS lupus are predisposed to bacterial meningitis/viral encephalitis. CCU clinicians must be careful to be sure that the patient with an SLE flare with CNS manifestations does not have a superimposed acute bacterial meningitis or acute viral encephalitis (1,18,22,23).

Granulomatous angiitis of the CNS is an uncommon cause of aseptic meningitis. The fever and encephalopathy are the most common manifestations of granulomatous angiitis of the CNS, but the focal abnormalities including seizures and cranial nerve palsies may mimic bacterial meningitis. Systemic laboratory tests are unhelpful. The ESR is usually elevated. The CSF profile includes a lymphocytic predominance (usually < 200 cells/mm^3), a low CSF glucose may occur, and RBCs are rarely present. Such findings are also compatible with the diagnosis of HSV meningoencephalitis or aseptic meningitis. The diagnosis of granulomatous angiitis of the CNS is made by head CT/MRI imaging demonstrating vasculitic lesions in the CSF (22,23).

Behçet's disease is a multisystem disorder of unknown etiology characterized by oral aphthous ulcers, genital ulcers, eye findings, and neurological manifestations in up to one quarter of patients. CNS presentation of Behçet's may be the presenting finding in about 5% of patients. Neuro-Behçet's disease is characterized by fever, headache, and meningeal signs closely mimicking a bacterial process. Aseptic meningitis, meningoencephalitis, or encephalitis may also be present. The CSF profile is indistinguishable from aseptic viral meningitis/encephalitis. There are no distinguishing features on the electroencephalogram (EEG) or head CT/MRI imaging. The diagnosis of neuro-Behçet's disease is based on recognizing that the patient has Behçet's disease and has neurologic manifestations not attributable to another or superimposed process (19,23).

Neurosarcoidosis is a common manifestation of sarcoidosis. Signs of CNS sarcoid include headaches, mental confusion, and cranial nerve palsies. Any of the cranial nerves may be affected. Patients with sarcoidosis may often present with polyclonal gammopathy on serum protein electrophoresis, an elevated ESR, leukopenia and mild anemia, and increased levels of serum angiotensin converting enzyme. Chest X-ray shows one of the four stages of sarcoidosis ranging from bilateral hilar adenopathy to parenchymal reticular nodular fibrotic changes. In neurosarcoid, the CSF is usually abnormal. A lymphocytic pleocytosis (≤ 300 cells/mm) is usual. Protein levels in the CSF are usually elevated, and ~20% of patients have a decreased CSF glucose level. RBCs are not a feature of neurosarcoidosis. Aseptic meningitis with sarcoidosis may present as an acute meningitis mimicking/viral aseptic meningitis. Sarcoid meningoencephalitis is more chronic mimicking the chronic causes of meningitis due to acid fast bacilli or fungi. Patients usually have a history of sarcoidosis, which is a clue to the diagnosis. Diagnosis of neurosarcoidosis is a diagnosis of association and exclusion. Neurosarcoidosis occurs in the setting of systemic sarcoidosis and is characterized by a negative CSF gram stain and culture. Treatment is with corticosteroids/immunosuppressives (Table 3) (1,20,21,23).

CLINICAL AND LABORATORY FEATURES OF ACUTE BACTERIAL MENINGITIS

Overview

The clinical diagnosis of acute bacterial meningitis concerns differentiating it from its mimics as well as the viral/aseptic causes of meningitis. Patients with acute bacterial meningitis have a more fulminant course and tend to be more critically ill than those with a meningitis mimic or a virally mediated meningeal process. Many meningeal

Table 3 Mimics of Acute Bacterial Meningitis

Meningeal mimic	Differential features and diagnostic clues

Enteroviral meningitis	Seasonal distribution: summer
	Not as ill as bacterial meningitis, clinically
	Sore throat, facial/maculopapular rash, loose stools/diarrhea common
	CSF:
	  Gram stain: −
	  Lactic acid: normal (<3 mmol/L)

Partially treated bacterial meningitis (usually 2° to *Haemophilus influenzae*)	Previous antibiotic therapy
	Onset: subacute
	CSF:
	  Gram stain: +/−
	  Lactic acid: mildly ↑ (4–6 mmol/L)

HSV-1	Season: nonseasonal
	Presentation: dense/prolonged neurologic defects, encephalopathic/coma
	Historical: antecedent herpes labialis (not concurrent)
	EEG: temporal lobe focus
	Head MRI/CT scan: temporal lobe focus (negative early)
	CSF:
	  Gram stain: −
	  RBCs (negative early; present later)
	  ↑ PMNs (may be >90%)
	Glucose may be ↓/normal
	↑ Lactic acid ~ RBCs in CSF

Meningeal carcinomatosis	History: leukemias, lymphomas, carcinomas, or without known primary neoplasm
	Onset: subacute/afebrile
	Mental status changes: +/−
	Nuchal rigidity: +/−
	80% have cranial nerve involvement, (CNs III, IV, VI, VII, or VIII most common)
	CSF:
	  Gram stain: −
	  RBCs: ±
	  Protein: highly ↑
	  Lactic acid: variably ↑
	Cytology: abnormal in 90%

Amebic meningoencephalitis (*Naegleria fowleri*)	History: recent swimming in fresh water
	Onset: rapid
	Olfactory/gustatory abnormalities: early
	Head MRI/CT: mass lesions
	CSF:
	  RBCs: +
	  Glucose: ↓
	  Lactic acid: variably ↑
	  Gram stain: "motile WBCs" (ameba) on wet prep

(Continued)

Table 3 Mimics of Acute Bacterial Meningitis (*Continued*)

Meningeal mimic	Differential features and diagnostic clues

Brain abscess (with ventricular leak)	Source usually suppurative lung disease (bronchiectasis), cyanotic heart disease (R → L shunts), mastoiditis, dental abscess, etc.
	Head MRI/CT: mass lesions
	CSF: mimics bacterial meningitis (with ventricular leak)
	  Protein: highly ↑
	  Without leak: usually <200 WBCs
	  With leak:≤100,000 WBCs

Leptospirosis	Usually associated with severe leptospirosis (Weil's syndrome)
	Presentation: clinically ill, jaundiced, conjunctival suffusion, ↑SGOT/SGPT
	CSF:
	  Bacterial profile
	  CSF: bilirubin ↑
	  RBCs: +

Tuberculosis/fungal meningitis	Presentation: acute, usually with evidence of primary infection. Lung lesions not always apparent in TB (chest X-ray negative in 50%)
	Basilar meningitis
	Fundi: characteristic choroidal tubercles
	CNS: unilateral CN VI abducens palsy,
	MRI/CT scans: hydrocephalus/arachnoiditis
	CSF:
	  WBCs: <500
	  PMNs (early); lymphs (later)
	  Glucose: ↓ (may be normal)
	  RBCs: ↑
	  TB smear/culture + ~80%
	Serial CSFs:
	Over time ↓ glucose/↑ protein
	  Lactic acid: ↑ (variably elevated)

Neurosarcoidosis	History/signs of systemic sarcoidosis (bilateral hilar adenopathy/interstitial infiltrates, skin lesions, uveitis, erythema nodosum, arthritis, hypercalciuria, ↑ ACE levels)
	Nuchal rigidity: mild
	Cranial nerves: unilateral/bilateral CN VII (facial nerve palsy characteristic also CN palsies II, VII, VIII, IX, X)
	CSF:
	  Lymphs: ↑
	  Glucose: ↓
	  WBCs: <100
	RBCs: none (vs. TB or Ca)

SLE cerebritis	History/signs of SLE (pneumonitis, nephritis, skin lesions, cytoid bodies/cotton wool spots in fundi) seizures/encephalopathy: ±

(Continued)

Table 3 Mimics of Acute Bacterial Meningitis (*Continued*)

Meningeal mimic	Differential features and diagnostic clues

	CSF:
	    CSF ANA: +
	    CSF C$_4$: ↓

LCM	Seasonal distribution: fall
	History: hamster/mouse/rodent contact
	Presentation: biphasic "flu-like" illness
	    followed by recovery, then headache, fever,
	    mental confusion/meningismus, myalgias
	CBC:
	    WBCs: ↓
	    Platelets↓CSF: resembles aseptic meningitis
	        if glucose normal
	    Glucose: normal/↓
	    WBCs: >1000 lymphs

RMSF	Seasonal distribution: spring/fall; woods/
	    animal exposure
	Onset: sudden with severe headache, myalgias,
	    and mild nuchal rigidity
	Conjunctival suffusion, periorbital edema/
	    edema of dorsum of hands/feet, wrists/
	    ankles rash
	CSF:
	    WBCs: <100 lymphs
	    Lactic acid: normal/slightly ↑
	    Glucose: normal/↓
	    Protein: ↑ (variably)

Mycoplasma meningoencephalitis	History: mycoplasma CAP
	Presentation: nonexudative pharyngitis, otitis/
	    bullous myringitis, loose stools/diarrhea,
	    erythema multiforme
	Cold agglutinin titers: >1:512
	CSF:
	    Culture for mycoplasma: ±

Abbreviations: CSF, cerebrospinal fluid; CNS, central nervous system; SLE, systemic lupus erythematosus; PMNs, polymorphonuclear leukocytes; LCM, lymphocytic choriomeningitis; RMSF, Rocky Mountain spotted fever; HSV, Herpes simplex virus; ACE, angiotensin converting enzyme; SGOT, serum glutamate oxaloacetate transaminase; SGPT, serum glutamate pyruvate transaminase; EEG, electroencephalogram; MRI, magnetic resonance imaging; CT, computed tomography.
Source: From Ref. 6.

pathogens have associated systemic manifestations, which, if appreciated and related to the CNS findings, make the diagnosis of the underlying condition relatively straightforward. However, in spite of an analysis of predisposing factors, host defense defects, age of the patient, and history of systemic disorders and cutaneous findings, the diagnosis of meningitis remains based on the analysis of CSF findings. Analysis of the CSF obtained by lumbar puncture is critical in ruling in the diagnosis of acute bacterial meningitis, as well as ruling out viral or noninfectious causes of meningitis (22,24).

Predicting the Pathogen in Acute Bacterial Meningitis

Normal hosts with acute bacterial meningitis may or may not have a variety of historical epidemiologic clues as well as physical findings that may suggest a particular organism. Patients with chronic meningitis are diagnostic not therapeutic problems and are not included in this chapter concerned primarily with the diagnosis and management of patients in the CCU with acute bacterial meningitis. In compromised hosts, the diagnosis of acute bacterial meningitis depends on correlating the underlying disorder with its host defense defect, which predicts the meningeal pathogen. Compromised hosts with impaired cellular-mediated immunity (CMI) usually present with chronic rather than bacterial meningitis. Such patients presenting with acute bacterial meningitis should be viewed as normal hosts from the standpoint of pathogen predictability, i.e., the underlying disorder is not responsible for their meningitis. If a patient who has an organ transplant or HIV, for example, is involved in an outbreak of meningococcal meningitis, the underlying disorder does not predispose the patient to this pathogen. With acute bacterial meningitis, compromised hosts with impaired CMI are afflicted with the same infectious diseases as are normal hosts. Compromised hosts are not exempt from the spectrum of infectious diseases that affect immunocompetent hosts. Compromised hosts with defects in humoral immunity (HI) or those with combined CMI and HI defects, e.g., chronic lymphatic leukemia, are predisposed to meningitis due to encapsulated organisms, *Streptococcus pneumoniae, Haemophilus influenzae*, or *Klebsiella pneumoniae* (Tables 4 and 5) (1–5,24).

Diagnostic Workup in Acute Bacterial Meningitis

The critical laboratory test in acute bacterial meningitis is analysis of the CSF. In acute bacterial meningitis, there is usually a pleocytosis of the CSF. In acute bacterial meningitis, the cells in the CSF are nearly all PMNs. As the meningeal infection is treated, the number of PMNs decreases, and there is a parallel rise in the number of CSF lymphocytes. Bacterial meningitis begins with a PMN predominance and ends with a lymphocytic predominance. Other CNS infections, e.g., tuberculosis, viral infections, fungal infections, syphilis, etc., may all present initially with a pleocytosis with a PMN predominance. These disorders are characterized by a lymphocytic CSF pleocytosis but initially may present with a PMN predominance. Importantly, with the exception of HSV-1, ≥90% PMNs in the CSF initially always indicate an acute bacterial meningitis. A PMN predominance of <90% is compatible with a wide variety of CNS pathogens and does not, of itself, indicate a bacterial etiology. In patients with fever and nuchal rigidity, a lumbar puncture should always be performed before a head CT/MRI scan is obtained. Patients with bacterial meningitis are acutely ill and have a potentially rapidly fatal disorder. To waste valuable time obtaining a head CT/MRI can result in a fatal outcome. Fear of supratentorial herniation is the main reason why head imaging studies are done before lumbar puncture, which is appropriate if a mass lesion is suspected, but not if the diagnosis includes acute bacterial meningitis. Far more people will die from a delay in therapy than have died from supratentorial herniation (Tables 6–9) (1–3,24–26).

The CSF Profile in Acute Bacterial Meningitis

The evaluation of the CSF is the definitive diagnostic test in patients with acute bacterial meningitis. Microscopic examination of the CSF by Gram stain provides rapid information regarding the CSF cellular response as well as the concentration morphology/arrangement of potential neuropathogenic bacteria. The typical "purulent profile" in the CSF of bacteria causing acute meningitis includes an early PMN

Table 4 Host–Pathogen Association in Meningitis

Host	Pathogen
Sinopulmonary function	*Streptococcus pneumoniae*
	Haemophilus influenzae
	Neisseria meningitidis
Elderly	*H. influenzae*
	Listeria monocytogenes
	Brain abscess (2° dental focus)
Sickle cell disease	*S. pneumoniae*
	Salmonella
	N. meningitidis
	H. influenzae
Splenectomy	*S. pneumoniae*
	H. influenzae
	N. meningitidis
	Klebsiella pneumoniae
HIV	HIV
	CMV
	Toxoplasma
	L. monocytogenes
	Nocardia sp.
	Cryptococcus neoformans
	TB/MAI
	Lymphomas
Complement deficiencies	*S. pneumoniae*
	N. meningitidis
CSF leak	*S. pneumoniae*
IVDAs	*Staphylococcus aureus*
	Gram-negative bacilli
Alcoholism/cirrhosis	*S. pneumoniae*
	Klebsiella
	TB
Hypogammaglobulinemia	*S. pneumoniae*
	H. influenzae
	N. meningitidis
	Enteroviruses
VA/VP shunts	*Staphylococcus epidermidis*
	S. aureus
	Gram-negative bacilli
Recurrent meningitis (usually 2° to immune/anatomic defects)	*S. pneumoniae*
	H. influenzae
	N. meningitidis
	Noninfectious CNS diseases SLE
	Neurosarcoidosis
	Neuro-Behçet's
	CNS granulomatosis
	Vasculitis
ABE	*S. pneumoniae*
	S. aureus
Brain abscess	Anaerobes
	Citrobacter (children)
	S. aureus
	Gram-negative enteric bacilli

Abbreviations: IVDAs, IV drug abusers; VA, ventriculo-atrial; VP, ventriculo-peritoneal; ABE, acute bacterial endocarditis; CMV, cytomegalovirus; CNS, central nervous system; SLE, systemic lupus erythematosus; MAI, mycobacterium arium-intracellulare.
Source: From Ref. 6.

Table 5 Complications of Meningitis

Conditions	Associated organisms
Deafness/hearing loss	*Haemophilus influenzae*
	Neisseria meningitidis
	TB
	RMSF
	Mumps
Seizures	*Streptococcus pneumoniae* (early)
	H. influenzae
	Group B streptococci
	Neurosarcoidosis
	HSV-1
	Histoplasmosis
	TB
	Brain abscess
Subdural effusions	*H. influenzae*
	S. pneumoniae
Septic arthritis	*N. meningitidis*
	Staphylococcus aureus
Hemiplegia	*S. pneumoniae*
Cerebral-vein thrombosis	*H. influenzae* (associated Jacksonian seizures)
Hydrocephalus	*H. influenzae*
	TB
	Neurosarcoidosis
	Group B streptococci
Cranial nerve abnormalities	*N. meningitidis* (CN VI, VII, VIII)
	Tuberculosis (CN VI)
	Sarcoidosis (CN VII)
	Meningeal carcinomatosis (multiple CNs)
Herpes labialis	*N. meningitidis*
	S. pneumoniae
Panophthalmitis	*N. meningitidis*
	S. pneumoniae
	H. influenzae
Purpura/petechiae or shock	*N. meningitidis*
	S. pneumoniae
	Listeria monocytogenes
	S. aureus

Abbreviations: RMSF, Rocky Mountain spotted fever; HSV, herpes simplex virus.
Source: From Ref. 6.

predominance, a decreased CSF glucose, a variabilitated CSF protein, no RBCs, and a highly elevated CSF lactic acid level. The positivity of the CSF gram stain depends on the concentration and type of organism present. The CSF gram stain is negative half the time with *L. monocytogenes* meningitis, for example, but the organism is virtually always culturable from the CSF. With acute bacterial meningitis due to the meningococcus, no organisms may be seen on CSF Gram stain, even in the presence of overwhelming infection due to autolysis by the organism. The CSF may appear turbid or cloudy due to the abundance of WBCs present. Organisms may not be visible on the CSF gram stain, but culture is invariably positive for *Neisseria meningitidis*. The typical purulent profile of acute bacterial meningitis may also be

Table 6 Central Nervous System Infections in Normal Versus Compromised Hosts

CNS infection in normal hosts
  Usually *acute* onset of signs and symptoms of meningitis
  Single pathogen
  Predictable pathogen based on epidemiology, patient age, head and neck/CNS anatomic
    abnormalities, and host defense defects
  Meningitis or *encephalitis* most frequent manifestation of CNS infection
CNS infection in compromised hosts
  Subacute/indolent onset of signs and symptoms of CNS infection
  Single or *sequential pathogens*
  Pathogen determined by type of immune defect and degree/duration of immunosuppression
  Encephalitis or mass lesions (brain abscess) most common manifestations of CNS infection

Abbreviation: CNS, central nervous system.

present in patients with early tuberculous or fungal meningitis, but more typically present as subacute/chronic meningitis (1,5).

The various causes of viral/aseptic meningitis are uniformly associated with a normal CSF glucose with a few important exceptions. The presence of a normal CSF glucose in a patient with suspected meningitis argues strongly against a bacterial tuberculous or fungal etiology and suggests a viral or noninfectious mimic of meningitis. The viruses that are capable of decreasing the CSF glucose include HSV, lymphocytic choriomeningitis, mumps, and occasionally enteroviruses. With these exceptions aside, a normal CSF glucose virtually excludes a bacterial etiology of acute bacterial meningitis (1,5).

Table 7 Central Nervous System Pathogens and Disorders Associated with Impaired B-Lymphocyte–Mediated Humoral Deficiency

Disorders associated with impaired B-lymphocyte function/humoral immunity
Multiple myeloma
B-cell lymphoma
  Splenic infarcts
  Advanced age
  Infiltrative diseases of the spleen
  Splenectomy
Waldeström's macroglobulinemia
Hereditary immunoglobulin deficiencies
CLL
IgA deficiency
Hyposplenia/decreased splenic function
  Sickle cell anemia
  Alcoholic liver disease
  Inflammatory bowel disease
  Rheumatoid arthritis

CNS pathogens associated with impaired B-lymphocyte function/humoral immunity

Common	Uncommon	Rare
Streptococcus pneumoniae	*Neisseria meningitidis*	*Pseudomonas aeruginosa*
Hemophilus influenzae	*Klebsiella pneumoniae*	Echovirus
		Poliovirus

Abbreviations: CNS, central nervous system; IgA, immunoglobulin A; CLL, chronic lymphatic leukemia.
Source: From Ref. 30.

Table 8 Central Nervous System Pathogens and Disorders Associated with Impaired
T-Lymphocyte/Macrophage-Mediated Cellular Immunity

Disorders associated with impaired T-lymphocyte/macrophage-mediated cellular Immunity
HIV/AIDS
Lymphoreticular malignancies
  Hodgkin's lymphoma
Chronic immunosuppressive
  therapy
    Organ transplantation (bone
      marrow, renal, cardiac,
      pancreatic, hepatic, etc.)
Chronic corticosteroid therapy
  Collagen vascular diseases
  Systemic vasculitis
  Chronic renal failure
  Rheumatoid ailments
CMV

CNS pathogens associated with impaired T-lymphocyte/macrophage-mediated cellular immunity

Common	Uncommon	Rare
Listeria	*Mycobacterium tuberculosis*	PML
Nocardia	Brucellosis	*Strongyloides stercoralis*
Cryptococcus neoformans	*Aspergillus*	*Toxicara canis*
CMV	*Mucor*	*Pneumocystis (carinii)jiroveci*
HSV		*Pseudallescheria boydii*
VZV		

Abbreviations: CNS, central nervous system; CMV, cytomegalovirus; VZV, varicella zoster virus; HSV, Herpes simplex virus; PML, progressive multifocal leukoencephalopahy.
Source: From Ref. 30.

RBCs are not a feature of acute bacterial meningitis, and should suggest an alternate explanation for the patient's symptoms. Excluding a traumatic tap, CNS leaking aneurism, etc., RBCs in the CSF limit diagnostic possibilities to *L. monocytogenes*, amebic meningoencephalitis, leptospirosis, tuberculous meningitis, HSV, and anthrax. RBCs in the CSF can also decrease the CSF glucose and increase the CSF lactic acid. The abnormalities in CSF glucose and lactic acid are proportional to the number of RBCs present in the CSF, and can account for mild to moderate abnormalities in these two CSF parameters (1,5).

The white blood cell response in the CSF typically is early and brisk with bacterial meningitis. Many CNS infections characteristically associated with a lymphocytic predominance often present acutely with a PMN predominance, i.e., TB, fungi, syphilis, viruses, etc. With the exception of HSV-1, only acute bacterial meningitis presents with a CSF PMN count ≥90%. Patients with partially treated meningitis have a mixed picture with both PMNs and lymphocytes as well as a moderately decreased glucose versus the profoundly decreased glucose and untreated acute bacterial meningitis, and will have CSF lactic acid levels that are intermediate between aseptic/viral meningitis and acute bacterial meningitis. The clinician uses not only the CSF gram stain but analyzes the patient's clinical information integrating the CSF findings of the number of white cells in relationship to the PMN predominance glucose levels, CSF lactic acid levels, and the presence or absence of RBCs in the absence of trauma to correctly analyze CSF findings (Tables 10 and 11) (1,5,27,28).

Table 9 Diagnostic Approach in Compromised Hosts with Symptoms/Signs of Central Nervous System Infection

Syndrome presentation	Diagnostic procedures	Comments
Meningeal signs	LP with CSF: 　WBC cell count/ 　　differential 　RBC count 　Glucose/protein 　Lactic acid 　Cytology 　Bacterial signs/culture 　AFB fungal smears/culture	Determine host defense defect 　to predict most likely CNS 　pathogens Rule out mimics of meningitis Empiric therapy is based on 　CSF findings
Encephalitis/ 　encephalopathy or 　mass lesion	Head CT/MRI: 　To rule out cerebritis 　To rule out mass lesions 　To rule out hydrocephalus 　To rule out CNS hemorrhage Lumbar puncture if papilledema 　not present: 　WBC cell count/differential 　Glucose/protein/RBCs 　Lactic acid 　Cytology 　Bacterial strains/culture 　AFB fungal smears/culture	Determine host defense defect 　to predict most likely CNS 　pathogens Rule out noninfectious causes 　by history/physical exam, 　and CT/MRI appearance Specific therapy based on tissue 　diagnosis, or empiric therapy 　for the most likely diagnostic 　possibility

Abbreviations: CNS, central nervous system; CSF, cerebrospinal fluid; MRI, magnetic resonance imaging, CT, computed tomography; AFB, acid-fast bacilli; LP, lumbar puncture.

The Critical Importance of the CSF Lactic Acid in the Diagnosis of Meningitis

In the diagnosis of acute bacterial meningitis, the CSF lactic acid levels are second only to the CSF gram stain as a rapid and reliable indicator of acute bacterial meningitis. It has been said that the CSF lactic acid levels offer no information that cannot be inferred from CSF glucose levels. This is not the case. The CSF glucose levels and CSF lactic acid levels are inversely proportioned to each other. As the CSF glucose decreases, the CSF lactic acid increases. With successful treatment, the CSF lactic acid levels and CSF glucose levels are the first to normalize. It takes days for the initial PMN predominance in the CSF to become lymphocytic, and a lymphocytic pleocytosis may persist in the CSF for weeks after clinical resolution of the patient's bacterial meningitis. The CSF lactic acid level decreases more rapidly and acutely than does the CSF glucose. For example, if a patient has *S. aureus* and acute bacterial endocarditis, and has seeded the CSF resulting in an early purulent meningitis, the CSF lactic acid level will be elevated before the Gram stain is positive or the CSF glucose levels have dropped. The CSF lactic acid test is invaluable in separating viral from bacterial meningitis as well as for identifying patients with partially treated meningitis (1,29–33).

　　CSF lactic acid levels are also useful in assessing the significance of RBCs in the CSF in patients with a decreased CSF glucose. If the diagnosis is between HSV-1 and *L. monocytogenes* meningitis, in *L. monocytogenes* meningoencephalitis, CSF lactic

Table 10 Cerebrospinal Fluid Gram Stain Clues in Acute Bacterial Meningitis

Purulent CSF/no organisms seen	Clear CSF/no organisms seen
Neisseria meningitidis	Viral meningitis
Streptococcus pneumoniae	Tuberculous/fungal meningitis
	Neurosarcoidosis meningitis
	Early bacterial meningitis
	Partially treated bacterial meningitis
Cloudy CSF/without WBCs	Meningitis in leukopenic host
S. pneumoniae	Meningeal carcinomatosis
Gram-positive bacilli	Brain abscess
Listeria monocytogenes	Parameningeal infection
Pseudomeningitis (*Bacillus,*	Bland emboli (2° to SBE)
Corynebacterium)	Cerebritis
	Neuroborreliosis
Gram-negative bacilli	LCM
Haemophilus influenzae (small	Viral meningitis
encapsulated, pleomorphic) enteric	*Listeria monocytogenes*
aerobic gram-negative bacilli	HIV
(larger, unencapsulated)	Syphilis
	Leptospirosis
Gram-positive cocci	Gram-negative cocci
Group A, B streptococci (pairs and chains)	*N. meningitidis*
S. pneumoniae (pairs)	Mixed organisms/polymicrobial
Staphylococcus aureus (clusters)	Pseudomeningitis
Staphylococcus epidermidis VA/VP shunt	Brain abscess with meningeal leak
infections only (clusters)	VP shunt infection
	Disseminated *Strongyloides stercoralis*
	Meningitis (2° to penetrating
	head trauma)

Abbreviations: CSF, cerebrospinal fluid; VA, ventriculo-atrial; VP, ventriculo-peritoneal; LCM, lymphocytic choriomeningitis; SBE, subacute endocarditis.

acid levels will be highly elevated, i.e., ≥ 6 mmol/dL, whereas the CSF lactic acid levels will be normal/near normal in HSV-1. A normal CSF lactic acid level in the absence of RBCs from a trauma or traumatic tap is the best way to differentiate aseptic from septic meningitis. If the Gram stain is negative and CSF lactic acid levels are normal, then the clinician can confidently wait for CSF cultures to be reported as negative during the next one to three days. No empiric antimicrobial therapy is needed if the CSF lactic acid level is normal and the CSF Gram stain is normal. CSF lactic acid levels may be obtained serially to determine if antimicrobial therapy of the meningitis is effective, and also may be used at the end of therapy as a test of cure (Fig. 1) (1,31,32).

Other CSF Tests

Another test that has been used to differentiate aseptic/viral meningitis from bacterial meningitis is the C-reactive protein (CRP). CSF CRP is elevated in bacterial meningitis but is not elevated in viral/aseptic meningitis, and is a useful adjunctive diagnostic test.

Other CSF parameters have been used, i.e., lactate dehydrogenase (LDH) to differentiate the various types of meningeal pathogens, but lack sensitivity and specificity. The CSF antigen tests, i.e., counter immunoelectrophoresis (CIE) techniques of the

Table 11 Differential Diagnosis of Cerebrospinal Fluid with a Negative Gram Stain

Predominantly PMNs/decreased glucose	RBCs
Partially treated bacterial meningitis	Traumatic tap
Listeria monocytogenes	Posterior fossa syndrome
HSV-1	HSV-1
Tuberculosis (early)	CNS bleed/tumor
Syphilis (early)	*Listeria monocytogenes*
Neurosarcoidosis	Leptospirosis
Parameningeal infection	TB meningitis
Septic emboli (2° to ABE)	Amebic *Naegleria fowleri* meningoencephalitis
Amebic meningoencephalitis	Predominantly lymphs/normal glucose
Naegleria fowleri	Partially treated bacterial meningitis
Syphilis (early)	Neurosarcoidosis
Posterior fossa syndrome	Neuroborreliosis
CSF lactic acid	HIV
<3 mmol/L	Leptospirosis
Aseptic "viral" meningitis	RMSF
Parameningeal infections	Viral meningitis
<3 mmol/L	Bland emboli (2° to SBE)
Partially treated meningitis	Parameningeal infection
RBCs	TB/fungal meningitis
TB/fungal meningitis	Neuropsittacosis
>6 mmol/L	Meningeal carcinomatosis
Bacterial meningitis	Predominantly lymphs/decreased glucose
CSF protein	Partially treated bacterial meningitis
Elevated (any CNS infection/ inflammation)	LCM
	Enteroviral meningitis
Very highly elevated	*Listeria monocytogenes*
Brain tumor	Mumps
Brain abscess	Leptospirosis
TB with subarachnoid block	TB/fungal meningitis
Multiple sclerosis	Neurosarcoidosis
	Meningeal carcinomatosis
	CSF eosinophilia
	CNS vasculitis
	NSAIDS
	Coccidioidomycosis
	Neuropsittacosis
	CNS lymphomas
	VA/VP shunts
	Interventional contrast materials

Abbreviations: CSF, cerebrospinal fluid; HSV, herpes simplex virus; CNS, central nervous system; ABE, acute bacterial endocarditis; LCM, lymphocytic choriomeningitis; SBE, subacute endocarditis; PMNs, polymorphonuclear leukocytes; RMSF, Rocky Mountain spotted fever; VA, ventriculo-atrial; VP, ventriculo-peritoneal; NSAIDs, nonsteroidal inflammatory drugs.

CSF, are generally unhelpful. The problems with the CSF CIE assays are a lack of sensitivity and specificity. When a CNS pathogen is demonstrated by Gram stain and culture, and there is no question about the diagnosis, the CIE is not infrequently negative. There are other tests that are useful in selected CNS disorders. The CSF C_4 level is decreased, and diagnostic of SLE meningitis/cerebritis although clonal bands in the CSF may be present in SLE as well as multiple sclerosis. Cytology of the CSF

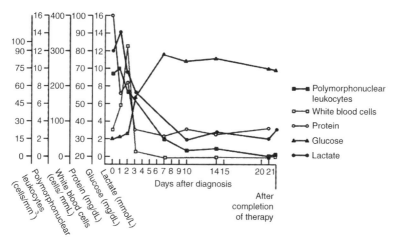

Figure 1 Temporal relationships of cerebrospinal fluid lactic acid levels in bacterial meningitis. *Source*: From Refs. 6, 31, 32.

may indicate meningeal carcinomatosis, which may mimic acute bacterial meningitis (28–30).

Other tests are useful in the CSF for selected pathogens. PCR technique is useful to make the diagnosis of enteroviral aseptic meningitis or HSV aseptic meningitis. PCR is also useful to diagnose acute tuberculous meningitis (1,5,28–30).

Radiologic Tests

Neuroimaging tests are primarily valuable for ruling out the mimics of acute bacterial meningitis. In acute bacterial meningitis, head CT/MRI scans are of limited value and are done primarily to rule out parameningeal suppurative focus or brain abscess, or systemic mimics of meningitis. As mentioned previously, lumbar puncture takes precedence over neuroimaging if the diagnosis of acute bacterial meningitis is being considered. The EEG is primarily useful in diagnosing encephalitis and is nondiagnostic in acute bacterial meningitis. The main use for EEG is in the early diagnosis of herpes meningoencephalitis because of the propensity of HSV-1 to localize in the frontal temporal lobe. EEG abnormalities are diffuse with most causes of acute viral encephalitis, but are localized very early with HSV-1 meningoencephalitis, which is an important diagnostic clue to its presence (1–5).

EMPIRIC THERAPY OF ACUTE BACTERIAL MENINGITIS

Overview

Empiric therapy of acute bacterial meningitis depends upon demonstrating or predicting the CNS pathogens so that an appropriate antibiotic may be selected. If the pathogen can be demonstrated by gram stain or inferred from aspects of the history, epidemiological data, systemic laboratory tests, or physical findings, then an antibiotic with an appropriate spectrum can be selected to begin treatment. Early treatment with an appropriate antibiotic is crucial to the outcome in patients with acute bacterial meningitis.

Not only must the antimicrobial being selected to treat acute bacterial meningitis be effective against the pathogen, but it must reach bactericidal concentrations in the CSF with the usual "meningeal doses." Certain antibiotics achieve a therapeutic CNS concentration when being in the usual dose, e.g., chloramphenicol, TMP-SMX, doxycycline, minocycline, antituberculous drugs, etc., whereas others require higher than usual doses, i.e., "meningeal doses" to penetrate the CSF, e.g., cefepime, meropenem. Most other antimicrobials do not achieve sufficient CSF concentration with usual or even with high dosing, i.e., first/second-generation cephalosporins, vancomycin, amphotericin, etc (1–3).

After selecting a drug with the appropriate spectrum for the presumed neuropathogen and delivering the drug intravenously in a dose that will rapidly achieve bactericidal concentrations in the CSF, patients are ordinarily treated for a total of two weeks. The main determinants of antibiotic penetration of the CSF are antibiotic size and the lipid solubility characteristics of the antibiotic. In general, highly lipid soluble antibiotics penetrate the CSF in the presence or absence of inflammation. β-lactam antibiotics do not penetrate the CSF well in the absence of inflammation. Third- and fourth-generation cephalosporins given in "meningeal doses" do not penetrate the CNS well, but penetrate sufficiently well and have a sufficiently high degree of activity that they are effective against nearly all common neuropathogens except *Listeria* (34–38).

Listeria meningitis is ordinarily treated with "meningeal doses" of ampicillin, i.e., 2 g (IV) q4h, in penicillin tolerant patients. In patients with *Listeria* meningitis intolerant of penicillin, chloramphenicol or TMP-SMX may be used. For the treatment of staphylococcal meningitis due to methicillin-sensitive strains, "meningeal doses" of an antistaphylococcal penicillin, e.g., nafcillin, may be given as a 2 g (IV) q4h dose. Drugs used to treat methicillin-resistant strains of *S. aureus* causing acute bacterial meningitis include minocycline and linezolid. Vancomycin does not penetrate the CSF well. Vancomycin CSF concentrations are approximately 15% of simultaneous serum concentrations. Therefore at the usually used dose of 1 g (IV) q12h (15 mg/kg/day), CSF concentrations may be inadequate. If vancomycin is selected to treat CNS methicillin-resistant *S. aureus* (MRSA) infections, then either 3 to 60 mg/day of vancomycin is necessary, or the usual dose of vancomycin [15 mg/kg/day (IV)] may be supplemented with 20 mg of intrathecally administered vancomycin daily. Linezolid and minocycline penetrate the CNS well and achieve therapeutic concentrations. Because bactericidal antibiotics are preferred in CNS infections, linezolid is preferred over minocycline for MRSA CNS infections (1,35–37).

The treatment of shunt-related infections usually requires shunt removal and the administration of an antibiotic that has a high degree of activity against *Staphylococcus epidermidis* or *S. aureus* (depending upon the pathogen isolated that penetrates the CSF in therapeutic concentrations). In patients with meningitis secondary to open CNS trauma, the antibiotics selected should have a high degree of aerobic gram-negative bacillary coverage as well as sufficient antistaphylococcal activity (1–5,35,39).

The preferred drugs for each pathogen causing meningitis are presented in tabular form here (Table 12).

The use of steroids as an adjunctive measure to treat acute bacterial meningitis remains controversial. Steroids have long been used together with antituberculous therapy in acute tuberculous meningitis, but there is relatively little information on the use of steroids in the treatment of acute bacterial meningitis in adults. Steroids have been shown to be beneficial in the treatment of meningitis in children due to *H. influenzae* but have been limited to *H. influenzae*. Because steroids affect blood/brain barrier permeability, if used they should be given after antimicrobial therapy has been initiated (36,40,41).

Table 12 Empiric Therapy of Central Nervous System Infections Acute Bacterial Meningitis

Subset	Usual pathogens	Preferred IV therapy	Alternate IV therapy	IV-to-PO switch
Normal host	*Neisseria meningitidis, Haemophilus influenzae, Streptococcus pneumoniae*	Ceftriaxone 2 g (IV) q12h × 2 wk	Meropenem 2 g (IV) q8h × 2 wk or cefotaxime 3 g (IV) q6h × 2 wk or ceftizoxime 3 g (IV) q6h × 2 wk	Chloramphenicol 500 mg (PO) q6h × 2 wk
Elderly or malignancy	*Listeria monocytogenes* (plus usual meningeal pathogens in normal hosts)	Before culture results: ceftriaxone 2 g (IV) q12h × 2 wk plus ampicillin 2 g (IV) q4h × 2 wk After culture results *Listeria present:* ampicillin 2 g (IV) q4h × 2 wk *Listeria* not present: treat as normal host	After culture results *Listeria* present: ampicillin 2 g (IV) q4h × 2 wk or chloramphenicol 500 mg (IV) q6h × 2 wk *Listeria* not present: treat as normal host	For Listeria meningitis only: TMP-SMX 5 mg/kg (PO) q6h × 2 wk or chloramphenicol 500 mg (PO) q6h × 2 wk For usual meningeal pathogens: chloramphenicol 500 mg (PO) q6h × 2 wk

Condition	Usual pathogens	Therapy	Therapy	Therapy
CNS shunt infections (VA shunts)[a] (treat initially for MSSA; if later, identified as MRSA, MSSE, or MRSE, treat accordingly)	*Staphylococcus aureus, Staphylococcus epidermidis* (coagulase negative staphylococci)	MSSA/MSSE: cefotaxime or ceftizoxime 3 g (IV) q6h[a] or linezolid 600 mg (IV) q12h[a] MRSA/MRSE: linezolid 600 mg (IV) q12h[a]	MSSA/MSSE: meropenem 2 g (IV) q8h × 2 wk[a] or cefepime 2 g (IV) q8h[a] MRSA/MRSE: vancomycin 1 g (IV) q12h[a] plus 20 mg (IT) q24h until shunt removal	MSSA/MRSE: linezolid 600 mg (PO) q12h[a] MSSA/MRSA: minocycline 100 mg (PO) q12h[a] or linezolid 600 mg (PO) q12h[a] TMP-SMX 5 mg/kg (PO) q6h × 2 wk after shunt removal
CNS shunt infections (VP shunts)[b]	*E. coli, K. pneumoniae, Enterobacter*	Ceftriaxone 2 g (IV) q12h × 2 wk after shunt removal or ceftizoxime or cefotaxime 3 g (IV) q6h × 2 wk after shunt removal	Meropenem 2 g (IV) q8h × 2 wk after shunt removal. TMP-SMX 5 mg/kg (IV) q6h × 2 wk after shunt removal	

Note: Duration of therapy represents total time IV or IV + PO. Most patients on IV therapy able to take PO therapy should be switched to PO therapy after clinical improvement.

[a]Remove central nervous system shunt as soon as possible.

[b]Treat for 1 wk after shunt removal.

Abbreviations: MSSA/MRSA, methicillin-sensitive/resistant *Staphylococcus aureus*; MSSE/MRSE, methicillin-sensitive/resistant *Staphylococcus epidermidis*; CNS, central nervous system; VA, ventriculo-atrial; VP, ventriculo-peritoneal; TMP-SMX, trimethroprim-sulfamethoxazole.

Source: From Ref. 35.

Repeat Lumbar Puncture

The diagnosis of acute bacterial meningitis rests on analysis of the CSF and demonstration of the putative organism in the CSF by gram stain or culture. Corroborative evidence includes a PMN predominance in the CSF, a decreased CSF glucose, and a highly increased CSF lactic acid level. A repeat lumbar puncture is indicated if the patient has not responded to therapy within 72 hours. If the antibiotic is ineffective, the CFS profile will remain relatively unchanged and most importantly, the CSF lactic acid levels will have not decreased. CSF lactic acid levels decrease rapidly with appropriate antimicrobial therapy, and CSF glucose levels also quickly return to normal. If the patient is clinically not responding to antimicrobial therapy and the repeat lumbar puncture shows the same or only slightly increased CSF glucose levels with the same or only slightly decreased lactic acid levels, then the clinician should reassess the antimicrobial regimen (1,5,31).

Reevaluation of the antibiotic should include a reassessment of its spectrum, degree of activity, dosage, and CNS penetration, to determine if a change in therapy is warranted. The only CNS infection that may present with acute bacterial meningitis that would change quickly as the result of appropriate therapy would be a brain abscess that has ruptured into the ventricular system. Such a large number of organisms released from the brain abscess into the CSF would be overwhelming to the host and in spite of appropriate antimicrobial therapy would not change the CSF parameters within three days without drainage of the brain abscess. There is no need to repeat the lumbar puncture if the patient is responding to therapy, suggesting that the proper antibiotic has been chosen and given in the correct dose, and that it is effectively cidal at CNS concentrations resulting in a rapid clinical response as well as a rapid response to the key CSF parameters of the lactic acid/CSF glucose (1–5).

REFERENCES

1. Schlossberg D. Infections of the Nervous System. New York: Springer-Verlag, 1990.
2. Scheld WM, Whitley RJ, Durack DT. Infections of the Central Nervous System. New York: Raven Press, 1991.
3. Tunkel AR. Bacterial Meningitis. Philadelphia: Lippincott Williams & Wilkins, 2001.
4. Roos KL. Central Nervous System Infectious Diseases and Therapy. New York: Marcel Dekker, Inc., 1997.
5. Wood M, Anderson M. Neurologic Infection. London: W.B. Saunders, 1988.
6. Cunha BA. Meningitis. In: Schlossberg D, ed. Central Nervous System Infections. Springer-Verlag, Berlin, 1990:3–24.
7. Thomas K, Hasbun R, Jekel J, Quagliarello VJ. The diagnostic accuracy of Kernig's and Brudzinski's signs in a prospective cohort of adults with suspected meningitis. Clin Infect Dis 2002; 35:46–52.
8. Attia J, Hatala R, Cook DJ, Wong JG. Does this adult patient have acute meningitis? JAMA 1999; 282:175–181.
9. Swartz MN. Bacterial meningitis—a view of the past 90 years. N Engl J Med 2004; 351: 1826–1828.
10. Roos KL. Pearls and pitfalls in the diagnosis and management of the central nervous system in infectious diseases. Semin Neurol 1998; 18:185–196.
11. Spanos A, Harrell FE Jr., Durack DT. Differential diagnosis of acute meningitis. An analysis of the predictive value of initial observation. JAMA 1989; 262:2700–2707.
12. Short WR, Tunkel AR. Changing epidemiology of bacterial meningitis in the United States. Curr Infect Dis Rep 2000; 2:327–331.

13. Schuchat A, Robinson K, Wenger JD, et al. Bacterial meningitis in the United States in 1995. N Engl J Med 1997; 337:970–976.

14. Eisenstein L, Calio F, Cunha BA. Herpes simplex virus type 1 (HSV-1) aseptic meningitis. Heart Lung 2004; 33:196–197.

15. Hasbun R. The acute aseptic meningitis syndrome. Curr Infect Dis Rep 2000; 2:345–351.

16. Moris G, Garcia-Monco JC. The challenge of drug-induced aseptic meningitis. Arch Intern Med 1999; 159:1185–1194.

17. Chaudry HJ, Cunha BA. Drug-induced aseptic meningitis. Postgrad Med 1991; 90:65–70.

18. Sanna G, Bertolaccini ML, Mathieu A. Central nervous system lupus: a clinical approach to therapy. Lupus 2003; 12:935–942.

19. Hadfield MG, Aydin F, Lippman HR, et al. Neuro-Behçet's disease. Clin Neuropathol 1997; 16:55–60.

20. James DG, Williams WJ. Sarcoidosis and Other Granulomatous Disorders. Philadelphia: WB Saunders, 1985.

21. Sharma OP. Sarcoidosis. In: Clinical Management. London: Butterworths, 1984.

22. Warnatz K, Peter HH, Schumacher M, et al. Infectious CNS disease as a differential diagnosis in systemic rheumatic diseases: three case reports and a review of the literature. Ann Rheum Dis 2003; 62:50–57.

23. Carsons SE, Belilos E. Mimics of central nervous system infections. In: Cunha BA, ed. Infectious Diseases in Critical Care Medicine. New York: Marcel Dekker, 1998:181–189.

24. Quagliarello VJ, Scheld WM. New perspectives on bacterial meningitis. Clin Infect Dis 1993; 17:603–610.

25. Durand ML, Calderwood SB, Weber DJ, et al. Acute bacterial meningitis in adults. A review of 493 episodes. N Engl J Med 1993; 328:21–28.

26. Hasbun R, Abrahams J, Jekel, Quagliarello VJ. Computed tomography of the head before lumbar puncture in adults with suspected meningitis. N Engl J Med 2001; 345:1727–1733.

27. Pruitt AA. Nervous system infections in patients with cancer. Neurol Clin 2003; 21:193–219.

28. Dropcho EJ. Remote neurologic manifestations of cancer. Neurol Clin 2002; 20:85–122.

29. Fishman RA. Cerebrospinal Fluid in Diseases of the Nervous System. 2nd ed. Philadelphia: WB Saunders, 1992.

30. Cunha BA. Central nervous system infections in the compromised host: a diagnostic approach. Infect Dis Clin North Am 2001; 15:567–590.

31. Bailey EM, Domenico P, Cunha BA. Bacterial versus viral meningitis. The importance of CSF lactic acid. Postgrad Med 1990; 88:217–223.

32. Cunha BA. The usefulness of CSF lactic acid levels in central nervous system infections with decreased cerebrospinal fluid glucose. Clin Infect Dis 2004; 39:1260–1261.

33. Latcha S, Cunha BA. *Listeria monocytogenes* meningoencephalitis—the diagnostic importance of the CSF lactic acid. Heart Lung 1994; 23:177–179.

34. Quagliarello VJ, Scheld WM. Treatment of bacterial meningitis. N Engl J Med 1997; 336: 708–716.

35. Cunha BA. Antibiotic Essentials. (5th Ed) Royal Oak, MI: Physicians' Press, 2006.

36. Aronin SI. Bacterial meningitis: principles and practical aspects of therapy. Curr Infect Dis Rep 2000; 2:337–344.

37. Aronin SI. Current pharmacotherapy of pneumococcal meningitis. Expert Opin Pharmacother 2002; 3:121–129.

38. Aronin SI, Peduzzi P, Quagliarello VJ. Community-acquired bacterial meningitis: risk stratification for adverse clinical outcome and effect of antibiotic timing. Ann Intern Med 1998; 129:862–869.

39. Gardner P, Leipzig T, Phillips P. Infections of central nervous system shunts. Med Clin North Am 1985; 69:297–314.

40. Girgis NI, Farid Z, Mikhail IA, et al. Dexamethasone treatment for bacterial meningitis in children and adults. Pediatr Infect Dis J 1989; 8:848–851.

41. McIntyre PB, Berkey CS, King SM, et al. Dexamethasone as adjunctive therapy in bacterial meningitis. A meta-analysis of randomized clinical trials since 1988. JAMA 1997; 278: 925–931.

6

Encephalitis and Its Mimics in the Critical Care Unit

Burke A. Cunha

*Infectious Disease Division, Winthrop-University Hospital, Mineola, and
State University of New York School of Medicine, Stony Brook, New York, U.S.A.*

INTRODUCTION

Encephalitis is usually due to a viral infection of the brain and is most often of viral etiology. Encephalitis presents as encephalopathy, i.e., with mental confusion. Meningitis is characterized by meningeal irritation and nuchal rigidity without mental confusion and is usually due to bacteria. Viral encephalitis is characterized by mental confusion, but nuchal rigidity is not a feature of the infection. Some organisms, i.e., *Mycoplasma pneumoniae*, *Listeria monocytogenes*, may present as meningoencephalitis or encephalitis. Patients with meningoencephalitis present with both mental confusion and nuchal rigidity. Patients are usually admitted to the critical care unit (CCU) with the diagnosis of encephalitis and some become encephalopathic while in the CCU. The main diagnostic problem in the CCU is to differentiate noninfectious from infectious causes as well as to identify the treatable causes of acute encephalopathy (1–4).

The commonest cause of encephalopathy in the CCU setting is drug induced. In patients being admitted from the community with mental confusion, the diagnostic challenge in the CCU is to differentiate infectious and noninfectious diseases with an encephalopathic component from the patient with encephalitis. Excluding drug-induced encephalopathy, most of the systemic disorders that have an encephalopathic component may be suspected on the basis of extra central nervous system (CNS) symptoms, signs, or findings that point to the underlying cause of the patients encephalopathy. After arriving at any presumptive diagnosis of encephalitis, the clinician then should begin appropriate empiric therapy for treatable disorders. After eliminating nonviral causes of encephalitis, the clinician must decide whether the patient has herpes simplex encephalitis, the only treatable cause of encephalitis versus encephalitis due to another virus. Supportive care is the key in encephalitis patients in the CCU. Supportive measures should be continued to provide them time to recover, if they can, from their viral encephalitis. Unlike acute bacterial meningitis where the main problem in the CCU is to determine appropriate empiric antimicrobial therapy based on clinical findings, cerebrospinal fluid (CSF) profile, and the gram stain of the CSF, in encephalitis, the main problem is diagnosis because only few causes of viral encephalitis are treatable, i.e., herpes-simplex virus-1 (HSV-1), varicella zoster virus (VZV), and cytomegalovirus (CMV) (1–4).

MIMICS OF ENCEPHALITIS IN THE CCU

Nonviral Infectious Mimics of Acute Viral Encephalitis

Viral encephalitis is caused by neurotropic viruses. These neurotropic viruses affect the cortical function of the brain, which is manifested as mental confusion clinically and as focal/diffuse electrical abnormalities in the electroencephalogram (EEG). Most bacteria that cause meningitis do not cause encephalitis, but a few species cause a combination of meningitis and encephalitis, i.e., meningoencephalitis. The only organisms that cause this commonly are *M. pneumoniae*, *L. monocytogenes*, and *Legionella* species (Table 1) (1,2).

L. monocytogenes Meningoencephalitis/Encephalitis

L. monocytogenes may cause a variety of infections but the primary CNS manifestation is that of meningitis or meningoencephalitis. Usually there are no systemic clues to the presence of *Listeria* CNS infection. However, *L. monocytogenes* meningitis or meningoencephalitis occurs in compromised hosts with impaired T-lymphocyte function and in elderly patients. *L. monocytogenes* is also the most common cause of meningitis in patients with malignancies. The only clue to the presence of *L. monocytogenes* is the cause of meningoencephalitis is in the CSF profile. In the CSF, patients with viral encephalitis usually have a variably elevated pleocytosis predominantly lymphocytic in nature. RBCs in the CSF may be of some help in differentiating *Listeria* from other causes of encephalitis (5,6).

Any acute bacterial or viral process effecting the CSF may present initially with a predominantly polymorphonuclear (PMN) pleocytosis. Most patients present with a lymphocytic predominance, but HSV-1 occasionally may present with over 90% PMNs in the CSF differential. Other viral etiologies may present with a PMN predominance but never exceeding 90% PMNs in the CSF, which is characteristic

Table 1 Mimics of Acute Encephalitis

Nonviral infectious causes	Noninfectious causes
Listeria monocytogenes	Toxic/metabolic encephalopathy
Mycoplasma pneumoniae	Hepatic encephalopathy
Legionella species	Collage vascular diseases
Neuroborreliosis	SLE cerebritis
Rocky Mountain spotted fever	CNS granulomatous angitis
Subacute bacterial endocarditis	CVA/intracranial hemorrhage
	Primary CNS lymphomas
	CNS metastases
	Bronchogenic carcinoma, squamous cell carcinoma, small cell carcinoma, breast carcinoma, lymphoma
	Acute psychosis

Abbreviations: SLE, systemic lupus erythematosus; CNS, central nervous system; CVA, cerebral vascular accident.
Source: From Refs. 1–4.

of acute bacterial meningeal pathogens. The CSF profile for *L. monocytogenes* typically is that of mononuclear predominance. The CSF glucose typically is normal. The CSF glucose may be decreased in mumps, lymphocytic choriomeningitis, and in some cases of enteroviral meningitis, but these organisms do not present as encephalitis. The only viral etiology of encephalitis that may present with a decreased CSF glucose is HSV-1 encephalitis (5,7).

In viral encephalitis, the protein is variably elevated and protein levels in the CSF of *L. monocytogenes* are variable as well and, therefore, this parameter is unhelpful diagnostically. Red blood cells (RBC) are present in the CSF excluding traumatic tap and other causes of CSF hemorrhage or leaking Berry/mycotic aneurysms. Therefore, RBC in the CSF excluding the exceptions mentioned points to HSV-1 or *L. monocytogenes* as the cause of the patient's encephalopathy. The CSF lactic acid is useful in the exclusionary sense in viral encephalitis, because CSF lactic acid levels are normal with viral infections of the CNS. The sole exception again is HSV-1 encephalitis, which may be associated with increased lactic acid levels. The increased CSF lactic acid HSV-1 encephalitis may either be due to/proportional to the RBCs present in the CSF. Excluding a large number of RBCs in the CSF, the CSF lactic acid levels in HSV-1 encephalitis should be normal/near normal. In contrast, *L. monocytogenes* meningoencephalitis CSF lactic acid levels should be low as in bacterial meningitis and lower out of proportion to the few RBCs that may be present with *L. monocytogenes* (8,9). The diagnosis of *L. monocytogenes* meningoencephalitis is made presumptively by demonstrating gram-positive bacilli in the gram stain of the CSF, which is positive in about half of cases. *L. monocytogenes*, however, is culturable from the CSF in virtually all cases, which confirms the diagnosis. *L. monocytogenes* meningoencephalitis may mimic viral encephalitis, i.e., West Nile encephalitis (WNE) (8–11).

Mycoplasma pneumoniae Meningoencephalitis/Encephalitis

M. pneumoniae is predominantly an infection of the respiratory tract without CNS manifestations, i.e., meningoencephalitis. *M. pneumoniae* meningoencephalitis is uncommon but is a distinct clinical entity. Patients with *M. pneumoniae* meningoencephalitis are those that have other extrapulmonary manifestations of *M. pneumoniae* infection. Aside from CSF involvement in a patient with *M. pneumoniae* infection, the feature that is most closely associated with *M. pneumoniae* meningoencephalitis is a highly elevated cold agglutinin titer. Approximately, three quarters of *M. pneumoniae* community–acquired pneumonias (CAPs) are with initial/transient increase in cold agglutinins. Of the patients with increased cold agglutinin titers, most patients with *M. pneumoniae* CAP will have cold agglutinin titers ≥1:64. A patient with CAP and a cold agglutinin titer ≥1:64 should be considered as having *M. pneumoniae* CAP until proven otherwise. Patients with *M. pneumoniae* meningoencephalitis will have cold agglutinin titers ≥1:512, usually in the thousands. Cold agglutinin titers of this order of magnitude are unusual in *Mycoplasma* CAP without CNS involvement. The diagnosis of *Mycoplasma* meningoencephalitis is suggested by the very highly elevated cold agglutinin titers as well as the extra-pulmonary manifestations of *Chlamydia pneumoniae* CAP.

The extra-pulmonary manifestations of *C. pneumoniae* CAP include otitis/bullous myringitis, nonexudative pharyngitis, *Erythema multiforme*, or watery diarrhea. Patients suspected of having *M. pneumoniae*, i.e., those with CAP with one or more of the extra-pulmonary findings described and highly elevated cold agglutinin titers should have specific tests to confirm the diagnosis. *M. pneumoniae* may be cultured on viral media from oropharyngeal secretions. Alternately, serological

Table 2 Clinical Features of Legionnaires' Disease

Organ involvement in legionnaires	Common features	Uncommon features	Argues
Clinical Features			
CNS	Headache mental confusion/dullness lethargy	Dizziness	Meningeal signs seizures
HEENT	None	Vertigo	Sore throat, ear pain, bullous myringitis, and otitis media
Cardiac	Relative bradycardia	Legionella endocarditis	Emboli to heart, joints, lungs, spleen, and CNS
GI	Loose stools/watery diarrhea	Abdominal pain	Hepatic tenderness and peritoneal signs
Renal	↑ Creatinine	Acute renal failure	CVA tenderness and chronic renal failure
Laboratory Tests			
CSF	Normal	Mild pleocytosis	RBCs, ↓ glucose, and ↑ lactic acid
WBC count (blood)	Leukocytosis	Leukopenia	Thrombocytosis and thrombocytopenia
Gram stain (sputum)	Few mononuclear cells and no bacteria	PMN predominance or mixed flora	Purulent sputum and single predominant organism
Pleural fluid	Exudative pattern	↑ WBCs	RBCs, ↓ pH, and ↓ glucose
SGOT/SGPT	Mildly elevated (<2×normal)	Moderately elevated (>2×normal)	Markedly elevated (>10×normal)
Urine analysis	Microscopic hematuria	Proteinuria, myoglobulinuria	Gross hematuria, pyuria, and hemoglobinuria

Abbreviations: CN, cranial nerve; CNS, central nervous system; CSF, cerebrospinal fluid; CVA, costovertebral angle; GI, gastrointestinal; HEENT, head, eyes, ears, nose and throat; RBC, red blood cell; SBE, subacute bacterial endocarditis; WBC, white blood cell; SGOT, serum glutamate oxaloacetate transaminase; SGPT, serum glutamate pyruvate transaminase.

diagnosis is made by demonstrating elevated IgM titer with or without an elevated IgG *M. pneumoniae* enzyme linked immunosorbent assay (ELISA) titer enzyme linked immunosorbent assay (5,12).

Legionnaires' Disease

Legionnaires' disease is an infection caused by any species of *Legionella* and is a systemic infection that predominantly affects the lungs. Legionnaires' disease, as with other atypical causes of CAP, is characterized by its particular pattern of extra-pulmonary organ involvement. In patients with *Legionella* CAP, CNS manifestations are frequent and include varying levels of consciousness, headache, and, most commonly, encephalopathy manifested my mental confusion. The characteristic pattern of extra-pulmonary organ involvement with *Legionella*, in addition to CNS findings, includes heart, liver, renal, and gastrointestinal involvement (Table 2). *Legionella* infections do not have upper respiratory tract or skin manifestations. The main cardiac manifestation of *Legionella* is relative bradycardia, i.e., a pulse temperature deficit (excluding patients on beta-blocker therapy, with arrhythmias, or pacemaker-induced rhythms). Gastrointestinal involvement is characterized by watery diarrhea as with *M. pneumoniae*. Hepatic involvement is manifested by an early mild/transient increase in the serum transaminases. In patients with atypical CAPs a slightly increased SGOT/SGPT limits diagnostic possibilities to Legionnaires' disease, Q fever, or psittacosis. CAP due to Q fever or psittacosis present with severe headache as the primary CNS manifestation but rarely, if ever, with encephalopathy. A low serum sodium secondary to syndrome of inappropriate ADH (SIADH) is common in patients with *Legionella* as well as any patient with a pulmonary/CNS process, although frequently *Legionella* is nonspecific and diagnostically unhelpful. Other laboratory tests pointing to *Legionella* are an elevated creatine phosphokinase (CPK) or creactive protein (CRP) of more than 30. Urinalysis may show otherwise unexplained microscopic hematuria. Increased cold agglutinins are not a feature of Legionnaires' disease and, if present, argue strongly against the diagnosis.

Because coinfections are exceedingly rare, high cold agglutinins ≥1:64 in a patient with atypical CAP should point to *M. pneumoniae* and not a co-infection with *Mycoplasma* and *Legionella*. Relative bradycardia is also not a feature of *M. pneumoniae*, which is a constant finding in those with Legionnaires' disease with or without CNS manifestations. The clinical syndromic diagnosis of *Legionella* is based on finding one or more of the extra-pulmonary clinical or laboratory findings mentioned and, if present, should prompt specific diagnostic testing. *Legionella* may be diagnosed early before treatment by direct fluorescent antibody (DFA) or respiratory secretions. Serologically, *Legionella* may be demonstrated by an increased IgM titer or a fourfold or greater increase between acute and convalescent IgG titers. *Legionella pneumophila* (serotype 01) may be diagnosed by the urinary antigen test. *Legionella* antigenuria is often negative early in the infectious process when the patient is in the CCU and is only positive with *L. pneumophila* serogroup 01. *Legionella* antigenuria becomes positive over time, persists for weeks after the infection, and is of more use later in the course of infection/convalescence when a retrospective diagnosis is desired. In the critical care setting, a negative initial *Legionella* titer or a negative *Legionella* antigen determination does not rule out *Legionella*. The presumptive diagnosis of *Legionella* is based on the clinical syndrome suggested by the characteristic pattern of organ involvement and laboratory tests described (Table 3) (5,14).

NONINFECTIOUS MIMICS OF ACUTE VIRAL ENCEPHALITIS

Toxic/Metabolic Encephalopathy

The most common cause of noninfectious acute encephalopathy in the CCU are related to acute metabolic/toxic encephalopathy usually due to one or more medications. Patients with toxic/metabolic abnormalities have no findings to suggest that an infectious etiology and toxic/metabolic encephalopathy is largely a diagnosis of exclusion. Computed tomography (CT)/magnetic resonance imaging (MRI) scans of the head are negative, and the EEG is unremarkable/nonspecific. CSF findings in toxic/metabolic encephalopathy usually contain <5 white blood cells/hpf and typically do not have an elevated protein, decreased glucose, or elevated CSF lactic acid level. Microbiologically, the CSF gram stain and culture are negative for

Table 3 Causes of Relative Bradycardia

Infectious	Noninfectious
Legionella	β-Blockers
Psittacosis	Diltiazem
Q fever	Verapamil
Typhoid fever	CNS lesions
Typhus	Lymphomas
Babesiosis	Factitious fever
Malaria	Drug fever
Leptospirosis	
Yellow fever	
Dengue fever	
Viral hemorrhagic fevers	
Rocky Mountain spotted fever	

Abbreviation: CNS, central nervous system.
Source: From Ref. 13.

neuropathogenic bacteria. Hepatic encephalopathy in patients with advanced liver disease frequently precipitates their admission to the CCU. Hepatic encephalopathy is a cause of the patients, altered mental status and is based on history and physical findings that point to chronic advanced liver disease. The diagnosis of hepatic encephalopathy is suggested by fetor hepaticus asterixis hyperventilation in addition to the stigmata of chronic alcohol-induced liver disease. Highly increased serum ammonia levels support the diagnosis of hepatic encephalopathy. Clinicians should be aware that patients with cirrhosis have impaired B->T-lymphocyte function which may predispose them to pneumonia or bacterial meningitis superimposed on their on hepatic encephalopathy. Lumbar puncture should be obtained, if possible, using plating/clotting factors infusions prelumbar puncture because such patients often have coagulopathy related to their hepatic dysfunction. Lumbar puncture with analysis of the CSF gram stain/cultures is the only way to definitely rule out a coexisting bacterial process that could easily be masked by the superimposed hepatic encephalopathy (Table 4) (1–3).

CNS Hemorrhage CVA

Patients in the CCU due to a massive cerebral vascular accident (CVA) or a massive intracranial hemorrhage may be suspected on the basis of neurologic findings. CNS hemorrhage or CVA may be confirmed by head CT or MRI scans. Lumbar puncture will reveal a bloody CSF in patients with CNS hemorrhage that communicates with the ventricles. CSF gram stain and culture will be negative, but in patients with intracranial hemorrhage, there will be a CSF pleocytosis and a variably elevated protein. The CSF glucose may be decreased in proportion to the RBCs present. RBCs in the CSF actively metabolize glucose and decrease the CSF glucose via this mechanism. The CSF lactic acid will also be elevated in direct proportion to the number of red cells present, but the negative CSF gram stains/culture will rule out an infectious etiology (1–3).

MISCELLANEOUS OTHER DISORDERS

SLE Cerebritis

There a variety of miscellaneous disorders that may present with mental confusion. Most of these are collagen vascular diseases, e.g., systemic lupus erythematosus (SLE)

Table 4 Noninfectious Mimics of Acute Encephalitis

Disorder	CSF findings	Other findings
Primary CNS lymphomas	+ Cytology ↑ Protein ± RBCs ↓ Glucose Normal/↑ lactic acid (~RBCs)	Mass lesion on head CT/MRI + HIV serology
Metastatic lymphoma to CNS	+ Cytology ↑ Protein ± RBCs ↓ Glucose N/↑ lactic acid (~RBCs)	Primary lymphoma
Metastases to CNS	+ Cytology	CXR central mass lesion (± cavitation with squamous cell carcinoma)
Squamous/small cell bronchogenic carcinoma	↑ Protein ± RBCs ↓ Glucose N/↑ lactic acid (~RBCs)	↑ Ca^{++} (with squamous cell carcinoma) Clubbing/Hypertrophic Pulmonary Osteoarthropathy (HPO) SVC/IVC syndrome + Bone marrow cytology with (small/squamous cell carcinomas)
Breast carcinoma	+ Cytology ↑ Protein ± RBCs ↓ Glucose N/↑ lactic acid (~RBCs)	History/presence of breast cancer
Other carcinomas	+ Cytology ↑ Protein ± RBCs ↓ Glucose N/↑ lactic acid (~RBCs)	History/presence of extra CNS primary malignancy
Massive intracerebral hemorrhage	↑↑↑ RBCs/bloody tap ↓ Glucose ↑ Lactic acid (~RBCs)	
SLE cerebritis	Lymphocytic pleocytosis ± ↓ Glucose ± ↓ Lactic acid ↓ CSF, C_4	History/features of SLE Evidence of SLE flare (↓ WBC count, ↓ C_3, ↑ ferritin)
Granulomatous CNS angitis	No pleocytosis N glucose N lactic acid	+ Head CT Magnetic Resonance Angiograhm (MRA) + Brain biopsy
Toxic/metabolic	No pleocytosis N glucose No RBCs N lactic acid	Multiple medications (opiates, narcotics, sedatives, etc.)

(*Continued*)

Table 4 Noninfectious Mimics of Acute Encephalitis (*Continued*)

Disorder	CSF findings	Other findings
Hepatic encephalopathy	No pleocytosis N glucose No RBCs N lactic acid	History/presence of severe/ advanced liver disease ↑ Ammonia levels

Abbreviations: CNS, central nervous system; CSF, cerebrospinal fluid; HIV, human immunodeficiency virus; RBC, red blood cell; SLE, systemic lupus erythematosus; WBC, white blood cell; CXR, chest X-ray; HPO, hypertrophic pulmonary osteoarthropathy.
Source: From Refs. 1–4.

or various causes of cerebral vasculitis. Among the collagen vascular diseases with CNS manifestations, SLE is the most common. Behçet's disease, sarcoidosis, antiphospholipid syndrome, and Sjögren's occasionally mimic meningitis but not encephalitis. Lupus cerebritis among the collagen vascular diseases is the most likely to mimic encephalitis. The possibility of lupus cerebritis is suggested by the patient's history, i.e., a long-standing history of lupus with multisystem manifestations. Lupus cerebritis may be diagnosed from head CT/MRI appearance showing bilateral abnormalities over the surface of both hemispheres. The diagnosis of lupus cerebritis may be confirmed by demonstrating decreased C_4 level in the CSF. Lupus cerebritis usually occurs as part of a SLE flare. SLE flare is suggested by the presence of leukopenia, decreased complement levels, or an increased ferritin level. SLE may also present with psychosis, seizure, or CVA (5,15,16).

CNS Vasculitis

Among the vasculitides that have CNS manifestations are periarteritis nodosa, Churg–Strauss granulomatosis, CNS angitis, and temporal arteritis. Patients with these disorders usually present with headache mimicking meningitis rather than encephalitis. Of this group, granulomatous CNS angiitis involving the leptomeninges may present with encephalitis. Diagnosis is by CT angiography or brain biopsy. The erythrocyte sedimentation rate (ESR) is highly elevated, and the serological tests for other collagen vascular diseases, e.g., SLE are negative. Neurologic involvement with sarcoidosis is infrequent but occurs in 5% to 10% of cases. The most common manifestation of neurosarcoidosis is chronic basilar meningitis. Cranial neuropathy, most frequently central seventh nerve palsy, with optic nerve involvement is the characteristic finding in neurosarcoidosis. Neurosarcoidosis may also present as AIDS or septic meningitis but encephalitis is rarely, if ever, a feature of neurosarcoidosis (1,15,17,18).

CNS Malignancies

Primary or metastatic disease to the CNS often presents as mental confusion. Primary CNS lymphoma occurs in patients with severely impaired T-cell function, e.g., human immunodeficiency virus (HIV). It is difficult in such patients without imaging to differentiate the encephalopathy due to HIV from HIV with superimposed CNS lymphoma. With HIV encephalopathy, the head CT/MRI shows no mass lesions, but with HIV and CNS lymphoma, there are mass lesions seen with neuroimaging studies. A variety of neoplasms metastasizes to the CNS and may present with encephalopathy. Common among these are the bronchogenic carcinomas, particularly squamous cell carcinoma and small cell carcinoma. Breast carcinoma is a frequent cause of CNS metastases. Patients with a history of breast cancer and encephalopathy should be viewed as potentially having encephalopathy due to CNS metastases. Metastatic lymphomas are also a common cause of metastatic disease to the CNS that present with mental confusion. Although virtually any tumor may metastasize to the CNS, other malignancies do so only rarely. The suspicion of CNS metastases based on a tumor is based on history, and the diagnosis may be confirmed by cytology of the CSF and/or brain biopsy. West Nile encephalitis (WNE) may also occur in patients with cancer, mimicking CNS metastases (19–21).

VIRAL CAUSES OF ACUTE ENCEPHALITIS IN THE CCU

The viruses responsible for acute encephalitis may be classified in several ways. Acute encephalitis may be classified as either being transmitted or not transmitted by arthropod vectors. Encephalitic viruses may also be classified according to season of peak occurrence, i.e., those having a seasonal, e.g., arboviruses, or nonseasonal occurrence, e.g., HSV-1 encephalitis. The viruses causing acute encephalitis have been named according to their original location, i.e., Powassan virus, West Nile virus (WNE), etc., of their isolation or their host, i.e., the equine encephalitides. Other neurotropic viruses causing encephalitis include the agent of Colorado tick fever, rabies, etc. The viruses causing acute encephalitis have many different physiochemical characteristics, come from different families, and are transmitted differently to humans. They also differ in their rapidity of onset, severity, and lethality. Encephalitis viruses may also be considered clinically as those that cause only encephalitis, e.g., HSV-1 and those that cause encephalitis with other extra CNS findings, e.g., WNV with encephalitis plus flaccid paralysis. In compromised hosts with impaired T-cell immunity, Epstein–Barr virus (EBV), human herpes virus-6 (HHV-6) and CMV may present with encephalitis. As there are only a limited number of antiviral agents effective against all the viral etiologies of viral encephalitis, drugs are available only for HSV and CMV. The clinical diagnostic approach in the CCU has a twofold purpose. The first clinical task is to eliminate disorders that may mimic encephalitis. The clinicians then can treat the few underlying disorders that are nonviral and for which there is effective therapy, e.g., *Listeria, Legionella*, and *M. pneumoniae* meningoencephalitis. The last task faced by the clinician is to try and differentiate the treatable causes of viral encephalitis, e.g., HSV or CMV, from the other nontreatable causes of viral encephalitis (Tables 5–8) (1–5,23–45).

CLINICAL DIAGNOSTIC APPROACH

Treatable Noninfectious Mimics of Viral Encephalitis

Among the noninfectious mimics of encephalitis, hepatic encephalopathy, SLE cerebritis, granulomatous CNS angiitis, some types of metastatic carcinomas to the CNS, and metastatic lymphomas to the CNS may be responsive to treatment. Other noninfectious mimics of encephalitis that are usually not responsive to therapeutic interventions are massive CVAs/intracranial hemorrhage.

Table 5 Causes of Acute Viral Encephalitis

HSV-1/HSV-2
VZV
HIV
Arboviruses
  US
    Western equine
    Eastern equine
    St. Louis
    California group
    Venezuelan equine
    Powassan
    Colorado tick fever
    West Nile virus
Influenza A
LCM
Enteroviruses
CMV[a]
Mumps
Measles
Rubella
EBV
Adenoviruses
Toxoplasma gondii[a]
Rabies

[a]Only in human immunodeficiency virus, organ transplants.
Abbreviations: HSV-1/HSV-2, herpes simplex types 1 and 2; VZV, varicella-zoster virus; HIV, human immunodeficiency virus; LCM, lymphocytic choriomeningitis; CMV, cytomegalovirus; EBV, Epstein–Barr virus.
Source: From Refs. 1–5.

Table 6 Geographical Distribution of Acute Arboviral Encephalitis

North America	EEE
	WEE
	StLE
	CE
	LAC
	POW
	WNE
South America	VEE
	EEE
	StLE
Eastern Europe	TBE
Africa	WNE
Asia	JE
	RSSE
	WNE
Australia	MVE

Abbreviations: EEE, eastern equine encephalitis; WEE, western equine encephalitis; StLE, St. Louis encephalitis; CE, California encephalitis; LAC, La Crosse; POW, Powassan; WNE, West Nile encephalitis; VEE, Venezuelan equine encephalitis; TBE, European tick-borne encephalitis; JE, Japanese B encephalitis; RSSE, Russian spring-summer encephalitis; MVE, Murray Valley encephalitis.
Source: From Refs. 1–3, 54.

Table 7 Clinical Features of Arbovirus Encephalitis

Viral type	Age group affected	Seizures	Other neurologic findings	Nonneurologic findings	Laboratory findings
CE	Children ≤10 yrs	+	Behavioral changes; focal signs in 20%	Nausea and vomiting common	↑ WBC count
EEE	Children and adults (70% mortality)	+	Most severe encephalitis; rapidly progressing severe encephalitis 1 wk or less; sequelae common in children not adults	Facial/extremity edema in some	Only virus with cloudy CSF peripheral leukocytosis; PMNs predominant (≥1000 cells/mm³ common); ↓ CSF glucose
WEE	Children and adults	−	Mild encephalitis; sequelae rare but severe	Tremors of tongue, hands, feet prominent	Normal WBC count
VEE	Children and adults	−	Mild encephalitis; no sequelae; recovery ≤1 wk	Pharyngitis, nausea, vomiting, diarrhea common; adenopathy in 30%	Profound leukopenia/lymphopenia
SLE	Adults (≥60 yrs)	+ (epidemics of "summer-stroke")	Resolves in ≤2 wks; no sequelae	Nausea/vomiting precedes encephalitis; urinary symptoms (dysuria in 20%); tongue/extremity tremors	↑ WBC; SIADH in 20%
CTF	Children (<15 yrs; history of tick bite in 90%)	−	None	"Camel-back fever curve"; abdominal pain and vomiting; splenomegaly, conjunctival suffusion, maculopapular rash in some	Marked leukopenia

(Continued)

Table 7 Clinical Features of Arbovirus Encephalitis (*Continued*)

Viral type	Age group affected	Seizures	Other neurologic findings	Nonneurologic findings	Laboratory findings
POW	Children (≤15 yrs)	+	Focal paralysis; meningeal signs	None	Normal WBC count
JE	Children (≤15 yrs; 40% mortality)	−	Weakness; extrapyramidal signs	None	Normal WBC count
WNE	Elderly	−	Weakness; tremors Parkinson's Disease Chorioretinitis	±Rash	Leukopenia; lymphopenia; ↑ferritin ↑amylase/lipase

Abbreviations: CE, California encephalitis group; EEE, Eastern equine encephalitis; WEE, Western, equine encephalitis; VEE, Venezuelan equine encephalitis; SLE, St. Louis encephalitis; CTF, Colorado tick fever; WNE, West Nile encephalitis; POW, Powassan encephalitis; JE, Japanese encephalitis; CSF, Cerebrospinal-spinal fluid; SIADH, syndrome of inappropriate antidiuretic hormone.
Source: From Refs. 1–4.

Table 8 Encephalitis Associations

Clinical clues	Type of encephalitis suggested
Chorioretinitis	WWE
Tongue tremors	SLE, WEE
Zoster ophthalmicus/contralateral hemiplegia	VZV
Annular rash (erythema migrans)	Lyme disease
Erythema multiforme	HSV, *Mycoplasma pneumoniae*
Vesicular rash	VZV, HSV (herpes labialis)
Maculopapular rash	Lupus cerebritis, measles, rubella, HIV, EBV, CTF, WNE
Petechial rash	RMSF, arboviral or hemorrhagic fever, CTF, arboviruses
Very rapid onset and prominent myalgias	Arboviruses
Posterior cervical adenopathy	SLE, VEE, HIV, CMV, toxoplasmosis, trypanosomiasis, LGV
"Stroke" with fever	Subacute bacterial endocarditis with emboli, lupus cerebritis
Diarrhea	Enteroviruses, VEE, Legionnaire's disease, Whipple's disease, *M. pneumoniae*
Pharyngitis	EBV, CMV, toxoplasmosis, enteroviruses, HIV, (secondary to CMV), *Candida,* VEE, rabies, *M. pneumoniae*, Lyme disease
Pneumonia	Adenovirus, *M. pneumoniae*, influenza, Legionnaire's disease, HIV (secondary to PCP), pertussis
Seizures	Lupus cerebritis, primary and secondary CNS malignancies, CE, EEE, Powassan, HSV, VEE
Tremors	WNE
Coma	Rabies, HSV, Reye's syndrome, CTF, VEE, WNE
Ataxia	EBV, SLE, tertiary syphilis, measles, VZV, echovirus 9
Epididymo-orchitis	Mumps, EBV, CTF

Abbreviations: CE, California encephalitis; CMV, cytomegalovirus; CNS, central nervous system; CTF, Colorado tick fever; EBV, Epstein–Barr virus; HIV, human immunodeficiency virus; HSV, herpes-simplex virus; SLE, systemic lupus erythematosus; VEE, Venezuelan equine encephalitis; VZV, varicella zoster virus; WEE, western equine encephalitis; WNE, West Nile encephalitis; RMSF, Rocky Mountain spotted fever; LGV, lympho granulomatous venereum; PCP, *Pneumocystis (carinii) jiroveci* pneumonia; EEE, Eastern equine encephalitis. *Source*: From Refs. 1–5, 23–45.

NONVIRAL INFECTIOUS MIMICS OF ACUTE ENCEPHALITIS IN THE CCU

All of the nonviral infectious mimics of encephalitis are amenable to antimicrobial therapy, i.e., *L. monocytogenes*, *M. pneumoniae*, and *Legionella* species. As with the noninfectious mimics of encephalitis, the clue to the diagnosis of the cause of the encephalopathy is usually apparent from the history, physical, and routine laboratory/radiology tests. With *L. monocytogenes* encephalopathy, meningoencephalitis/encephalitis may be the only clinical feature making the diagnosis possible and only by CSF gram stain/culture (8–11).

M. pneumoniae and *Legionella* as typical pneumonias have one or more extra-pulmonary findings, which, if recognized, should suggest the diagnosis. In a patient with CAP and ill-defined infiltrates on the chest X-ray without relative bradycardia, and encephalopathy with a nonexudative pharyngitis, otitis, or *E. multiforme* may have *M. pneumoniae*. Even if these findings are not present, ill-defined infiltrates in a normal host with meningoencephalitis should cause the clinician to order cold agglutinin titers or perform a bedside agglutination disassociation test. The bedside cold agglutination disassociation test is positive if the cold agglutinin titer present is ≥1:64. If this is positive, serum cold agglutinin titers can be ordered and the actual titers can be determined. An elevated bedside cold agglutination disassociation test also should prompt the clinician to order specific serological testing for *Mycoplasma*, i.e., *M. pneumoniae* IgM ELISA titer (1,5,12).

The diagnosis of *Legionella* in a patient with encephalopathy and CAP is suggested by the presence of relative bradycardia, mild early/transient increase in serum transaminases, and mild early/transient decrease in the serum phosphorous, with/without microscopic hematuria. Any combination of these findings in a patient with encephalopathy and CAP should prompt specific *Legionella* diagnostic testing, i.e., sputum direct fluorescent antibody (DFA), *Legionella* serology, and *Legionella* urinary antigen determinations (1,5,14).

TREATABLE CAUSES OF ACUTE ENCEPHALITIS IN THE CCU

The first priority in the diagnostic approach is to identify treatable/reversible causes of encephalopathy, both infectious and noninfectious. After the treatable and non-treatable mimics of acute encephalitis are eliminated from further diagnostic consideration, the next task is to try and identify HSV or VZV encephalitis in a normal host or CMV or *Toxoplasma gondii* encephalitis in the compromised host with impaired cell-mediated immunity (CMI).

The most straightforward diagnosis is VZV-associated encephalopathy, because it is associated with readily apparent cutaneous manifestations. In nondisseminated VZV, zoster involving the dermatomes closest to the CNS are those most likely to be associated with VZV encephalopathy. Lumbar puncture shows a lymphocytic pleo-cytosis with a normal CSF glucose and lactic acid with a variably elevated protein level (Table 5) (45–52).

ACUTE ENCEPHALITIS IN NORMAL HOSTS

HSV-1 Encephalitis

The single most important viral cause of acute encephalitis amenable to treatment to identify is HSV encephalitis. HSV encephalitis has no seasonal distribution, does not have a positive arthropod/zoonotic contact history, and has no geographical distri-bution. When these factors are absent in the history in a patient presenting with acute encephalitis, then HSV-1 encephalitis should be the main diagnostic considera-tion. Patients with HSV encephalitis have early and dense neurological deficits. Some patients have a mild course of encephalitis when treatment has begun early but they will not be in the CCU. Patients admitted to the CCU with HSV-1 ence-phalitis will have substantial neurological defects. There are no specific clues from the history in a patient with HSV encephalitis except within the previous two weeks having had herpes labialis. Patients with HSV encephalitis often have a recent history of herpes labialis, but importantly, the lesions are not present at the time the patient presents with encephalitis.

The presumptive diagnosis of HSV-1 encephalitis is suggested by the EEG, which shows focal activity in the area of the temporal lobe. Excluding HHV-6 encephalitis, every other cause of encephalitis has nonfocal findings on the EEG. Because HHV-6 encephalitis is rare and HSV-1 is so common, the findings of focality on EEG should suggest HSV-1 encephalitis until proven otherwise. The head computed tomography (CT)/magnetic resonance imaging (MRI) shows focal abnormalities in the temporal region, but these changes occur after the EEG changes and may not be visible on imaging studies initially. The severity of HSV encephalitis is proportional to the degree of parenchymal damage visualized on the head CT/MRI.

The CSF in HSV-1 encephalitis is abnormal, but the findings are relatively nonspecific. HSV-1 encephalitis is the great neurologic imitator. It is not uncommon to find an initial PMN predominance early in the process. HSV-1 encephalitis is the only viral CNS infection that may be associated with $\geq 90\%$ of PMNs in the CSF. Subsequently, the CSF pleocytosis changes from a predominance of PMNs to a lymphocytic pleocytosis. In the CSF, RBCs may not be present initially but become present subsequently and are proportional to the degree of parenchymal damage. The CSF lactic acid in HSV-1 encephalitis is directly proportional to the number of red cells present in the CSF. The protein is variably elevated. HSV-1 is one of the few neurotropic viruses that may lower the CSF glucose. Focal EEG or head CT/MRI abnormalities and RBCs in the CSF with mild elevations of the CSF lactic acid should prompt the clinician to obtain a polymerase chain reaction (PCR) determination for herpes in the CSF. Empiric therapy should be started with acyclovir as soon as the diagnosis is entertained and should not wait for confirmation by CSF PCR (1,6,53).

Varicella Zoster Virus Encephalitis

VZV encephalitis may complicate localized/dermatomal VZV of the head/neck or may be secondary to disseminated VZV. Patients that have VZV and develop encephalitis should be considered as having VZV-associated encephalitis until proven otherwise. Unlike HSV-1 encephalitis where there are no cutaneous clues to the cause of the patient's encephalopathy, the characteristic vesicular lesions of VZV are the key clue to the diagnosis. The main diagnostic problem is that many physicians fail to appreciate the CNS manifestations of head/neck dermatomal VZV and do not appreciate the relationship between the skin lesions and the patient's encephalopathy. A lumbar puncture in patients with VZV encephalitis reveals a CSF which has a viral profile. The CSF findings in VZV usually reveal a modest lymphocytic pleocytosis with a normal CSF glucose, variably elevated CSF protein, a normal CSF lactic acid, and no RBCs. Head CT/MRI scans reveal no abnormalities. The diagnosis of VZV encephalitis is clinical (Table 9) (1,45).

ACUTE ENCEPHALITIS IN COMPROMISED HOSTS

CMV Encephalitis

In the compromised host with severely impaired CMI due to decreased lymphocyte function, opportunistic infections of the CSF are common. Among these, the most important causes are CMV and toxoplasmosis. CMV encephalitis may occur in HIV patients or immunosuppressed organ transplants patients. CMV encephalitis should be considered in the differential diagnosis in patients with impaired CMI but there are no clinical features, which would suggest a specific diagnosis except

Table 9 Differential Diagnosis of the Causes of Meningoencephalitis/Encephalitis Responsive to Antimicrobial Therapy

Causes of meningoencephalitis/ encephalitis	Clinical features	
	CSF findings	Non-CSF findings
Listeria monocytogenes	Monocytic/lymphocytic pleocytosis ↓ Glucose + RBCs ↑ Lactic acid/(not ~RBCs) + Gram stain(50%+) (100%+)/culture	History/presence of malignancy (especially lymphoreticular malignancies)
Legionella	Mild/no pleocytosis N glucose N lactic acid N protein	CAP + relative bradycardia ↑ SGOT/SGPT ↓ PO$_4$
Mycoplasma pneumoniae	N/↓ glucose N lactic acid N/variably increased protein	CAP + no relative bradycardia N LFTs ↑↑↑ Cold agglutinin titers
HSV-1 encephalitis	PMNs/lymphocytic pleocytosis ± ↓ glucose ↑ lactic acid (~ to RBCs) - Gram stain/culture N/variably increased protein + PCR for HSV-1	Recent history of herpes labialis (not concurrent)
VZV encephalitis	Lymphocytic pleocytosis N glucose N lactic acid N/variably increased protein	Recent dermatomal head/neck VZV Recent disseminated VZV

Abbreviations: CAP, community-acquired pneumonia; CSF, cerebrospinal fluid; HSV, herpes-simplex virus; RBC, red blood cell; VZV, varicella zoster virus; N, normal; LFT, liver function test.
Source: From Refs. 1–5, 53.

in patients with CMV retinitis. The funduscopic appearance of CMV retinitis is that of diffuse white exudates superimposed on the retina that have a "tomato soup" appearance. The EEG scan shows nonfocal bilateral hemispheric abnormalities, which are nonspecific. Changes include periventricular abnormalities with variable degrees of enhancement. The diagnosis of CMV encephalitis is suggested by obtaining semiquantitative CMV antigen levels in the serum, which were highly elevated, indicating an active infection. Alternately, a CSF PCR for CMV may be obtained. However, patients with severely impaired CMI may not express a serological response and IgM antibody titers may be negative. CMV encephalitis occurs in HIV patients with CD4 counts < 50 cells/mm^3 (1,3,53,54).

Toxoplasmosis Encephalitis

There are no specific findings on the EEG or head CT/MRI, which suggests *T. gondii* encephalitis. Patients with *T. gondii* encephalitis will have an elevated *T. gondii* IgG titer, which may be the only clue to the patient's encephalopathy. Aside from having an IgG toxoplasmosis titer, patients with *T. gondii* encephalitis usually do not have concomitant pneumonia. Head CT/MRI shows mass lesions which are often multiple and indistinguishable from primary CNS lymphoma or tuberculosis. Characteristic of *T. gondii* CNS lesions are their location. Most lesions are at the corticomedullary junction and baso ganglia. Edema and mass effect are common with these multiple CNS *T. gondii* lesions (53,54).

There are a variety of other viral infectious diseases that may have an encephalopathic component. EBV, HHV-6, and others may in normal hosts present with an infectious mono-like illness, which may or may not be accompanied by mental confusion. Encephalopathy is rare with EBV, CMV, and HHV-6 in normal hosts, but it does occur. As with most causes of acute viral encephalitis or disorders that mimic acute encephalitis, clues to the diagnosis are derived from the epidemiology and associated physical and laboratory findings, which point to the cause of the patient's encephalopathy. There is no specific therapy for EBV, CMV, or HHV-6 encephalitis in immunocompetent hosts (1–3,54).

THERAPEUTIC APPROACH

Treatment of Nonviral Mimics of Acute Viral Encephalitis

Patients diagnosed with SLE cerebritis or CNS angiitis should be treated with vasculitis doses of steroids. The care for intracerebral hemorrhage or CVA is supportive. The treatment of toxic metabolic encephalopathy or drug-induced encephalopathy involves discontinuing the medication and treating underlying metabolic abnormalities to reverse the patients, altered mental status. The therapeutic approach to these and other disorders that may present with encephalopathy involves removing/correcting the underlying cause.

TREATMENT OF INFECTIOUS MIMICS OF VIRAL ENCEPHALITIS

The infectious diseases most likely mimicking acute viral encephalitis are amenable to specific therapy. The treatment of *L. monocytogenes* meningoencephalitis in the penicillin-tolerant patient is with meningeal doses of ampicillin. In penicillin-intolerant patients, trimethoprim-sulfametoxozole (TMP-SMX) or chloramphenicol is usually effective. Treatment for *Listeria* meningoencephalitis is usually for two weeks. The treatment of *Mycoplasma* meningoencephalitis or Legionnaires' disease requires antimicrobial therapy, which is effective in the lung as well as the CNS. Although it has not been shown that there is direct invasion of the CSF in either *Mycoplasma*- or Legionella-induced CNS disease, it would seem prudent to use an antimicrobial, which is effective in both CNS and extra-CNS sites of infection. Of the antibiotics effective against *Mycoplasma* and *Legionella*, quinolones, macrolides, and tetracyclines have the advantage of CNS penetration. Of the tetracyclines, doxycycline and minocycline achieve therapeutic concentrations in the CSF as well as the lung and would be preferred agents in *Mycoplasma* or *Legionella* infections with CNS manifestations. Toxoplasma encephalitis occurs exclusively in patients with severely impaired CMI, i.e., organ transplants, HIV, etc. Toxoplasma encephalitis may be treated with clindamycin, sulfadiazine pyrimethamine, or TMP-SMX (1,53).

TREATMENT OF ACUTE VIRAL ENCEPHALITIS

Excluding HSV-1, VZV, and CMV encephalitis, the therapy of other causes of acute viral encephalitis is supportive in the CCU. Recovery of CNS function is difficult to predict, and patients' vital functions should be supported until it is clear if the process is reversible or terminal. CMV encephalitis occurs in patients with markedly impaired T-lymphocyte function, i.e., HIV, organ transplants, etc. and does not occur in normal hosts. Treatment for CMV encephalitis is with ganciclovir or valganciclovir. After initial therapy, life-long suppression is required in survivors.

HSV-1 and VZV encephalitis are the causes of viral encephalitis most amenable to specific antiviral therapy. HSV-1 should be treated as soon as the diagnosis is suspected from historical laboratory or X-ray findings. Mild encephalopathy seen in early HSV infection is readily reversible with early treatment with acyclovir or an acyclovir derivative. In HSV encephalitis, which presents with dense neurological deficits, RBCs in the CSF, frontotemporal EEG abnormalities, or frontal/temporal lobe destruction, head CT/MRI is much less responsive to therapy. Patients presenting with severe HSV-1 encephalitis usually have a poor prognosis and, if they survive, frequently have serious neurological sequelae. Treatment is ordinarily with acyclovir for 10 to 14 days. The treatment of VZV encephalitis is with the same drug also for the 10 to 14 days in duration (1,53).

REFERENCES

1. Boos J, Esiri MM. Viral Encephalitis in Humans. Washington: ASM Press, 2003.
2. Ho M. Acute viral encephalitis. In: Vinken PJ, Bruyn GW, eds. Handbook of Clinical Neurology. Infections of the Nervous System. Part II. Vol. 34. New York: North Holland Publishing, 1978:63–82.
3. Wood M, Anderson M. Neurologic Infections. London: W.B. Saunders, 1988.
4. Cunha BA. Encephalitis. Infect Dis Pract 1989; 12:1–12.
5. Cunha BA. The diagnosis and therapy of acute bacterial meningitis. In: Schlossberg D, ed. Central Nervous System Infections. Berlin: Springer-Verlag, 1990:3–24.
6. Cunha BA. The usefulness of CSF lactic acid levels in central nervous system infections with decreased cerebrospinal fluid glucose. Clin Infect Dis 2004; 39:1260–1261.
7. Latcha S, Cunha BA. *Listeria monocytogenes* meningoencephalitis–the diagnostic importance of the CSF lactic acid. Heart Lung 1994; 23:177–179.
8. Bailey EM, Domenico P, Cunha BA. Bacterial or viral meningitis? Measuring lactate CSF can help you know quickly. Postgrad Med 1990; 88:217–219.
9. Cunha BA. The diagnostic significance of the CSF lactic acid. Infect Dis Pract 1997; 21:57–60.
10. Mylonakis E, Hohmann EL, Calderwood SB. Central nervous system infection with *Listeria monocytogenes*. 33 years' experience at a general hospital and review of 776 episodes from the literature. Medicine (Baltimore) 1998; 77:313–336.
11. Cunha BA, Filozov A, Reme P. *Listeria monocytogenes* encephalitis mimicking West Nile encephalitis. Heart Lung 2004; 33:61–64.
12. Bitnun A, Ford-Jones E, Blaser S, et al. *Mycoplasma pneumoniae* encephalitis. Semin Pediatr Infect Dis 2003; 14:96–107.
13. Cunha BA. Diagnostic significance of relative bradycardia. Infect Dis Prac 1997; 21:38–40.
14. Cunha BA. Clinical Diagnosis of Legionnaire's Disease. Sem Resp Infect 1998; 13:116–127.
15. Warnatz K, Peter HH, Schumacher M, et al. Infectious CNS disease as a differential diagnosis in systemic rheumatic diseases: three case reports and a review of the literature. Ann Rheum Dis 2003; 62:50–57.

16. Sanna G, Bertolaccini ML, Mathieu A. Central nervous system lupus: a clinical approach to therapy. Lupus 2003; 12:935–942.

17. Hadfield MG, Aydin F. Lippman HR, et al. Neuro-Behçet's disease. Clin Neuropathol 1997; 16:55–60.

18. Carsons SE, Belilos E. Mimics of central nervous system infections. In: Cunha BA, ed. Infectious Diseases in Critical Care Medicine. New York: Marcel Dekker Inc., 1998:181–189.

19. Jeyakumar A, Hindenburg A, Minnaganti VR, Cunha BA. West Nile encephalitis mimicking central nervous system metastases from small cell lung cancer. Am J Med 2003; 9:594–595.

20. Dropcho EJ. Remote neurologic manifestations of cancer. Neurol Clin 2002; 20:85–122.

21. Pruitt AA. Nervous system infections in patients with cancer. Neurol Clin 2003; 21:193–219.

22. Cunha BA. Eastern equine encephalitis. Infect Dis Pract 1996; 20:75–79.

23. Roos KL. Encephalitis. Neurol Clin 1999; 17:813–833.

24. Whitley RJ, Gnann JW. Viral encephalitis: familiar infections and emerging pathogens. Lancet 2002; 359:507–513.

25. Redington JJ, Tyler KL. Viral infections of the nervous system, 2002: update on diagnosis and treatment. Arch Neurol 2002; 59:712–718.

26. Kennedy PG. Viral encephalitis: causes, differential diagnosis, and management. J Neurol Neurosurg Psychiatry 2004; 75:10–15.

27. Gutierrez KM, Prober CG. Encephalitis. Identifying the specific cause is a key to effective management. Postgrad Med 1998; 103:123–125, 129–130, 140–143.

28. Chaudhuri A, Kennedy PG. Diagnosis and treatment of viral encephalitis. Postgrad Med J 2002; 78:575–583.

29. Kizilkilic O, Karaca S. Influenza-associated encephalitis-encephalopathy with a reversible lesion in the splenium of the corpus callosum: case report and literature review. Am J Neurolradiol 2004; 25:1863–1864.

30. Studahl M. Influenza virus and CNS manifestations. J Clin Virol 2003; 28:225–232.

31. Portegies P, Corssmit N. Epstein–Barr virus and the nervous sytem. Curr Opin Neurol 2000; 13:301–304.

32. Liebert UG. Measles virus infections of the central nervous system. Intervirology 1997; 40:176–184.

33. Volpi A. Epstein–Barr virus and human herpesvirus type 8 infections of the central nervous system. Herpes 2004; 11:120–127.

34. Dewhurts S. Human herpesvirus type 6 and human herpesvirus type 7 infections of the central nervous system. Herpes 2004; 11:95–104.

35. Soto-Hernandez JL. Human herpesvirus 6 encephalomyelitis. Emerg Infect Dis 2004; 10:1700–1702.

36. Dumpis U, Crook D, Oksi J. Tick-borne encephalitis. Clin Infect Dis 1999; 28:882–890.

37. McJunkin JE, Khan RR, Tsai TF. California-LaCrosse encephalitis. Infect Dis Clin North Am 1998; 12:83–93.

38. Tiroumourougane SV, Raghave P, Srinivasan S. Japanese viral encephalitis. Postgrad Med J 2002; 78:205–215.

39. Gholam BI, Puksa S, Provias JP. Powassan encephalitis: a case report with neuropathology and literature review. CMAJ 1999; 161:1419–1422.

40. Cunha BA. West Nile Encephalitis. Clinical diagnostic and prognostic indicators in compromised hosts. Clinical Infectious Disease 2006; 42:117.

41. Solomon T. Flavivirus encephalitis. N Engl J Med 2004; 351:370–378.

42. Cunha BA. Differential diagnosis of West Nile encephalitis. Curr Opin Infect Dis 2004; 17:413–420.

43. Cunha BA, Minnaganti VR, Johnson DH, Klein NC. Profound and prolonged lymphopenia in West Nile encephalitis. Clin Infect Dis 2000; 31:1116–1117.

44. Cunha BA, Sachdev B, Canario D. Serum ferritin levels in West Nile encephalitis. Clin Microbiol Infect 2004; 10:184–186.

45. Arvin AM, Gershon AA. Varicella-Zoster Virus. United Kingdom: Cambridge University Press, 2000.
46. Maschke M, Kastrup O, Diener HC. CNS manifestations of cytomegalovirus infections: diagnosis and treatment. CNS Drugs 2002; 16:303–315.
47. Cinque P, Marenzi R, Ceresa D. Cytomegalovirus infections of the nervous system. Intervirology 1997; 40:85–97.
48. Montoya JG, Liesenfeld O. Toxoplasmosis. Lancet 2004; 363:1965–1976.
49. Collazos J. Opportunistic infections of the CNS in patients with AIDS: diagnosis and management. CNS Drugs 2003; 17:869–887.
50. Levitz RE. Herpes simple encephalitis: a review. Heart Lung 1998; 27:209–212.
51. Eisenstein L, Calio F, Cunha BA. Herpes simplex virus type 1 (HSV-1) aseptic meningitis. Heart Lung 2004; 33:196–197.
52. Cunha BA. Antibiotic Essentials 5th Ed. Michigan: Physician's Press, 2006.
53. Roos KL. Pearls and pitfalls in the diagnosis and management of central nervous system in infectious diseases. Semin Neurol 1998; 18:185–196.

7

Severe Head and Neck Infections in the Critical Care Unit

Franco Paradisi and Giampaolo Corti
Infectious Disease Unit, University of Florence School of Medicine, Florence, Italy

OVERVIEW

Introduction

The availability of a lot of new antimicrobials for successful therapy of many infections generated a widespread euphoria in the past, so that "most experts believe that by the year 2000 viral and bacterial infections will have disappeared from our life" (1). The recent and current epidemiology has totally put an end to that enthusiasm. Due to a series of phenomena such as immune suppression, bacterial resistance to antibiotics, migratory flows, and so on, infectious diseases are still an important challenge in the third millennium.

Among them, severe head and neck infections (HNIs) include a heterogeneous variety of deep fascial space infections (in the facial, suprahyoid, and infrahyoid regions) and other cervical infections (suppurative parotitis and thyroiditis, peritonsillar abscess, and acute epiglottitis), and some intracranial suppurative complications (brain abscess, subdural empyema, epidural abscess, and septic thrombophlebitis) that can follow cervical infections as well as pericranial infections (mastoiditis, otitis, and sinusitis).

All those infections were much more common and frequently fatal in the preantibiotic era, when they challenged physicians' ability to make an early and correct diagnosis and treatment by the available means. In the past, HNIs most frequently followed oropharyngeal, tonsillar, or sinusal infections, whereas currently they are generally the consequence of a dental infection or secondary to either animal or human bite wounds, traumatic or surgical injuries, or irradiation of malignancies.

Epidemiology

The availability of potent and effective antibiotics and vaccines has fortunately reduced both incidence and severity of HNIs: for example, the mortality rate of Ludwig's angina and peritonsillar abscess was greater than 50% in the preantibiotic era and is less than 5% currently (2), and similarly the mortality rate of septic cavernous sinus thrombophlebitis and other complications (i.e., rupture of the internal carotid artery) has markedly decreased from virtually 100% to less than 30% (3). The mortality rate of brain abscess and subdural empyema has decreased from approximately 50% and virtually 100% in the preantibiotic era to the current 5% to 10% and 10% to 20% rates, respectively (4).

In the same way, the improvement of radiologic techniques with the availability of computed tomography (CT) scanning and magnetic resonance imaging (MRI) for both early diagnosis and postoperative follow-up has greatly contributed to the reduced mortality rate of intracranial suppurative infections; for example, the mortality rate of brain abscess has decreased from 44% before advent of CT scanning to approximately zero following its introduction (5).

Moreover, the scenario of invasive infections caused by *Haemophilus influenzae*—such as meningitis, epiglottitis, and others—has notably changed since the introduction of conjugate vaccine anti–*H. influenzae* type b (Hib) among preschool-aged children in 1988. So, between 1987 and 1997 the incidence of Hib invasive infections dramatically declined by 97% in children aged less than five years, whereas it remained stable among adults and children aged greater than or equal to five years (6).

MICROBIOLOGY

Most Relevant Pathogens

The microbiology of severe HNIs, and in particular of cervical infections, presents a series of features that can be summarized as follows:

- The etiology is very complex and typically polymicrobial, as it generally reflects the indigenous flora of the oral cavity, upper respiratory tract, and certain parts of the head and neck.
- Among such autochthonous microflora, aerobes and anaerobes, gram-positives and gram-negatives, cocci and bacilli, and even spirochetes can be present.
- Globally, anaerobes outnumber aerobes by an 8–10:1 ratio (7).
- As a group, bacterial agents of severe HNIs are opportunists that invade the deep tissues of the head and neck in the presence of breaks on the mucosal surfaces (i.e., for infections or trauma). Moreover, invasiveness is favored by synergic interactions between bacterial species, adherence properties of certain bacteria, local conditions (pH and oxygen tension), and predisposing factors (age, diet, smoking, oral hygiene, immune suppression, hospitalization, and previous antibiotic therapy) (8).
- Unique microbial niches are characteristically observed, although a few streptococcal species are by far predominant among the oral flora (*Streptococcus mutans* and *S. sanguis* on the gingival crevice and dental plaque, and *Streptococcus salivarius* and *S. mitior* on the tongue and in the saliva). However, *Actinomyces* on the gingival crevice, *Corynebacterium* and *Lactobacillus* on the dental plaque, and *Peptostreptococcus* and *Veillonella* in the saliva are numerous as well (9).
- *Streptococcus pyogenes* is prevalent in pharyngeal and tonsillar tissue infections, and staphylococci (in particular, *Staphylococcus aureus*) of the cutaneous flora are important in the genesis of suppurative parotitis and thyroiditis.
- Aerobic gram-negative bacilli are uncommon in normal adults, but they can be prominent in patients with risk factors (advanced age, frequent hospitalization, and severe underlying conditions) (10).

The etiology of intracranial suppurations (brain and epidural abscess, subdural empyema, and septic thrombophlebitis) is typically polymicrobial as well, with the participation of aerobic and anaerobic, gram-positive and gram-negative, and bacillary and coccal microorganisms. However, in contrast to the previously cited HNIs, some microorganisms (i.e., *Streptococcus pneumoniae*) can play an increasing role as a consequence of the spread from a contiguous focus of infection, most often the middle ear and paranasal sinuses. Importantly, the efficacy of antibiotic therapy can be limited by the poor penetration of most antibacterial agents into the central nervous system, making these severe infections frequently devastating.

Bacterial Resistance to Antibiotics

Soon after the introduction of antimicrobial agents into clinical practice, it appeared clear that bacteria could possess the capacity to acquire resistance to antibiotics. Penicillin was first used in 1941, but by 1944 *S. aureus* was able to destroy it by means of penicillinase (11), and by the end of 1940s the majority of strains were resistant (12). As early as in 1955, Maxwell Finland observed that "changes in the susceptibilities of strains of various species to the different antibiotics perhaps reflect the effects of the extensive use of any given antimicrobial agents and the susceptibility of different bacteria to the same and to different agents" (13).

Currently, antibiotic resistance among a number of microorganisms is one of the most important causes of therapeutic failure in every part of the world. In particular, as far as the United States is concerned, a comprehensive national surveillance study has recently found a worrisome increase in resistance between the period 1997–2001 and the year 2002; for example, *Pseudomonas aeruginosa* isolates that are resistant to third-generation cephalosporins, imipenem, and quinolones increased by 22%, 32%, and 37%, respectively, whereas methicillin-resistant *S. aureus* (MRSA) and vancomycin-resistant enterococci increased by 13% and 11%, respectively (14). A concise but exhaustive overview of resistance issues targeted to bacteria that produce HNIs seems to be quite pertinent.

Staphylococcus aureus

If, by the mid-1970s, 85% to 95% of both community and hospital isolates of *S. aureus* were resistant to penicillin (15), the emergence and spread of MRSA is much more recent. Methicillin was introduced into clinical practice in 1960, but the first methicillin-resistant strain was reported as early as 1961 (16), and the first nosocomial outbreak of MRSA infection dates back to 1968 (17). In U.S. hospitals, a 12-fold increase of the isolation rate of MRSA (from 2.4% to 29%) was observed between 1975 and 1991 (18), and the percentage reached 42% at the end of the millennium (19). In European hospitals, the MRSA prevalence varies from less than 1% in Scandinavian countries to more than 30% to 40% in Britain and Mediterranean countries (20), and similarly high rates have been recently found in Africa (South Africa, 39%) and Asia (Malaysia, 49%) (21).

However, the epidemiology of *S. aureus* is changing, as MRSA is increasingly recovered in nursing homes, where in Wisconsin it rose from 18% in 1997 to 51% in 2002 (22), but it is emerging also in the community (23,24). In 1980, the first community-acquired outbreak of MRSA was reported by the Centers for Disease Control among drug abusers (25), and the proportion of community-associated MRSA isolates increased in San Francisco from 7% in 1993 to 29% in 1999 (19).

During 2004, a number of papers have been published on clusters of community-onset MRSA infections (mostly of skin and soft tissues) in many parts of the United States (26–30), including outbreaks among military trainees, jail inmates, and football players (31–33).

The epidemiology of *S. aureus* has been further complicated since 1997 by the reporting of clinical strains (named vancomycin-intermediate *S. aureus* VISA) with reduced susceptibility to vancomycin (34) that until then was considered the last resource for therapy of multiresistant *S. aureus* infections, as it had been always effective in vitro. Some experts compared that finding with the Roman Emperor Julius Caesar's surprise in discovering his adopted son, Brutus, among conspirators ("You, my son, as well?") (35), and the report of the first fully vancomycin-resistant *S. aureus* (VRSA) isolate followed after a few years (36). Fortunately, large surveillance studies have found percentages of VISA that were either negligible (<0.1%) (37) or just equal to 0 (38), and until now only papers describing a single case or small outbreaks (39) have been published in some parts of the world. Even the feared dissemination of isolates that were heterointermediately resistant to vancomycin (hVISA), initially observed in Japanese hospitals (40), has not subsequently come true, as the prevalence of these strains has been recently found to be low (4.3%) in the Far East, whereas neither VISA nor VRSA was isolated (41).

Also, one must consider that many VISA or hVISA isolations were reported from patients with confounding factors such as inadequate vancomycin levels, severe underlying conditions, presence of foreign devices, or undrained abscesses (42).

Streptococcus pyogenes

Despite more than 60 years of extensive and frequently indiscriminate use of penicillin and its derivatives, *S. pyogenes* remains extremely susceptible to these antibiotics; no clinical isolate that was resistant to penicillin has been identified to date. Some of the most likely explanations for this unique phenomenon are (i) beta-lactamases may not be expressed or may be toxic to the microorganisms; (ii) low-affinity penicillin-binding proteins either are not expressed or make bacteria nonviable; (iii) circumstances favorable for the development of resistance have not yet occurred; and (iv) mechanisms for or barriers to genetic transfer of resistance are inefficient (43).

Either a macrolide or clindamycin is recommended as alternative treatment for patients allergic to beta-lactams (44). As opposed to penicillin, the increased clinical consumption of erythromycin and its derivatives has been related to increased resistance of *S. pyogenes* to all macrolides, primarily in Spain and Finland (45,46). Indeed, a significant class effect exists among macrolides, because the constitutive MLS$_B$ phenotype of erythromycin resistance (target modification) determines high-level and cross-resistance to macrolides, lincosamides, and streptogramin B, whereas the other mechanism (drug efflux, i.e., M phenotype) confers low-level resistance to 14- (clarithromycin, dirithromycin, and roxithromycin) and 15-membered (azithromycin) macrolides only (47).

Currently, erythromycin-resistant *S. pyogenes* (ERSP) is present worldwide, primarily in Southern Europe (20–25%) and in the Far East (average 18.3%), as evidenced by the results of a multinational surveillance program named PROTEKT that was carried out during the years 1999 and 2000 (Fig. 1). Clindamycin resistance was present only in ERSP strains and ranged from zero in Australia and North America to 51% in Western Europe (38). An even more recent (2001–2002) update of the same study targeted to the United States confirms a low prevalence of ERSP (6%) that is homogeneous through all the states, varying from 4.3% in the

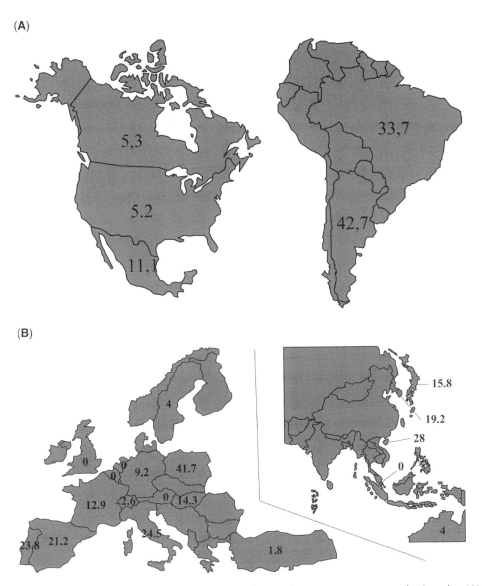

Figure 1 Prevalence (%) of erythromycin-resistant *Streptococcus pyogenes* in America (**A**), Europe, and the Far East (**B**). *Source*: From Ref. 38.

southwestern states to 7% in the northwestern and southcentral ones; the rate of clindamycin resistance continues to be negligible (0.6%) (48).

Streptococcus pneumoniae

Pneumococci were among the most highly penicillin-susceptible bacteria throughout the first quarter-century of penicillin use. The first clinical penicillin-resistant pneumococcal (PRP) strain was isolated in 1967 from a patient in Papua, New Guinea (49), and during the following 10 years sporadic reports on PRP clinical strains from various parts of the world were published. The subsequent event in the epidemiology of antibiotic-resistant pneumococci was the 1977 South African outbreak of pneumococcal disease caused by multiresistant strains, which were shown to have greatly increased minimal inhibitory concentrations (MIC) not only for penicillin, but also for many other drugs (50).

The current epidemiology of PRP is worrisome worldwide. In the United States, the rate of penicillin-nonsusceptible strains [both intermediate (MIC 0.12–1 µg/mL) and resistant (MIC ≥2 µg/mL)] varies from 25.7% in the Northcentral states to 44.3% in the Southcentral ones (Fig. 2) (48). The most recent problem with PRP is the emergence of very high-level penicillin resistance (MIC ≥8 µg/mL), whose prevalence increased across the United States from 0.56% in 1995 to 0.87% in 2001 ($p = 0.03$) (51). The epidemiology of penicillin-nonsusceptible strains is very heterogeneous in Europe, as their frequency is high in France (56.7%), Greece (36.4%), and Spain (54.5%) and low in Germany (9.1%), Italy (12.4%), and the United Kingdom (6.7%) (52).

Macrolide resistance is generally increasing among both penicillin-susceptible and penicillin-resistant strains, with variations between geographic areas: in the United States, from 22.4% in the northwestern states to 34.7% in the southcentral ones (53); in Europe, from 10% to 20% in Germany, Greece, and the United Kingdom to 30% to 40% in Italy and Spain, and to more than 50% in France (52). All these high rates of antibiotic resistance are correlated with outpatient antibiotic use (54,55).

Haemophilus influenzae

H. influenzae was uniformly susceptible to ampicillin until the early 1970s, when the first beta-lactamase-producing (BLP) strains appeared. Today, production of plasmid-mediated beta-lactamases is by far the most common mechanism by which

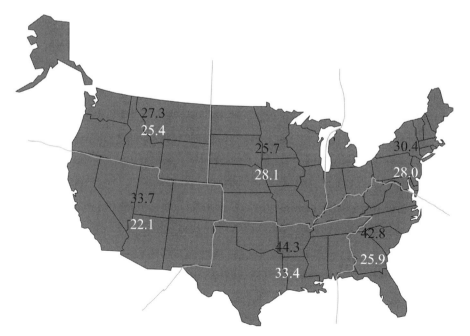

Figure 2   Prevalence (%) of penicillin-resistant *Streptococcus pneumoniae* (*black numbers*) and beta-lactamase-producing *Haemophilus influenzae* (*white numbers*) in the United States. *Source*: From Ref. 48.

H. influenzae acquires resistance to aminopenicillins and partly to former oral cepha-losporins, remaining almost invariably susceptible to beta-lactam/beta-lactamase inhibitor combinations and third-generation cephalosporins.

In the United States, the rate of BLP *H. influenzae* varies from 22.1% in the southwestern states to 33.4% in the southcentral ones (Fig. 2) (48).The epidemiology of BLP *H. influenzae* is very heterogeneous in Europe, as their prevalence is high in France (33.1%), moderate in Spain (19.1%) and the United Kingdom (13.9%), and low in Germany (8.1%), Greece (6.2%), and Italy (8%) (52).

Enteric Gram-Negative Bacilli

Members of the family Enterobacteriaceae are a heterogeneous group of aerobic gram-negative bacilli that include both multiresistant microorganisms (*Enterobacter* spp., *Serratia* spp., and indole-positive *Proteus*) and less "difficult-to-treat" bacteria (*Escherichia coli*, *Klebsiella* spp., and *Proteus mirabilis*), all of which are important agents of infection in the hospital environment and in the immunosuppressed patient. However, even in *E. coli*, in *Klebsiella* spp., and, to a lesser degree, in *P. mirabilis* new resistance determinants have eventually emerged, in particular because of the increasing resistance to third-generation cephalosporins that is mediated by extended-spectrum beta-lactamases (ESBLs). These transferable enzymes conferring resistance to oxymino beta-lactams (third-generation cephalosporins and monobac-tams) and making carbapenems as the therapeutic option of choice were first reported two decades ago in gram-negative bacilli from Europe (56) and, after a few years, from the United States as well (57), and they eventually spread worldwide.

Large ongoing surveillance studies provide us with an updated overview of the global resistance prevalence. The production of ESBLs is currently more frequent in Europe than in North America and more common among *Klebsiella* spp. than among *E. coli* strains (58). For instance, the MYSTIC Programme found ESBL-positive *Klebsiella* isolates in U.S. hospitals to be 6.6% in 2001 and 8.6% in 2003, and simultaneously ESBL-positive *E. coli* decreased from 7.1% to 2.1% (59,60). Between 1997 and 2000, the same multinational study showed that in European hos-pitals the ESBL rate among *E. coli* and *Klebsiella* spp. was 22.1%, with higher values in the eastern countries (29.9%) than in the northern and southern ones and higher percentages among *Klebsiella* spp. (32.8%) than among *E. coli* (14.4%) (61). Between 2001 and 2002, the PEARLS study showed a lower ESBL prevalence among noso-comial pathogens, which was higher in Southern Europe for both *Klebsiella* spp. (25.7%) and *E. coli* (6.6%) than in Northern Europe (5.2% and 1.4%, respectively) (62). At the same time, ESBLs have appeared and spread in *P. mirabilis* as well, reach-ing a prevalence rate of approximately 15% (63).

Resistance associated with the production of chromosomally mediated (AmpC) cephalosporinases among some "difficult-to-treat" Enterobacteriaceae (*Enterobacter* spp. and *Serratia* spp.) is a more widespread and worrying problem than the ESBL-mediated resistance. In Europe, ceftazidime resistance has been observed in 34% of *Enterobacter* spp., 20% of *Citrobacter* spp., and 12% of *Serratia* spp. strains (64), whereas in U.S. hospitals resistance to third-generation cephalosporins among *Enter-obacter* spp. is as high as 20.3%, reaching 26.6% in the intensive care unit (14).

Anaerobes

Like common aerobic bacteria, anaerobes have showed increasing antimicrobial resistance in the recent years as well, primarily with microorganisms of the

Bacteroides fragilis group. For example, in the United States a significant increase in both the geometric mean MICs and the resistance rates for clindamycin and cephamycins (cefoxitin) was observed between 1990 and 1996 (65).

Among the mechanisms of beta-lactam resistance displayed by anaerobes, i.e., production of beta-lactamases, alteration of penicillin-binding proteins, and blocking of the drug penetration into the bacterial cell, the first one is by far the most important (66). The first BLP *B. fragilis* isolate was described by Garrod in 1955 (67), but BLP strains were subsequently found in other *Bacteroides* spp., *Fusobacterium* spp., and *Clostridium* spp.

To date, more than 95% of *B. fragilis* strains are BLP and, therefore, resistant to penicillin and aminopenicillins in both the United States and Europe (68), whereas imipenem, beta-lactam/beta-lactam inhibitor combinations (piperacillin/tazobactam), and metronidazole maintain an in vitro efficacy that is superior to 97% (69). Increasing resistance is showed by *B. fragilis* and *Peptostreptococcus magnus* to clindamycin (13%) and by *Peptostreptococcus anaerobius* to amoxicillin/clavulanate (10%), whereas other both gram-negative (*Prevotella* spp., *Fusobacterium nucleatum*, and *Porphyromonas* spp.) and gram-positive (*Peptostreptococcus micros*) anaerobes are still exquisitely susceptible to beta-lactams, clindamycin, and metronidazole (68).

CLINICAL PRESENTATION OF DEEP FASCIAL SPACE INFECTIONS

These "space infections" most frequently derive from odontogenic foci and include infections of the facial (buccal, canine, masticator, and parotid spaces), suprahyoid (lateral pharyngeal, sublingual, and submandibular spaces), and infrahyoid (pretracheal and retropharyngeal spaces) regions.

Infections of the Facial Region

Infections of the Buccal, Canine, and Masticator Spaces

They generally arise from molar teeth (buccal and masticator spaces) or from maxillary incisor or canine teeth (canine space) and present as major, painful swelling of the relative area: cheek for buccal space, upper lip and canine fossa for canine space, and mandibular region for masticator space. Systemic signs and symptoms are mostly absent. Trismus can be prominent in infections of the masticator space.

The involvement of the temporal space can spread to the whole hemiface including the orbit and produce severe pain and complications (optic neuritis and ocular nerve palsy).

Infection of the Parotid Space

It most often complicates a masseteric space infection with severe pain and swelling of the angle of the jaw, chills, and fever. In turn, it can spread into the infrahyoid region and then into the posterior mediastinum.

Infections of the Suprahyoid Region

Infection of the Lateral Pharyngeal Space

It generally complicates an odontogenic infection or, more rarely, an upper respiratory tract infection (mastoiditis, otitis, parotitis, pharyngitis, and tonsillitis) and can affect either the anterior (prestyloid) or the posterior (retrostyloid) compartment. Infection of the anterior space is mostly suppurative and produces high fever with chills, trismus, marked pain, dysphagia, swelling below the angle of the mandible, and medial bulging of the pharyngeal wall.

Patients with infection of the posterior space are septic and can present severe complications such as dysphagia, edema of the larynx, involvement of the internal carotid artery (erosion and aneurysm formation), and thrombophlebitis of the internal jugular vein. The latter can in turn spread and complicate with metastatic abscesses of bones, brain, joints, liver, lungs, and other sites, and with right-sided endocarditis.

Infections of the Sublingual and Submandibular Spaces

These infections usually occur from mandibular incisor teeth (sublingual) and from the second and third mandibular molar teeth (submandibular), and they present as erythematous and tender swelling of the mouth floor with elevation of the tongue, pain and swelling of the submylohyoid space, and minimal trismus.

Ludwig's angina is a bilateral infection of both sublingual and submandibular spaces that begins in the floor of the mouth and then rapidly and contiguously spreads as an indurated cellulitis without abscess formation and lymphatic involvement. Clinically, the patient presents with a brawny swelling of submandibular spaces and an enlargement of the tongue that can make eating, swallowing, and even breathing very difficult; fever and other systemic toxicities are generally present and often severe. Ludwig's angina and other submandibular space infections can rapidly spread to the neck and thoracic regions such as the laryngeal space (edema of the neck and glottis, stridor, cyanosis, and asphyxiation), the retropharyngeal space, and then the mediastinum (Fig. 3).

Infections of the Infrahyoid Region

Infections of the pretracheal and retropharyngeal spaces arise most commonly from penetrating trauma caused by instrumentation or foreign bodies (i.e., chicken bones). Alternatively, the infection of the retropharyngeal space can occur from distant sites (odontogenic and peritonsillar infections) via the lymphatics. Both infections present with systemic (high fever and chills) and local manifestations (dysphagia, dyspnea); they can complicate with asphyxiation and spread into the mediastinum, where acute necrotizing mediastinitis is characterized by a mortality rate as high as 25%.

Further signs and symptoms of retropharyngeal involvement include neck stiffness, regurgitation, and pain, swelling, and bulging of the posterior pharyngeal wall. Hemorrhage and thrombosis of the jugular vein are other possible complications of this localization (9).

CLINICAL PRESENTATION OF OTHER CERVICAL INFECTIONS

Suppurative Parotitis

Acute bacterial parotitis primarily affects immunosuppressed (dehydrated, elderly, and malnourished) or postoperative patients or subjects with predisposing factors (sialolithiasis, parotid trauma). A tender and painful erythematous swelling around the ear suddenly begins and extends to the angle of the mandible with high fever and

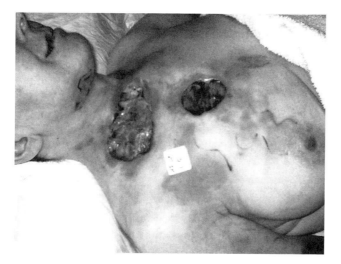

Figure 3 Abscess of the right parotid and submandibular spaces following abscess of the third mandibular molar tooth, and complicated by necrotizing fasciitis of the neck, right supraclavear, and anterior thoracic regions. The patient—a 61-year-old woman with rheumatoid arthritis—was in chronic suppression therapy with the steroid methylprednisolone and the cytotoxic methotrexate. Cultures of both needle aspirate and bioptic specimen from the skin lesions grew numerous colonies of a *Streptococcus anginosus* strain which was sensitive to beta-lactams and resistant to macrolides and clindamycin (personal observation).

chills. This infection can complicate with septicemia, osteomyelitis of the contiguous bones, massive swelling of the neck with asphyxiation, and spread to the infrahyoid region and, consequently, to the posterior mediastinum.

Although staphylococci are by far more prevalent, gram-negative bacilli and anaerobes (*Fusobacterium* spp., peptostreptococci, pigmented *Prevotella* and *Porphyromonas*, and *Propionibacterium acnes*) can cause suppurative parotitis as well (70).

Suppurative Thyroiditis

It can result from hematogenous dissemination or from adjacent sites of infection and is facilitated by predisposing conditions such as goiter, adenoma, or thyroglossal fistula. Thyroiditis can affect one or both lobes and presents as the classical signs of inflammation (erythema, pain, tenderness, and warmth), dysphagia, dysphonia, and systemic toxicity (high fever and chills). Thyroid function tests are mostly normal.

In addition to *S. aureus*, aerobic streptococci and secondarily, gram-negative anaerobes and peptostreptococci can be isolated from patients with suppurative thyroiditis (71).

Peritonsillar Abscess

In the antibiotic era, this suppurative complication of streptococcal tonsillopharyngitis is luckily infrequent and primarily affects young adults. The abscess is generally monolateral and produces high fever, sore throat, dysphagia, trismus, and cervical lymphadenitis. As a complication, airway obstruction or lateral pharyngeal space infection can emerge.

Non-A beta-hemolytic streptococci, *S. aureus*, and anaerobes are other putative agents of peritonsillar abscess.

Acute Epiglottitis

Acute epiglottitis is a nonsuppurative infection of supraglottic structures and epiglottis that can cause a severe airway obstruction. It is very difficult to diagnose in
younger children, whereas older pediatric and adult patients present with sore throat
followed by odynophagia, fever, stridor, and muffled voice. The respiratory obstruction is announced by the appearing of cyanosis and bradycardia and must be treated
by very expert health care workers (physicians and nurses) in a hospital emergency
department.

In developed countries, the incidence of acute epiglottitis has considerably
declined in children since the introduction of the Hib vaccine in the late 1980s to
early 1990s, whereas in the same period it has dramatically increased in adults. In
Israel, for instance, its mean annual incidence rose from 0.88 per 100,000 adult population in 1986—1990 to 2.1 in 1991—1995 and to 3.1 in 1996—2000 ($p < 0.001$). This
increase appeared to be unrelated to *H. influenzae* but related to other bacterial
pathogens (*S. pneumoniae*, *S. aureus*, and *Klebsiella pneumoniae*) (72).

DIAGNOSIS OF CERVICAL INFECTIONS

Laboratory Tests

A moderate to severe leukocytosis with left shift can be found in the vast majority of
deep fascial space and other cervical infections, along with an elevation of the main
laboratory indices of inflammation (erythrocyte sedimentation rate, C-reactive protein, and fibrinogenemia).

The etiologic diagnosis of infection is very important in order to begin a targeted
antibiotic therapy as soon as possible. Special care must be taken for a correct
documentation of anaerobic infections:

- An appropriate collection of specimens, such as needle aspiration of liquid,
  pus, or tissue—which is preferred to swabs,
- An expeditious transportation of specimens to the microbiology laboratory, within 30 minutes if possible, under anaerobic conditions, and
- A careful cultivation in the laboratory—are all of crucial importance for a
  successful isolation of anaerobes.

In addition to culture methods, the Gram stain for direct microscopic examination can provide useful and early information on the etiology of infection (73).

Radiology

In an era of newer and more sensitive and specific diagnostic tools, standard X ray is
of limited value for radiologic diagnosis of cervical infections, although it can be
helpful in selected cases, provided that the patient is in the sitting position with
the neck hyperextended and in inspiration, if possible. So, radiographic views of the
lateral neck demonstrate soft tissue swelling and gas collection within necrotic tissue
in a number of deep fascial space infections; in addition, cervical lordosis and
compression or deviation of tracheal air can be evident in retropharyngeal space

infections, whereas enlargement of the epiglottis, thickening of the aryepiglottic folds, and ballooning of the hypopharynx are classical signs of acute epiglottitis (74).

Ultrasonography can provide further information on gas and, primarily, fluid collections.

CT scanning and MRI are extremely useful in localizing the infection and differentiating an abscess from cellulitis. It shows hypodensity and, in the presence of an abscess, the typical ring enhancement of the inflammatory mass following injection of contrast (Fig. 4) (75).

Radionuclide scanning (technetium bone and gallium- or indium-labeled white blood cells) is particularly helpful for diagnosis of osteomyelitis of the jaws or mandible.

THERAPY OF CERVICAL INFECTIONS

For a proper management of severe cervical infections, both medical (antibiotic) and surgical (debriding, drainage, etc.) therapies are generally required as soon as possible.

The duration of antimicrobial therapy is a critical issue. Normally, antibiotics should be continued for two or three weeks, but if one considers the possible etiologic role of anaerobes, which often produce chronic infections, four weeks of treatment seem to be a reasonable duration.

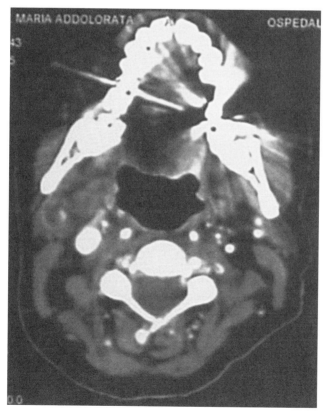

Figure 4 Computed tomography scanning of a 1.5 cm abscess of the right submandibular space (same case as Fig. 3) showing the hypodense center surrounded by the ring enhancement following injection of contrast (personal observation).

Table 1 Criteria Applicable for Switch from Intravenous to Oral
Antibiotic Therapy

Clinically stable patient, who is capable of assuming oral drugs
Identical or similar drug in both parenteral and oral formulations
Documented clinical efficacy after oral administration
High oral bioavailability
No gastrointestinal abnormalities
Good safety
No interactions

The availability of oral antibiotics for switch therapy is another important consideration. After an initial period of parenteral therapy, when a series of conditions are encountered (Table 1) the passage to the oral route of administration for some antibiotics (amoxicillin/clavulanate, chloramphenicol, clindamycin, and metronidazole) is desirable (76).

Empiric Antibiotic Therapy

In the field of antimicrobial chemotherapy for bacterial infections, targeted therapy is the gold standard for a number of reasons, but it is often difficult to obtain an etiologic diagnosis; so physicians must develop an empiric therapy based on the knowledge of both epidemiology of infections and characteristics of antibiotics. Moreover, antimicrobial therapy is initially always empiric, waiting for the results of microbiologic cultures.

Factors to be considered in choosing initial antibiotic therapy are summarized in Table 2 .

The antibacterial spectrum of antibiotics available for therapy of both aerobic and anaerobic infections is shown in Table 3. In summary, beta-lactam/beta-lactamase inhibitor combinations, carbapenems, and, to a lesser degree, cephamycins possess the broadest spectrum of antibacterial activity, being effective against both the main aerobic and anaerobic agents of cervical infections. On the other hand, penicillin is the drug of choice only against non–beta-lactamase–producing anaerobes. Among drugs that are effective against anaerobes, chloramphenicol, clindamycin, metronidazole, and, limitedly to gram-positive bacteria, glycopeptides (vancomycin) can be considered, but only in combination with an antimicrobial agent active against aerobes and as an alternative to the previously cited beta-lactams for allergic patients.

Table 2 Factors to be Considered for an Appropriate Choice of
Antibiotic Therapy

Bactericidal activity
Efficacy against both aerobic and anaerobic microorganisms
No or little ability to induce bacterial resistance
No or little effect on the normal flora
Favorable pharmacokinetics (high drug levels in the infected site)
Good compliance
Minor toxicity
No significant drug interactions
Low costs

Table 3 Aerobic and Anaerobic Antibacterial Spectrum of Some Antibiotics

	Enterobacteriaceae	Gram-positive cocci (no MRSA)	Bacteroides fragilis	Other gram-negative anaerobes	Peptostreptococci	Clostridia
Penicillin	−	+	−	+/+++	+++	+++
Ureido- and carboxy-penicillins	++	++	+	++	+++	+++
Penicillin/beta-lactamase inhibitor	+++	+++	+++	+++	+++	+++
Cephamycins	++	++	+++	+++	+++	++
Carbapenems	+++	+++	+++	+++	+++	+++
Chloramphen.	+	++	+++	+++	+++	+++
Clindamycin	−	++/+++	++	+++	+++	+++
Glycopeptides	−	+++	−	−	+++	+++
Metronidazole	−	−	+++	+++	++	+++

Abbreviation: MRSA, methicillin-resistant *Staphylococcus aureus*.

Table 4 Antibiotic Therapy of Selected Cervical Infections

Infection	Prevalent etiology	Antibiotic therapy
Suppurative parotitis or thyroiditis	*Staphylococcus aureus*	Oxacillin (nafcillin) 2 g every 4 hrs[a] ± rifampin 600 mg every 24 hrs
Peritonsillar abscess	*Streptococcus pyogenes*	Penicillin G, 4 mU every 4 hrs
Acute epiglottitis	*Haemophilus influenzae*	Cefotaxime 2 g every 8 hrs Ceftriaxone 2 g every 24 hrs

[a]Replace oxacillin (nafcillin) with vancomycin in areas with a high prevalence of methicillin-resistant *Staphylococcus aureus.*

Because of their peculiar etiology, some cervical infections require a peculiar antimicrobial treatment (Table 4).

Targeted Antibiotic Therapy

Obviously, the choice of antimicrobial agents for therapy of infections is simplified when culture results are available. In this case, ecologic and economic issues must influence the selection.

Indeed, a narrow-spectrum antibiotic such as penicillin G and oxacillin (nafcillin) is preferable as it induces bacterial resistance with a lower frequency than other drugs do (semisynthetic penicillins, cephalosporins, and carbapenems) and, last but not least, it is much cheaper.

Schedules of targeted antimicrobial therapy for cervical infections are suggested in Table 5, whereas the different antibiotic dosages are summarized in Table 6.

Table 5 Targeted Therapy of Cervical Infections

Microorganism	Suggested therapy	Alternative therapy
Methicillin-susceptible *Staphylococcus aureus*	Oxacillin (nafcillin) ± rifampin	Vancomycin ± rifampin
Methicillin-resistant *S. aureus*	Vancomycin ± rifampin	Linezolid
All streptococci	Penicillin G	Vancomycin
Penicillin-susceptible *Streptococcus pneumoniae*	Penicillin G	Chloramphenicol
Penicillin-intermediate *S. pneumoniae*	High-dose ceftriaxone (cefotaxime)	Vancomycin ± rifampin
Penicillin-resistant *S. pneumoniae*	High-dose ceftriaxone (cefotaxime) + vancomycin	Vancomycin ± rifampin
Clostridia	Penicillin G	Chloramphenicol
Haemophilus influenzae	Ceftriaxone (cefotaxime)	Cotrimoxazole
Enterobacteriaceae	Broad-spectrum cephalosporin[a]	Ciprofloxacin, meropenem
Non-BLP gram-negative anaerobes	Penicillin G	Metronidazole
BLP gram-negative anaerobes	Metronidazole	Clindamycin
Actinomyces spp.	Penicillin G	Clindamycin
Nocardia asteroides	Cotrimoxazole	Imipenem + amikacin

[a]Cefotaxime, ceftriaxone, and cefepime.
Abbreviation: BLP, beta-lactamase-producing.

Table 6   Antibiotic Dosages for Therapy of Cervical Infections

Penicillin G, 4 mU every 4 hrs
Oxacillin (nafcillin), 2 g every 4 hrs
Ampicillin/sulbactam, 3 g every 6 hrs
Amoxicillin/clavulanate, 2.2 g every 8 hrs
Ticarcillin/clavulanate, 3.1 g every 6 hrs
Piperacillin/tazobactam, 4.5 g every 8 hrs
Imipenem, 500 mg every 6 hrs
Meropenem, 1 g every 8 hrs
Cefotetan, 2 g every 12 hrs
Cefoxitin, 2 g every 6 hrs
Cefotaxime, 2 g every 8 hrs
Ceftriaxone, 2 g every 24 hrs
Cefepime, 2 g every 12 hrs
Chloramphenicol, 500 mg every 6 hrs
Clindamycin, 900 mg every 8 hrs
Metronidazole, 500 mg every 6 hrs
Cotrimoxazole, 30 mg/kg every 8 hrs
Rifampin, 600 mg every 24 hrs
Linezolid, 600 mg every 12 hrs
Ciprofloxacin, 400 mg every 12 hrs
Amikacin, 15 mg/kg every 24 hrs
Vancomycin, 500 mg every 6 hrs

Adjunctive Therapy

Surgical therapy plays a role in changing the local environment in order to prevent bacterial (primarily anaerobic) proliferation. This is possible promptly and early by

- Debriding necrotic tissue
- Decompressing soft tissues and closed spaces (i.e., sinuses)
- Draining abscesses
- Relieving obstructions

Other adjunctive therapies (e.g., hyperbaric oxygen) can be useful in individual cases (77).

In infections that can be associated with airway obstruction (Ludwig's angina and acute epiglottitis), a well-timed maintenance of an adequate airway is often required, even by an artificial control; under these circumstances, tracheostomy is generally less traumatic and safer than intubation.

CLINICAL PRESENTATION OF INTRACRANIAL SUPPURATIVE INFECTIONS

Brain Abscess

Predisposing factors to brain abscess and related microbiology are shown in Table 7. The most frequent pathogenetic mechanism for the formation of brain abscess is the spread from a contiguous focus of infection, primarily otitis media and mastoiditis in the extreme ages and sinusitis in the 10- to 30-year age group, and secondarily odontogenic infections. Other mechanisms include hematogenous dissemination from a

Table 7 Predisposing Factors to Brain Abscess and Related Microbiology

Predisposing factor	Preferred localization	Microbiology
Otitis media, mastoiditis	Temporal lobe, cerebellum	Aerobic and anaerobic streptococci, *Bacteroides, Prevotella,* Enterobacteriaceae
Sinusitis	Frontal lobe	Streptococci, *Bacteroides, Haemophilus influenzae,* Enterobacteriaceae, *Staphylococcus aureus*
Dental infection	Frontal and temporal lobes	Anaerobes (streptococci, *Bacteroides, Prevotella, Fusobacterium*)
Pulmonary infection (lung abscess, pleural empyema, cystic fibrosis, bronchiectasis)	Multiple and multiloculated	Anaerobes (streptococci, *Bacteroides, Prevotella, Fusobacterium*), *Actinomyces, Nocardia asteroides*
Cyanotic congenital heart disease (tetralogy of Fallot, transposition of the great vessels)		Streptococci, *H. influenzae*
Bacterial endocarditis		*S. aureus,* streptococci
Post-traumatic (cranial fracture, foreign body, dog bite), postneurosurgical		*S. aureus,* streptococci, Enterobacteriaceae, clostridia
Immune suppression (no HIV infection)		Enterobacteriaceae, *Aspergillus, Candida, Mucorales, N. asteroides*

distant focus of infection (mainly pulmonary), trauma or postneurosurgical proce-dures, and cryptogenic origin (the latter in approximately 20% of cases, although many of these are associated with dental infections) (78). Importantly, in up to 30% of all brain abscesses no obvious source of infection can be determined for a certainty (79).

The onset of symptoms can be abrupt or insidious, with hemicranial or gener-alized headache being the benchmark, present in approximately three-quarters of patients. Most clinical manifestations are caused by brain space–occupying lesions: altered mental status and focal neurologic deficits in more than 50% of cases, nausea, vomiting, and seizures in less than 50%, and nuchal rigidity and papilledema in a minority of patients. Fever is present in approximately half the cases, whereas the classical triad fever, headache, and focal neurologic signs are currently observed in less than 50% of patients (80).

The localization of the abscess obviously modifies the clinical picture. So, frontal lesions most frequently cause headache, lethargy, and other mental status changes; temporal abscesses produce homonymous headache, hemianopsia, and possibly apha-sia; and cerebellar masses determine ataxia, dysmetria, intention tremor, nystagmus, and vomiting. Patients with brain stem abscess generally present with headache, dysphagia, facial weakness, hemiparesis, and vomiting (81).

Subdural Empyema

As in the case of brain abscess, the most frequent pathogenetic mechanism for the formation of subdural empyema is the spread from a contiguous focus of infection, primarily frontal or ethmoidal sinusitis (50–80%) and secondarily otitis media and mastoiditis (10–20%), dental, facial, or scalp infections. Other mechanisms include posttraumatic or postneurosurgical localization and hematogenous dissemination from a distant focus of infection, mainly from the pulmonary district (5%) (82). Consequently, microbiology of subdural empyema consists of pneumococci, *H. influenzae*, Enterobacteriaceae, staphylococci, both anaerobic (peptostreptococci) and microaerophilic (*S. anginosus, S. constellatus*, and *S. intermedius*) streptococci, and *B. fragilis* (83).

Subdural empyema is a rapidly progressive, life-threatening clinical condition most frequently observed in young men and localized over the convexity of the hemisphere. The clinical picture includes symptoms and signs of

- General involvement: high fever with chills
- Increased intracranial pressure: headache (initially localized and, subsequently, often generalized), vomiting, papilledema, altered mental condition, risk of herniation, and death
- Meningeal irritation: nuchal rigidity, positive Kernig's, Brudzinski's, and/or Lasegue's signs
- Focal neurologic signs: most commonly hemiparesis/hemiplegia, but even disphasia, hemianesthesia, ipsilateral hemianopsia, mydriasis, ocular palsies, cerebellar signs (ataxia, dysmetria, and nystagmus), and either focal or generalized seizures (84)

The complications of subdural empyema, such as venous sinus thrombosis and brain abscess, are potentially devastating (85).

Subdural empyema resulting from complications of craniotomy is usually subacute, with a protracted course and a frequent absence of focal neurologic signs (86).

Epidural Abscess

The pathogenesis and microbiology of epidural abscess are generally identical to those aforementioned for subdural empyema, with virtually all cases following frontal sinusitis, mastoiditis, or craniotomy (87).

The onset of epidural abscess is generally insidious and masked by the preexisting sinusal or mastoid infection. The clinical picture, essentially comprised of headache, is much more indolent than in subdural empyema, unless deeper intracranial extension (with major neurologic signs) or abscess enlargement (with signs of elevated intracranial pressure) develops. Osteomyelitis of the overlying bone is often present (88).

Septic Intracranial Thrombophlebitis

Suppurative thrombophlebitis of venous sinuses usually follows infection of the paranasal sinuses, middle ear, mastoid, face, or oropharynx, and it secondarily complicates other intracranial infections, and occasionally it can spread from more distant sites (i.e., pulmonary). Clinical presentation, microbiology, and sinuses affected vary with predisposing factors.

Sinusitis and infections of the face or mouth promote septic thrombosis of the cavernous sinus, which is caused by streptococci, Enterobacteriaceae, staphylococci, and anaerobes. The altered venous drainage produces periorbital edema, hexophthalmos, papilledema, visual loss, and headache, whereas dysfunction of the third to sixth cranial nerve determines diplopia, ocular palsies, ptosis and proptosis, photophobia, lachrymation, chemosis, reduced pupillary reactivity and corneal reflex, and weakness of ocular muscles. Meningismus and change in mental status can be present, and fever is prominent. The onset is generally acute or chronic in cases secondary to facial infection or sinusitis, respectively.

Thrombophlebitis of the lateral sinus is most often associated with otitis media and mastoiditis, and etiologic agents include streptococci, Enterobacteriaceae, and anaerobes. Patients predominantly complain of headache, fever, and, because of the ear involvement, earache with edema over the mastoid (Griesinger's sign), vertigo, and vomiting. The frequent fifth and sixth nerve palsy produces homonymous facial pain with altered sensation and lateral rectus muscle weakness (Gradenigo's syndrome). Papilledema and other signs of increased intracranial pressure appear if the contralateral sinus is also compromised.

Septic thrombosis of the superior sagittal sinus can complicate an infection of the face or scalp and cause bilateral leg weakness followed by arm weakness, and increased intracranial pressure with hydrocephalus, papilledema, and altered mental status.

Finally, thrombophlebitis of the petrosal sinuses can derive from otitis media or mastoiditis and produce Gradenigo's syndrome (89).

DIAGNOSIS OF INTRACRANIAL SUPPURATIVE INFECTIONS

Laboratory Tests

An elevation of white blood cell count, erythrocyte sedimentation rate, and C-reactive protein is generally encountered in patients with brain abscess, subdural empyema, or epidural abscess. Blood cultures are positive only in 30% of patients (90), but they should always be collected, even in the absence of fever, as these noninvasive procedures can provide information of fundamental importance. Indeed, a significant percentage of cases can be polymicrobial in nature (91).

Lumbar puncture is contraindicated because of the risk of cerebral herniation. Moreover, there is recent evidence that lumbar puncture can cause cerebral venous thrombosis by decreasing blood flow velocity in veins or dural sinus (92). Lastly, even if performed, lumbar puncture only gives aspecific information: increased opening pressure, elevated protein concentration, slightly reduced or normal glucose concentration, and moderate neutrophil pleocytosis. Cerebrospinal fluid (CSF) culture can be positive in up to 40% of patients (90,93).

As for cervical infections, the etiologic diagnosis is very important in order to begin a targeted antibiotic therapy as soon as possible. The most appropriate surgical techniques for collecting purulent material are described below (see Section "Adjunctive therapy").

Radiology

The advent of cross-sectional imaging (CT and MRI) has revolutionized the diagnosis of intracranial suppurative infections and made angiographic and radionuclide techniques obsolete because of its high sensitivity and specificity (94). However, it is important to remember that concomitant steroid therapy can decrease the sensitivity of those newer radiologic methods.

Brain Abscess

In patients with brain abscess, CT scanning typically shows a round lesion with a hypodense center and a peripheral ring-enhancement capsule after injection of the contrast, surrounded by an usually large, hypodense area of cerebral edema. The sensitivity of CT is greater than 95%, whereas its specificity is a little lower, as the characteristic lesion appears with neoplasms, brain infarction, and hematomas as well. Further CT findings in the case of brain abscess include nodular enhancement and low attenuation zones, primarily in the early cerebritis phase. Other important uses of CT scanning include the follow-up of abscesses and the guidance for stereotactic aspiration in order to obtain material for microbiologic diagnosis.

MRI is even more sensitive and specific than CT, particularly for early detection of cerebritis, satellite lesions, and brain edema. T_1-weighted images display a typically hypointense center of the abscess and an isointense to mildly hyperintense capsule that becomes resolutely hyperintense following administration of the contrast agent gadolinium (Fig. 5); T_2-weighted images show a hyperintense center and a hypointense capsule of the abscess with a surrounding area of edema as a marked high signal intensity (Fig. 6) (95).

In the case of inconclusive results with both CT and MRI, scintigraphy with ^{111}In-radiolabeled leukocytes can be useful because of their tendency to accumulate in zones of active inflammation. This technique is highly accurate, giving false-positive results only in the presence of necrotic neoplasms and false-negative results after the concomitant use of steroids (96).

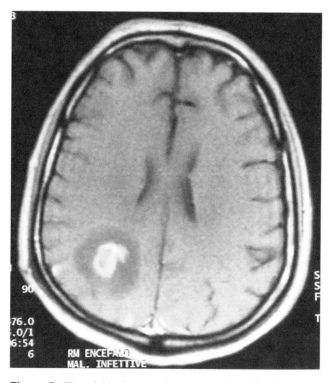

Figure 5 T_1-weighted magnetic resonance imaging (MRI) of a right occipital abscess showing a hypointense center with a hyperintense capsule following administration of the contrast agent gadolinium and hypointense surrounding edema (personal observation).

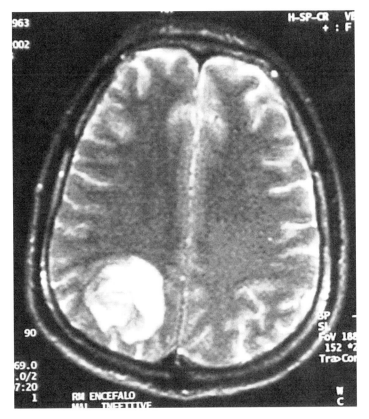

Figure 6 T$_2$-weighted MRI of a right occipital abscess (same case as Fig. 5) showing a hyperintense center with a hypointense capsule of the abscess and a hyperintense area of surrounding edema (personal observation).

Subdural Empyema and Epidural Abscess

In subjects with subdural empyema, CT scanning with contrast shows a hypodense, sometimes multiloculated area that is often associated with displacement of the adjacent structures due to mass effect and is surrounded by an intense enhancement (Fig. 7). MRI with gadolinium contrast is currently the procedure of choice as it is morphologically superior to CT, primarily in identifying small fluid collections, empyemas of the base or along the falx cerebri, or the infrequent localizations in the posterior fossa (Figs. 8–10) (97).

Also in epidural abscess, MRI with gadolinium enhancement is superior to CT, revealing the epidural collection of pus as a thick, superficial, and limited zone of reduced density (98).

Septic Intracranial Thrombophlebitis

Both CT scanning and MRI typically reveal filling defects in the sinus vessels, with MRI being considerably more sensitive and specific. Newer noninvasive imaging techniques with angiography (CT and MRI venography) have demonstrated a higher sensitivity in showing the typical filling defects and are more and more used for both initial evaluation and follow-up control (99).

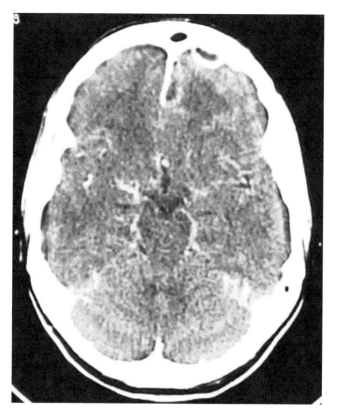

Figure 7 Computed tomography scanning of a left frontal subdural empyema with extension to the left side of the anterior falx cerebri that is slightly displaced to right. The hypodense center is surrounded by an intense enhancement. This patient is a 17-year-old girl with subdural empyema following left frontal, ethmoidal, and mascellar sinusitis (personal observation).

In all these infections, the usefulness of both CT and MRI also consists of evaluating adjacent structures (paranasal sinuses, middle ear, and mastoid) and detecting concomitant cerebral edema and infarction, hemorrhage, etc. (Fig. 11).

THERAPY OF INTRACRANIAL SUPPURATIVE INFECTIONS

As in the case of severe cervical infections, urgent medical and surgical therapy is generally required (except for septic thrombophlebitis) in order to (i) facilitate abscess sterilization by antibiotics; (ii) provide purulent material for bacterial cultures; and (iii) control increased intracranial pressure. However, in selected patients, especially those with epidural abscess or with an early and/or small (no larger than 2.5 cm) brain abscess or subdural empyema, it is possible to use antibiotics alone, provided that antimicrobial therapy is prolonged up to 12 weeks, and noninvasive imaging (MRI) is repeated in order to control the evolution of infection. Multiple and/or deep-sided abscesses, concomitant meningitis, and preexisting conditions that increase surgical risk are important contraindications to surgery (100).

In the field of suppurative intracranial infections, it is of fundamental importance that antibiotics are not only active against the putative pathogens, but even

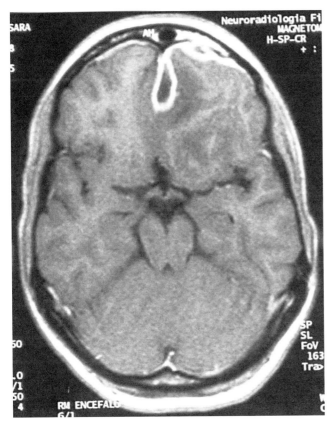

Figure 8 T_1-weighted MRI of left frontal multiloculated subdural empyema (same case as Fig. 7) showing a hypointense center with a hyperintense capsule following administration of the contrast agents gadolinium, a hypointense surrounding edema, and displacement of the adjacent structures (personal observation).

capable of penetrating the abscess or empyema. Antibiotic penetration of the blood–brain barrier (BBB) is even more variable than penetration of the blood–CSF barrier, and it is affected by a number of factors such as molecular weight, lipid solubility, level of ionization, protein binding, and drug interactions (101). The following considerations can be made:

- Among broad-spectrum agents, aminoglycosides have a very poor penetration of the BBB, whereas beta-lactams [in particular, third- and fourth-generation cephalosporins and carbapenems (meropenem)] generally achieve fair to good concentrations, provided that high doses are used;
- Among antibiotics that are active against anaerobes, chloramphenicol and, first of all, metronidazole, penetrate the BBB better than clindamycin does;
- Among agents that are effective against difficult-to-treat gram-positive cocci, the drug concentrations achievable with glycopeptides (vancomycin) cannot be sufficiently high, especially if corticosteroids are concomitantly used, whereas the new oxazolidinones (linezolid) penetrate the BBB very well, although they are only bacteriostatic.

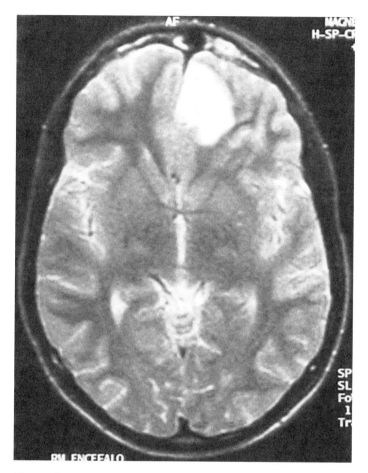

Figure 9 T$_2$-weighted MRI of left frontal multiloculated subdural empyema showing a hyperintense center with a hypointense capsule of the abscess, and a large hyperintense area of surrounding edema displacing the adjacent structures (personal observation).

Also the duration of antimicrobial therapy is a critical issue. A six- to eight-week course of high-dose parenteral antibiotics has traditionally been recommended, often followed by oral therapy for two to six months, although the efficacy of this long additional therapeutic period has not been demonstrated. Three- to four-week courses are believed to be generally appropriate for patients undergoing surgical excision of the abscess. The rare brain abscesses caused by *Nocardia asteroides* should be treated for up to one year (79).

Empiric Antibiotic Therapy

Once purulent material has been collected for microbiologic as well as histopathologic purposes, empiric antimicrobial therapy should be started based on the predisposing conditions and related microbiology (Table 8). In the vast majority of cases, the combination of a beta-lactam antibiotic (penicillin G or, better, a third-generation cephalosporin) with an antianaerobic (metronidazole) agent is a very effective and safe treatment (102).

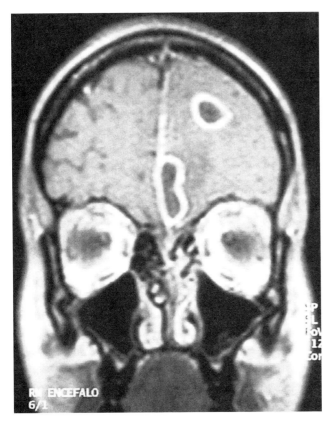

Figure 10 T$_1$-weighted MRI of left frontal multiloculated subdural empyema complicated by brain abscess in coronal projection (personal observation).

Vancomycin and linezolid are the preferred antistaphylococcal agents in patients allergic to penicillins and where a methicillin-resistant strain is likely (see Section "Bacterial Resistance to Antibiotics"), otherwise oxacillin (or nafcillin) must be preferred.

Targeted Antibiotic Therapy

The same considerations and schedules of targeted antimicrobial therapy for cervical infections (see above and Table 6) are valid for intracranial suppurative complications as well. However, suggested daily dosages of third-generation cephalosporins and meropenem are higher than normal: cefotaxime, 8 g in four doses; ceftriaxone, 4 g in two doses; and meropenem, 6 g in three doses.

Adjunctive Therapy

Surgical drainage is required for most patients with brain abscess, subdural empyema, and epidural abscess. Either stereotactic CT-guided aspiration after burr hole placement or complete excision after craniotomy may be performed. Currently, the latter procedure is no longer preferred, primarily in early cases, because of the availability of accurate and safe aspiration techniques; however it is of choice in particular cases, i.e., posterior fossa localization, multiloculated or not resolving abscesses, or where

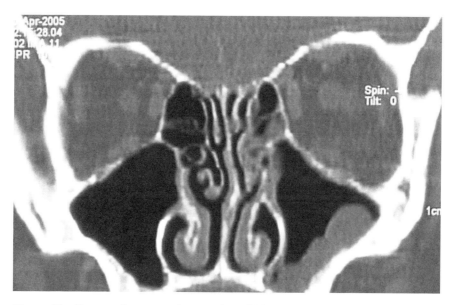

Figure 11 Computed tomography scanning of left ethmoidal and mascellar sinusitis complicated by left subdural empyema (same case as Fig. 7). Inflammatory effusion can be seen both
along the alveolar border of the left mascellar sinus and in the left ethmoidal cells (personal
observation).

Table 8 Empiric Antibiotic Therapy of Suppurative Intracranial Infections

Predisposing condition	Probable organisms	Suggested initial regimen
Sinusitis, otitis media, mastoiditis	Aerobic, microaerophilic, and anaerobic streptococci, gram-negative anaerobes, *Staphylococcus aureus*, Enterobacteriaceae	Broad-spectrum cephalosporin[a] + metronidazole ± vancomycin[b]
Trauma, cranial surgery	Staphylococci (often methicillin-resistant), Enterobacteriaceae	Broad-spectrum cephalosporin[a,c] + vancomycin
Dental infection	All anaerobes, streptococci	Penicillin G + metronidazole
Pulmonary infection	Gram-negative anaerobes, streptococci, *Actinomyces, Nocardia asteroides*	Penicillin G + metronidazole ± cotrimoxazole[d]
Bacterial endocarditis	Staphylococci, streptococci	Vancomycin + gentamicin
Congenital heart disease	Streptococci, *Haemophilus influenzae*	Broad-spectrum cephalosporin[a]
Unknown		Broad-spectrum cephalosporin[a] + metronidazole ± vancomycin

[a]Cefotaxime, ceftriaxone, cefepime.
[b]If methicillin-resistant *Staphylococcus aureus* is suspected.
[c]Ceftazidime or cefepime if *Pseudomonas aeruginosa* is suspected.
[d]If *Nocardia asteroides* is suspected.

aspiration has failed (103,104). Concomitant surgical therapy of the primary infection (sinusitis, otitis media, and mastoiditis) can be necessary as well.

The use of corticosteroids (a short course of dexamethasone at the dosage of 0.15 mg/kg of body weight every six hours) for control of increased intracranial pressure and its life-threatening complications (i.e., cerebral herniation) remains controversial: reduced antibiotic entry into the abscess, impaired clearance of certain pathogens, and delay in the encapsulation process are important clues that argue against their use. Antiepilectic drugs (carbamazepine, phenytoin, and phenobarbital) are generally appropriate in order to prevent the appearance or recurrence of seizures, even after surgery (79).

In patients with septic intracranial thrombophlebitis, the use of anticoagulants has always been controversial, but based upon recent limited evidence, anticoagulation appears to be safe, associated with a potential reduction in the risk of death, and not complicated by significant thrombocytopenia or major hemorrhage (105). Preliminary results indicate that thrombolytic agents can have a promising role in adjunctive therapy of septic intracranial thrombophlebitis, but randomized controlled trials are needed in order to verify their efficacy and safety in this field (106).

REFERENCES

1. Time Magazine. February 25, 1966.
2. Chow AW. Life-threatening infections of head, neck, and upper respiratory tract. In: Hall JB, Schmidt GA, Wood LDHM, eds. Principles of Critical Care. 2nd ed. New York: McGraw-Hill, 1998:887–902.
3. Chow AW. Life-threatening infections of the head and neck. Clin Infect Dis 1992; 14(5): 991–1002.
4. Heilpern KL, Lorber B. Focal intracranial infections. Infect Dis Clin North Am 1996; 10(4):879–898.
5. Rosenblum ML, Joff JT, Norman D, et al. Decreased mortality from brain abscesses since advent of computed tomography. J Neurosurg 1978; 49(5):658–668.
6. Progress toward eliminating *Haemophilus influenzae* type b disease among infants and children—United States, 1987–1997. MMWR 1998; 47(46):993–998.
7. Roscoe DL, Chow AW. Normal flora and mucosal immunity of the head and neck. Infect Dis Clin North Am 1988; 2(1):1–19.
8. Yao ES, Lamont RJ, Leu SP, et al. Interbacterial binding among strains of pathogenic and commensal oral bacterial species. Oral Microbiol Immunol 1996; 11(1):35–41.
9. Chow AW. Infections of the oral cavity, neck, and head. In: Mandell GL, Bennett JE, Dolin R, eds. Mandell, Douglas, and Bennett's Principles and Practice of Infectious Diseases. Vol. 1, 5th ed. Philadelphia: Churchill Livingstone, 2000:689–702.
10. Valenti WM, Trudell RB, Bentley DW. Factors predisposing to oropharyngeal colonization with gram-negative bacilli in the aged. N Engl J Med 1978; 298(20):1108–1111.
11. Kirby W. Extraction of a highly potent penicillin inactivator from penicillin resistant staphylococci. Science 1944; 99:452–453.
12. Barber M, Rozwadowska-Dowzenko M. Infection by penicillin-resistant staphylococci. Lancet 1948; 2(6530):641–644.
13. Finland M. Changing patterns of resistance of certain common pathogenic bacteria to antimicrobial agents. N Engl J Med 1955; 252(14):570–580.
14. National Nosocomial Infections Surveillance (NNIS) System Report. Data summary from January 1992 through June 2003, issued August 2003. Am J Infect Control 2003; 31(8):481–498.

15. Chambers HF. The changing epidemiology of *Staphylococcus aureus*? Emerg Infect Dis 2001; 7(2):178–182.

16. Jevons MP. "Celbenin"-resistant staphylococci. Br Med J 1961; Vol. 1(5219):124–125.

17. Barrett FF, McGehee RF, Finland M. Methicillin-resistant *Staphylococcus aureus* at Boston City Hospital: bacteriologic and epidemiologic observations. N Engl J Med 1968; 279(9):441–448.

18. Panlilio AL, Culver DH, Gaynes RP, et al. Methicillin-resistant *Staphylococcal aureus* in U.S. hospitals, 1975–1991. Infect Control Hosp Epidemiol 1992; 13(10):582–586.

19. Charlebois ED, Perdreau-Remington F, Kreiswirth B, et al. Origins of community-acquired strains of methicillin-resistant *Staphylococcus aureus*. Clin Infect Dis 2004; 39(1): 47–54.

20. Tiemersma EW, Bronzwaer SLAM, Lyytikäinen O, et al. Methicillin-resistant *Staphylococcus aureus* in Europe, 1999–2002. Emerg Infect Dis 2004; 10(9):1627–1634.

21. Zinn CE, Westh H, Rosdahl VT, et al. An international multicenter study of antimicrobial resistance and typing of hospital *Staphylococcus aureus* isolates from 21 laboratories in 19 countries or states. Microb Drug Resist 2004; 10(2):160–168.

22. Drinka PJ, Gauerke C, Le D. Antimicrobial use and methicillin-resistant *Staphylococcus aureus* in a large nursing home. J Am Med Dir Assoc 2004; 5(4):256–258.

23. Rosenberg J. Methicillin-resistant *Staphylococcus aureus* (MRSA) in the community: who's watching? Lancet 1995; 346(8968):132–133.

24. Palavecino E. Community-acquired methicillin-resistant *Staphylococcus aureus* infections. Clin Lab Med 2004; 24(2):403–418.

25. Centers for Disease Control. Community-acquired methicillin-resistant *Staphylococcus aureus* infections—Michigan. MMWR 1981; 30(16):185–187.

26. Dietrich DW, Auld DB, Mermel LA. Community-acquired methicillin-resistant *Staphylococcus aureus* in Southern New England children. Pediatrics 2004; 113(4):347–352.

27. Baggett HC, Hennessy TW, Rudolph K, et al. Community-onset methicillin-resistant *Staphylococcus aureus* associated with antibiotic use and the cytotoxin Panton-Valentine leukocidin during a furunculosis outbreak in rural Alaska. J Infect Dis 2004; 189(9): 1565–1573.

28. Buckingham SC, McDougal MK, Cathey LD, et al. Emergence of community-associated methicillin-resistant *Staphylococcus aureus* at a Memphis, Tennessee children's hospital. Pediatr Infect Dis J 2004; 23(7):619–624.

29. Centers for Disease Control and Prevention. Community-associated methicillin-resistant *Staphylococcus aureus* infections in Pacific islanders—Hawaii, 2001–2003. MMWR 2004; 53(33):767–770.

30. Stemper ME, Shukla SK, Reed KD. Emergence and spread of community-associated methicillin-resistant *Staphylococcus aureus* in rural Wisconsin, 1989 to 1999. J Clin Microbiol 2004; 42(12):5673–5680.

31. Campbell KM, Vaughn AF, Russell KL, et al. Risk factors for community-associated methicillin-resistant *Staphylococcus aureus* infections in an outbreak of disease among military trainees in San Diego, California, in 2002. J Clin Microbiol 2004; 42(9):4050–4053.

32. Baillargeon J, Kelley MF, Leach CT, et al. Methicillin-resistant *Staphylococcus aureus* infection in the Texas prison system. Clin Infect Dis 2004; 38(9):e92–e95.

33. Kazakova SV, Hageman JC, Matava M, et al. A clone of methicillin-resistant *Staphylococcus aureus* among professional football players. N Engl J Med 2005; 352(5): 468–475.

34. Hiramatsu K, Hanaki H, Ino T, et al. Methicillin-resistant *Staphylococcus aureus* clinical strain with reduced vancomycin susceptibility. J Antimicrob Chemother 1997; 40(1): 135–136.

35. Waldvogel FA. New resistance in *Staphylococcus aureus*. N Engl J Med 1999; 340(7): 556–557.

36. Centers for Disease Control and Prevention. *Staphylococcus aureus* resistant to vancomycin—United States, 2002. MMWR 2002; 51(26):565–567.

37. Diekema DJ, Pfaller MA, Schmitz FJ, et al. Survey of infections due to *Staphylococcus* species: frequency of occurrence and antimicrobial susceptibility of isolates collected in the United States, Canada, Latin America, Europe, and the Western Pacific region for the SENTRY Antimicrobial Surveillance Program, 1997–1999. Clin Infect Dis 2001; 32(suppl 2):S114–S132.

38. Cantón R, Loza E, Morosini MI, et al. Antimicrobial resistance among isolates of *Streptococcus pyogenes* and *Staphylococcus aureus* in the PROTEKT antimicrobial surveillance programme during 1999–2000. J Antimicrob Chemother 2002; 50(suppl S1): 9–24.

39. Mallaval F-O, Carricajo A, Delavenna F, et al. Detection of an outbreak of methicillin-resistant *Staphylococcus aureus* with reduced susceptibility to glycopeptides in a French hospital. Clin Microbiol Infect 2004; 10(5):459–461.

40. Hiramatsu K, Aritaka N, Hanaki H, et al. Dissemination in Japanese hospitals of strains of *Staphylococcus aureus* heterogeneously resistant to vancomycin. Lancet 1997; 350(9092): 1670–1673.

41. Song J-H, Hiramatsu K, Suh JY, et al. Emergence in Asian countries of *Staphylococcus aureus* with reduced susceptibility to vancomycin. Antimicrob Agents Chemother 2004; 48(12):4926–4928.

42. Goldstein FW, Kitzis MD. Vancomycin-resistant *Staphylococcus aureus*: no apocalypse now. Clin Microbiol Infect 2003; 9(8):761–765.

43. Horn DL, Zabriskie JB. Why have group A streptococci remained susceptible to penicillin? Report on a symposium. Clin Infect Dis 1998; 26(6):1341–1345.

44. Bisno AL, Stevens DL. *Streptococcus pyogenes* (including streptococcal toxic shock syndrome and necrotizing fasciitis). In: Mandell GL, Bennett JE, Dolin R, eds. Mandell, Douglas, and Bennett's Principles and Practice of Infectious Diseases. Vol. 2. 5th ed. Philadelphia: Churchill Livingstone, 2000:2101–2117.

45. Granizo JJ, Aguilar L, Casal J, et al. *Streptococcus pyogenes* resistance to erythromycin in relation to macrolide consumption in Spain (1986–1997). J Antimicrob Chemother 2000; 46(6):959–964.

46. Bergman M, Huikko S, Pihlajamäki M, et al. Effect of macrolide consumption on erythromycin resistance in *Streptococcus pyogenes* in Finland in 1997–2001. Clin Infect Dis 2004; 38(9):1251–1256.

47. Prieto J, Calvo A, Gómez-Lus ML. Antimicrobial resistance: a class effect? J Antimicrob Chemother 2002; 50(suppl S2):7–12.

48. Brown SD, Rybak MJ. Antimicrobial susceptibility of *Streptococcus pneumoniae, Streptococcus pyogenes* and *Haemophilus influenzae* collected from patients across the USA, in 2001–2002, as part of the PROTEKT US study. J Antimicrob Chemother 2004; 54(suppl S1):i7–i15.

49. Hansman D, Bullen MM. A resistant pneumococcus. Lancet 1967; 2(7509):264–265.

50. Jacobs MR, Koornhof HJ, Robins-Browne RM, et al. Emergence of multiply resistant pneumococci. N Engl J Med 1978; 299(14):735–740.

51. Schrag SJ, McGee L, Whitney CG, et al. Emergence of *Streptococcus pneumoniae* with very-high-level resistance to penicillin. Antimicrob Agents Chemother 2004; 48(8): 3016–3023.

52. Jones ME, Blosser-Middleton RS, Critchley IA, et al. In vitro susceptibility of *Streptococcus pneumoniae, Haemophilus influenzae* and *Moraxella catarrhalis*: a European multicenter study during 2000–2001. Clin Microbiol Infect 2003; 9(7):590–599.

53. Farrell DJ, Jenkins SG. Distribution across the USA of macrolide resistance and macrolide resistance mechanisms among *Streptococcus pneumoniae* isolates collected from patients with respiratory tract infections: PROTEKT US 2001–2002. J Antimicrob Chemother 2004; 54(suppl S1):i17–i22.

54. Bronzwaer SLAM, Cars O, Buchholz U, et al. A European study on the relationship between antimicrobial use and antimicrobial resistance. Emerg Infect Dis 2002; 8(3): 278–282.

55. Albrich WC, Monnet DL, Harbarth S. Antibiotic selection pressure and resistance in *Streptococcus pneumoniae* and *Streptococcus pyogenes*. Emerg Infect Dis 2004; 10(3):514–517.
56. Shah PM, Stille W. *Escherichia coli* and Klebsiella pneumoniae strains more susceptible to cefoxitin than to third generation cephalosporins. J Antimicrob Chemother 1983; 11(6):597–598.
57. Jacoby GA, Medeiros AA, O'Brien TF, et al. Broad-spectrum, transmissible beta-lactamases. N Engl J Med 1988; 319(11):723–724.
58. Winokur PL, Canton R, Casellas JM, et al. Variations in the prevalence of strains expressing an extended-spectrum beta-lactamase phenotype and characterization of isolates from Europe, the Americas, and the Western Pacific region. Clin Infect Dis 2001; 32(suppl 2):S94–S103.
59. Rhomberg PR, Jones RN, Sader HS, et al. Results from the Meropenem Yearly Susceptibility Test Information Collection (MYSTIC) Programme: report of the 2001 data from 15 United States medical centres. Int J Antimicrob Chemother 2004; 23(1):52–59.
60. Rhomberg PR, Jones RN, Sader HS, et al. Antimicrobial resistance rates and clonality results from the Meropenem Yearly Susceptibility Test Information Collection (MYSTIC) Programme: report of the year five (2001). Diagn Microbiol Infect Dis 2004; 49(4): 273–281.
61. Jones RN, Pfaller MA, the MYSTIC Study Group. Antimicrobial activity against strains of *Escherichia coli* and *Klebsiella* spp. with resistance phenotypes consistent with an extended-spectrum β-lactamase in Europe. Clin Microbiol Infect 2003; 9(7):708–712.
62. Bouchillon SK, Johnson BM, Hoban DJ, et al. Determining incidence of extended-spectrum β-lactamase producing Enterobacteriaceae, vancomycin-resistant *Enterococcus faecium* and methicillin-resistant *Staphylococcus aureus* in 38 centers from 17 countries: the PEARLS study 2001–2002. Int J Antimicrob Agents 2004; 24(2):119–124.
63. Mutnick AH, Turner PJ, Jones RN. Emerging antimicrobial resistance among *Proteus mirabilis* in Europe: report from the MYSTIC Program (1997–2001). J Chemother 2002; 14(3):253–258.
64. Pfaller MA, Jones RN, MYSTIC Study Group (Europe). Antimicrobial susceptibility of inducible AmpC β-lactamase-producing Enterobacteriaceae from the Meropenem Yearly Susceptibility Test Information Collection (MYSTIC) Programme, Europe 1997–2000. Int J Antimicrob Agents 2002; 19(5):383–388.
65. Snydman DR, Jacobus NV, McDermott LA, et al. Multicenter study of in vitro susceptibility of the *Bacteroides fragilis* group, 1995 to 1996, with comparison of resistance trends from 1990 to 1996. Antimicrob Agents Chemother 1999; 43(10):2417–2422.
66. Nord CE. Mechanisms of β-lactam resistance in anaerobic bacteria. Rev Infect Dis 1986; 8(suppl 5):S543–S548.
67. Garrod LP. Sensitivity of four species of *Bacteroides* to antibiotics. Br Med J 1955; 2(4955):1529–1531.
68. Koeth LM, Good CE, Appelbaum PC, et al. Surveillance of susceptibility patterns in 1297 European and US anaerobic and capnophilic isolates to co-amoxiclav and five other antimicrobial agents. J Antimicrob Chemother 2004; 53(6):1039–1044.
69. Hedberg M, Nord CE, ESCMID Study Group on Antimicrobial Resistance in Anaerobic Bacteria. Antimicrobial susceptibility of *Bacteroides fragilis* group isolates in Europe. Clin Microbiol Infect 2003; 9(6):475–488.
70. Brook I. Acute bacterial suppurative parotitis: microbiology and management. J Craniofac Surg 2003; 14(1):37–40.
71. Brook I. Microbiology and management of acute suppurative thyroiditis in children. Int J Pediatr Otorhinolaryngol 2003; 67(5):447–451.
72. Berger G, Landau T, Berger S, et al. The rising incidence of adult acute epiglottitis and epiglottic abscess. Am J Otolaryngol 2003; 24(6):374–383.
73. Brook I. Anaerobic bacteria in upper respiratory tract and other head and neck infections. Ann Otol Rhinol Laryngol 2002; 111(5 Pt 1):430–440.

74. Rotta AT, Wiryawan B. Respiratory emergencies in children. Respir Care 2003; 48(3): 248–258.

75. Lee SS, Schwartz RH, Bahadori RS. Retropharyngeal abscess: epiglottitis of the new millennium. J Pediatr 2001; 138(3):435–437.

76. Jewesson P. Cost-effectiveness and value of an IV switch. Pharmacoeconomics 1994; 5(suppl 2):20–26.

77. Brook I. Management of anaerobic infection. Expert Rev Anti-infect Ther 2004; 2(1): 89–94.

78. Wispelwey B, Dacey RG Jr., Scheld WM. Brain abscess. In: Scheld WM, Whitley RJ, Durack DT, eds. Infections of the Central Nervous system. 2nd ed. Philadelphia: Lippincott-Raven, 1997:463–493.

79. Mathisen GE, Johnson JP. Brain abscess. Clin Infect Dis 1997; 25(4):763–779.

80. Tunkel AR, Wispelwey B, Scheld WM. Brain abscess. In: Mandell GL, Bennett JE, Dolin R, eds. Mandell, Douglas, and Bennett's Principles and Practice of Infectious Diseases. Vol. 1. 5th ed. Philadelphia: Churchill Livingstone, 2000:1016–1028.

81. Tunkel AR, Scheld WM. Bacterial infections of the central nervous system. In: Hall JB, Schmidt GA, Wood LDHM, eds. Principles of Critical Care. 2nd ed. New York: McGraw-Hill, 1998:853–870.

82. Dill SR, Cobbs CG, McDonald CK. Subdural empyema: analysis of 32 cases and review. Clin Infect Dis 1995; 20(2):372–386.

83. Nathoo N, Nadvi SS, van Dellen JR. Intracranial subdural empyemas in the era of computed tomography: a review of 699 cases. Neurosurgery 1999; 44(3):529–536.

84. Bleck TP, Greenlee JE. Subdural empyema. In: Mandell GL, Bennett JE, Dolin R, eds. Mandell, Douglas, and Bennett's Principles and Practice of Infectious Diseases. Vol. 1. 5th ed. Philadelphia: Churchill Livingstone, 2000:1028–1031.

85. Krauss WE, McCormick PC. Infections of the dural spaces. Neurosurg Clin North Am 1992; 3(2):421–433.

86. Bockova J, Rigamonti D. Intracranial empyema. Pediatr Infect Dis J 2000; 19(8): 735–737.

87. Dolan RW, Chowdhury K. Diagnosis and treatment of intracranial complications of paranasal sinus infections. J Oral Maxillofac Surg 1995; 53(9):1080–1087.

88. Bleck TP, Greenlee JE. Epidural abscess. In: Mandell GL, Bennett JE, Dolin R, eds. Mandell, Douglas, and Bennett's Principles and Practice of Infectious Diseases. Vol. 1. 5th ed. Philadelphia: Churchill Livingstone, 2000:1031–1034.

89. Bleck TP, Greenlee JE. Suppurative intracranial phlebitis. In: Mandell GL, Bennett JE, Dolin R, eds. Mandell, Douglas, and Bennett's Principles and Practice of Infectious Diseases. Vol. 1. 5th ed. Philadelphia: Churchill Livingstone, 2000:1034–1036.

90. Tattevin P, Bruneel F, Clair B, et al. Bacterial brain abscesses: a retrospective study of 94 patients admitted to an intensive care unit (1980 to 1999). Am J Med 2003; 115(2): 143–146.

91. Bernardini GL. The diagnosis and management of brain abscess and subdural empyema. Curr Neurol Neurosci Rep 2004; 4(6):448–456.

92. Canhao P, Batista P, Falcao F. Lumbar puncture and dural sinus thrombosis—a causal or casual association? Cerebrovasc Dis 2005; 19(1):53–56.

93. Yang SY. Brain abscess: a review of 400 cases. J Neurosurg 1981; 55(5):794–799.

94. Osenbach RK, Loftus CM. Diagnosis and management of brain abscess. Neurosurg Clin North Am 1992; 3(2):403–420.

95. Zimmerman RA, Girard NJ. Imaging of intracranial infections. In: Scheld WM, Whitley RJ, Durack DT, eds. Infections of the Central Nervous System. 2nd ed. Philadelphia: Lippincott-Raven Publishers, 1997:923–944.

96. Rehncrona S, Brismar J, Holtas S. Diagnosis of brain abscess with indium-111 labeled leukocytes. Neurosurgery 1985; 16(1):23–36.

97. Greenlee JE. Subdural empyema. Curr Treat Options Neurol 2003; 5(1):13–22.

98. Bleck TP. Imaging in the diagnosis of CNS infections. In: Mandell GL, Bennett JE, Dolin R, eds. Mandell, Douglas, and Bennett's Principles and Practice of Infectious Diseases Updates. Vol. 4. 4th ed. New York: Churchill Livingstone, 1995:1–13.

99. Schwarz S, Daffertshofer M, Schwarz T, et al. Current controversies in the diagnosis and management of cerebral venous and dural sinus thrombosis. Nervenarzt 2003; 74(8): 639–653.

100. Carpenter JL. Brain stem abscesses: cure with medical therapy, case report, and review. Clin Infect Dis 1994; 18(2):219–226.

101. Yogev R, Bar-Meir M. Management of brain abscesses in children. Pediatr Infect Dis J 2004; 23(2):157–159.

102. Jansson AK, Enblad P, Sjolin J. Efficacy and safety of cefotaxime in combination with metronidazole for empirical treatment of brain abscesses in clinical practice: a retrospective study of 66 consecutive cases. Eur J Clin Microbiol Infect Dis 2004; 23(1):7–14.

103. Shahzadi S, Lozano AM, Bernstein M, et al. Stereotactic management of bacterial brain abscess. Can J Neurol Sci 1996; 23(1):34–39.

104. De Falco R, Scarano E, Cigliano A, et al. Surgical treatment of subdural empyema: a critical review. J Neurosurg Sci 1996; 40(1):53–58.

105. Stam J, De Bruijn SF, DeVeber G. Anticoagulation for cerebral sinus thrombosis. Cochrane Database Syst Rev 2002; (4):CD002005.

106. Canhao P, Falcao F, Ferro JM. Thrombolytics for cerebral sinus thrombosis: a systematic review. Cerebrovasc Dis 2003; 15(3):159–166.

8

Severe Community-Acquired Pneumonia in the Critical Care Unit

Burke A. Cunha

Infectious Disease Division, Winthrop-University Hospital, Mineola, and State University of New York School of Medicine, Stony Brook, New York, U.S.A.

INTRODUCTION

Severe community-acquired pneumoniae (CAP) can present as mild, moderate, or severe pneumonia. Patients with severe CAP require hospital admission and usually are admitted to the critical care unit (CCU). Patients with severe CAP in the CCU are those with compromised respiratory function requiring ventilatory support. The clinical presentation of severe CAP occurs in both normal and compromised hosts. In immunocompetent patients, severe CAP is severe because of the underlying cardiopulmonary status of the patient. Although some pathogens are inherently more virulent than others, e.g., *Legionella* is more virulent than *Moraxella catarrhalis*, clinical severity is primarily determined by host rather than microbial factors. A patient with good cardiopulmonary function may present with severe CAP with Legionnaires' disease, and a patient with severe chronic obstructive pulmonary disease (COPD) with *M. catarrhalis* CAP will present as a severe pneumonia. Patients with asplenia, although not strictly normal hosts, are usually considered as a variant of normal host. Patients with various degrees of hyposplenism if they have pneumonia, usually present as severe CAP. In contrast, compromised hosts in the usual sense refer to patients with congenital or acquired severe immune defects, e.g., human immunodeficiency virus (HIV) (1–3).

As patients presenting with severe CAP may occur in normal or compromised patients, and due to a variety of diseases, the clinical approach depends on determining the pre-admission cardiopulmonary status, degree of splenic dysfunction, and identifying the disorders associated with specific immune defects. This analysis of host defense defects is usually done by history combined with the chest X-ray appearance and arterial blood gas determinations (1,4).

Empiric therapy depends upon predicting the usual pathogens related to specific immune defects in compromised hosts. Antimicrobial coverage in normal hosts with impaired cardiopulmonary function is the same as in normal hosts with normal cardiopulmonary function. A cardinal principle of empiric antimicrobial therapy in the CCU is that severe CAP is treated the same as nonsevere CAP in terms of antibiotic selection. Patients with severe CAP in the CCU are initially treated intravenously. Therapy is usually continued as the diagnostic workup is in progress. Therapy for severe pneumonia is usually two to three weeks in total (5,6).

DETERMINANTS OF SEVERE CAP

Microbial Factors

Microorganisms causing CAP exhibit a spectrum of clinical severity ranging from mild to severe. The clinical spectrum of *Streptococcus pneumoniae* CAP ranges from mild in young ambulatory adults, to fulminating, overwhelming sepsis in asplenics. *M. catarrhalis* in a patient with severe COPD presents as severe CAP. Because of advanced lung disease and even low virulence organisms, e.g., *M. catarrhalis* may decrease already compromised respiratory function. Host factors, not microbial virulence are the key determinants of severe CAP.

Secondary bacteremias reflect the bacteremic potential of the organism and are not per se a marker of clinical severity. Bacteremia frequently accompanies *S. pneumoniae* or *Haemophilus influenzae* CAP and is not related to severity (7,8).

Pulmonary Factors

Elderly adults with decreased lung function have diminished pulmonary reserve, readily compromised by superimposed pneumonia. The added burden of CAP easily causes respiratory decompensation. In patients with advanced lung disease and borderline pulmonary function, any organism causing CAP may manifest as severe CAP. The functional capacity of the lungs is a key determinant of severe CAP (1,3,4).

Cardiac Factors

If cardiac function is borderline, cardiac decompensation is frequent in patients with CAP. The fever of pneumonia that increases heart rate per minute may be enough to precipitate congestive heart failure (CHF). Heart rate increases 10 beats/min for every degree (Fahrenheit) of temperature elevation above normal. Fever often precipitates CHF, increasing the apparent clinical severity of pneumonia. Cardiac decompensation also results in diminished oxygenation secondary to decreased ejection fraction in patients with CAP. Decreases in pO_2 in patients with advanced cardiac disease can adversely affect cardiac function (1,4).

Cardiopulmonary Factors

Heart and lungs are physiologically interrelated and decompensation in one will adversely affect the other. Elderly patients often have both lung and heart disease. Elderly patients with CAP and limited cardiopulmonary reserve, usually present as severe CAP requiring critical care admission/ventilatory support (1–4).

CLINICAL APPROACH TO SEVERE CAP

Normal Hosts

Normal hosts presenting with CAP are invariably those with impaired cardiac or respiratory function. The most common clinical conditions included are CHF, cardiomyopathy, or severe valvular disease among the cardiac causes. The most

Table 1 Determinants of Severe Community-Acquired Pneumonia

Pathogen related factors	*Host defense factors*
Inoculum size	Impaired B-lymphocyte function (HI)
Highly virulent organisms	Disorders associated with ↓ HI
Streptococcus pneumoniae	SLE
Klebsiella pneumoniae	Multiple myeloma
Francilla tularensis	Cirrhosis
Bacillus anthracis	Hyposplenia
Avain influenza	Asplenia
Pulmonary factors	Impaired T-lymphocyte function (CMI)
Decreased functional lung capacity	Disorders associated with ↓ CMI
(emphysema)	T-cell lymphomas
Advanced lung disease	High dose/chronic steroid therapy
(chronic bronchitis)	Immunosuppressive therapy
	HIV
Cardiac factors	Impaired combined B/T lymphocyte function
CHF	Disorders associated with ↓ HI/CMI
Severe valvular disease	CLL
Cardiomyopathy	SLE with flare
CAD	SLE with flare/immunosuppressive therapy
	Advanced age
Systemic factors	
Advanced age (CNS/esophageal	
dysfunction)	
Hepatic insufficiency	
Uremia	

Abbreviations: HI, humoral immunity; CMI, cellular mediated immunity; CHF, congestive heart failure; SLE, systemic lupus erythematous; HIV, human immunodeficiency virus; CNS, central nervous system; CAD, coronary artery disease; CLL, chronic lymphocytic leukemia.

common respiratory causes are COPD, bronchiectasis, interstitial pulmonary disease, and pulmonary fibrosis. These conditions are readily recognizable by history because these are, in the main, chronic conditions. The analysis of the chest X-ray pattern also complements the history and physical examination in determining the nature and severity of impaired lung and/or cardiac function. Importantly, if the clinical presentation of severe CAP in the CCU occurs in patients with good cardiopulmonary function, the clinician should analyze the patient from the perspective of having an immune defect to explain the severity of the clinical presentation (Table 1) (1,4).

Determining Probable Pathogens by Recognizing Disorders with Specific Immune Defects

In compromised hosts presenting with CAP, the clinician should determine whether the patient is likely to have a common or unusual pathogen causing pneumonia. Compromised hosts, like normal patients, may be infected with the usual array of community-acquired pathogens, but may present as severe CAP due to their underlying defect. Compromised patients with disorders that are associated with specific immune defects predispose to a narrow, not wide, range of potential pathogens causing pneumonia. Physicians often reason in error because the patient is a compromised host and the range of pathogens is wide. In point of fact, it is narrow because the range of pathogens is limited by the host-specific immune defect. For example, patients with multiple myeloma who have CAP are particularly prone to develop CAP due to encapsulated typical bacterial pathogens not viruses, Rickettsia, or parasitic infections. If the clinician has determined by history or laboratory tests that the patient has multiple myeloma, then the pathogens are predictable and are not extensive or unusual. The clinical approach, therefore, rests on the relationship between the disorders, which determines the immune defect. The immune defect in turn determines the range of potential pathogens. The range of potential pathogens determines what is antimicrobial coverage for the immunocompromised patient with severe CAP in the CCU (9,10).

Disorders Associated with Impaired HI

The disorders associated with impaired B-lymphocyte function are those that decrease humoral immunity (HI). Regardless of the disorder with underlying B-lymphocyte defect, the pathogens predisposed to by impaired B-lymphocyte function are the same. The pathogens causing pneumonia associated with impaired HI are the encapsulated pulmonary pathogens, i.e., *S. pneumoniae* and *H. influenzae*. The disorders that commonly encounter the clinical practice associated with impaired HI include hyposplenia/asplenia, multiple myeloma, alcoholic cirrhosis, systemic lupus erythematous (SLE), and CLL (a combined B/T-lymphocyte disorder with primarily impaired HI). There is insufficient time for pneumonia to develop in these critically ill patients with overwhelming sepsis. The more common clinical scenarios are patients with various degrees of hyposplenism that do not present with sepsis and do have sufficient time to present as severe CAP. The pathogen range of hyposplenic function may be inferred from either X-ray evidence of intra-abdominal pathology decreasing splenic blood flow or displacing function parenchyma of the spleen. The degree of hyposplenism may be inferred from the complete blood count (CBC) by noting the concentration of Howell-Jolly bodies in the peripheral smear. The number of Howell-Jolly bodies is inversely proportional to the degree of splenic function. The most common clinical presentation of hyposplenism is an "apparently normal" host with good cardiopulmonary function that presents inexplicably with severe CAP. Severe CAP is not a random occurrence, but always has an underlying cardiopulmonary or immunologic explanation. Patients with multiple myeloma or CLL may be diagnosed by previous history, findings on the peripheral blood smear/bone marrow examination, as well as other specific diagnostic studies. Patients presenting with CAP and hypotension/shock have either impaired splenic function, influenza, and *S. aureus* pneumonia, or CAP with an unrelated systemic disorder causing hypotension/shock. Normal hosts with CAP do not present with hypotension/shock (Tables 2 and 3) (1,2,4,11–16).

Disorders Associated with Impaired CI

Patients with impaired cellular immunity (CI) or cell-mediated immunity (CMI) are those with impaired T-lymphocyte or macrophage function. Impaired disorders associated with impaired CMI predispose to intracellular pathogens, i.e., viruses, *Rickettsiae*, systemic mycoses, and intracellular bacteria. However, the entire range of potential pathogens that may affect patients with impaired CMI are not those that are frequently associated with pneumonia, i.e., Herpes simplex virus, cytomegalovirus (CMV), Rocky Mountain Spotted fever, *Listeria*, etc. The systemic mycoses causing pneumonias may occur in normal hosts after inhalation exposure, e.g., histoplasmosis

Table 2 Diagnostic Approach to CAP with Hypotension/Shock

Infectious causes	Noninfectious plus infectious causes
CAP with hyposplenia	MI with CAP
CAP with asplenia	GI bleed with CAP
Severe human Avian influenza	Pancreatitis with CAP
Post-influenza S.aures	Severe lung disease with CAP
(MSSA/CA-MRSA)	Severe CAD, cardiomyopathy, valvular
	disease with CAP

Abbreviations: CAP, community-acquired pneumonia; CAD, coronary artery disease; CA-MRSA, community acquired MRSA.
Source: From Refs. 1, 4.

may occur after endogenous reactivation in the presence of decreased CMI. Therefore, the usual pathogens associated with pneumonia in patients with decreased CMI are *Pneumocystis* (carinii) *jiroveci* (PCP) pneumonia, CMV pneumonia, and *Legionella* pneumonia. The most commonly encountered conditions associated with decreased CMI include chronic high dose corticosteroid therapy, immunosuppressive therapy, organ transplants, and HIV. As mentioned previously, CLL is an example of an acquired combined B/T-lymphocyte defect with moderately impaired CMI (6,17).

Disorders Associated with Both Impaired Humoral and CI

Most of the disorders that have combined defects excluding CLL are those that represent an underlying B-lymphocyte disorder combined with a drug that decreases CMI. Common examples include inflammatory bowel disease treated with monoclonal antibody therapy, various arthritis treated with steroids or immunosuppressives, etc. A good example of appreciating the subtleties of layered and combined immune defects is in the patient who presents with SLE. SLE itself is a pure B-lymphocyte defect. Patients with SLE that flare resemble CLL and have a predominantly impaired HI with a component of decreased CMI. Lastly, patients with SLE with flare and receiving therapy with corticosteroids/immunosuppressive therapy represent predominantly a T-lymphocyte defect not unlike transplant patients. The infectious disease consultant can be invaluable in assessing patients with multiple or combined defects in the CCU setting, because an accurate assessment defines differential diagnostic possibilities and points to appropriate empiric therapy. It would be superficial to consider all SLE patients as those having pure lymphocyte defects because the patients with flare and/or immunosuppressive therapy change radically the nature of the host defense effects (1,4,17).

Table 3 Disorders Associated with Functional/Anatomic Hyposplenia

Splenectomy	Ulcerative colitis
Congenital asplenia	Celiac disease
Splenic atrophy	Amyloidosis
Impaired splenic blood flow	Graft versus host disease
Sickle cell anemia	Rheumatoid arthritis
Hemoglobin SC disease	SLE
Infiltrative disorders of the spleen	Cirrhosis

Abbreviations: SLE, systemic lupus erythematous.
Source: From Refs. 1, 4.

CLINICAL APPROACH TO SEVERE CAP BY CHEST X-RAY PATTERN AND DEGREE OF HYPOXEMIA

Patients that are normal hosts without significant pre-existing lung disease usually present with segmental or lobar defects with or without pleural effusion. Pleural effusion is dependent upon the pathogen and would be most common with Group A streptococci CAP and less common with *H. influenzae* CAP and uncommon with *S. pneumoniae* CAP. Ill-defined infiltrates due to atypical organisms, i.e., *Mycoplasma pneumoniae*, only present as severe CAP in patients with host defense defects. *Legionella* may affect normal or patients with impaired CMI and presents characteristically as a rapidly progressive bilateral asymmetric pulmonic process. It is the behavior of the infiltrates rather than the location or description of the infiltrates per se that suggests the possibility of *Legionella* CAP.

Excluding *Legionella* bilaterality, bilateral pulmonary infiltrates, which are primarily perihilar and interstitial, are not a feature the common typical or atypical pulmonary pathogens. Bilateral interstitial infiltrates suggest an intracellular pathogen, e.g., PCP or CMV, etc. Bilateral interstitial infiltrates presenting as severe pneumonia that are not a mimic of pneumonia are always due to intracellular pathogens, either viruses or PCP, that typically is an infection of the interstitium causing an oxygen diffuse defect across the alveolar membrane. A combination of bilateral perihilar interstitial infiltrates, hypoxemia, and a $\downarrow$ DLco/$\uparrow$ A-a gradient (>30) all point to an interstitial process typical of PCP or CMV. There are many noninfectious mimics of pneumonia that may present with bilateral infiltrates that are not on an infectious basis. The common mimics of pneumonia encountered in the CCU include acute pulmonary edema, multiple pulmonary emboli/infarcts, lupus pneumonitis, pulmonary vasculitis, pulmonary drug effects, bronchiolitis obliterans–organizing pneumonia (BOOP), pulmonary leukostasis, pulmonary hemorrhage, and acute respiratory distress syndrome (ARDS). It is of critical importance to remember that with the exception of viral pneumonia and PCP, the pathogens presenting as severe CAP are not caused by the pathogens presenting with severe CAP. Severe bacterial pneumonias, fungal pneumonias, and Rickettsial pneumonias may be accompanied by impressive pulmonary infiltrates but are *not* accompanied by profound diffusion defects, i.e., $\downarrow$ pO$_2$/$\downarrow$ DLco/$\uparrow$ A-a gradient (>30) (Table 4) (6,18).

Disorders Associated with Decreased PMN Function

Most disorders associated with neutropenia are the result of chemotherapy. When the peripheral PMN count drops below $1\,K/mm^3$, the probability of infection increases greatly. Patients with neutropenia are predisposed to *Pseudomonas aeruginosa* bacteremia or Candidemia. Patients with prolonged neutropenia also are predisposed to *Aspergillus* and other fungal infections. Patients with neutropenia do not ordinarily present with pneumonia even though their PMN counts are very low, but present with bacteremia or fungemia (6,19).

Severe CAP Accompanied by Cavitation

The presence of cavitation on the chest X-ray or computed tomography chest scan is an important diagnostic clue to the etiology of the pulmonic infectious process. Pneumonias with cavitation tend to be severe because they represent a necrotic invasive pulmonary process. Severe CAP that presents with cavitation may be

Table 4 Diagnostic Approach to Bilateral Diffuse Pulmonary Infiltrates

Without oxygen diffusion defect (N/↓ pO$_2$/N A-a gradient)	With profound oxygen diffusion defect (↓↓↓ pO$_2$/↑ A-a gradient >30)
Aspiration pneumonia	PCP
Pulmonary edema/LHF	CMV
Pulmonary hemorrhage	HSV-1
Typical bacterial pneumonitis	HHV-6
Atypical bacterial pneumonitis	Influenza
Advanced pulmonary tuberculosis	RSV
Fungal pneumonias	ARDS
Rickettsial pneumonias	BOOP
Parasitic pneumonias[a]	
Radiation pneumonitis	
Pulmonary drug reaction	
Noncardiogenic pulmonary edema	
Leukostasis	

[a]Excluding PCP.
Abbreviations: ARDS, acute respiratory distress syndrome; BOOP, bronchiolitis obliterans–organizing pneumonia; CMV, cytomegalovirus; HSV, herpes simplex virus; PCP, *Pneumocystis (carinii) jiroveci* pneumonia; LHF, left heart failure; HHV, human herpes virus; RSV, respiratory syncytial virus.
Source: From Ref. 6.

approached clinically by the rapidity of the cavitary process. Cavitation within 72 hours in a patient with pneumonia is limited to *S. aureus* or *S. aeruginosa* pneumonias. Patients with *S. aureus* pneumonias are almost always those that follow viral influenza pneumonia. The presentation of influenza pneumonia is that of a viral pneumonia or may be accompanied simultaneously by pulmonary infiltrates usually due to *S. aureus*. The third clinical presentation of viral pneumonia is for an initial viral influenza presentation followed by a period of improvement followed subsequently by superimposed focal or segmental pneumonia usually due to *S. pneumoniae* or *H. influenzae*. Therefore, in a patient who presents with viral influenza pneumonia during the influenza season, the chest X-ray is unremarkable even though oxygen diffusion defects are present but pulmonary infiltrates are virtually absent in the early phases. If such a patient has pulmonary infiltrates, then a superimposed bacterial pneumonia is the working diagnosis. Because *S. pneumoniae* and *H. influenzae* usually follow a period of improvement and are not accompanied by cavitation, the diagnostic possibilities of an influenza presentation with rapid cavitation within 24 hours limit the diagnosis to superimposed *S. aureus* pneumonia. *Pseudomonas* pneumonia is rare and nearly always fatal, and it occurs only in the setting of chronic bronchiectasis or cystic fibrosis. Normal hosts do not present with *P. aeruginosa* CAP. Patients presenting with bilateral interstitial infiltrates and a diffusion defect may have a noninfectious disorder, i.e., BOOP or ARDS. If the etiology of the infiltrate is infectious, the differential diagnosis is limited to PCP or viral causes. One of the common clinical scenarios in a nonorgan transplant patient presenting with CAP is a HIV patient with PCP/CMV. In transplant patients or those with impaired CI, CMV pneumonia may present as an isolated clinical entity as severe CAP. However, in the HIV patient, PCP is the predominant cause of the patient's diffusion defect and CMV is a secondary or suppressed pathogen, which may be demonstrated as an incidental finding in three quarters of the patients with PCP and HIV. The bystander role of CMV is indicated by the fact that if the PCP is treated in an HIV patient, the patient gets well and the CMV does not require separate treatment as it does in a transplant patient with CMV pneumonia (1,17).

Cavitation occurring after three to five days points to *K. pneumoniae* as the pathogen. *K. pneumoniae* occurs almost exclusively in patients with chronic alcoholism. Therefore, the clinical history plus the speed of cavitation will point to the diagnosis, which is easily confirmed by gram stain/culture of the sputum and/or blood cultures. The *K. pneumoniae* CAP typically presents as severe CAP. Cavitation after five to seven days is associated with aspiration pneumonia. Such patients will not present as severe CAP unless the aspiration is bilateral and massive, or if the aspiration is more limited but superimposed upon limited pulmonary function. These patients usually present with pneumonia that becomes more severe as cavitation becomes apparent after the first week of hospitalization. In massive bilateral aspiration, severe CAP is the usual clinical presentation (19,20).

Empiric Therapy for CAP

Appropriate empiric therapy depends upon identifying the most likely pathogen in the patient presenting with severe CAP in the CCU. The pathogen is determined primarily by host factors. The presentation of severity may be manifested by focal and segmental infiltrates unaccompanied by diffusion defect or bilateral interstitial infiltrates with or without accompanying oxygen diffusion defect. The patient's history is important in identifying previously diagnosed disorders that are associated with specific immune defects that, combined with the X ray presentation and the presence or absence of profound hypoxemia, helps limit differential diagnosis possibilities (10,21–23).

A patient presenting with severe CAP, who is apparently a normal host with focal or segmental infiltrates, should be treated for the usual typical and atypical pathogens causing CAP. Therapy should be started as soon as the diagnosis of CAP is made (20,24).

Normal hosts presenting with near normal chest X-ray and profound hypoxemia should be considered as having viral influenza or PCP. If the severe pneumonia occurs during influenza season, then influenza is a likely, diagnostic possibility. If the CAP occurs during spring, summer, or fall, then PCP is likely, particularly if accompanied by isolated cytopenias. PCP is becoming more common as more people in the general population develop HIV. PCP is an HIV-defining illness and is not an infrequent pulmonary presentation for HIV. The influenza patient is treated with antivirals, and antimicrobial therapy is not needed unless there is simultaneous infection with *S. aureus* or subsequent infection due to *S. pneumoniae* or *H. influenzae*. PCP should be treated initially with TMP-SMX or pentamidine accompanied by steroids as the diagnostic work up is in progress. Patients who are on steroids or immunosuppressive therapy, as well as organ transplants, may present with focal or segmental pneumonias that are not accompanied by diffusion defects. Bacterial pathogens should be covered empirically in these patients, even though the diagnostic work up proceeds to exclude such causes as *Aspergillus*. Because the number of fungal pathogens is extensive, a tissue biopsy is needed upon which to base specific antifungal therapy. Immunosuppressed patients/organ transplants presenting with bilateral symmetrical interstitial infiltrates may be approached in two categories, i.e., those with an oxygen diffusion defect and those without an oxygen diffusion defect. In such patients, the absence of a diffusion defect suggests pulmonary hemorrhage,

Table 5 Clinical Approach to Community-Acquired Pneumoniae in Compromised Hosts

Host defense defect	Infiltrate	Onset	Oxygen diffusion defect: ↓ pO₂/ ↑ A-a gradient (>30)	Diagnostic test	Likely diagnosis	Empiric therapy
None/ ↓ HI	Focal/segmental	Acute	−	Sputum/blood cultures	Typical/atypical pneumonia	"Respiratory quinolone" or β-lactam+doxycycline
↓ CMI	Focal/segmental	Acute	−	Sputum/blood cultures	Typical/atypical pneumonia	"Respiratory quinolone" or β-lactam+doxycycline
	Bilateral diffuse	Acute	+	Cysts in trans bronchial biopsy	PCP	TMP-SMX atoragone, or pentamidine
				BAL + for CMV cytology	CMV	Ganciclovir or valgangciclovir
				Sputum DFA	Influenza A	Oseltamivir + either amantadine or rimantadine
↓ HI/CMI	Focal/segmental	Subacute/chronic	−	Sputum + for AFB	Tuberculosis	INH, rifampin, ethambutol, PZA
				Lung biopsy	Nocardia	TMP-SMX or minocycline
				Lung biopsy	Aspergillus	Caspofungin or voriconazole
	Bilateral diffuse	Subacute/chronic	+	Sputum DFA or serology or cytology on bronchoscopy	HSV-1, CMV, RSV, HHV-6	HSV (acyclovir), CMV (ganciclovir or valgansadovir), RSV (ribaririn).

Abbreviations: HI, humoral immunity; CMI, cellular mediated immunity; CMV, cytomegalovirus; HSV, herpes simplex virus; AFB, acid-fast bacilli; PCP, BAL, bronchoalveolar lavage; DFA, direct fluorescent antibody; RSV, respiratory syncytial virus; HHV, human herpes virus; PZA, pyrazinamide; TMP-SMX, trimethoprim-sulfametoxozole.

Source: From Refs. 1, 6, 20.

pulmonary embolus, or another noninfectious process. In this patient group, with bilateral infiltrates accompanied by a profound oxygen diffusion defect, viral pneumonias and PCP are the most likely diagnostic infectious possibilities. Noninfectious causes of oxygen defects and bilateral pulmonary infiltrates include BOOP and ARDS, which should be relatively straightforward diagnoses (Table 5) (6,17,20).

In conclusion, the clinician should not use a "shot gun" approach to treating patients with severe CAP, because of the mistaken notion that there are many diagnostic possibilities. The diagnostic process is concerned with limiting diagnostic possibilities to one or two possible etiologies based on a syndromic analysis of the history, physical, and laboratory abnormalities, as well as the chest X-ray appearance and the presence or absence of an oxygen diffusion defect. Except in patients with decreased CMI, focal or segmental defects may be treated the same as in normal hosts with antibiotics that are active against typical and atypical pathogens. No unusual organisms will be missed using this approach. Patients with decreased CMI are more complex and may also present with the pathogens that affect the normal population. If patients with decreased CMI present with an acute, severe CAP, then the same therapeutic approach is used as in normal patients, i.e., use an antibiotic, e.g., respiratory quinolone or combination therapy that is effective against both typical and atypical pathogens. Usually the focal and segmental infiltrates in patients with decreased CMI are subacute or chronic, and they do not usually become diagnostic problems in the setting of severe CAP. The patients developing focal infiltrates due to *Aspergillus* do so over weeks rather than days.

Clinicians should be aware of the noninfectious mimics of pneumonia both in the normal and compromised hosts. The mimics of pneumonia can usually be excluded by history and routine laboratory tests. Transbronchial or open lung biopsy is necessary when analysis fails or the patient is not responding to appropriate antimicrobial therapy. Compromised hosts respond more slowly than normal hosts to appropriate therapy. Normal hosts with severe CAP may show improvement in three to five days, but compromised hosts may take a week or more to show improvement. The duration of therapy in compromised hosts is necessarily longer because of their impaired host defenses. Normal hosts are usually treated for 10 to 14 days, whereas pneumonias in the compromised host are often treated for two to three weeks (20–22).

The prognosis in CAP is a function of the same determinants that make CAP severe, i.e., host factors. Delay in therapy can make the prognosis worse (25–30).

REFERENCES

1. Cunha BA. Severe community-acquired pneumonia: determinants of severity and approach to therapy. Infect Med 2005; 22:53–58.
2. Moine P, Vercken J-P, Chevret S, et al. Severe community-acquired pneumonia. Chest 1994; 105:1487–1495.
3. Lim WS, van der Eerden M, et al. Defining community acquired pneumonia severity on presentation to hospital: an international derivation and validation study. Thorax 2003; 58:377–382.
4. Cunha BA. Severe community-acquired pneumonia. Crit Care Clin 1998; 14:105–118.
5. Recognizing and managing severe community-acquired pneumonia. Br J Hosp Med. 2006; 67:76–78.
6. Cunha BA. Pulmonary infections in the compromised host. Infect Dis Clin 2001; 16:591–612.

7. van Riemsdijk, van Overbeeke IC, van den Berg B. Severe Legionnaire's disease requiring intensive care treatment. Neth J Med 1996; 49:185–188.
8. Janssens JP, Gauthey L, Hermmann F, et al. Community-acquired pneumonia in older patients. J Am Geriatr Soc 1996; 44:539–544.
9. Dean NC, Silver MP, Bateman KA, et al. Decreased mortality after implementation of a treatment guideline for community-acquired pneumonia. Am J Med 2001; 110:451–457.
10. Cunha BA. Community-acquired pneumonias: reality revisited. Am J Med 2000; 108: 436–437.
11. Wara DW. Host defense against *Streptococcus pneumoniae*: the role of the spleen. Rev Infect Dis 1981; 3:299.
12. Cunha BA. Infections in acutely ill non-leukopenic compromised hosts with diabetes mellitus, SLE, asplenia, or on steroids. Crit Care Clin 1998; 8:263–282.
13. Gopal V, Bisno AL. Fulminant pneumococcal infection in "normal" asplenic hosts. Arch Intern Med 1977; 137:1526.
14. Cunha BA. Community-acquired pneumonias in SLE. J Crit Illness 1997; 13:779–783.
15. Jong GM, Hsiue TR, Chen CR, et al. Rapidly fatal outcome of bacteremic *Klebsiella* pneumonia in alcoholics. Chest 1995; 107:214–217.
16. Johnson DH, Cunha BA. Infections in alcoholic cirrhosis. Infect Dis Clin 2001; 16:363–372.
17. Cunha BA. Community-acquired pneumonia in HIV patients. Clin Infect Dis 1999; 28: 410–411.
18. Cunha BA. Severe community-acquired pneumonia. J Crit Illness 1997; 12:711–721.
19. Cunha BA. Differential diagnosis of pneumonia. In: Brandstetter R, Cunha BA, Keretsky M, eds. The Pneumonias. New Jersey: Medec Books, Oradell:1993.
20. Cunha BA, Essentials of Antimicrobial Therapy (5th Ed) Birmingham, Michigan: Physicians Press, 2006.
21. Cunha BA. Empiric therapy of community-acquired pneumonia. Chest 2004; 125:1913–1919.
22. Cunha BA. Antibiotic treatment of severe community-acquired pneumonia. Semin Respir Crit Care Med 2000; 21:61–69.
23. Cunha BA. Clinical relevance of penicillin resistant *Streptococcus pneumoniae*. Semin Respir Infect 2002; 17:204–214.
24. Heath CH, Grove DI, Looke DF. Delay in appropriate therapy of *Legionella* pneumonia associated with increased mortality. Eur J Clin Microbiol Infect Dis 1996; 5:286–290.
25. MacFarlane JT, Finch RG, Ward MJ, et al. Hospital study of adult community-acquired pneumonia. Lancet 1982; 2:255–258.
26. Klimek JJ, Ajemian E, Fontecchio S, et al. Community-acquired bacterial pneumonia requiring admission to hospital. Am J Infect Control 1983; 11:79–82.
27. Leroy O, Santré C, Beuscart C, et al. A five-year study of severe community-acquired pneumonia with emphasis on prognosis in patients admitted to an intensive care unit. Intensive Care Med 1995; 21:24–31.
28. Angus DC, Marrie TJ, Obrosky DS, et al. Severe community-acquired pneumonia. Am J Respir Crit Care Med 2002; 166:717–723.
29. Martinez FJ. Monotherapy versus dual therapy for community-acquired pneumonia in hospitalized patients. Clin Infect Dis 2004; 38:328–340.
30. Cunha BA. Empiric antibiotic therapy for community-acquired pneumonia: guidelines for the perplexed? Chest 2004; 125:1913–1921.

9
Nosocomial Pneumonia in the Critical Care Unit

Emilio Bouza
Clinical Microbiology and Infectious Diseases Department, Hospital General Universitario "Gregorio Marañón," Universidad Complutense, Madrid, Spain

Almudena Burillo
Department of Clinical Microbiology, Hospital Madrid-Montepríncipe, Madrid, Spain

María V. Torres
Clinical Microbiology and Infectious Diseases Department, Hospital General Universitario "Gregorio Marañón," Universidad Complutense, Madrid, Spain

OVERVIEW

Introduction

Nosocomial pneumonia or hospital-acquired pneumonia (HAP) is defined as pneumonia that appears 48 hours or more after hospitalization. In this definition, it is assumed that the patient was not incubating the causative microorganism when admitted to the hospital. Patients with HAP may be managed in a ward or when the illness is severe in the intensive care unit (ICU). Ventilator-associated pneumonia (VAP) refers to pneumonia that begins and develops after endotracheal intubation (1,2). However, a patient who has just undergone tracheotomy yet is not on a ventilator is similarly susceptible to VAP. Thus, a more appropriate term would be "endotracheal-tube-associated pneumonia." In this chapter we have opted, nevertheless, to use the traditional term.

Epidemiology

HAP is currently the second most common nosocomial infection in North America and is associated with a high morbidity and mortality. Although HAP is not a reportable illness, the available data indicate that it occurs at a rate of 5 to 10 cases per 1000 hospital admissions, and that this rate is 6- to 20-times higher in patients subjected to mechanical ventilation (3,4). Nevertheless, the incidence density of VAP varies widely depending on the case definition of pneumonia and the hospital population evaluated. Numbers of reported episodes per 1000 days of ventilation are: 34.5 after major heart surgery (5), 26 in a burns ICU (6), 18.7 in a pediatric ICU (7), and between 8.0 (8) and 46.3 (9) in mixed medical/surgical ICUs. In the most recent report of the Centers for Disease Control National Nosocomial Infection Surveillance System it is stated that surgery and trauma ICUs have the highest VAP rates (mean 15.2/1000 ventilator days), followed by medical ICUs (mean VAP rate 4.9), coronary ICUs (mean VAP rate 4.4), and surgical ICUs (mean VAP rate 9.3) (10).

The incidence of VAP in mechanically ventilated patients rises as the time of ventilation is prolonged. Early during the course of a hospital stay, the incidence of VAP is highest, with estimates of 3% per day during the first five days of ventilation, 2% per day from days 5 to 10, and 1% per day thereafter (11). Approximately half of all VAP episodes occur within the first four days of mechanical ventilation. The intubation process itself carries a risk of infection such that when acute respiratory failure is noninvasively managed, the rate of nosocomial pneumonia is lower (12–16).

The overall mortality rate for HAP may be as high as 30% to 70%, but many critically ill patients with HAP die of their underlying disease rather than of pneumonia. VAP-related mortality has been estimated at 33% to 50% in several case-matched studies. Increased mortality rates have been attributed to the factors: bacteremia, especially that caused by *Pseudomonas aeruginosa* or *Acinetobacter* spp., medical rather than surgical illnesses, and ineffective antibiotic therapy (17–19).

As well as being the leading cause of nosocomial mortality, VAP is the leading cause of nosocomial morbidity. Secondary bacteremia and empyema have been reported to occur in 4% to 38% and 5% to 8% of cases, respectively. On average, the hospital stay of VAP patients is extended for 4 to 13 days (median 7.6 days). Current estimates indicate that this additional length of stay generates a cost of $20,000 to $40,000 per case of HAP or VAP in the ICU.

PATHOGENESIS

The pathogenesis of HAP and VAP is linked to two separate, but related, processes: colonization of the aerodigestive tract with pathogenic bacteria and aspiration of contaminated secretions.

For VAP to occur, the delicate balance between host defenses and microbial invasion has to be upset, allowing pathogens to colonize the lower respiratory tract (20).

In healthy subjects, the oropharynx is colonized by generally nonpathogenic microorganisms including *Streptococcus viridans*, *Streptococcus pneumoniae*, several anaerobes, and occasionally *Haemophilus influenza*, yet it is rare to find opportunistic gram-negative rods such as *P. aeruginosa* and *Acinetobacter* spp. Several factors have been reported to contribute to the pathogenesis of VAP such as the severity of the underlying disease, prior surgery, exposure to antibiotics, as well as the use of invasive respiratory equipment (2,21–30). Oropharyngeal and tracheal colonization by *P. aeruginosa* and enteric gram-negative bacilli have been related to the length of hospital stay and the severity of the underlying disease (26).

The main route of VAP infection is oropharyngeal colonization by normal flora or by exogenous pathogens acquired in the ICU. Typical sources of these pathogens are the hands of medical staff or contaminated respiratory equipment, water, or air.

Once the oropharynx has been invaded, microorganisms may reach the lower respiratory tract and lungs through several mechanisms. The main portals of bacterial entry into the lungs are *oropharyngeal pathogen aspiration* or the leakage of bacteria-containing secretions around the endotracheal cuff. The stomach and sinuses may act as potential reservoirs for nosocomial pathogens colonizing the oropharynx, but their relative role is largely unknown and could depend on the patient population or the changing natural history and management of VAP.

Microaspiration is common even in healthy individuals. Approximately 45% of healthy subjects aspirate during sleep, and the rate of aspiration is higher in patients with reduced levels of consciousness. Factors promoting aspiration include a generally reduced level of consciousness, a diminished gag reflex, abnormal swallowing for any reason, delayed gastric emptying, or decreased gastrointestinal motility. Reflux and aspiration of nonsterile gastric contents is also a possible mechanism of pathogen entry into the lungs.

The risk of pneumonia is determined by the type and quantity of bacteria colonizing the oropharynx (31). Hospitalized patients may become colonized with aerobic gram-negative bacteria within several days of admission, and as many as 75% of severely ill patients will be infected within 48 hours (32). In addition, the near sterility of the stomach and upper gastrointestinal tract may be disrupted by alterations in gastric pH due to illness, medication, or enteric feeding. Much attention has therefore been paid to the possible detrimental effects of ulcer prophylaxis regimens that raise the gastric pH (29,30).

Orotracheal intubation diminishes the natural defense mechanisms of the respiratory tract affecting mechanical factors (ciliated epithelium and mucus), humoral factors (antibody and complement), and cellular factors (polymorphonuclear leukocytes, macrophages, lymphocytes, and their respective cytokines).

The dorsal decubitus position is more conducive to microaspiration. The use of a nasogastric tube obstructs the ostia of the facial sinuses. The sinuses may then act as an infection reservoir causing the cardias to remain permanently open and inducing gastroesophagic reflux (33–35).

The formation of a biofilm on the endotracheal tube could help sustain tracheal colonization, and this mechanism is also thought to play a role in late-onset VAP caused by resistant organisms.

In summary, most cases of *endemic* VAP are acquired through the aspiration of microorganism-containing oropharyngeal, gastric, or tracheal secretions around the cuffed endotracheal tube into the normally sterile lower-respiratory tract.

On the contrary, the most common source of *epidemic* VAP infection is contaminated respiratory treatment equipment, bronchoscopes, medical aerosols, water (e.g., *Legionella*), or air (e.g., *Aspergillus*).

Direct inoculation of pathogens through ventilation devices is possible if no preventive measures are taken. Bacterial contamination of equipment was able to account for several VAP outbreaks in the 1970s, although today's improved hygiene has meant that this route is only responsible for a few isolated outbreaks. Water condensing in the ventilation circuit is a potential source of contamination and several preventive measures are specifically recommended (see below) to avoid the risk of contamination via this route (2,22–25,27).

The *inhalation of pathogens* such as viruses, fungi (*Aspergillus* spp.), or even *Legionella* spp. from the environment (2,15,22) has also been described.

Pneumonia can also be acquired by the *spread* of infection from adjacent infected tissue such as the pleura or mediastinum, but this occurs very rarely.

Bacterial translocation from the gastrointestinal tract is another pathogenic mechanism described for VAP. The intestinal wall of critically ill patients loses its capacity to prevent the systemic absorption of bacteria and toxins. This in turn leads to impaired intestinal function, promoting the invasion of the blood system with intestinal pathogens and causing bacteremia and thus metastatic infections (36,37).

The *hematogenous spread* of pathogens from intravascular catheters seems to be rare.

An exception to the idea that "pathogenesis always starts with oropharyngeal colonization" is the case of infection by *Pseudomonas* spp. The findings of several studies indicate that tracheal colonization by these pathogens may occur without previous oropharyngeal colonization (38–40).

MICROBIOLOGY

Although HAP and VAP are caused by a wide range of bacterial pathogens and some infections are polymicrobial [rates are especially high in patients with adult respiratory distress syndrome (ARDS)], viral or fungal pathogens are rarely the causative agents in immunocompetent patients. Sixty percent of nosocomial pneumonias are caused by gram-negative bacilli, representing six of the seven most frequently identified pathogens: *P. aeruginosa* (17%), *Staphylococcus aureus* (16%), *Enterobacteriaceae* (11%), *Klebsiella* spp. (7%), *Escherichia coli* (6%), *H. influenzae* (6%) and *Serratia marcescens* (5%) (41). Moreover, in some hospitals, *Acinetobacter* spp. are starting to account for a significant number of cases of nosocomial pneumonia (42–44).

Gram-positive cocci, such as *S. aureus*, particularly methicillin-resistant *S. aureus* (MRSA) represent another source of infection. The detection of an increased load of oropharyngeal commensals (viridans group streptococci, coagulase-negative staphylococci and *Corynebacterium* spp.) in distal bronchial specimens is difficult to interpret, but it is not generally considered that they could cause pneumonia. Rates of polymicrobial infection are highly variable although they seem to be on the increase and are particularly high in patients with ARDS (22,23,25,45–51).

In a series of 104 patients over 75 years of age with severe pneumonia, El-Solh et al. identified *S. aureus* (29%), enteric gram-negative rods (15%), *S. pneumoniae* (9%), and *Pseudomonas* spp. (4%) as the pathogens most commonly responsible for nursing-home–acquired pneumonia (47). Generally, both nonventilated and ventilated patients show similar bacteriology and infection is usually provoked by multidrug-resistant pathogens (MDR) such as MRSA, *P. aeruginosa, Acinetobacter* spp., and *K. pneumoniae*. Pneumonia due to *S. aureus* is more common in patients with diabetes mellitus, head trauma, and ICU patients (4,47,52,53). *P. aeruginosa* is a frequent pathogen in patients with severe chronic obstructive pulmonary disease (COPD) and those with prior hospitalization, prolonged intubation (more than eight days), and prior exposure to antibiotics (54). Infection with *Acinetobacter baumannii* has been related to specific risk factors (55) including neurosurgery, ARDS, head trauma, and large-volume pulmonary aspiration.

MDR-related VAP rates have recently undergone a dramatic increase in hospitalized patients. These pathogens are more likely to infect patients with late-onset HAP and VAP. The following risk factors for colonization and infection with MDR pathogens have been identified (2,19,56–59):

1. Antimicrobial therapy in the preceding 90 days
2. A length of hospital stay of five days or more
3. An existing high incidence of resistance to antibiotics in the hospital area or unit

4. Risk factors for health-care–associated pneumonia
   a. Hospitalization for two days or more in the preceding 90 days
   b. Residence in a nursing home or extended care facility
   c. Home infusion therapy (including antibiotics)
   d. Chronic dialysis within the previous 30 days
   e. Home wound care
   f. Family member with a multidrug-resistant infection
5. Immunosuppressive disease and/or therapy

Today, the role of anaerobic bacteria is still under investigation (60). In one report, anaerobes were isolated from 23% of patients with VAP diagnosed by quantitative culture methods (45). The authors of this study highlighted that the anaerobes recovered mirrored the bacteriology of the oropharynx and that only in four patients were they the only microorganism isolated. No anaerobic bacterium was found in blood or associated with necrotizing disease. In a more recent study, however, no anaerobes could be recovered using the same culture methods in 143 patients strictly followed during 185 episodes of VAP (61). Collectively, these and other findings point to an unlikely role of anaerobes in VAP or late-onset HAP. Their role in patients with poor dentition could, however, be more significant.

Early-onset and late-onset disease can be distinguished using quantitative culture methods of diagnosis. When pneumonia develops within four or five days of admission (or intubation), microorganisms associated with community-acquired pneumonia are isolated with some frequency. In contrast, when disease develops after five days, few pathogens associated with community-acquired pneumonia are recovered and gram-negative bacilli and *S. aureus* are the main agents detected. Although indicators of late-onset disease, these bacteria can also cause early-onset pneumonia, especially in patients with severe comorbidities under recent antimicrobial treatment, making the distinction between early-onset and late-onset disease more difficult. As mentioned above, a longer period of mechanical ventilation and antimicrobial therapy will increase the risk of infection by MDR pathogens.

Fungal pathogens are uncommon in immunocompetent hosts. Nosocomial *Aspergillus* spp. infection should warn of airborne transmission by spores related to an environmental source, such as contaminated hospital air ducts. Recently, a high rate of hospital-acquired *Aspergillus* pneumonia was observed in patients with COPD under therapy with antibiotics and high-dose corticosteroids (62). *Candida albicans* or other *Candida* species are often detected in endotracheal aspirates (EA), but usually indicate airway colonization rather than pneumonia and antifungal treatment is rarely necessary (63–67).

Within the categories described, the causes of nosocomial pneumonia also vary considerably according to geographic, temporal, and intra-hospital factors. The use of up-to-date local epidemiologic ICU data on endemic pathogens can help select the most appropriate empirical antibiotic regimen and infection control strategies.

Table 1 lists the conditions that may predispose a patient to acquire VAP attributable to a specific pathogen.

HAP and VAP of viral cause is also rare in immunocompetent hosts. Outbreaks of HAP and VAP due to viruses, such as influenza, parainfluenza, adenovirus, measles, and respiratory syncitial virus have usually been seasonal. Influenza, parainfluenza, adenovirus, and respiratory syncitial virus account for 70% of all nosocomial viral pneumonias. The diagnosis of these viral infections is often made by rapid antigen testing and viral cultures or serological assays. Influenza A is probably

Table 1 Risk Factors for Ventilator-Associated Pneumonia Attributable to a Specific Microorganism

Risk factor	Responsible microorganism
Aspiration	Anaerobic microorganisms
Abdominal surgery	Anaerobic microorganisms
IV drug abuse	
Coma	*Staphylococcus aureus*
Diabetes mellitus	
Chronic renal failure	
Prolonged ICU or hospital stay	*Pseudomonas aeruginosa*
Antimicrobial therapy	*Acinetobacter* spp.
	Stenotrophomonas maltophilia
	Enterobacter spp.
	Methicillin-resistant *S. aureus*
Chronic obstructive pulmonary disease	*Pseudomonas aeruginosa*
Age >65 yr	
Hypoalbuminemia <2.5 g/dL	
Nonresolving pneumonia	
Immunocompromise	*Candida* spp.
Isolated outbreaks	*Aspergillus* spp.
	Mucor spp.

Abbreviation: ICU, intensive care unit.

the most common viral cause of HAP in adult patients and predisposes the patient to secondary bacterial infection (2,68–72).

The role of herpes simplex virus (HSV) as a causative agent of VAP is presently under discussion. In a prospective study performed at our center, HSV was isolated from respiratory secretions in 6.4% of all patients not fulfilling VAP criteria and in 13.4% of those who did fulfill these criteria (Bouza E et al. Unpublished observations). However, the role of HSV in pneumonia is yet far from clear.

RISK FACTORS

Several risk factors have been linked to nosocomial pneumonia through univariate and multivariate analysis of prospective and retrospective data (11,22,60,73–84). The elderly and moderately to severely ill are especially at risk. In these subjects, respiratory tract function is impaired, lung volume is diminished, and airway clearance may be reduced. Trauma, surgery, medications, and respiratory therapy devices may additionally impair the capacity of the lungs to ward off infection.

Notwithstanding, the most significant risk factor for nosocomial pneumonia is mechanical ventilation. In effect, the terms nosocomial pneumonia and VAP are often used interchangeably. It has been described that when an endotracheal tube is introduced, many lines of host defense are bypassed such that microorganisms gain direct access to the lower respiratory tract (22,75,79,81). Further, as the tube is inserted, possible damage to the tracheal mucosa will allow pathogens to achieve a foothold. Table 2 provides additional risk factors listed by category for both VAP and pneumonia occurring in both ventilated and more mixed nonventilated hospital populations.

Table 2 Risk Factors for Nosocomial Pneumonia and Ventilator-Associated Pneumonia

Category	Unventilated or wide range of hospital patients	Mechanically ventilated patients
Host-related	Advanced age, severe illness, trauma/head injury, poor nutritional status, coma, impaired airway reflexes, neuromuscular disease	Advanced age, chronic lung disease, severe illness, reduced consciousness or coma, organ failure, severe head trauma, shock, blunt trauma, burns, stress ulceration
Device-related	Endotracheal intubation, nasogastric tube, bronchoscopy	Prolonged mechanical ventilation, reintubation or self-extubation, ventilator circuit changes at intervals <48 hrs, emergent intubation after trauma, PEEP, tracheostomy
Drug-related	Immunosuppression therapy	Prior antimicrobial therapy, antacid or H_2 blocker therapy, barbiturate therapy after head trauma
Miscellaneous	Thoracic or upper abdominal surgery, prolonged surgery, prolonged hospitalization, large-volume aspiration	Thoracic or upper abdominal surgery; gross aspiration of gastric contents, supine head position, fall-winter season

Abbreviations: H_2, histamine type 2; PEEP, positive end-expiratory pressure.
Source: From Refs. 2,11,22,28–30,60,74,75,79–105.

The risk factors identified by Croce et al. (106) to predict VAP in a review of admissions to a trauma center over a 28-month period were: penetrating wounds, a high Glasgow Coma Scale score, spinal cord injury, the coexistence of emergent laparotomy, a high Injury Severity Score and number of blood units transfused in the resuscitation room, and the place of initial intubation.

PREVENTION

Understanding the dual pathogenesis of VAP (colonization of the aerodigestive tract with pathogenic bacteria and their subsequent aspiration) has allowed the development of several VAP prevention strategies. These education-based programs have shown that the occurrence of VAP can be reduced by as much as 50% or more (107) if measures that prevent colonization and aspiration are implemented. These measures are based on avoiding or improving the specific risk factors identified to promote VAP in studies involving multivariate analysis.

In 2003, a revised set of recommendations for the prevention of nosocomial pneumonia was published by the Hospital Infection Control Practices Advisory Committee (HICPAC) of the Centers for Disease Control and Prevention (2). As before, its key components are (i) staff education and infection surveillance, (ii) preventing the transmission of microorganisms, and (iii) modifying host risk factors for infection.

VAP prevention strategies strive to minimize invasive mechanical ventilation and reduce airway contamination from endogenous (oropharynx, stomach, and sputum retention) and exogenous sources.

Effective infection control measures, hand hygiene, and patient isolation to reduce cross-infections are routine mandatory practices (2,29,88,104,108). Recommended practices are the surveillance of ICU infections to identify and quantify endemic and new MDR pathogens, and the acquiring of recent data on which to base infection monitoring and antimicrobial therapy in patients with suspected HAP or another nosocomial infection (2,28,29,71,88,104,108–111).

The time of invasive ventilatory support and therefore the risk of VAP can be reduced by noninvasive ventilatory support (112) and protocol-driven weaning (113). Reintubation also increases the risk of VAP (2,23,29,30,102,114–116).

In high-risk populations, early tracheostomy in patients predicted to require prolonged mechanical ventilation has been proposed as a preventive strategy and shown to reduce the incidence of VAP (117).

The use of orotracheal intubation and orogastric tubes rather than nasotracheal intubation and nasogastric tubes has been reported to prevent nosocomial sinusitis and to reduce the risk or VAP, although a direct link has not been demonstrated (2,29,30,86,104,118).

Good oral hygiene can reduce the load of infective microorganisms in the oropharynx and can be a cost-effective way of preventing VAP (119). The use of oral chlorhexidine has served to avoid ICU-acquired HAP in selected subsets of patients such as those undergoing coronary bypass, but its routine use is not recommended until more data become available (120–123). Unfortunately, sponge toothettes, despite being ineffective at plaque removal, are the only tools used today for oral care in ICUs (124). Selective decontamination of the digestive tract (SDD) using topical antimicrobial agents for oral decontamination and the use of SDD to prevent gastric colonization in critically ill, mechanically ventilated, or ICU patients appear to reduce the incidence of VAP (22,75,122,125–127), although the widespread use of antimicrobial prophylaxis is not recommended.

The infective organism load of the stomach can increase when the pH of the stomach contents is lowered. Thus, H_2 blockers and sucralfate, although this latter medication does not induce stomach acidity to the same degree, are risk factors for VAP (128) and unsuitable in patients with a high risk of gastrointestinal bleeding (129). Impairing gastroesophageal reflux reduces the risk of aspiration. Accordingly, a semirecumbent position (87,90–93,130–132) and the use of an inflated esophageal balloon (in patients with a nasogastric tube and enteral feeding tube) during mechanical ventilation (133) can reduce gastroesophageal reflux and the possible bronchial aspiration of gastric contents.

When in use in an individual patient, the breathing circuit (i.e., ventilator tubing and exhalation valve and the attached humidifier) should not be routinely changed. The circuit should be replaced only when visibly soiled or not working properly (2).

Compared to open endotracheal suction systems, closed systems reduce cross-contamination between the bronchial system and gastric juices (134) but increase colonization rates of ventilator tubing with multidrug-resistant microorganisms (135). There is no increase in VAP frequency (135); however, closed endotracheal suction systems may be in fact associated with lower rates of VAP relative to open systems (134). No recommendation is made, nonetheless, as to the preferential use of one system over the other in the HICPAC guidelines (2,136,137).

Closed suction systems do not have to be changed every day (138,139), and a policy of weekly changes of the in-line suction catheter offers substantial cost savings with no significant increase in the incidence of VAP (140). Adequate sputum clearance above the endotracheal cuff is essential if VAP is to be minimized. Subglottic suctioning is effective at removing secretions above the endotracheal cuff (2,35,87,136), but may damage the bronchial mucosa (141) and does not appear to prevent late-onset VAP (142). Endotracheal tube cuff pressure should be higher than 20 cmH$_2$O to prevent leakage of bacterial pathogens around the cuff into the lower respiratory tract (143,144).

Good humidification is important for sputum clearance (145), although passive as opposed to active humidification devices have been related to a lower VAP incidence (139,146).

Kinetic beds may be useful for secretion clearance and to reduce VAP (147). It is difficult to avoid airway contamination from exogenous sources, but changing ventilators only for infection control and not allowing the build up of condensation in the ventilator circuit can minimize contamination (139). Contaminated condensates should be carefully emptied from ventilator circuits and their entry into the endotracheal tube or in-line medication nebulizer should be avoided (144,148,149).

Silver-coated endotracheal tubes have been reported to reduce the incidence of *Pseudomonas* pneumonia in intubated dogs and to delay airway colonization in intubated patients, although patient subsets likely to benefit from this practice still need to be identified before the system can be applied on a large scale (150).

The daily interruption of sedation or its reduction, and avoiding agents that could depress the cough reflex have proved effective in the prevention of VAP (114).

Making sure there are adequate numbers of staff in the ICU will reduce length of stay, improve infection control practices, and reduce the duration of mechanical ventilation (115,116,151,152).

A selective transfusion policy should be adopted for the transfusion of red blood cells or other allogeneic blood products (20). Leukocyte-depleted red blood cell transfusion can help to reduce HAP in some patient populations (153–156).

Intensive insulin therapy to keep serum glucose levels in the range 80 to 100 mg/dL has been studied in ICU patients to reduce nosocomial bloodstream infection, duration of mechanical ventilation, ICU stay, morbidity, and mortality (157), but more studies are required before widespread recommendation.

Preventive measures are ineffective if not put into practice by all medical staff. Accordingly, multidisciplinary educational programs directed towards ICU staff that emphasize preventive strategies have been associated with decreased rates of VAP (139,158). For example, Babcock et al. (159) showed a 46% reduction in the VAP rate following a training program focusing on preventive measures.

Although not mentioned in the HICPAC guidelines, two further promising preventive measures are the implementation of protocols for ventilator management (160) and the use of antimicrobial agents in the ICU. Indeed, a ventilator management protocol was able to reduce the duration of ventilatory support and the incidence of VAP in a small study (116). In a French ICU, the results of a four-year study indicated that the rotation and restricted use of antibiotics reduced the frequency of VAP associated with multidrug-resistant bacteria; findings that have been subsequently confirmed (161,162). The proportions of VAP caused by methicillin-susceptible *S. aureus* increased from 40% to 60% and those of MDR gram-negative bacilli decreased from 61% to 49%. These findings warrant further investigation (Table 3).

A program started by the Institute for Healthcare Improvement (IHI), the "100,000 Lives Campaign," aims to enlist thousands of hospitals across the United States and abroad to implement changes in care that are known to prevent deaths (http://www.ihi.org/IHI/Programs/Campaign). This campaign seeks to reduce the number of avoidable deaths by 100,000 over an 18-month period that finishes

Table 3 Preventing Health Care–Associated Pneumonia

Recommendation	Category
Staff education and involvement in infection prevention	IA
Infection and microbiological surveillance	
Conduct surveillance for bacterial pneumonia	IB
Do not routinely perform surveillance cultures	II
Prevention of transmission of microorganisms	
Sterilization or disinfection and maintenance of equipment and devices	
General measures	
Thoroughly clean all equipment and devices to be disinfected or sterilized later	IA
Use steam sterilization or high-level disinfection for reprocessing semicritical equipment or devices. After disinfection, proceed with appropriate rinsing, drying, and packaging	IA
Use sterile water or isopropyl alcohol for rinsing reusable semicritical respiratory equipment and devices and dry	IB
Mechanical ventilators	
Do not routinely sterilize or disinfect internal machinery	II
Breathing circuits, humidifiers, and HME	
Change the breathing circuit only if visibly soiled or malfunctioning	IA
Breathing-circuit-tubing condensate: periodically drain and discard (use gloves for this procedure or to handle the fluid)	IB
Previously decontaminate hands	IA
Humidifier fluids: use sterile water to fill bubbling humidifiers	II
Ventilator breathing circuits with HMEs: change an HME only if visibly soiled or malfunctioning; do not change more frequently than every 48 hrs; do not routinely replace the breathing circuit attached to an HME while in use on a patient	II
Oxygen humidifiers: change the humidifier tubing only if visibly soiled or malfunctioning	II
Small-volume medication nebulizer	
Between treatments on the same patient: clean, disinfect, rinse with sterile water, and dry	IB
Use only sterile fluid for nebulization and dispense the fluid aseptically into the nebulizer	IA
Use aerosolized medications in single-dose vials	IB
Mist-tents: between uses on different patients these require sterilization or high-level disinfection; daily, on the same patient, they require low-level disinfection	II
Other devices used in association with respiratory therapy: between uses on different patients, sterilize or subject to high-level disinfection: portable respirometers, ventilator thermometers, and reusable hand-powered resuscitation bags	IB
Anesthesia machines and breathing systems or patient circuits	IB
The internal machinery of anesthesia equipment does not require routine sterilization or disinfection	IB
Between uses on different patients, clean reusable components of the breathing system or patient circuit and then sterilize or subject them to high-level disinfection in accordance with manufacturers' instructions	IB
Pulmonary-function testing equipment	
Do not routinely sterilize or disinfect internal machinery	II

(Continued)

Table 3 Preventing Health Care–Associated Pneumonia (*Continued*)

Recommendation	Category
Change the mouthpiece of a peak flow meter or the mouthpiece and filter of a spirometer between patients	II
Room-air humidifiers and faucet aerators	
Do not use large-volume room-air humidifiers that create aerosols unless they can be sterilized or subjected to high-level disinfection	II
If *Legionella* spp. are detected in the water of a transplant unit and until no longer detected by culture, remove faucet aerators from the unit	II
Prevention of person-to-person transmission of bacteria	
Standard precautions	
Hand hygiene: decontaminate hands before and after contact with a patient with an endotracheal or tracheostomy tube in place, and before and after contact with any respiratory device that is used on the patient, whether or not gloves are worn	IA
Gloving: wear gloves for handling respiratory secretions or objects contaminated with respiratory secretions of any patient	IB
Change gloves and decontaminate hands between contacts with different patients and between contacts with a contaminated body site and the respiratory tract of, or respiratory device on, the same patient	IA
Gowning: when soiling with respiratory secretions from a patient is anticipated, wear a gown and change it before providing care to another patient	IB
Care of patients with tracheostomy	
Perform tracheostomy under aseptic conditions	II
Change tracheostomy tubes aseptically wearing a gown, and replace the tube with one that has undergone sterilization or high-level disinfection	IB
Suctioning of respiratory tract secretions	
If an open suction system is employed, use a sterile single-use catheter	II
Use sterile fluid to remove secretions from the suction catheter if it is to be used for re-entry into the patient's lower respiratory tract	II
Modifying host risk factors for infection	
Increasing host defense against infection: administration of immune modulators	
Pneumococcal vaccination	
The 23-valent pneumococcal polysaccharide vaccine is recommended in persons aged >65 yr; in persons aged 5–64 yr with certain conditions (see Guideline) and in persons in long-term care facilities	IA
The 7-valent pneumococcal polysaccharide protein-conjugate vaccine is recommended in all children aged <2 yr and in children aged 24–59 mo with certain conditions	IB
Precautions for prevention of aspiration: as soon as the clinical indications for their use are resolved, remove all tubes (endotracheal, tracheostomy, or enteral) from patients	IB
Prevention of aspiration associated with endotracheal intubation	
Use noninvasive ventilation to reduce the need for and the duration of endotracheal intubation	II
Avoid repeat endotracheal intubation	II
Perform orotracheal rather than nasotracheal intubation	IB
If feasible, perform continuous or frequent intermittent suctioning of tracheal secretions that accumulate in the patient's subglottic area	II

(*Continued*)

Table 3 Preventing Health Care–Associated Pneumonia (*Continued*)

Recommendation	Category
Prevention of aspiration associated with enteral feeding	
Elevate the bed head rest to an angle of 30–45° for patients at high risk for aspiration pneumonia	II
Routinely verify appropriate placement of the feeding tube	IB
Prevention or modulation of oropharyngeal colonization	
Oropharyngeal cleaning and decontamination with an antiseptic agent	II
Use an oral chlorhexidine gluconate (0.12%) rinse during the perioperative period on adult patients who have undergone cardiac surgery	II
Prevention of postoperative pneumonia	
Instruct preoperative patients, especially those at high risk for contracting pneumonia, about taking deep breaths and ambulating as soon as medically indicated in the postoperative period	IB
Encourage all patients to take deep breaths, move about the bed, and ambulate unless medically contraindicated	IB
Use incentive spirometry on postoperative patients at high risk for developing pneumonia	IB
Other prophylactic measures for pneumonia	
Administration of antimicrobial agents other than SDD	Unresolved
Turning or rotational therapy	Unresolved

Note: Guidelines of the Centers for Disease Control and Prevention (Ref. 2).
Abbreviations: HICPAC, hospital infection control practices advisory committee; HME, heat-moisture exchangers; SDD, selective decontamination of the digestive tract.

in June 2006. A number of U.S. organizations, are now partners in this campaign. The program has started by implementing the following measures:

1. Deploy rapid response teams
2. Provide reliable, evidence-based care for acute myocardial infarction
3. Prevent adverse drug events
4. Prevent central line infections
5. Prevent surgical site infections
6. Prevent VAP

The IHI aims to prevent VAP by focusing on four components of care jointly denoted "the Ventilator Bundle." Care bundles are sets of best practices for managing a disease process. Individually these measures improve care, but when applied together they give rise to a substantial improvement. The scientific basis for each bundle component is sufficiently established to be considered the care standard. Hence, the IHI's ventilator bundle is a group of evidence-based practices that, when applied to all patients on mechanical ventilation, leads to a dramatic reduction in the rate of VAP.

The four measures comprising the ventilator bundle are:

1. Elevate the bed headrest (30–45°) so that the patient adopts a semi-recumbent position
2. Interrupt sedation daily and assess readiness to extubate daily
3. Prophylaxis for peptic ulcer disease
4. Prophylaxis for deep vein thrombosis unless contraindicated

The use of the ventilator bundle in the care of ventilated patients can markedly reduce the incidence of VAP. This reduction was estimated at 45% on average in a recent ICU collaborative improvement IHI project.

CLINICAL PRESENTATION AND DIAGNOSTIC TESTING

Establishing a Diagnosis of VAP

There is no single pathognomonic test that ensures or excludes the presence of VAP. Wide spectrum antimicrobial therapy should be started if there is reasonable suspicion and this can then be adjusted once the results of microbiological tests become available (22,163).

The American Thoracic Society and the Infectious Disease Society of America (20) recently defined VAP as the presence of new or progressing lung infiltrates plus clinical evidence that the infiltrates are of an infectious origin. The presence of infection is determined on the basis of two or more of the following data: fever greater than 38°C or hypothermia, leukocytosis or leukopenia, purulent secretions, and reduced oxygenation (164). In the absence of demonstrable pulmonary infiltrates, a diagnosis of infective tracheobronchitis is pursued (165).

Unfortunately, radiographic data from chest X rays show low sensitivity and specificity for diagnosing VAP (166–169). Radiological infiltrates are difficult to define and distinguish from other frequent conditions in this patient population. Moreover, they correlate poorly with computed tomography (CT) data and postmortem criteria. Lung infiltrates are also provoked by other causes such as atelectasis, pulmonary edema, pleural effusion, pulmonary hemorrhage, lung infarction, and ARDS (169). In a study comparing the use of portable chest X rays and CT scans, 26% of infiltrates detected by CT were missed by the portable chest X rays, particularly those located in lower lobes (170). This also occurs when we compare any gold standards such as the postmortem examination (164,168) and bronchoscopic examination (168,171–173).

CT has shown a sensitivity and a specificity of 53% and 63%, respectively, for the diagnosis of VAP (174). Ground glass infiltrates appeared to have a higher specificity but were found in only 45% of patients. Added to these limitations is interobserver variability in interpreting radiological observations (175).

The sensitivity of the use of other clinical data increases if only one criterion is considered sufficient, but this occurs at the expense of specificity, leading to significantly more antibiotic treatment (164). For patients with ARDS, suspicion of pneumonia should be high and even one of the clinical criteria described should prompt further diagnostic testing (176).

When clinical diagnoses of nosocomial pneumonia were compared to histopathologic diagnoses made at autopsy, pneumonia was diagnosed correctly in less than two-thirds of cases (177).

The Clinical Pulmonary Infection Score (CPIS) described by Pugin et al. (178) is a multifactorial system used to make a diagnosis of VAP. This method is based on assigning points to clinical, radiological, and physiological variables. In the original report, a score of ≥6 points was found to correlate well with a diagnosis of VAP. However, in subsequent studies, the sensitivity and specificity of the CPIS score proved not to be much improved over the subjective clinical approach unless the score includes microbiological information (rapid Gram stain or culture results) (Table 4) (179). Nonetheless, a clinical score of ≤6 is good at identifying a subset of patients

Table 4 Modified Clinical Pulmonary Infection Score

Criterion	Points		
	0	1	2
Temperature	$\geq$36.5°C to $\leq$38.4°C	$\geq$38.5°C to $\leq$38.9°C	$\leq$36°C to $\geq$39°C
Blood leukocytes (/μL)	$\geq$4,000 to $\leq$11,000	<4,000 or >11,000	<4,000 or >11,000 + bands (>500)
Tracheal secretions	Rare	Abundant	Abundant and purulent
Chest X ray infiltrates	None	Diffuse	Localized
PaO$_2$/FiO$_2$	>240 or ARDS		<240 and no ARDS
Microbiology	Negative		Positive

Abbreviation: ARDS, adult respiratory distress syndrome.

who either do not require antimicrobial therapy for VAP or, when antibiotics are pre-scribed, is amenable to a short course (three days) of treatment, provided the patient remains clinically stable and with a nonincreased score three days later (180).

Confirming the Etiology

Although the presence of clinical signs should raise a suspicion of VAP, confirming the diagnosis is much more difficult because clinical variables are of no use for defin-ing the microbiologic etiology of pneumonia. For an etiologic diagnosis of VAP, a lower respiratory tract culture and a quantitative bacterial culture are needed. The threshold bacterial count depends on the type of specimen collected (more or less dilution of the original respiratory secretions), the collection method, and the sam-pling time (whether there has been a recent change or not in antimicrobial therapy) (20). Growth below the threshold is assumed to be due to colonization or contamina-tion. This type of information has been used as a basis for decisions about whether to start antibiotic therapy, which pathogens are responsible for infection, which antimi-crobial agents to use, and whether to continue therapy (181,182).

Today, the most common methods of sampling the lower respiratory tract are endotracheal aspirates (EA), protected brush samples (PBS), and bronchoalveolar lavage (BAL). No single method is considered better than any other including bronchoscopic versus non bronchoscopic sampling (165,183–190).

It is essential that the laboratory is informed of the type of sample submitted to adequately process the sample and interpret the results (20). Nonetheless, in a survey of different sampling techniques, Ruiz et al. (185) found no differences in rates of diagnoses, changing of antimicrobial treatment due to etiologic findings, length of ICU stay and of mechanical ventilation, and crude 30-day or adjusted mortality.

Quantitative cultures were found to be especially useful for diagnosing VAP in patients with a low or equivocal clinical suspicion of infection (186,187). Fagon et al. performed a multicenter, randomized, uncontrolled trial to evaluate the effects on clinical outcome and antibiotic use of the two approaches "clinical" versus "bacteri-ological" to diagnose VAP and select the initial treatment for this condition (188). These authors concluded that the invasive management strategy was significantly associated with fewer deaths at 14 days, earlier improvement of organ dysfunction, and less use of antibiotics.

Blood cultures are not very useful for diagnosing VAP (189,190). Overall, their sensitivity is less than 25% and, when positive, the organisms detected could largely correspond to an extrapulmonary source, even if VAP is also present (191). Blood cultures are mainly useful for diagnosing extrapulmonary infections or detecting respiratory pathogens in patients with *borderline* respiratory sample cultures (191–193).

Value of Rapid Gram Stain

A reliable tracheal aspirate Gram stain can be used to decide upon initial empirical antimicrobial therapy (194), and infrequently gives rise to inappropriate treatment (22,188). A negative tracheal aspirate in a patient without a recent change in antibiotics (within 72 hours) has strong negative predictive value (94%) for VAP (195).

Value of Cultures

The etiologic cause of pneumonia is determined by microscopy examination of an endotracheal aspirate (EA) culture (196–198). From a practical standpoint, quantitative culture counts between 100 to 1000 cfu/mL for protected specimen brush (PSB) specimens and between 1000 and 10000 cfu/mL for (BAL) broncho-alveolar lavage specimens should be considered probably positive for VAP and are an indication for antibiotic treatment (199). Counts of $\geq$100,000 cfu/mL in blind, aspirated, undiluted tracheal secretions suggest infection rather than colonization (196).

Several technical considerations can affect the results of quantitative cultures, and may explain why the reported accuracy of invasive methods varies so widely. Methodological issues responsible for the inconsistent results of published studies have been summarized in a meta-analysis (200). One of the most frequent problems is the dilution of BAL, which could minimize bacterial counts. This occurs particularly in patients with severe COPD. Knowledge of the extent of dilution can dramatically increase the value of quantitative cultures. The recent starting or a change in antibiotic therapy is among the main factors causing false negative quantitative cultures, especially if the start or change occurs in the preceding 24 to 72 hours (187,201). Thus, all cultures should be obtained prior to treatment. If this is not possible, then a change in the diagnostic threshold could be useful (163,201). For BAL, the use of a threshold 10-fold lower than usual may avoid some false negative results in patients given antibiotics before testing.

Assessment of Response

Along with the findings of semiquantitative tracheal aspirates, the patient response should be assessed on day 3 of therapy (202). By this time, fever resolves, the PaO_2/FiO_2 is >250 mmHg, and a normal white blood cell count is found in 73.3%, 74.7%, and 53.3% of patients, by this time, fever resolve is 73.3% of patients, the PaO_2/FiO_2 is >250 mm Hg is 74.7% of patients and a normal white blood cell count is found in 53.3% of patients (54). Other authors report that infection variables resolve after antimicrobial therapy in patients with VAP by day 6 (203). Resolution of radiologic opacities and clearance of secretions occur at a median time of 14 and 6 days, respectively (54). However, failure to improve after 48 hours of therapy occurs in 65% of ARDS patients (54). Thus, ARDS significantly delays the clinical response to

Table 5 Performance of the Different Culture Methods for the Diagnosis of Ventilator-Associated Pneumonia

Diagnostic technique	Cutoff	Sensitivity	Specificity	References
Conventional				
Tracheal aspirates	10^5 cfu/mL	80% (60–97)	62% (41–74)	(196,207–209)
Tracheal aspirates	10^6 cfu/mL	66% (38–82)	78% (72–85)	(198,210,211)
BAL	10^4 cfu/mL	73% (42–93)	82% (45–100)	(199,212–217)
Protected specimen brush	10^3 cfu/mL	66% (33–100)	90% (50–100)	(215–217)
Plugged telescopic catheter	10^3 cfu/mL	72% (54–100)	82% (58–93)	(207,218,219)
Blind				
Tracheal aspirates	10^5 cfu/mL	94%	50%	(220)
Bronchial suction	10^3–10^4 cfu/mL	74–97%	74–100%	(221)
Mini BAL	10^3–10^4 cfu/mL	63–100%	66–100%	(220,221)
Protected specimen brush	10^3 cfu/mL	66% (54–98)	91% (57–100)	(209,221,222)
Protected telescopic catheter	10^3 cfu/mL	65%	83%	(220)

Note: Range given in parenthesis.
Abbreviations: cfu, colony forming units; BAL, bronchoalveolar lavage.

treatment in critically ill patients with VAP, although temperature is still the earliest resolution variable in this group of patients. Reassessment is necessary in patients who show no clinical improvement by day 3, whereas for those showing a good response, it may be possible to design an abbreviated course of therapy (204).

Prompt empirical therapy for all patients suspected of having VAP should be balanced with the need to limit antimicrobial misuse in ICUs. The reassessment of the patient's situation on the basis of culture results is another major principle. In patients with positive cultures, therapy can be tailored in terms of quality and duration. In patients with negative cultures, the need to continue with antimicrobial drugs should be promptly reassessed. Discontinuation of antimicrobial agents is presently recommended in patients with a stable condition although in deteriorating or critically ill patients, it is difficult to make this decision.

The Value of Surveillance

Several research teams have addressed the issue of whether routine systematic surveillance of EA cultures may serve as a predictive diagnostic tool for VAP, although results have been contradictory (5,205,206). In a study performed at our center, the pathogens present in surveillance cultures taken prospectively on a twice-weekly basis did not correlate well with cultures obtained on diagnosis of VAP (5).

Table 5 summarizes the performance of the different culture methods for the diagnosis of VAP.

Table 6 Initial Empirical Antibiotic Treatment for Ventilator-Associated Pneumonia According to the Potential Pathogens

Potential pathogen	Recommended AB	Dosing
No known risk factors for MDR pathogens, early onset, and any disease severity		
S. pneumoniae	Ceftriaxone or	2 g/day IV–IM
H. influenzae	Levofloxacin	500 mg/day IV–PO
MSSA	Moxifloxacin or	400 mg/day PO
Antibiotic sensitive gram-negative bacilli (E. coli, K. pneumoniae,	Ciprofloxacin or	750 mg/12 hr PO or 400 mg/12 hr IV
Enterobacter spp., Proteus spp., S. marcescens)	Ampicillin/sulbactam or	1.5–3 g/6 hr IV
	Ertapenem	1 g/day IV–IM

Potential pathogen	Combination AB therapy	Dosing
Risk factors for MDR pathogens, late-onset, and any disease severity		
Pathogens above and P. aeruginosa	Antipseudomonal cephalosporin	cefepime 1–2 g/8–12 hr IV;
K. pneumoniae ESBL	or	ceftazidime 2 g/8 hr IV
Acinetobacter spp.	Antipseudomonal carbapenem	impipenem 500 mg/6 hr or 1 g/8 hr IV;
	or	meropenem 1 g/8 hr
	β-lactam/β-lactamase inhibitor	4.5 g/6 hr piperacillin-tazobactam
	plus	
	Antipseudomonal fluorquinolone	ciprofloxacin 400 mg/8 hr IV;
	or	levofloxacin 750 mg/day
	Aminoglycoside	amikacin, 20 mg/kg/day, single dose
		gentamicin, 7 mg/kg/day, single dose
		tobramycin, 7 mg/kg/day, single dose
MRSA	Linezolid	600 mg/12 hr IV
	or	
	Vancomycin	15 mg/kg/12 hr IV

Abbreviations: AB, antibiotic; MRSA, methicillin-resistant *S. aureus*; MDR, multidrug-resistant pathogens; MSSA, methicillin-sensitive *S.aureus*; ESBL, extended-spectrum beta-lactam mases.

ANTIMICROBIAL TREATMENT

Selecting an Empirical Regimen

When trying to overcome severe infection, cardiovascular support and measures to improve hemodynamics and oxygenation are critical (54). The most important lesson learned in the last decade on the management of VAP is probably that delaying effective antimicrobial therapy in these patients increases mortality (50,108,111,223), length of stay, and costs (224).

As soon as there is clinical suspicion of VAP, adequate antibiotics should be administered to increase the likelihood of an early reduction in the bacterial load.

The first step is to decide whether a patient carries a low or high risk of having a MDR pathogen. The main risk factors for a MDR pathogen are (i) five or more days of prior hospitalization or mechanical ventilation, (ii) exposure to antibiotics in the preceding 90 days, (iii) a high incidence of antimicrobial resistance in the specific hospital unit, and (iv) comorbidities such as use of corticosteroids, head trauma, and lung structural disease among others (20,55–57,59,225–229).

Patients with none of these risk factors can start therapy with reduced-spectrum drugs such as ceftriaxone, a fluorquinolone (levofloxacin, moxifloxacin), ampicillin/sulbactam, or ertapenem. If the patient has any of the risk factors for a MDR pathogen then a two to three drug regimen should be started, including an anti-*Pseudomonas* beta-lactam agent (cefepime or ceftazidime, or piperacillin/tazobactam or imipenem or meropenem), a second anti-*Pseudomonas* agent (aminoglycoside or anti-*Pseudomonas* fluoroquinolone such as ciprofloxacin or levofloxacin) plus a broad-spectrum agent against gram-positive microorganisms (linezolid or vancomycin) (Table 6). Treatment should be started immediately after obtaining adequate samples for microbiological diagnosis.

Treatment Based on Knowledge of the Etiologic Microorganism

A key issue in the antimicrobial treatment of VAP is the de-escalation of treatment once microbiological information becomes available. We have already mentioned that antimicrobial agents should be discontinued when appropriate culture results are negative.

Once 24 to 48 hours has passed, information on the number and type of microorganisms growing in culture should be available. Depending on whether there is a lack of gram-negative microorganisms or one of gram-positive microorganisms, the specific drug against the corresponding microorganisms can be withdrawn even before the identity and susceptibility of the etiologic agent is known.

The microorganisms that deserve most attention are MRSA, *P. aeruginosa*, and *A. baumannii*.

Vancomycin is presently the standard agent against MRSA, although both industry-sponsored clinical trials and data from individual centers have consistently reported clinical failure rates of 40% or greater, at least using a standard dose. New evidence suggests that vancomycin failure could be related to inadequate dosing (230,231) and some authors argue that trough levels of around 15 mg/L are needed (232), although the success of this strategy requires confirmation in clinical trials. The addition of rifampin, aminoglycosides, or other drugs has achieved little improvement (233).

The use of new antimicrobial agents against MRSA has also been explored. Thus, quinupristin-dalfopristin has generated worse results than vancomycin (230).

Linezolid, an oxazolidinone antimicrobial agent, is active against MRSA and achieves better tissue penetration than vancomycin, but is bacteriostatic rather than bactericidal (234,235). However, a combined analysis of the results of two randomized trials comparing linezolid with vancomycin for the treatment of nosocomial pneumonia (each in combination with aztreonam for gram-negative coverage) suggests a therapeutic advantage for linezolid (236). In a further analysis of a subset of patients with MRSA VAP, linezolid was associated with a significantly higher probability of bacterial eradication, clinical cure, and hospital survival (237). Despite higher costs, linezolid therapy for MRSA VAP was attributed an absolute mortality benefit of 22%, which translates into five patients as the number-needed-to-treat to save one life (237). This has led linezolid to become recommended therapy for MRSA VAP (20).

Further agents presently under investigation include tigecycline, a new glycylglycine antimicrobial derived from tetracyclines. Tigecycline has an extremely broad spectrum of action against gram-positive, gram-negative, and anaerobic pathogens, with the exception of *Pseudomonas* (238). Its role in VAP is currently being evaluated in a phase III clinical trial.

Pneumonia due to *P. aeruginosa* in ventilated patients is frequently a recurrent disease caused most of the time by several relapsing infections (239). Frequently, the pathogens are MDR such that no single antibiotic is active against all isolates. Empirical therapy includes the combination of two drugs active against *P. aeruginosa* to improve the chances of successful early treatment. Once the susceptibility pattern is known, many physicians prefer combination therapy with a beta-lactam agent plus either an aminoglycoside or an anti-*Pseudomonas* fluoroquinolone, based on early findings related to patients with bloodstream infections (240). There is presently, however, no evidence that combination therapy has any benefit over monotherapy in patients with VAP or other forms of nosocomial pneumonia (241–243). Moreover, the combined regime was even found to fail at avoiding the development of resistance during therapy (242). In select patients with infections caused by MDR strains, aerosolized colistin has proved beneficial as supplemental therapy (244).

A. baumannii is a nonfermenter gram-negative rod, which has been held responsible for the recent rise in VAP. It is intrinsically resistant to many antimicrobial agents, and the agents found to be most active against them are the carbapenems, sulbactam, and polymyxins (42,54). In effect, intravenous carbapenem is today the treatment of choice for MDR isolates (245). In patients with strains resistant to carbapenems, intravenous colistin has been successfully used (43).

Adequate Dosing

To ensure the best outcome for patients, it is essential that the dosing of initial antibiotics for suspected MDR pathogens is adequate (235). All too often, agents are initially underdosed. For example, vancomycin should not be routinely given at a dose of 1 g q12h, but rather the dose should be calculated by weight in mg/kg (a dose that needs adjusting for renal impairment). Retrospective pharmacokinetic modeling has suggested that the failures described for vancomycin could be the result of inadequate dosing. Many physicians aim for a trough vancomycin concentration of at least 15 mg/L, although, as mentioned in the previous section, the success of this strategy has not been prospectively confirmed.

Some antibiotics penetrate well and achieve high local concentrations in the lungs, whereas others do not. For example, most beta-lactam antibiotics achieve less than 50% of their serum concentration in the lungs, whereas fluoroquinolones and linezolid attain equivalent or higher concentrations than blood levels in bronchial secretions.

Table 7 shows how to adjust the antibiotic dose in patients with renal impairment.

Aerosolized Antibiotics

All patients with VAP should initially receive antibiotics intravenously, but conversion to oral/enteral therapy may be possible in certain responding patients. The direct aerosol delivery of antibiotics is not considered as a standard therapy either for prophylaxis or for the treatment of lower respiratory tract infections (246).

In the past, aminoglycosides and polymyxins were the most common agents used in aerosols.

In a prospective randomized trial, the use of intravenous therapy was compared to the same treatment plus aerosolized tobramycin. The results of this trial suggest no better clinical outcome, but bacterial cultures of the lower respiratory tract were more rapidly eradicated (246b).

At present aerosolized antimicrobial therapy is mainly limited to MDR pathogens for which no other treatment exists, such is the case of MDR *P. aeruginosa* and *A. baumannii*, which are treated with intratracheal colistin (244).

Monotherapy or Combination Therapy

When considering the use of a single antimicrobial agent or combined therapy, we first need to make the distinction between the use of multiple antimicrobial agents in the initial empirical regimen (to ensure that a highly resistant pathogen is covered by at least one drug) and that of combination therapy continued intentionally after the pathogen is known to be susceptible to both agents. The former use of combination therapy is uniformly recommended, whereas the latter use remains controversial. Two meta-analyses have recently explored the value of combination antimicrobial therapy in patients with sepsis (243) and gram-negative bacteremia (247). No benefits of combination therapy were shown, and nephrotoxicity in patients with sepsis or bacteremia increased. However, in the subset of bacteremic patients infected with *P. aeruginosa*, combination therapy (usually a beta-lactam and an aminoglycoside) reduced the risk of mortality by half. A trend towards improved survival has been previously observed with aminoglycoside-including, but not with quinolone-including combinations (8). Combination therapy could therefore be beneficial in patients with severe, antimicrobial-resistant infections. Whether this benefit is due to more reliable initial coverage or to a synergistic effect is unclear. The present general consensus is to use combination therapy with an aminoglycoside for the initial five days in patients with VAP caused by gram-negative bacilli (20,162). However, the nephrotoxicity of aminoglycosides limits the use of these agents.

Duration of Therapy

The ideal length of antibiotic therapy is still under debate. In a prospective randomized clinical trial, Chastre et al. (248) demonstrated that an eight-day antibiotic regimen is comparable to a 15-day regimen in terms of mortality, superinfections, and relapse of VAP. A seven-day treatment course was described as safe, effective,

Table 7 Antibiotic Dose Adjustment in Renal Impairment

Antibiotic	CrCl (mL/min)	Dose adjustment
Amicacin	≥40	15 mg/kg/24 hrs
	30–39	15 mg/kg/36 hrs
	20–29	15 mg/kg/48 hrs
	<20	7.5 mg/kg × 1 and consult kinetics
Ampicillin/ sulbactam	>30	Normal dose IV q6 hrs
	15–30	Normal dose IV q12 hrs
	<15	Normal dose IV q24 hrs
Cefepime	>60	No adjustment
	30–60	1–2 g/24 hrs
	11–29	500 mg to 1 g/24 hrs
	<11	250–500 mg/24 hrs
Ceftazidime	>50	1–2 g/8 hrs
	10–50	1–2 g/12 hrs
	<10	1 g/24–48 hrs
Ceftriaxone		Adults with both kidney and liver failure should not receive more than 2 g/24 hrs
Ciprofloxacin	>50	750 mg/12 hrs PO 400 mg/12 hrs IV
	10–50	250–500 mg/12 hrs PO 400 mg/18 hrs IV
	<10	250–500 mg/18 hrs PO 400 mg/24 hrs IV
Ertapenem	>31	No adjustment
	≤30	500 mg/24 hrs IV–IM
Gentamicin	≥50	5 mg/kg/24 hrs
	30–49	5 mg/kg/36 hrs
	20–29	5 mg/kg/48 hrs
	<20	2 mg/kg × 1 and consult kinetics
Imipenem	≥71	≥70 kg: 500 mg/6 hrs
		60–69 kg: 500 mg/8 hrs
		50–59 kg: 250 mg/6 hrs
		40–49 kg: 250 mg/6 hrs
		30–39 kg: 250 mg/8 hrs
	41–70	≥70 kg: 500 mg/8 hrs
		60–69 kg: 250 mg/6 hrs
		50–59 kg: 250 mg/6 hrs
		40–49 kg: 250 mg/8 hrs
		30–39 kg: 125 mg/6 hrs
	21–40	≥70 kg: 250 mg/6 hrs
		60–69 kg: 250 mg/8 hrs
		50–59 kg: 250 mg/8 hrs
		40–49 kg: 250 mg/12 hrs
		30–39 kg: 125 mg/8 hrs
	6–20	≥70 kg: 250 mg/12 hrs
		60–69 kg: 250 mg/12 hrs
		50–59 kg: 250 mg/12 hrs
		40–49 kg: 250 mg/12 hrs
		30–39 kg: 125 mg/12 hrs
		Patients with CrCl ≤5mL/min should not receive imipenem/ cilastatin unless dialysis is programmed within 48 hrs. These patients may be at an increased risk of seizures

(*Continued*)

Table 7 Antibiotic Dose Adjustment in Renal Impairment (*Continued*)

Antibiotic	CrCl (mL/min)	Dose adjustment
Levofloxacin	>50	500 mg/24 hrs
	20–49	500 mg/48 hrs
	<20	500 mg × 1, then 250 mg/48 hrs
Linezolid	No adjustment	
Meropenem	>50	No adjustment
	26–50	Normal dose q12 hrs
	10–25	50% normal dose q12 hrs
	<10	50% normal dose q24 hrs
Moxifloxacin	No adjustment	
Piperacillin–	>40	No adjustment
tazobactam	20–40	4.5 g/8 hrs
	<20	4.5 g/12 hrs
Tobramycin	≥50	5 mg/kg/24 hrs
	30–49	5 mg/kg/36 hrs
	20–29	5 mg/kg/48 hrs
	<20	2 mg/kg × 1 and consult kinetics
Vancomycin	>50	15 mg/kg/12 hrs
	10–50	1 g/3–10 days
	<10	1 g/5–10 days

Note: CrCl calculated using the formula: males: $[(140 - age) \times IBW]/[SrCr \times 72]$ where age is the age in years, IBW, the ideal body weight in kg, IBW in men = 50 kg + 2.3 kg/in. of height over 60 in., IBW in women = 45.5 kg + 2.3 kg/in. of height over 60 in., SrCr = serum creatinine in mg/dL, females = CrCl (males) × 0.85.
Abbreviation: CrCl, creatinine clearance.

and less likely to promote the growth of resistant organisms in patients who are clinically improving. Patients with VAP caused by nonfermenting gram-negative bacilli, including *P. aeruginosa* given eight days of antimicrobial therapy had no less favorable outcomes but had a higher infection-recurrence rate compared to those receiving 15 days of treatment (40.6% *vs.* 25.4%; difference; 15.2%, 90% CI: 2.9–26.6). This was not found in patients with VAP caused by MRSA, in whom infection recurrence was 14.3% and 19% for the 8- and 15-day courses of antibiotics, respectively (90% CI: 9.9–0.4). Most authors agree, nevertheless, that the length of treatment should be tailored to suit each patient (227).

Resolution patterns can help optimize the duration of antibiotic therapy. Thus, after 48 hours of defervescence and resolution of hypoxemia, antibiotic therapy can be withdrawn (54). In patients with ARDS, fever is the main clinical variable used to evaluate the response to therapy.

Examining the Causes of Treatment Failure

Treatment failure should be assessed to simultaneously determine both the pulmonary/extrapulmonary and infectious/noninfectious causes of a failed response. The etiology of treatment failure can be ascribed to three possible causes (i) inadequate antibiotic treatment; (ii) concomitant foci of infection; or (iii) a noninfectious origin of disease (249). In a study designed to establish the causes of nonresponse to treatment in VAP patients in an ICU performed by Ioanas et al. (250), of a total of

71 patients, 44 (62%) were described as nonresponders. In 64% of these nonresponders, at least one cause of nonresponse was identified: inappropriate treatment (23%), superinfection (14%), concomitant foci of infection (27%), and noninfectious origin (16%). The remaining nonresponding patients underwent septic shock, multiple organ dysfunction, or had acute respiratory distress syndrome. In this type of situation, we would recommend the following basic tests: further respiratory sampling using invasive techniques; central lines should be checked and removed if necessary and surveillance cultures taken (251); urine cultures; echocardiography; and ultrasonographic examination of the abdomen. Further examinations could include CT scans of the sinuses, CT scan of the chest (to check for pulmonary embolism or abscess and empyema formation), and CT scan of the abdomen.

REFERENCES

1. Niederman MS. Guidelines for the management of respiratory infection: why do we need them, how should they be developed, and can they be useful? Curr Opin Pulm Med 1996; 2(3):161–165.
2. Tablan OC, Anderson LJ, Besser R, et al. Guidelines for preventing health-care–associated pneumonia, 2003: recommendations of CDC and the Healthcare Infection Control Practices Advisory Committee. MMWR Recomm Rep 2004; 53(RR-3):1–36.
3. Vincent JL, Bihari DJ, Suter PM, et al. The prevalence of nosocomial infection in intensive care units in Europe. Results of the European Prevalence of Infection in Intensive Care (EPIC) Study. EPIC International Advisory Committee. JAMA 1995; 274(8):639–644.
4. Richards MJ, Edwards JR, Culver DH, et al. Nosocomial infections in medical intensive care units in the United States. National Nosocomial Infections Surveillance System. Crit Care Med 1999; 27(5):887–892.
5. Bouza E, Perez A, Munoz P, et al. Ventilator-associated pneumonia after heart surgery: a prospective analysis and the value of surveillance. Crit Care Med 2003; 31(7):1964–1970.
6. Santucci SG, Gobara S, Santos CR, et al. Infections in a burn intensive care unit: experience of seven years. J Hosp Infect 2003; 53(1):6–13.
7. Abramczyk ML, Carvalho WB, Carvalho ES, et al. Nosocomial infection in a pediatric intensive care unit in a developing country. Braz J Infect Dis 2003; 7(6):375–380.
8. Fowler RA, Flavin KE, Barr J, et al. Variability in antibiotic prescribing patterns and outcomes in patients with clinically suspected ventilator-associated pneumonia. Chest 2003; 123(3):835–844.
9. Rosenthal VD, Guzman S, Crnich C. Device-associated nosocomial infection rates in intensive care units of Argentina. Infect Control Hosp Epidemiol 2004; 25(3):251–255.
10. National Nosocomial Infections Surveillance (NNIS) System Report, data summary from January 1992 through June 2004, issued October 2004. Am J Infect Control 2004; 32(8):470–485.
11. Cook DJ, Walter SD, Cook RJ, et al. Incidence of and risk factors for ventilator-associated pneumonia in critically ill patients. Ann Intern Med 1998; 129(6):433–440.
12. Brochard L, Mancebo J, Wysocki M, et al. Noninvasive ventilation for acute exacerbations of chronic obstructive pulmonary disease. N Engl J Med 1995; 333(13):817–822.
13. Antonelli M, Conti G, Rocco M, et al. A comparison of noninvasive positive-pressure ventilation and conventional mechanical ventilation in patients with acute respiratory failure. N Engl J Med 1998; 339(7):429–435.
14. Hilbert G, Gruson D, Vargas F, et al. Noninvasive ventilation in immunosuppressed patients with pulmonary infiltrates, fever, and acute respiratory failure. N Engl J Mcd 2001; 344(7):481–487.
15. Rello J, Ollendorf DA, Oster G, et al. Epidemiology and outcomes of ventilator-associated pneumonia in a large US database. Chest 2002; 122(6):2115–2121.

16. Ibrahim EH, Ward S, Sherman G, et al. A comparative analysis of patients with early-onset versus late-onset nosocomial pneumonia in the ICU setting. Chest 2000; 117(5): 1434–1442.

17. Rello J, Ausina V, Ricart M, et al. Impact of previous antimicrobial therapy on the etiology and outcome of ventilator-associated pneumonia. Chest 1993; 104(4):1230–1235.

18. Heyland DK, Cook DJ, Griffith L, et al. The Canadian Critical Trials Groups. The attributable morbidity and mortality of ventilator-associated pneumonia in the critically ill patient. Am J Respir Crit Care Med 1999; 159(4 Pt 1):1249–1256.

19. Fagon JY, Chastre J, Hance AJ, et al. Nosocomial pneumonia in ventilated patients: a cohort study evaluating attributable mortality and hospital stay. Am J Med 1993; 94(3):281–288.

20. Niederman S, Craven DE, et al. Guidelines for the management of adults with hospital-acquired, ventilator-associated, and healthcare-associated pneumonia. Am J Respir Crit Care Med 2005; 171(4):388–416.

21. Anonymous Coliform organisms in the pharynx. Lancet 1970; 1(7637):75.

22. Chastre J, Fagon JY. Ventilator-associated pneumonia. Am J Respir Crit Care Med 2002; 165(7):867–903.

23. Celis R, Torres A, Gatell JM, et al. Nosocomial pneumonia. A multivariate analysis of risk and prognosis. Chest 1988; 93(2):318–324.

24. Torres A, Aznar R, Gatell JM, et al. Incidence, risk, and prognosis factors of nosocomial pneumonia in mechanically ventilated patients. Am Rev Respir Dis 1990; 142(3): 523–528.

25. Craven DE, Steger KA. Epidemiology of nosocomial pneumonia. New perspectives on an old disease. Chest 1995; 108(suppl 2):1S–16S.

26. Johanson WG Jr., Pierce AK, Sanford JP, et al. Nosocomial respiratory infections with gram-negative bacilli. The significance of colonization of the respiratory tract. Ann Intern Med 1972; 77(5):701–706.

27. Stout J, Yu VL, Vickers RM, et al. Potable water supply as the hospital reservoir for Pittsburgh pneumonia agent. Lancet 1982; 1(8270):471–472.

28. Pittet D, Hugonnet S, Harbarth S, et al. Effectiveness of a hospital-wide programme to improve compliance with hand hygiene. Infection Control Programme. Lancet 2000; 356(9238):1307–1312.

29. Kollef MH. The prevention of ventilator-associated pneumonia. N Engl J Med 1999; 340(8):627–634.

30. Craven DE, Steger KA. Nosocomial pneumonia in mechanically ventilated adult patients: epidemiology and prevention in 1996. Semin Respir Infect 1996; 11(1):32–53.

31. Garrouste-Orgeas M, Chevret S, Arlet G, et al. Oropharyngeal or gastric colonization and nosocomial pneumonia in adult intensive care unit patients. A prospective study based on genomic DNA analysis. Am J Respir Crit Care Med 1997; 156(5):1647–1655.

32. Scheld WM. Developments in the pathogenesis, diagnosis and treatment of nosocomial pneumonia. Surg Gynecol Obstet 1991; 172(suppl):42–53.

33. Cameron JL, Reynolds J, Zuidema GD. Aspiration in patients with tracheostomies. Surg Gynecol Obstet 1973; 136(1):68–70.

34. du Moulin GC, Paterson DG, Hedley-Whyte J, et al. Aspiration of gastric bacteria in antacid-treated patients: a frequent cause of postoperative colonisation of the airway. Lancet 1982; 1(8266):242–245.

35. Valles J, Artigas A, Rello J, et al. Continuous aspiration of subglottic secretions in preventing ventilator-associated pneumonia. Ann Intern Med 1995; 122(3):179–186.

36. Niederman MS. Gram-negative colonization of the respiratory tract: pathogenesis and clinical consequences. Semin Respir Infect 1990; 5(3):173–184.

37. Inglis TJ, Sherratt MJ, Sproat LJ, et al. Gastroduodenal dysfunction and bacterial colonisation of the ventilated lung. Lancet 1993; 341(8850):911–913.

38. Niederman MS, Mantovani R, Schoch P, et al. Patterns and routes of tracheobronchial colonization in mechanically ventilated patients. The role of nutritional status in colonization of the lower airway by Pseudomonas species. Chest 1989; 95(1):155–161.

39. Cardenosa Cendrero JA, Sole-Violan J, Bordes Benitez A, et al. Role of different routes of tracheal colonization in the development of pneumonia in patients receiving mechanical ventilation. Chest 1999; 116(2):462–470.

40. Berthelot P, Grattard F, Mahul P, et al. Prospective study of nosocomial colonization and infection due to *Pseudomonas aeruginosa* in mechanically ventilated patients. Intensive Care Med 2001; 27(3):503–512.

41. Guideline for prevention of nosocomial pneumonia. Centers for Disease Control and Prevention. Respir Care 1994; 39(12):1191–1236.

42. Montero A, Corbella X, Ariza J. Clinical relevance of *Acinetobacter baumannii* ventilator-associated pneumonia. Crit Care Med 2003; 31(10):2557–2559.

43. Garnacho-Montero J, Ortiz-Leyba C, Jimenez-Jimenez FJ, et al. Treatment of multidrug-resistant *Acinetobacter baumannii* ventilator-associated pneumonia (VAP) with intravenous colistin: a comparison with imipenem-susceptible VAP. Clin Infect Dis 2003; 36(9): 1111–1118.

44. Garnacho J, Sole-Violan J, Sa-Borges M, et al. Clinical impact of pneumonia caused by *Acinetobacter baumannii* in intubated patients: a matched cohort study. Crit Care Med 2003; 31(10):2478–2482.

45. Dore P, Robert R, Grollier G, et al. Incidence of anaerobes in ventilator-associated pneumonia with use of a protected specimen brush. Am J Respir Crit Care Med 1996; 153(4 Pt 1):1292–1298.

46. Yu VL, Kroboth FJ, Shonnard J, et al. Legionnaires' disease: new clinical perspective from a prospective pneumonia study. Am J Med 1982; 73(3):357–361.

47. El-Solh AA, Sikka P, Ramadan F, et al. Etiology of severe pneumonia in the very elderly. Am J Respir Crit Care Med 2001; 163(3 Pt 1):645–651.

48. El-Solh AA, Aquilina AT, Dhillon RS, et al. Impact of invasive strategy on management of antimicrobial treatment failure in institutionalized older people with severe pneumonia. Am J Respir Crit Care Med 2002; 166(8):1038–1043.

49. Lim WS, Macfarlane JT. A prospective comparison of nursing home acquired pneumonia with community acquired pneumonia. Eur Respir J 2001; 18(2):362–368.

50. Luna CM, Vujacich P, Niederman MS, et al. Impact of BAL data on the therapy and outcome of ventilator-associated pneumonia. Chest 1997; 111(3):676–685.

51. Torres A, Puig de la Bellacasa J, Xaubet A, et al. Diagnostic value of quantitative cultures of bronchoalveolar lavage and telescoping plugged catheters in mechanically ventilated patients with bacterial pneumonia. Am Rev Respir Dis 1989; 140(2):306–310.

52. Fridkin SK, Edwards JR, Tenover FC, et al. Antimicrobial resistance prevalence rates in hospital antibiograms reflect prevalence rates among pathogens associated with hospital-acquired infections. Clin Infect Dis 2001; 33(3):324–330.

53. Rello J, Torres A, Ricart M, et al. Ventilator-associated pneumonia by *Staphylococcus aureus*. Comparison of methicillin-resistant and methicillin-sensitive episodes. Am J Respir Crit Care Med 1994; 150(6 Pt 1):1545–1549.

54. Vidaur L, Sirgo G, Rodriguez AH, et al. Clinical approach to the patient with suspected ventilator-associated pneumonia. Respir Care 2005; 50(7):965–974.

55. Baraibar J, Correa H, Mariscal D, et al. Risk factors for infection by *Acinetobacter baumannii* in intubated patients with nosocomial pneumonia. Chest 1997; 112(4): 1050–1054.

56. Trouillet JL, Chastre J, Vuagnat A, et al. Ventilator-associated pneumonia caused by potentially drug-resistant bacteria. Am J Respir Crit Care Med 1998; 157(2):531–539.

57. Gaynes R. Health care—associated bloodstream infections: a change in thinking. Ann Intern Med 2002; 137(10):850–851.

58. Niederman MS, Mandell LA, Anzueto A, et al. Guidelines for the management of adults with community-acquired pneumonia. Diagnosis, assessment of severity, antimicrobial therapy, and prevention. Am J Respir Crit Care Med 2001; 163(7):1730–1754.

59. Rello J, Sa-Borges M, Correa H, et al. Variations in etiology of ventilator-associated pneumonia across four treatment sites: implications for antimicrobial prescribing practices. Am J Respir Crit Care Med 1999; 160(2):608–613.

60. Mayhall CG. Nosocomial pneumonia. Diagnosis and prevention. Infect Dis Clin North Am 1997; 11(2):427–457.

61. Marik PE, Careau P. The role of anaerobes in patients with ventilator-associated pneumonia and aspiration pneumonia: a prospective study. Chest 1999; 115(1):178–183.

62. Bouza E, Guinea J, Pelaez T, et al. Workload due to *Aspergillus fumigatus* and significance of the organism in the microbiology laboratory of a general hospital. J Clin Microbiol 2005; 43(5):2075–2079.

63. el-Ebiary M, Torres A, Fabregas N, et al. Significance of the isolation of *Candida* species from respiratory samples in critically ill, non-neutropenic patients. An immediate post-mortem histologic study. Am J Respir Crit Care Med 1997; 156(2 Pt 1):583–590.

64. Krasinski K, Holzman RS, Hanna B, et al. Nosocomial fungal infection during hospital renovation. Infect Control 1985; 6(7):278–282.

65. Lentino JR, Rosenkranz MA, Michaels JA, et al. Nosocomial aspergillosis: a retrospective review of airborne disease secondary to road construction and contaminated air conditioners. Am J Epidemiol 1982; 116(3):430–437.

66. Loo VG, Bertrand C, Dixon C, et al. Control of construction-associated nosocomial aspergillosis in an antiquated hematology unit. Infect Control Hosp Epidemiol 1996; 17(6):360–364.

67. Gage AA, Dean DC, Schimert G, et al. Aspergillus infection after cardiac surgery. Arch Surg 1970; 101(3):384–387.

68. Hall CB, Douglas RG Jr. Nosocomial influenza infection as a cause of intercurrent fevers in infants. Pediatrics 1975; 55(5):673–677.

69. Graman PS, Hall CB. Epidemiology and control of nosocomial viral infections. Infect Dis Clin North Am 1989; 3(4):815–841.

70. Pachucki CT, Pappas SA, Fuller GF, et al. Influenza A among hospital personnel and patients. Implications for recognition, prevention, and control. Arch Intern Med 1989; 149(1):77–80.

71. Evans ME, Hall KL, Berry SE. Influenza control in acute care hospitals. Am J Infect Control 1997; 25(4):357–362.

72. Hoffman PC, Dixon RE. Control of influenza in the hospital. Ann Intern Med 1977; 87(6):725–728.

73. Lode HM, Schaberg T, Raffenberg M, et al. Nosocomial pneumonia in the critical care unit. Crit Care Clin 1998; 14(1):119–133.

74. Craven DE, Steger KA. Hospital-acquired pneumonia: perspectives for the healthcare epidemiologist. Infect Control Hosp Epidemiol 1997; 18(11):783–795.

75. Bonten MJ, Kollef MH, Hall JB. Risk factors for ventilator-associated pneumonia: from epidemiology to patient management. Clin Infect Dis 2004; 38(8):1141–1149.

76. Bruchhaus JD, McEachern R, Campbell GD Jr. Hospital-acquired pneumonia: recent advances in diagnosis, microbiology and treatment. Curr Opin Pulm Med 1998; 4(3):180–184.

77. Morehead RS, Pinto SJ. Ventilator-associated pneumonia. Arch Intern Med 2000; 160(13): 1926–1936.

78. Combes A, Figliolini C, Trouillet JL, et al. Factors predicting ventilator-associated pneumonia recurrence. Crit Care Med 2003; 31(4):1102–1107.

79. Fleming CA, Balaguera HU, Craven DE. Risk factors for nosocomial pneumonia. Focus on prophylaxis. Med Clin North Am 2001; 85(6):1545–1563.

80. Tejada Artigas A, Bello Dronda S, Chacon Valles E, et al. Risk factors for nosocomial pneumonia in critically ill trauma patients. Crit Care Med 2001; 29(2):304–309.

81. Lynch JP III. Hospital-acquired pneumonia: risk factors, microbiology, and treatment. Chest 2001; 119(suppl 2):373S–384S.

82. Ibrahim EH, Tracy L, Hill C, et al. The occurrence of ventilator-associated pneumonia in a community hospital: risk factors and clinical outcomes. Chest 2001; 120(2):555–561.

83. Arozullah AM, Khuri SF, Henderson WG, et al. Development and validation of a multifactorial risk index for predicting postoperative pneumonia after major noncardiac surgery. Ann Intern Med 2001; 135(10):847–857.

84. Cook DJ, Kollef MH. Risk factors for ICU-acquired pneumonia. JAMA 1998; 279(20): 1605–1606.

85. Chevret S, Hemmer M, Carlet J, et al. Incidence and risk factors of pneumonia acquired in intensive care units. Results from a multicenter prospective study on 996 patients. European Cooperative Group on Nosocomial Pneumonia. Intensive Care Med 1993; 19(5):256–264.

86. Rouby JJ, Laurent P, Gosnach M, et al. Risk factors and clinical relevance of nosocomial maxillary sinusitis in the critically ill. Am J Respir Crit Care Med 1994; 150(3):776–783.

87. Kollef MH. Prevention of hospital-associated pneumonia and ventilator-associated pneumonia. Crit Care Med 2004; 32(6):1396–1405.

88. Bonten MJ. Controversies on diagnosis and prevention of ventilator-associated pneumonia. Diagn Microbiol Infect Dis 1999; 34(3):199–204.

89. Pawar M, Mehta Y, Khurana P, et al. Ventilator-associated pneumonia: Incidence, risk factors, outcome, and microbiology. J Cardiothorac Vasc Anesth 2003; 17(1):22–28.

90. Torres A, Serra-Batlles J, Ros E, et al. Pulmonary aspiration of gastric contents in patients receiving mechanical ventilation: the effect of body position. Ann Intern Med 1992; 116(7):540–543.

91. Orozco-Levi M, Torres A, Ferrer M, et al. Semirecumbent position protects from pulmonary aspiration but not completely from gastroesophageal reflux in mechanically ventilated patients. Am J Respir Crit Care Med 1995; 152(4 Pt 1):1387–1390.

92. Davis K Jr., Johannigman JA, Campbell RS, et al. The acute effects of body position strategies and respiratory therapy in paralyzed patients with acute lung injury. Crit Care 2001; 5(2):81–87.

93. Drakulovic MB, Torres A, Bauer TT, et al. Supine body position as a risk factor for nosocomial pneumonia in mechanically ventilated patients: a randomised trial. Lancet 1999; 354(9193):1851–1858.

94. Pingleton SK, Hinthorn DR, Liu C. Enteral nutrition in patients receiving mechanical ventilation. Multiple sources of tracheal colonization include the stomach. Am J Med 1986; 80(5):827–832.

95. Ibrahim EH, Mehringer L, Prentice D, et al. Early versus late enteral feeding of mechanically ventilated patients: results of a clinical trial. J Parenter Enteral Nutr 2002; 26(3): 174–181.

96. Craven DE, Driks MR. Nosocomial pneumonia in the intubated patient. Semin Respir Infect 1987; 2(1):20–33.

97. Heyland DK, Drover JW, MacDonald S, et al. Effect of postpyloric feeding on gastroesophageal regurgitation and pulmonary microaspiration: results of a randomized controlled trial. Crit Care Med 2001; 29(8):1495–1501.

98. Niederman MS, Craven DE. Devising strategies for preventing nosocomial pneumonia—should we ignore the stomach? Clin Infect Dis 1997; 24(3):320–323.

99. Bonten MJ, Gaillard CA, de Leeuw PW, et al. Role of colonization of the upper intestinal tract in the pathogenesis of ventilator-associated pneumonia. Clin Infect Dis 1997; 24(3):309–319.

100. Prod'hom G, Leuenberger P, Koerfer J, et al. Nosocomial pneumonia in mechanically ventilated patients receiving antacid, ranitidine, or sucralfate as prophylaxis for stress ulcer. A randomized controlled trial. Ann Intern Med 1994; 120(8):653–662.

101. Cook D, Guyatt G, Marshall J, et al. Canadian Critical Care Trials Group. A comparison of sucralfate and ranitidine for the prevention of upper gastrointestinal bleeding in patients requiring mechanical ventilation. N Engl J Med 1998; 338(12):791–797.

102. Torres A, Gatell JM, Aznar E, et al. Re-intubation increases the risk of nosocomial pneumonia in patients needing mechanical ventilation. Am J Respir Crit Care Med 1995; 152(1):137–141.

103. Weinstein RA. Nosocomial infection update. Emerg Infect Dis 1998; 4(3):416–420.

104. Weinstein RA. Epidemiology and control of nosocomial infections in adult intensive care units. Am J Med 1991; 91(3B):179S–184S.

105. Bergmans DC, Bonten MJ, van Tiel FH, et al. Cross-colonisation with *Pseudomonas aeruginosa* of patients in an intensive care unit. Thorax 1998; 53(12):1053–1058.
106. Croce MA, Tolley EA, Fabian TC. A formula for prediction of posttraumatic pneumonia based on early anatomic and physiologic parameters. J Trauma 2003; 54(4): 724–729; discussion 729–730.
107. Zack JE, Garrison T, Trovillion E, et al. Effect of an education program aimed at reducing the occurrence of ventilator-associated pneumonia. Crit Care Med 2002; 30(11): 2407–2412.
108. Kollef MH, Sherman G, Ward S, et al. Inadequate antimicrobial treatment of infections: a risk factor for hospital mortality among critically ill patients. Chest 1999; 115(2): 462–474.
109. Haley RW, Culver DH, White JW, et al. The efficacy of infection surveillance and control programs in preventing nosocomial infections in US hospitals. Am J Epidemiol 1985; 121(2):182–205.
110. Haley RW, Morgan WM, Culver DH, et al. Update from the SENIC project. Hospital infection control: recent progress and opportunities under prospective payment. Am J Infect Control 1985; 13(3):97–108.
111. Iregui M, Ward S, Sherman G, et al. Clinical importance of delays in the initiation of appropriate antibiotic treatment for ventilator-associated pneumonia. Chest 2002; 122(1):262–268.
112. Wang C, Shang M, Huang K. Sequential non-invasive following short-term invasive mechanical ventilation in COPD induced hypercapnic respiratory failure. Zhonghua Jie He He Hu Xi Za Zhi 2000; 23(4):212–216.
113. Dries DJ, McGonigal MD, Malian MS, et al. Protocol-driven ventilator weaning reduces use of mechanical ventilation, rate of early reintubation, and ventilator-associated pneumonia. J Trauma 2004; 56(5):943–951; discussion 951–942.
114. Kress JP, Pohlman AS, O'Connor MF, et al. Daily interruption of sedative infusions in critically ill patients undergoing mechanical ventilation. N Engl J Med 2000; 342(20): 1471–1477.
115. Needleman J, Buerhaus P, Mattke S, et al. Nurse-staffing levels and the quality of care in hospitals. N Engl J Med 2002; 346(22):1715–1722.
116. Marelich GP, Murin S, Battistella F, et al. Protocol weaning of mechanical ventilation in medical and surgical patients by respiratory care practitioners and nurses: effect on weaning time and incidence of ventilator-associated pneumonia. Chest 2000; 118(2): 459–467.
117. Moller MG, Slaikeu JD, Bonelli P, et al. Early tracheostomy versus late tracheostomy in the surgical intensive care unit. Am J Surg 2005; 189(3):293–296.
118. Holzapfel L, Chastang C, Demingeon G, et al. A randomized study assessing the systematic search for maxillary sinusitis in nasotracheally mechanically ventilated patients. Influence of nosocomial maxillary sinusitis on the occurrence of ventilator-associated pneumonia. Am J Respir Crit Care Med 1999; 159(3):695–701.
119. van Nieuwenhoven CA, Buskens E, Bergmans DC, et al. Oral decontamination is cost-saving in the prevention of ventilator-associated pneumonia in intensive care units. Crit Care Med 2004; 32(1):126–130.
120. DeRiso AJ II, Ladowski JS, Dillon TA, et al. Chlorhexidine gluconate 0.12% oral rinse reduces the incidence of total nosocomial respiratory infection and nonprophylactic systemic antibiotic use in patients undergoing heart surgery. Chest 1996; 109(6): 1556–1561.
121. Abele-Horn M, Dauber A, Bauernfeind A, et al. Decrease in nosocomial pneumonia in ventilated patients by selective oropharyngeal decontamination (SOD). Intensive Care Med 1997; 23(2):187–195.
122. Bergmans DC, Bonten MJ, Gaillard CA, et al. Prevention of ventilator-associated pneumonia by oral decontamination: a prospective, randomized, double-blind, placebo-controlled study. Am J Respir Crit Care Med 2001; 164(3):382–388.

123. Pugin J, Auckenthaler R, Lew DP, et al. Oropharyngeal decontamination decreases incidence of ventilator-associated pneumonia. A randomized, placebo-controlled, double-blind clinical trial. JAMA 1991; 265(20):2704–2710.

124. Grap MJ, Munro CL, Ashtiani B, et al. Oral care interventions in critical care: frequency and documentation. Am J Crit Care 2003; 12(2):113–118; discussion 119.

125. D'Amico R, Pifferi S, Leonetti C, et al. Effectiveness of antibiotic prophylaxis in critically ill adult patients: systematic review of randomised controlled trials. BMJ 1998; 316(7140): 1275–1285.

126. van Nieuwenhoven CA, Buskens E, van Tiel FH, et al. Relationship between methodological trial quality and the effects of selective digestive decontamination on pneumonia and mortality in critically ill patients. JAMA 2001; 286(3):335–340.

127. Lingnau W, Berger J, Javorsky F, et al. Changing bacterial ecology during a five-year period of selective intestinal decontamination. J Hosp Infect 1998; 39(3):195–206.

128. Bornstain C, Azoulay E, De Lassence A, et al. Sedation, sucralfate, and antibiotic use are potential means for protection against early-onset ventilator-associated pneumonia. Clin Infect Dis 2004; 38(10):1401–1408.

129. Dodek P, Keenan S, Cook D, et al. Evidence-based clinical practice guideline for the prevention of ventilator-associated pneumonia. Ann Intern Med 2004; 141(4):305–313.

130. Tulleken JE, Spanjersberg R, van der Werf TS, et al. Semirecumbent position in intensive care patients. Lancet 2000; 355(9208):1013–1014.

131. van Saene HK, de la Cal MA, Petros AJ. Semirecumbent position in intensive care patients. Lancet 2000; 355(9208):1012–1013.

132. Roggla G, Roggla M. Semirecumbent position in intensive care patients. Lancet 2000; 355(9208):1012; author reply 1013.

133. Orozco-Levi M, Felez M, Martinez-Miralles E, et al. Gastro-oesophageal reflux in mechanically ventilated patients: effects of an oesophageal balloon. Eur Respir J 2003; 22(2):348–353.

134. Rabitsch W, Kostler WJ, Fiebiger W, et al. Closed suctioning system reduces cross-contamination between bronchial system and gastric juices [table of contents]. Anesth Analg 2004; 99(3):886–892.

135. Topeli A, Harmanci A, Cetinkaya Y, et al. Comparison of the effect of closed versus open endotracheal suction systems on the development of ventilator-associated pneumonia. J Hosp Infect 2004; 58(1):14–19.

136. Mahul P, Auboyer C, Jospe R, et al. Prevention of nosocomial pneumonia in intubated patients: respective role of mechanical subglottic secretions drainage and stress ulcer prophylaxis. Intensive Care Med 1992; 18(1):20–25.

137. Kollef MH, Skubas NJ, Sundt TM. A randomized clinical trial of continuous aspiration of subglottic secretions in cardiac surgery patients. Chest 1999; 116(5):1339–1346.

138. Darvas JA, Hawkins LG. The closed tracheal suction catheter: 24 hour or 48 hour change? Aust Crit Care 2003; 16(3):86–92.

139. Hess DR, Kallstrom TJ, Mottram CD, et al. Care of the ventilator circuit and its relation to ventilator-associated pneumonia. Respir Care 2003; 48(9):869–879.

140. Stoller JK, Orens DK, Fatica C, et al. Weekly versus daily changes of in-line suction catheters: impact on rates of ventilator-associated pneumonia and associated costs. Respir Care 2003; 48(5):494–499.

141. Berra L, De Marchi L, Panigada M, et al. Evaluation of continuous aspiration of subglottic secretion in an in vivo study. Crit Care Med 2004; 32(10):2071–2078.

142. Safdar N, Crnich CJ, Maki DG. The pathogenesis of ventilator-associated pneumonia: its relevance to developing effective strategies for prevention. Respir Care 2005; 50(6): 725–741.

143. Rello J, Sonora R, Jubert P, et al. Pneumonia in intubated patients: role of respiratory airway care. Am J Respir Crit Care Med 1996; 154(1):111–115.

144. Cook D, De Jonghe B, Brochard L, et al. Influence of airway management on ventilator-associated pneumonia: evidence from randomized trials. JAMA 1998; 279(10):781–787.

145. Hess D. Prolonged use of heat and moisture exchangers: why do we keep changing things? Crit Care Med 2000; 28(5):1667–1668.
146. Kola A, Eckmanns T, Gastmeier P. Efficacy of heat and moisture exchangers in preventing ventilator-associated pneumonia: meta-analysis of randomized controlled trials. Intensive Care Med 2005; 31(1):5–11.
147. Ahrens T, Kollef M, Stewart J, et al. Effect of kinetic therapy on pulmonary complications. Am J Crit Care 2004; 13(5):376–383.
148. Craven DE, Goularte TA, Make BJ. Contaminated condensate in mechanical ventilator circuits. A risk factor for nosocomial pneumonia? Am Rev Respir Dis 1984; 129(4): 625–628.
149. Craven DE, Lichtenberg DA, Goularte TA, et al. Contaminated medication nebulizers in mechanical ventilator circuits. Source of bacterial aerosols. Am J Med 1984; 77(5): 834–838.
150. Diaz E, Rodriguez AH, Rello J. Ventilator-associated pneumonia: issues related to the artificial airway. Respir Care 2005; 50(7):900–909.
151. Brook AD, Ahrens TS, Schaiff R, et al. Effect of a nursing-implemented sedation protocol on the duration of mechanical ventilation. Crit Care Med 1999; 27(12):2609–2615.
152. Thorens JB, Kaelin RM, Jolliet P, et al. Influence of the quality of nursing on the duration of weaning from mechanical ventilation in patients with chronic obstructive pulmonary disease. Crit Care Med 1995; 23(11):1807–1815.
153. Hebert PC, Wells G, Blajchman MA, et al. Canadian Critical Care Trials Group. A multicenter, randomized, controlled clinical trial of transfusion requirements in critical care. Transfusion Requirements in Critical Care Investigators. N Engl J Med 1999; 340(6): 409–417.
154. Vamvakas EC, Carven JH. Exposure to allogeneic plasma and risk of postoperative pneumonia and/or wound infection in coronary artery bypass graft surgery. Transfusion 2002; 42(1):107–113.
155. Vamvakas EC, Carven JH. Transfusion and postoperative pneumonia in coronary artery bypass graft surgery: effect of the length of storage of transfused red cells. Transfusion 1999; 39(7):701–710.
156. Leal-Noval SR, Marquez-Vacaro JA, Garcia-Curiel A, et al. Nosocomial pneumonia in patients undergoing heart surgery. Crit Care Med 2000; 28(4):935–940.
157. van den Berghe G, Wouters P, Weekers F, et al. Intensive insulin therapy in the critically ill patients. N Engl J Med 2001; 345(19):1359–1367.
158. Salahuddin N, Zafar A, Sukhyani L, et al. Reducing ventilator-associated pneumonia rates through a staff education programme. J Hosp Infect 2004; 57(3):223–227.
159. Babcock HM, Zack JE, Garrison T, et al. An educational intervention to reduce ventilator-associated pneumonia in an integrated health system: a comparison of effects. Chest 2004; 125(6):2224–2231.
160. Macintyre NR. Ventilator-associated pneumonia: the role of ventilator management strategies. Respir Care 2005; 50(6):766–773.
161. Gruson D, Hilbert G, Vargas F, et al. Strategy of antibiotic rotation: long-term effect on incidence and susceptibilities of Gram-negative bacilli responsible for ventilator-associated pneumonia. Crit Care Med 2003; 31(7):1908–1914.
162. Gruson D, Hilbert G, Vargas F, et al. Rotation and restricted use of antibiotics in a medical intensive care unit. Impact on the incidence of ventilator-associated pneumonia caused by antibiotic-resistant gram-negative bacteria. Am J Respir Crit Care Med 2000; 162(3 Pt 1):837–843.
163. Niederman MS, Torres A, Summer W. Invasive diagnostic testing is not needed routinely to manage suspected ventilator-associated pneumonia. Am J Respir Crit Care Med 1994; 150(2):565–569.
164. Fabregas N, Ewig S, Torres A, et al. Clinical diagnosis of ventilator associated pneumonia revisited: comparative validation using immediate post-mortem lung biopsies. Thorax 1999; 54(10):867–873.

165. Rouby JJ, Martin De Lassale E, Poete P, et al. Nosocomial bronchopneumonia in the critically ill. Histologic and bacteriologic aspects. Am Rev Respir Dis 1992; 146(4): 1059–1066.

166. Andrews CP, Coalson JJ, Smith JD, et al. Diagnosis of nosocomial bacterial pneumonia in acute, diffuse lung injury. Chest 1981; 80(3):254–258.

167. Rubin SA, Winer-Muram HT, Ellis JV. Diagnostic imaging of pneumonia and its complications in the critically ill patient. Clin Chest Med 1995; 16(1):45–59.

168. Wunderink RG, Woldenberg LS, Zeiss J, et al. The radiologic diagnosis of autopsy-proven ventilator-associated pneumonia. Chest 1992; 101(2):458–463.

169. Meduri GU, Mauldin GL, Wunderink RG, et al. Causes of fever and pulmonary densities in patients with clinical manifestations of ventilator-associated pneumonia. Chest 1994; 106(1):221–235.

170. Beydon L, Saada M, Liu N, et al. Can portable chest x-ray examination accurately diagnose lung consolidation after major abdominal surgery? A comparison with computed tomography scan. Chest 1992; 102(6):1697–1703.

171. Winer-Muram HT, Rubin SA, Ellis JV, et al. Pneumonia and ARDS in patients receiving mechanical ventilation: diagnostic accuracy of chest radiography. Radiology 1993; 188(2):479–485.

172. Lefcoe MS, Fox GA, Leasa DJ, et al. Accuracy of portable chest radiography in the critical care setting. Diagnosis of pneumonia based on quantitative cultures obtained from protected brush catheter. Chest 1994; 105(3):885–887.

173. Wunderink RG. Radiologic diagnosis of ventilator-associated pneumonia. Chest 2000; 117(4 suppl 2):188S–190S.

174. Hahn U, Pereira P, Heininger A, et al. Value of CT in diagnosis of respirator-associated pneumonia. ROFO 1999; 170(2):150–155.

175. Fagon JY, Chastre J, Hance AJ, et al. Evaluation of clinical judgment in the identification and treatment of nosocomial pneumonia in ventilated patients. Chest 1993; 103(2): 547–553.

176. Delclaux C, Roupie E, Blot F, et al. Lower respiratory tract colonization and infection during severe acute respiratory distress syndrome: incidence and diagnosis. Am J Respir Crit Care Med 1997; 156(4 Pt 1):1092–1098.

177. Combes A, Figliolini C, Trouillet JL, et al. Incidence and outcome of polymicrobial ventilator-associated pneumonia. Chest 2002; 121(5):1618–1623.

178. Pugin J, Auckenthaler R, Mili N, et al. Diagnosis of ventilator-associated pneumonia by bacteriologic analysis of bronchoscopic and nonbronchoscopic "blind" bronchoalveolar lavage fluid. Am Rev Respir Dis 1991; 143(5 Pt 1):1121–1129.

179. Fartoukh M, Maitre B, Honore S, et al. Diagnosing pneumonia during mechanical ventilation: the clinical pulmonary infection score revisited. Am J Respir Crit Care Med 2003; 168(2):173–179.

180. Singh N, Rogers P, Atwood CW, et al. Short-course empiric antibiotic therapy for patients with pulmonary infiltrates in the intensive care unit. A proposed solution for indiscriminate antibiotic prescription. Am J Respir Crit Care Med 2000; 162(2 Pt 1):505–511.

181. Bonten MJ, Bergmans DC, Stobberingh EE, et al. Implementation of bronchoscopic techniques in the diagnosis of ventilator-associated pneumonia to reduce antibiotic use. Am J Respir Crit Care Med 1997; 156(6):1820–1824.

182. Croce MA, Fabian TC, Waddle-Smith L, et al. Utility of Gram's stain and efficacy of quantitative cultures for posttraumatic pneumonia: a prospective study. Ann Surg 1998; 227(5):743–751; discussion 751–745.

183. Kirtland SH, Corley DE, Winterbauer RH, et al. The diagnosis of ventilator-associated pneumonia: a comparison of histologic, microbiologic, and clinical criteria. Chest 1997; 112(2):445–457.

184. Wermert D, Marquette CH, Copin MC, et al. Influence of pulmonary bacteriology and histology on the yield of diagnostic procedures in ventilator-acquired pneumonia. Am J Respir Crit Care Med 1998; 158(1):139–147.

185. Ruiz M, Torres A, Ewig S, et al. Noninvasive versus invasive microbial investigation in ventilator-associated pneumonia: evaluation of outcome. Am J Respir Crit Care Med 2000; 162(1):119–125.

186. Heyland DK, Cook DJ, Marshall J, et al. Canadian Critical Care Trials Group. The clinical utility of invasive diagnostic techniques in the setting of ventilator-associated pneumonia. Chest 1999; 115(4):1076–1084.

187. Baker AM, Bowton DL, Haponik EF. Decision making in nosocomial pneumonia. An analytic approach to the interpretation of quantitative bronchoscopic cultures. Chest 1995; 107(1):85–95.

188. Fagon JY, Chastre J, Wolff M, et al. Invasive and noninvasive strategies for management of suspected ventilator-associated pneumonia. A randomized trial. Ann Intern Med 2000; 132(8):621–630.

189. Rello J, Mirelis B, Alonso C, et al. Lack of usefulness of blood cultures to diagnose ventilator-associated pneumonia. Eur Respir J 1991; 4(8):1020.

190. Chendrasekhar A. Are routine blood cultures effective in the evaluation of patients clinically diagnosed to have nosocomial pneumonia? Am Surg 1996; 62(5):373–376.

191. Luna CM, Videla A, Mattera J, et al. Blood cultures have limited value in predicting severity of illness and as a diagnostic tool in ventilator-associated pneumonia. Chest 1999; 116(4):1075–1084.

192. Ioanas M, Ferrer R, Angrill J, et al. Microbial investigation in ventilator-associated pneumonia. Eur Respir J 2001; 17(4):791–801.

193. Papazian L, Martin C, Albanese J, et al. Comparison of two methods of bacteriologic sampling of the lower respiratory tract: a study in ventilated patients with nosocomial bronchopneumonia. Crit Care Med 1989; 17(5):461–464.

194. Rumbak MJ, Bass RL. Tracheal aspirate correlates with protected specimen brush in long-term ventilated patients who have clinical pneumonia. Chest 1994; 106(2):531–534.

195. Blot F, Raynard B, Chachaty E, et al. Value of gram stain examination of lower respiratory tract secretions for early diagnosis of nosocomial pneumonia. Am J Respir Crit Care Med 2000; 162(5):1731–1737.

196. Woske HJ, Roding T, Schulz I, et al. Ventilator-associated pneumonia in a surgical intensive care unit: epidemiology, etiology and comparison of three bronchoscopic methods for microbiological specimen sampling. Crit Care 2001; 5(3):167–173.

197. Wu CL, Yang D, Wang NY, et al. Quantitative culture of endotracheal aspirates in the diagnosis of ventilator-associated pneumonia in patients with treatment failure. Chest 2002; 122(2):662–668.

198. Aucar JA, Bongera M, Phillips JO, et al. Quantitative tracheal lavage versus bronchoscopic protected specimen brush for the diagnosis of nosocomial pneumonia in mechanically ventilated patients. Am J Surg 2003; 186(6):591–596.

199. Timsit JF, Misset B, Goldstein FW, et al. Reappraisal of distal diagnostic testing in the diagnosis of ICU-acquired pneumonia. Chest 1995; 108(6):1632–1639.

200. Michaud S, Suzuki S, Harbarth S. Effect of design-related bias in studies of diagnostic tests for ventilator-associated pneumonia. Am J Respir Crit Care Med 2002; 166(10): 1320–1325.

201. Souweine B, Veber B, Bedos JP, et al. Diagnostic accuracy of protected specimen brush and bronchoalveolar lavage in nosocomial pneumonia: impact of previous antimicrobial treatments. Crit Care Med 1998; 26(2):236–244.

202. Luna CM, Blanzaco D, Niederman MS, et al. Resolution of ventilator-associated pneumonia: prospective evaluation of the clinical pulmonary infection score as an early clinical predictor of outcome. Crit Care Med 2003; 31(3):676–682.

203. Dennesen PJ, van der Ven AJ, Kessels AG, et al. Resolution of infectious parameters after antimicrobial therapy in patients with ventilator-associated pneumonia. Am J Respir Crit Care Med 2001; 163(6):1371–1375.

204. Niederman MS. The clinical diagnosis of ventilator-associated pneumonia. Respir Care 2005; 50(6):788–796.

205. Nopmaneejumruslers C, Chan CK. Is there a role for routine surveillance endotracheal aspirate cultures in the treatment of BAL-confirmed ventilator-associated pneumonia? Chest 2005; 127(2):425–427.

206. Michel F, Franceschini B, Berger P, et al. Early antibiotic treatment for BAL-confirmed ventilator-associated pneumonia: a role for routine endotracheal aspirate cultures. Chest 2005; 127(2):589–597.

207. Valencia Arango M, Torres Marti A, Insausti Ordenana J, et al. Diagnostic value of quantitative cultures of endotracheal aspirate in ventilator-associated pneumonia: a multicenter study. Arch Bronconeumol 2003; 39(9):394–399.

208. Fangio P, Rouquette-Vincenti I, Rousseau JM, et al. Diagnosis of ventilator-associated pneumonia: a prospective comparison of the telescoping plugged catheter with the endotracheal aspirate. Ann Fr Anesth Reanim 2002; 21(3):184–192.

209. Wood AY, Davit AJ II, Ciraulo DL, et al. A prospective assessment of diagnostic efficacy of blind protective bronchial brushings compared to bronchoscope-assisted lavage, bronchoscope-directed brushings, and blind endotracheal aspirates in ventilator-associated pneumonia. J Trauma 2003; 55(5):825–834.

210. Cook D, Mandell L. Endotracheal aspiration in the diagnosis of ventilator-associated pneumonia. Chest 2000; 117(4 suppl 2):195S–197S.

211. Jourdain B, Novara A, Joly-Guillou ML, et al. Role of quantitative cultures of endotracheal aspirates in the diagnosis of nosocomial pneumonia. Am J Respir Crit Care Med 1995; 152(1):241–246.

212. Torres A, El-Ebiary M. Bronchoscopic BAL in the diagnosis of ventilator-associated pneumonia. Chest 2000; 117(4 suppl 2):198S–202S.

213. Jourdain B, Joly-Guillou ML, Dombret MC, et al. Usefulness of quantitative cultures of BAL fluid for diagnosing nosocomial pneumonia in ventilated patients. Chest 1997; 111(2):411–418.

214. Sole Violan J, Rodriguez de Castro F, Caminero Luna J, et al. Comparative efficacy of bronchoalveolar lavage and telescoping plugged catheter in the diagnosis of pneumonia in mechanically ventilated patients. Chest 1993; 103(2):386–390.

215. Chastre J, Fagon JY, Bornet-Lecso M, et al. Evaluation of bronchoscopic techniques for the diagnosis of nosocomial pneumonia. Am J Respir Crit Care Med 1995; 152(1):231–240.

216. Marquette CH, Copin MC, Wallet F, et al. Diagnostic tests for pneumonia in ventilated patients: prospective evaluation of diagnostic accuracy using histology as a diagnostic gold standard. Am J Respir Crit Care Med 1995; 151(6):1878–1888.

217. Papazian L, Thomas P, Garbe L, et al. Bronchoscopic or blind sampling techniques for the diagnosis of ventilator-associated pneumonia. Am J Respir Crit Care Med 1995; 152(6 Pt 1):1982–1991.

218. Casetta M, Blot F, Antoun S, et al. Diagnosis of nosocomial pneumonia in cancer patients undergoing mechanical ventilation: a prospective comparison of the plugged telescoping catheter with the protected specimen brush. Chest 1999; 115(6):1641–1645.

219. Pham LH, Brun-Buisson C, Legrand P, et al. Diagnosis of nosocomial pneumonia in mechanically ventilated patients. Comparison of a plugged telescoping catheter with the protected specimen brush. Am Rev Respir Dis 1991; 143(5 Pt 1):1055–1061.

220. Mentec H, May-Michelangeli L, Rabbat A, et al. Blind and bronchoscopic sampling methods in suspected ventilator-associated pneumonia. A multicentre prospective study. Intensive Care Med 2004; 30(7):1319–1326.

221. Campbell GD Jr. Blinded invasive diagnostic procedures in ventilator-associated pneumonia. Chest 2000; 117(4 suppl 2):207S–211S.

222. Bello S, Tajada A, Chacon E, et al. Blind protected specimen brushing versus bronchoscopic techniques in the aetiolological diagnosis of ventilator-associated pneumonia. Eur Respir J 1996; 9(7):1494–1499.

223. Kollef MH, Ward S. The influence of mini-BAL cultures on patient outcomes: implications for the antibiotic management of ventilator-associated pneumonia. Chest 1998; 113(2):412–420.

224. Dupont H, Mentec H, Sollet JP, et al. Impact of appropriateness of initial antibiotic therapy on the outcome of ventilator-associated pneumonia. Intensive Care Med 2001; 27(2):355–362.
225. Rello J, Quintana E, Ausina V, et al. Risk factors for *Staphylococcus aureus* nosocomial pneumonia in critically ill patients. Am Rev Respir Dis 1990; 142(6 Pt 1):1320–1324.
226. Rello J, Ausina V, Ricart M, et al. Risk factors for infection by *Pseudomonas aeruginosa* in patients with ventilator-associated pneumonia. Intensive Care Med 1994; 20(3): 193–198.
227. Sandiumenge A, Diaz E, Bodi M, et al. Therapy of ventilator-associated pneumonia. A patient-based approach based on the ten rules of "The Tarragona Strategy". Intensive Care Med 2003; 29(6):876–883.
228. Ibrahim EH, Ward S, Sherman G, et al. Experience with a clinical guideline for the treatment of ventilator-associated pneumonia. Crit Care Med 2001; 29(6):1109–1115.
229. Trouillet JL, Vuagnat A, Combes A, et al. *Pseudomonas aeruginosa* ventilator-associated pneumonia: comparison of episodes due to piperacillin-resistant versus piperacillin-susceptible organisms. Clin Infect Dis 2002; 34(8):1047–1054.
230. Fagon J, Patrick H, Haas DW, et al. Nosocomial Pneumonia Group. Treatment of gram-positive nosocomial pneumonia. Prospective randomized comparison of quinupristin/dalfopristin versus vancomycin. Am J Respir Crit Care Med 2000; 161(3 Pt 1):753–762.
231. Malangoni MA, Crafton R, Mocek FC. Pneumonia in the surgical intensive care unit: factors determining successful outcome. Am J Surg 1994; 167(2):250–255.
232. Moise PA, Forrest A, Bhavnani SM, et al. Area under the inhibitory curve and a pneumonia scoring system for predicting outcomes of vancomycin therapy for respiratory infections by *Staphylococcus aureus*. Am J Health Syst Pharm 2000; 57:S4–S9.
233. Levine DP, Fromm BS, Reddy BR. Slow response to vancomycin or vancomycin plus rifampin in methicillin-resistant *Staphylococcus aureus* endocarditis. Ann Intern Med 1991; 115(9):674–680.
234. Lamer C, de Beco V, Soler P, et al. Analysis of vancomycin entry into pulmonary lining fluid by bronchoalveolar lavage in critically ill patients. Antimicrob Agents Chemother 1993; 37(2):281–286.
235. Conte JE Jr., Golden JA, Kipps J, et al. Intrapulmonary pharmacokinetics of linezolid. Antimicrob Agents Chemother 2002; 46(5):1475–1480.
236. Wunderink RG, Rello J, Cammarata SK, et al. Linezolid versus vancomycin: analysis of two double-blind studies of patients with methicillin-resistant *Staphylococcus aureus* nosocomial pneumonia. Chest 2003; 124(5):1789–1797.
237. Kollef MH, Rello J, Cammarata SK, et al. Clinical cure and survival in Gram-positive ventilator-associated pneumonia: retrospective analysis of two double-blind studies comparing linezolid with vancomycin. Intensive Care Med 2004; 30(3):388–394.
238. Anstead GM, Owens AD. Recent advances in the treatment of infections due to resistant *Staphylococcus aureus*. Curr Opin Infect Dis 2004; 17(6):549–555.
239. Rello J, Mariscal D, March F, et al. Recurrent *Pseudomonas aeruginosa* pneumonia in ventilated patients: relapse or reinfection? Am J Respir Crit Care Med 1998; 157(3 Pt 1): 912–916.
240. Hilf M, Yu VL, Sharp J, et al. Antibiotic therapy for *Pseudomonas aeruginosa* bacteremia: outcome correlations in a prospective study of 200 patients. Am J Med 1989; 87(5): 540–546.
241. Fink MP, Snydman DR, Niederman MS, et al. The Severe Pneumonia Study Group. Treatment of severe pneumonia in hospitalized patients: results of a multicenter, randomized, double-blind trial comparing intravenous ciprofloxacin with imipenem-cilastatin. Antimicrob Agents Chemother 1994; 38(3):547–557.
242. Cometta A, Baumgartner JD, Lew D, et al. Prospective randomized comparison of imipenem monotherapy with imipenem plus netilmicin for treatment of severe infections in nonneutropenic patients. Antimicrob Agents Chemother 1994; 38(6):1309–1313.

243. Paul M, Benuri-Silbiger I, Soares-Weiser K, et al. Beta lactam monotherapy versus beta lactam-aminoglycoside combination therapy for sepsis in immunocompetent patients: systematic review and meta-analysis of randomised trials. BMJ 2004; 328(7441):668.

244. Hamer DH. Treatment of nosocomial pneumonia and tracheobronchitis caused by multidrug-resistant *Pseudomonas aeruginosa* with aerosolized colistin. Am J Respir Crit Care Med 2000; 162(1):328–330.

245. Wood GC, Hanes SD, Croce MA, et al. Comparison of ampicillin-sulbactam and imipenem-cilastatin for the treatment of acinetobacter ventilator-associated pneumonia. Clin Infect Dis 2002; 34(11):1425–1430.

246. Palmer LB, Smaldone GC, Simon SR, et al. Aerosolized antibiotics in mechanically ventilated patients: delivery and response. Crit Care Med 1998; 26(1):31–39.

246b. Le Comte P, Poti IG, Clementi E, et al. Administration of tobramycin aerosols in patients with nasocomial pneumonia: a preliminary study. Presse Med 2000; 29(2): 76–78.

247. Safdar N, Handelsman J, Maki DG. Does combination antimicrobial therapy reduce mortality in Gram-negative bacteraemia? A meta-analysis. Lancet Infect Dis 2004; 4(8): 519–527.

248. Chastre J, Wolff M, Fagon JY, et al. Comparison of 8 versus 15 days of antibiotic therapy for ventilator-associated pneumonia in adults: a randomized trial. JAMA 2003; 290(19):2588–2598.

249. Cavalcanti M, Valencia M, Torres A. Respiratory nosocomial infections in the medical intensive care unit. Microbes Infect 2005; 7(2):292–301.

250. Ioanas M, Ferrer M, Cavalcanti M, et al. Causes and predictors of nonresponse to treatment of intensive care unit-acquired pneumonia. Crit Care Med 2004; 32(4):938–945.

251. Bouza E, Munoz P, Burillo A, et al. The challenge of anticipating catheter tip colonization in major heart surgery patients in the intensive care unit: Are surface cultures useful? Crit Care Med 2005; 33(9):1953–1960.

10

Pleural Empyema/Lung Abscess in the Critical Care Unit

John G. Bartlett

Department of Medicine, School of Medicine, Johns Hopkins University, Baltimore, Maryland, U.S.A.

INTRODUCTION

Pneumonia is a relatively common infection associated with a wide variety of microbes. Empyema and necrotizing pneumonia or lung abscess are relatively rare complications that are usually associated with relatively few pathogens. Many of these processes are indolent and chronic, but some are also acute and life threatening. The purpose of this chapter is to review empyema and lung abscess with particular attention to specific microbial associations and management guidelines.

EMPYEMA

The classic definition is "pleural pus." Subsequent alternative definitions are based on a leukocyte count exceeding $25,000/mm^3$ with a predominance of polymorphonuclear leukocytes or pleural fluid with microorganisms demonstrated by Gram stain and/or culture. The most recent and now well-accepted definition is a pleural fluid pH of ≤ 7.0 or lower (1,2).

Pathophysiology

The most common cause of empyema is simply extension of a bacterial infection of the lung to contiguous pleural space. This accounts for 40% to 60% in most series (3–9). Previous thoracic surgery accounts for the majority of nosocomial infections and represents 15% to 30% of cases. A third mechanism is extension from a subdiaphragmatic collection. Rare predisposing conditions are esophageal perforation, chest trauma with a hemothorax, extension from a perimandibular or neck space infection, and septicemia or thoracentesis with inadequate sterile technique.

Empyema is classically divided into three stages, which represent a continuum. This sequence dictates the findings on pleural fluid analysis and also the appropriate method of drainage (1,2). The initial stage is exudative with thin, free-flowing fluid with a small number of leukocytes, a pH above 7.2 and lactate dehydrogenase (LDH) below 1000 IU/L. At this stage microbial studies are generally negative, and antibiotic treatment at this stage usually stops progression. The second stage is the "fibropurulent stage" with pleural fluid showing a large number of polymorphonuclear leukocytes and fibrin. Pleural fluid analysis at this stage shows a pH < 7.2, LDH exceeding 1000 IU/L, low glucose, and positive Gram stain and culture for bacteria. Deposits of fibrin on the parietal and visceral pleural surfaces at the site of involvement result in loculation. The loculated collections make adequate drainage with chest tubes progressively difficult. The final stage is the "organizing stage" in which there is the production of a pleural peel of fibrous tissue. This is a chronic stage in which the exudate is thick pus, and the lung becomes entrapped.

Incidence

In the prepenicillin era empyema was said to complicate 10% to 20% of cases of pneumococcal pneumonia (10,11). It was a relatively late complication of untreated disease. Streptococcal empyema was also well described in the prepenicillin era and, in contrast to pneumococcal pneumonia, the empyema complication occurred early in the course of the disease (12,13). Since that time there has been a substantial decrease in the frequency of empyema so that this complication is now noted in only about 1% of cases of community-acquired pneumonia sufficiently severe to require hospitalization (14). The frequency of empyema as a complication of lung resection is reported at 1% to 5% (15,16). Most of these latter cases are associated with a bronchopleural fistula.

Diagnostic Studies

Pleural effusions may be caused by a number of infectious and noninfectious diseases. The infections include those due to mycobacteria, viruses, fungi, bacteria, and, on rare occasions, parasites. The noninfectious diseases include pulmonary embolism, postcardiotomy syndrome, collagen vascular disease (particularly systemic lupus erythematosus or rheumatoid effusions), malignancies, drug-induced pulmonary disease, congestive heart failure, and sympathetic effusions from subdiaphragmatic conditions such as pancreatitis or subphrenic abscess.

Routine tests recommended include pH determination, leukocyte count with differential, total protein, levels of LDH, glucose levels, and Gram stain and cultures for aerobic and anaerobic bacteria. Pleural collections that are grossly purulent generally require no studies beyond culture and Gram stain. A meta-analysis of multiple reports showed the pleural fluid pH had the highest diagnostic accuracy for identifying effusions that require drainage (17). The decision threshold in this analysis was 7.21 to 7.29. For tuberculosis effusions, adenosine deaminase (ADA) levels are particularly useful (18,19), but this diagnosis rests on recovery of *Mycobacterium tuberculosis* from sputum, pleural fluid, or pleural tissue. Demonstration of granulomas in pleural biopsies is suggestive (20). Bloody effusions with low ADA levels favor malignancy (21).

Bacteriology

Streptococcus pneumoniae

Bacteriology studies of empyema in the prepenicillin era showed *S. pneumoniae* accounted for 60% to 70% (Table 1) (10,11). The most comprehensive review was a summary of 5393 cases of pneumococcal pneumonia reported from 1926 to 1939, which included 286 with empyema for a frequency of 5.3% (11). The more recent

Table 1 Bacteriology of Empyema

Refs.	Period	Cases	Sterile (%)	*Streptococcus pneumoniae* (%)	Beta strep (%)	*Staphylococcus aureus* (%)	GNB (%)	Anaerobes (%)
(22)	1934–1939	3000	NS*	64	9	7	–	5
(23)	1932–1939	500	NS*	63	16	5	–	7
(24)	1950–1972	482	53	13	–	12	6	19
(25)	1971–1973	83	0	6	0	20	25	76
(5)	1970–1978	117	32	15	–	25	29	11
(6)	1984–1990	82	7	11	–	13	26	39
(8)	1989–1993	43	37	2	–	26	2	12
(3)	–	427	43	7	–	9	–	–

*NS, not stated.
Abbreviation: GNB, gram-negative bacilli.

studies have shown a substantial decline in the frequency of empyema as a complication of pneumococcal pneumonia presumably attributed to successful antimicrobial therapy. Most studies now show this organism accounts for only 5% to 10% of all cases (3–9). The largest recent report included 430 cases with the pneumococcus accounting for 7% (3). Most of these represent extension of pneumonia through contiguous pleural surfaces because *S. pneumoniae* is infrequently or almost never associated with pulmonary necrosis.

Mycobacteria

M. tuberculosis is a relatively common cause of pleural effusion and obviously an important diagnosis to establish (18–21). These are particularly common in developing countries, immigrants from these areas, and the presence of HIV infection. Many of these patients have very large pleural collections (26). Characteristic features of the fluid include high levels of ADA and a predominance of lymphocytes, and most respond to standard therapy for tuberculosis (18–21,26).

Streptococcus pyogenes

This organism accounted for 10% to 15% of empyema in the prepenicillin era and now is relatively rare as a cause of either pneumonia or empyema (12,13). One of the highly characteristic features is the predominance of this microbial pathogen in pediatric cases and the clinical course of infection, which shows rapid accumulations of pleural fluid and/or empyema, which presumably reflects the penchant of this organism to block lymphatics. The typical presentation is relatively rapid.

Anaerobic Bacteria

During the past two decades there has been substantial attention to the role of anaerobic bacteria in empyema, complicating aspiration pneumonia or lung abscess (1,24,25,27–29). The yield is highly variable, which presumably reflects variations in laboratory capability to detect oxygen-sensitive forms and the population studied. The yield in most recent series has ranged from 11% to 76% (1,3–9,24,25,27–29). The clinical clues to these infections are the presence of putrid pleural fluid, which is considered diagnostic of anaerobic infection and a Gram stain showing a polymicrobial flora or a Gram stain showing the unique morphologic characteristic of anaerobic gram-negative bacilli.

Staphylococcus aureus

S. aureus is by far the most frequent pathogen associated with nosocomial empyema and usually represents a complication of thoracic surgery (15,16). Many of these infections involve methicillin-resistant *S. aureus* (MRSA), which obviously has important implications regarding infection control and therapy. In the past several years there has been the recognition of a new variety of MRSA pulmonary infections associated with "community-acquired MRSA (CA-MRSA)," which is now referred to as the "USA300" strain (30–32). This is a devastating cause of necrotizing pneumonia that is commonly complicated by empyema formation and will be discussed more extensively in the section on lung abscess.

Bacillus anthracis

Inhalation anthrax is virtually always due to bioterrorism (30–32). The last case of naturally occurring inhalation anthrax in the United States was reported in 1976, and then there were the 11 cases resulting from bioterrorism in 2002. This organism is actually an infrequent cause of pneumonia per se, but is acquired by inhalation and is transported to hilar and mediastinal lymph nodes, where it produces toxins resulting in rapid progression to sepsis, the characteristic wide mediastinum on chest X-ray and shock. Large bloody pleural fluid collections are common; the average case is associated with pleural collections that average 1600 mL (30–32). In fact, chest compression has been thought to be an important contributing factor to death so that daily drainages are now considered an essential feature of management.

Clinical Features

The common features with empyema include fever, cough, sputum production, dyspnea and, in approximately 60% of patients, pleurisy. The physical exam demonstrates reduced breath sounds and dullness at the implicate site. It is not possible by physical exam to distinguish parapneumonic effusions and empyema. Chest X-rays show pleural effusions, which are common in pneumonia. It is often recommended that the lateral decubitus X-ray is important for detection for small pleural effusions (2); if the distance from the inside chest wall to the bottom of the lung measures over 10 mm a thoracentesis is commonly recommended but infrequently done in practice (33). Computed tomography (CT) will readily distinguish pleural collections from parenchymal infiltrates (34,35). There are multiple causes of pleural effusions, but empyema is quite rare as noted above.

Treatment

The three core principles of treatment are prompt antibiotics, complete evacuation of the pleural collection, and preservation of lung function.

Antibiotic Treatment

Antibiotic selection is obviously much simpler if an etiologic diagnosis is made on the basis of Gram stain and culture. Most antibiotics diffuse well into pleural fluid so that local installations are not required (36,37).

Thrombolytic Agents

Streptokinase and urokinase are often advocated for lysis of loculated effusions. A large controlled clinical trial with this method failed to demonstrate any benefit with installations of streptokinase. However, these results have been challenged by the suggestion that a subset of patients who were younger and had less complicated cases might benefit from this treatment (38). This report (38) showing a favorable outcome had a much smaller sample size (22 patients vs. 430 patients) but also used larger tubes (#24 or 28 French vs. #12 French), and tubes were placed under ultrasound guidance (Diacon AH). The method commonly advocated is instillation of 250,000 IU streptokinase given in 30 mL saline q12 h for six doses (3). Thus, no conclusions are available, and the reported experience is variable (3,9,38–42).

Drainage

The main issue in the management of empyemas is drainage, which has been the mainstay of treatment for 2000 years (43). Despite consensus on the importance of this issue there is substantial controversy about how it is actually done, and a recent guideline for empyema in children noted sparse evidence to support any specific tactic. In general, the recommendations are dictated by findings on chest X-rays or CT and analysis of pleural fluid, which indicates the stage of infection (2,22,23,44–55).

During the initial exudative phase (Table 2) the fluid is thin and free flowing, the lung is easily reexpanded, and the empyema may resolve simply with thoracentesis and antibiotic treatment: This may be augmented with repeated thoracentesis or tube thoracostomy drainage (49,51). The need for thoracostomy drainage increases with a lower pH and higher LDH. Nearly all patients with a pleural fluid pH below 7.2 require tube drainage, and nearly all with pH above 7.3 have resolution with appropriate antibiotics (2,44–48,52–54). The pleural fluid pH interval from 7.0 to 7.3 is arbitrary meaning repeated pleural fluid analyses and careful clinical observation along with antibiotic treatment. Tuberculous effusions usually respond to anti-TB therapy, but many advocate drainage of large collections to remove as much fluid as possible (26).

Table 2 Management Recommendations

Stage	Drainage
Early stage	Thoracentesis + antibiotics
pH < 7.2	
Glucose < 40 mg/dL	
LDH > 1000 IU/dL	
Protein > 2.5 g/dL	
WBC > 500/mm^3	
Fluid is serous or cloudy, free flowing	
Fibropurulent stage	Large-bore thoracostomy tube ± fibrinolytics
Thick fluid and positive cultures	
Organizing stage	Open thoracostomy
Organizing peel with entrapped lung	Mini-thoracotomy
	Thoracoscopic evacuation
	Decortication

Abbreviations: LDH, lactate dehydrogenase; WBC, white blood count.

The fibropurulent phase is associated with fluid that is too thick for drainage by thoracentesis necessitating thoracostomy, often with large-bore needles. The drainage may be facilitated by catheter placement under fluoroscopic, computed tomographic, or ultrasonic guidance (22,23,51,52). Closed drainage with suction is recommended if the fluid is thick, there is evidence of a bronchopleural fistula, or the pleural fluid is putrid. The thoracostomy tubes are left in place until the cavity is obliterated, and the yield of pleural drainage is less than $25\,mL/day$, any bronchopleural fistula is sealed, and fever has resolved. Failure to achieve these goals may indicate the requirement for chest tube positioning or reinsertion. Failure of the closed procedure often indicates the need for open drainage with rib resection or decortication.

Decisions regarding drainage procedure may be facilitated by the empyema severity score based on pleural fluid pH glucose and results of imaging—ultrasonography to localize loculated pleural fluid prior to aspiration or thoracostomy, or CT scan to detect a pleural peel (56). Factors indicating a possible need for surgery are failure to defeverse with antibiotics and thoracentesis and a severity of pleural disease score based on low pleural fluid pH, low glucose, moderate or severe scoliosis, presence of pleural peel, and infection due to anaerobes or gram-negative bacilli.

The initial surgical procedure is often a closed tube thoracostomy using ultrasound or CT guidance for tube placement. Fibrolytic agents are often instilled through the tubes, but their utility is not clearly established. The next stage for patients who do not respond is rib resection with open drainage, a procedure associated with substantial morbidity. A variant is the mini-thoracotomy, which involves a 5 cm incision and short segment rib resection (57).

The late organizing phase is characterized by an extensive collection of fibrous material or pleural peel and lung entrapment, which generally requires open thoracotomy or decortication (9,41,48). This procedure is done with open thoracotomy, debridement of the coagulum, careful excision of the peel, and assessment of lung expansion prior to closure. A variant recently introduced is decortication with video assistance to reduce morbidity.

Outcome

Studies from the prepenicillin era showed mortality rates of 7% to 41% with pneumococcal empyema (10,11). The mortality is obviously much lower in the current era associated with antibiotics and improved thoracic surgery but still reported at 8% to 20% (3–12,58,59). This includes studies published since 1984 (3,60). Factors that indicate a poor prognosis include chronic empyema, nosocomial empyema, advanced age, association with malignancy, and the presence of a bronchopleural fistula. Excluding patients with serious or ultimately lethal underlying conditions, the mortality rates are generally 3% to 6% (3,57). In many of these cases, the major difficulty is achieving adequate drainage. These cases are associated with long hospital stays and continuing controversies about the next step in the patient with persistent pleural collections.

LUNG ABSCESS

Introduction

Lung abscess results from necrosis of lung parenchyma. The term "necrotizing pneumonia" and "pulmonary gangrene" are sometimes used to indicate small pulmonary abscesses in contiguous areas of the lung. These represent a continuum and are

infections involving a relatively small number of pathogens that can cause this pathologic result. Thus, as with empyema, the tabulation of microbes that cause pneumonia
is legion; the number that cause pulmonary necrosis is a relatively short list.

Classification

A number of methods to classify lung abscess and either the terms or the definitions
have been used in the literature. Some of the standard terms that have been used during
the past 50 years include

- *Acute or chronic abscesses* with four to six weeks as the standard dividing
  line.
- *Primary versus secondary abscesses*; the former generally refers to abscesses
  in patients prone to aspiration or in healthy adults while secondary abscesses represent complications of a primary condition of the lung such as a
  neoplasm or HIV infection.
- *Nonspecific lung abscess* often refers to abscesses in which no likely pathogen is recovered from expectorated sputum; most of these are considered
  anaerobic infections.
- *Putrid lung abscess* indicates the offensive odor of sputum that is considered
  diagnostic of anaerobic infection.
- *Nosocomial lung abscess* in reference to those that occur during hospitalization and are usually due to nosocomial pathogens.

In an extensive experience with over 1000 reported cases of lung abscess in the
antibiotic era, approximately 80% were considered primary, 60% putrid, 40% nonspecific, and 40% chronic (61–68).

Clinical Features

Lung abscesses may be acute or chronic. Chronic abscesses are most likely to represent
microbacteria infections due to mycobacteria, anaerobic bacteria, and melioidosis.
The latter is a relatively common cause of pulmonary infections due to *Burkholderia
pseudomallei* in Asia; this is extremely rare in the United States except for occasional
immigrants. Acute lung abscess is usually associated with more virulent organisms such
as *Klebsiella* and *S. aureus*.

The usual clinical features of lung abscess include fever, fatigue, cough with sputum production, and sometimes pleurisy and/or hemoptysis. Chronic lung abscesses
are usually accompanied by weight loss and anemia. Approximately 60% of patients
with bacteriologically confirmed lung abscesses that are due to anaerobic bacteria
have putrid sputum, empyema fluid, or breath.

Evaluation

The characteristic feature on chest X-ray is a cavity in the pulmonary parenchyma
often with an air-fluid level within a pulmonary infiltrate. Lymphadenopathy suggests some specific conditions such as mycobacterial or fungal infection. CT is a
particularly sensitive method to detect lung abscess and provides good anatomic
definition. This also will clearly distinguish air-fluid levels in the pleural space from
those within the pulmonary parenchyma (68,69). Segmental location of the abscess is
important in the differential diagnosis. Anaerobic lung abscess due to aspiration

Table 3 Pulmonary Lesions with Appearance of Lung Abscess

Necrotizing infections of the lung
    Bacteria: anaerobic bacteria, microaerophilic/anaerobic streptococci (*Streptococcus milleri*), enteric GNB (esp. *Klebsiella*), *Pseudomonas aeruginosa*, *Staphylococcus aureus* (including MRSA USA 300)
    Less common: nocardia, actinomycosis, Rhodococcus, Legionella, *Pasteurella multocida*
Mycobacteria: *Mycobacterium tuberculosis*, *M. kansasii*, *M. avium-intracellulare*
Fungi: Coccidioidomycosis, Histoplasmosis, Blastomycosis, Aspergillus, Cryptococcus, Mucor
Parasite: *Entamoeba histolytica*, *Paragonimus westermani*, *Echinococcus*
Cavity
    Bland infarct ± infection
    Septic emboli
    Vasculitis: Wegner's granulomatosis, periarteritis nodosa
    Neoplasms: lung cancer, metastatic carcinoma, lymphoma
    Others: cysts, blebs, pneumatocele, sequestration, bronchiectasis, empyema

Abbreviation: MRSA, methicillin-resistant *Staphylococcus aureus*.

usually involves dependent pulmonary segments, the posterior segments of the upper lobe of superior segments of the lower lobes. These reflect the dependent pulmonary segments in the recumbent position. Tuberculosis favors the upper lobes.

There are a number of conditions to consider in the patient with an established or suspected abscess involving the pulmonary parenchyma as indicated in Table 3.

Detection of the etiologic agent is particularly important because these infections are often both severe and chronic so that pathogen-specific therapy is highly desired. A good pretreatment expectorated sputum is useful for Gram stain and culture; the diagnostic yield is generally excellent for detection of *S. aureus* and aerobic gram-negative bacilli, particularly *Klebsiella pneumoniae* or *Pseudomonas aeruginosa*. This specimen is not appropriate for anaerobic culture so that these organisms, the most common causes of lung abscess, must be treated empirically or there needs to be a diagnostic method which bypasses the contamination associated with specimens that traverse the upper airways. In former years this was done by transtracheal aspiration (TTA), which became the technique to define the etiology of aspiration pneumonia and lung abscess in the 1970s (58,59,70,71). The TTA has subsequently been abandoned. More recent studies have sometimes used quantitative cultures of bronchoscopic specimens, either bronchoalveolar lavage or use of the protected brush (72–75). The experience with this technique is quite variable, in part related to the need for specimens prior to antibiotic treatment, the deleterious effect of lidocaine on some fastidious anaerobes, the difficulty that many laboratories have in cultivating oxygen-sensitive bacteria, and inconsistent methods of specimen collection and processing. Thus, many authorities do not regard this as an appropriate method to either rule in or rule out anaerobic bacteria. An alternative method that is occasionally used is transthoracic aspiration in which there is needle aspiration of the abscess percutaneously.

Bacteriology

Anaerobic Bacteria

These are the organisms that represent normal flora of the oral cavity, primarily the gingiva crevice. They reach the lung by aspiration, usually in a host that is prone to aspiration due to decreased consciousness or dysphagia. The dominant isolates in these cases are *Peptostreptococcus* spp., *Prevotella melaninogenica*, and *Fusobacterium nucleatum* (58,59,70,71,76,77).

Staphylococcus aureus

This organism has been historically found primarily in pediatric patients, patients with influenza complicated by bacterial superinfections, injection drug users with tricuspid valve endocarditis with septic emboli to the lung, and with nosocomial pulmonary infections (78,79). More recently there has been a new syndrome attributed to "CA-MRSA," an epidemic strain referred to as "USA300" (80–84). The latter actually refers to a family of related strains, but those involved are a relatively homogeneous group that is characterized by the presence of genes for the Paton-Valentine Leukocidin, a possible virulence factor, and the mecIV element, which confers resistance to all betalactams (85). Many or most of these strains are sensitive to many antibiotics that are not generally found to be active in vitro with nosocomial strains of MRSA; these include trimethoprim-sulfamethoxazole, gentamicin, rifampin, and doxycycline. The clinical syndrome associated with this pathogen is usually devastating. Most of the patients are young, previously healthy adults, who acquire influenza and then have a rapid and fulminant course characterized by necrotizing pneumonia and shock. The putative is recovered from blood and/or respiratory secretions. The mortality rate is variously reported at 20% to 50% (80–84).

Klebsiella

Klebsiella has always been recognized as a possible pulmonary pathogen with a penchant to cause abscess (86,87). The classic description was in the prepenicillin era when the typical presentation was a debilitated host who presented with fever, cough, pleurisy, and sputum that looked like currant jelly and an X ray that showed an upper lobe infiltrate with the "bulging fissure sign"; this went on to cavitate. This form of *Klebsiella* pulmonary infection is rarely seen currently, but *Klebsiella* continues to be occasionally implicated in lung abscess, particularly in Taiwan where it is epidemic (87).

Miscellaneous Bacteria

Other agents implicated include nocardia (88,89) Legionella (90–92), *Streptococcus milleri* (93,94), *S. pyogenes* (95,96), *Rhodococcus equi* (97–100), *Fusobacterium necrophorum* (as a complication of Lemierre syndrome) (101–103), and *B. pseudomallei* (melioidosis) (104).

Treatment

Most patients respond to antibiotic treatment, and this is best if it is pathogen-specific. Tuberculosis is treated with the standard four drug regimen. *Klebsiella* generally responds to cephalosporin treatment, but in vitro sensitivity tests are desired, and *P. aeruginosa* is found primarily in the compromised host or the patient with structural disease of the lung; optimal therapy is controversial due to the debate concerning the need for one or two drugs directed against this pathogen (105,106). Long courses of a fluoroquinolone selected on the basis of in vitro activity in patients with HIV infection show high rates of failure, suggesting that alternative drugs may be preferred (106).

For infections involving *S. aureus* (USA300), most are MRSA, and the recommended treatment is either vancomycin combined with rifampin or linezolid combined with rifampin (25,26). Some strains are methicillin-sensitive and should be treated with oxycillin or nafcillin. Patients tend to do poorly despite seemingly adequate antibiotic treatment (80–84). It is possible that antibiotics directed against exotoxin production such as clindamycin or linezolid are important (81).

For abscesses involving anaerobic bacteria, penicillin and tetracyclines were the standard drugs in the 1950s and 1960s when these were referred to as nonspecific lung abscesses; most patients responded. More recent trials have shown that clindamycin is superior to penicillin in terms of time to defervescence, time to eradication of putrid sputum and overall response rates (107,108). Any betalactam–betalactamase inhibitor combination also appears to be successful in the great majority of cases (109,110). Metronidazole is active against virtually all anaerobic bacteria but has a relatively poor track record in the treatment of anaerobic lung infections (111–113). The presumed explanation is the potentially important role of microaerophilic and aerobic streptococci in these infections. This may be obviated by the addition of penicillin to metronidazole. The duration of treatment is arbitrary, and many patients relapse when the treatment is discontinued prematurely. Current recommendations are to treat for six weeks or, preferably, treat until the X ray is clear or shows only a small, stable residual scar.

Drainage is generally an essential component of managing abscesses, but this does not usually apply to lung abscess, which drains spontaneously by communication with the bronchus. There is an occasional attempt to facilitate drainage with physical therapy for postural drainage or bronchoscopy. Studies in the prepenicillin era showed bronchoscopic therapy had virtually no effect on outcome. For patients who fail to respond, thoracic surgery is occasionally required, usually in about 5% to 10% (114–117). The usual indications are failure of medical management and suspected neoplasm or hemorrhage. Failure to respond is usually associated with an extremely large abscess measuring greater than 6 cm in diameter, abscesses that have been present for prolonged periods, and those due to relatively resistant organisms such as *P. aeruginosa*. When surgery is performed, the usual procedure is a lobectomy or pneumonectomy. An alternative drainage option is drainage under computed tomographic guidance which has a modest but favorable reported experience.

Outcome

Patients with lung abscess due to anaerobic bacteria usually show decrease in fever within three to four days of initiating antibiotic treatment with complete defervescence over 7 to 10 days (27,62,64,107). Patients with fever lasting more than 7 to 14 days usually undergo bronchoscopy or other diagnostic intervention to better define the microbiology. CT scans may be particularly useful for anatomic definition to determine possible obstruction or adenopathy that would prompt an investigation for alternative pathogens such as TB or fungi. Mortality rates for lung abscess are usually reported at 5% to 15% but are much lower if there is no major underlying, ultimately fatal condition. A review of lung abscess cases in Japan showed a mortality of 2% in community-acquired cases and 67% for nosocomial infections (65).

REFERENCES

1. Bartlett JG. Bacterial infections of the pleural space. Semin Respir Infect 1988; 3:309.
2. Light RW. A new classification of Parapneumonic effusions and empyema. Chest 1995; 108:299.
3. Maskell NA, Davies CW, Nunn AJ, et al. U.K. Controlled trial of intrapleural streptokinase for pleural infection. N Engl J Med 2005; 352:865–874.
4. Mayo P. Early thoracotomy and decortication for nontuberculous empyema in adults with and without underlying disease: a 25-year review. Am Surg 1985; 51:230.
5. Benfield G. Recent trends in empyema thoracis. Br J Dis Chest 1981; 75:358.
6. Alfageme I, Munoz F, Pena N, Umbria S. Empyema of the thorax in adults: etiology, microbiologic findings, and management. Chest 1993; 103:839.
7. Wiedemann HP, Rice TW. Lung abscess and empyema. Semin Thorac Cardiovasc Surg 1995; 7:119.
8. LeMense GP, Strenge C, Sahn SA. Empyema thoracis: therapeutic management and outcome. Chest 1995; 107:1532.
9. deSousa A, Offner PJ, Moore EE, et al. Optimal management of complicated empyema. Am J Surg 2000; 180:507.
10. Finland M. The significance of pneumococcal types in disease, including types IV to XXXII (Cooper). Ann Intern Med 1939; 15:1531.
11. Heffron R. Pneumonia. Cambridge, MA: Harvard University Press, 1939:566–585.
12. Keefer C, Rantz L, Rammelkamp C. Hemolytic streptococcal pneumonia and empyema: a study of 55 cases with special reference to treatment. Ann Intern Med 1941; 14:1533.
13. Welch C, Tombridge T, Baker W, et al. Beta-hemolytic streptococcal pneumonia: report of an outbreak in a military population. Am J Med Sci 1961; 242:157.
14. Fine MJ, Smith MA, Carson CA, et al. Prognosis and outcomes of patients with community-acquired pneumonia. JAMA 1996; 275:134.
15. Deschamps C, Allen MS, Trastek VA, Pairolero PC. Empyema following pulmonary resection. Chest Surg Clin North Am 1994; 4:583.
16. Bernard A, Pillet M, Goudet P, Viard H. Antibiotic prophylaxis in pulmonary surgery: a prospective randomized double-blind trial of flash Cefuroxime versus forty-eight-hour Cefuroxime. J Thorac Cardiovasc Surg 1994; 107:896.
17. Heffner JE, Brown LK, Barbieri C, DeLeo JM. Pleural fluid chemical analysis in Parapneumonic effusions: a meta-analysis. Am J Respir Crit Care Med 1995; 151:1700.
18. Hiraki A, Aoe K, Eda R, et al. Comparison of six biological markers for the diagnosis of tuberculous pleuritis. Chest 2005; 125:987–989.
19. Diacon AH, Van de Wal BW, Wyser C, Smedema JP, et al. Diagnostic tools in tuberculous pleurisy: a direct comparative study. Eur Respir J 2003; 22:589–591.
20. Chapman SJ, Davies RJ. The management of pleural space infections. Respirology 2004; 9:4–11.
21. Villena V, Lopez-Encuentra A, Garcia-Lujan R, Echave-Sustaeta J, Martinez CJ. Clinical implications of appearance of pleural fluid at thoracentesis. Chest 2004; 125:156–159.
22. Yim AP, Ho JK, Lee TW, Chung SS. Thoracoscopic management of pleural effusions revisited. Aust NZ J Surg 1995; 65:308.
23. Hunnam GR, Flower CD. Radiologically-guided percutaneous catheter drainage of empyemas. Clin Radiol 1988; 39:121.
24. Sullivan K, O'Toole R, Fisher R, et al. Anaerobic empyema thoracis. Arch Intern Med 1973; 131:521.
25. Bartlett JG, Thadepalli H, Gorbach S, et al. Bacteriology of empyema. Lancet 1974; 1:338.
26. Porcel JM, Vives M. Etiology and pleural fluid characteristics of large and massive effusions. Chest 2003; 124:978–983.
27. Bartlett JG. Anaerobic bacterial infections of the lung and pleural space. Clin Infect Dis 1993; 16:S248.

28. Beerens H, Tahon-Castel M. Infection humaines a bacteries anarobes non-toxigenes. Brussels: Academiques Europeennes, 1965:92.
29. Kelly JW, Morris MJ. Empyema thoracis: medical aspects of evaluation and treatment. South Med J 1994; 87:1102.
30. Inglesby TV, O'Toole T, Henderson DA, et al. Anthrax as a biological weapon, 2002: updated recommendations for management. JAMA 2002; 288:1849.
31. Jernigan JA, Stephens DS, Ashford DA, et al. Anthrax Bioterrorism Investigation Team. Bioterrorism-related inhalational anthrax: the first 10 cases reported in the United States. Emerg Infect Dis 2001; 7:933–944.
32. Kyriacou DN, Stein AC, Yarnold PR, et al. Clinical predictors of bioterrorism-related inhalational anthrax. Lancet 2004; 364:449–452.
33. Sokolowski JW Jr., Burgher LW, Jones FL Jr., et al. Guidelines for thoracentesis and needle biopsy of the pleura. Am Rev Respir Infect 1988; 140:257.
34. Schabel SL. Imaging of pleural infections. Semin Respir Infect 1988; 3:298.
35. Levin DL, Klein JS. Imaging techniques for pleural space infections. Semin Respir Infect 1999; 14:31.
36. Teixeira LR, Sasse SA, Villarino MA, et al. Antibiotic levels in empyema fluid. Chest 2000; 117:1734.
37. Hughes CE, Van Scoy RE. Antibiotic therapy of pleural empyema. Semin Respir Infect 1991; 6:94.
38. Diacon AH, Theron J, Schuurmans MN, et al. Intrapleural streptokinase for empyema and complicated parapneumonic effusions. Am J Respir Crit Care Med 2004; 170:49.
39. Aye RW, Froese DP, Hill LD. Use of purified streptokinase in empyema and hemothorax. Am J Surg 1991; 37:371–374.
40. Light RW, Nguyen T, Mulligan ME, Sasse SA. The in vitro efficacy of varidase versus streptokinase or urokinase for liquefying purulent exudative material from locutated empyema. Lung 2000; 178:13.
41. Henke CA, Leatherman JW. Intrapleurally administered streptokinase in the treatment of acute loculated nonpurulent Parapneumonic effusions. Am Rev Respir Dis 1992; 45:680.
42. Pollak JS, Passik CS. Intrapleural urokinase in the treatment of loculated pleural effusions. Chest 1994; 105:868.
43. Miller JI Jr. The history of surgery of empyema, thora coplasty, eloesser flap and muscle flap transposition. Chest Surg Clin North Am 2000; 10:45.
44. Kearney SE, Davies CW, Davies RJ, Gleeson kFV. Computed tomography and ultra-sound in Parapneumonic effusions and empyema. Clin Radiol 2000; 55:542.
45. Sasse S, Nguyen T, Teixeira LR, Light R. The utility of daily therapeutic thoracentesis for treatment of early empyema. Chest 1999; 116:1703–1708.
46. Light RW, Rodriguez RM. Management of Parapneumonic effusions. Clin Chest Med 1998; 19:373–382.
47. Powell LL, Allen R, Brenner M, et al. Improved patient outcome after surgical treatment for loculated empyema. Am J Surg 2000; 179:1.
48. Chen LE, Langer JC, Dillon PA, et al. Management of late-stage Parapneumonic empyema. J Pediatr Surg 2002; 37:371–374.
49. Colice GL, Curtis A, Deslauriers J, et al. Medical and surgical treatment of Parapneumonic effusions: and evidence-based guideline. Chest 2001; 119:319.
50. Manuel Porcel J, Vives M, Esquerda A, Ruiz A. Usefulness of the British Thoracic Society and the American College of Chest Physicians guidelines in predicting pleural drainage of non-purulent parapneumonic effusions. Respir Med 2005 [Epub ahead of print].
51. Balfour-Lyn IM, Abrahamson A, Cohen G, et al. BTS guidelines for the management of pleural infection in children. Thorax 2005; 60:i1–i21.
52. O'Moore PV, Mueller PR, Simeone JF, et al. Sonographic guidance in diagnostic and therapeutic interventions in the pleural space. AJR 1987; 149:1.

53. Davies CH, Gleeson FV, Davies RJO. BTS guidelines on the management of pleural infection. Thorax 2003; 58:ii18–ii28.

54. Maskell NA, Davies CWH, Ghabe R, et al. Predictors of survival in patients with pleural infection but without cancer: results from MRC/BTS MIST Trial, ICTN 39138989. Thorax 2004; 59:ii40.

55. Cantin L, Chartrand-Lefebvre C, Lepanto L, et al. Chest tube drainage under radiological guidance for pleural effusion and Pneumothorax in a tertiary care university teaching hospital: review of 51 cases. Can Respir J 2005; 12:209–233.

56. Hoff SJ, Neblett WW III, Heller RM, et al. Parapneumonic empyema in childhood: selecting appropriate therapy. J Pediatr Surg 1989:659–663.

57. Raffensperger JG, Luck SR, Shkolnik A, Ricketts RR. Mini-thoracotomy and chest tube insertion for children with empyema. J Thorac Cardiovasc Surg 1982; 84:497–504.

58. Bartlett JG, Rosenblatt JE, Finegold SM. Percutaneous transtracheal aspiration in the diagnosis of anaerobic pulmonary infection. Ann Intern Med 1973; 79:535.

59. Bartlett JG, Gorbach SL, Tally FP, et al. Bacteriology and treatment of primary lung abscess. Am Rev Respir Dis 1974; 109:510.

60. Jess P, Brynitz S, Friis Moller A. Mortality in thoracic empyema. Scand J Thorac Cardiovasc Surg 1984; 18:85–87.

61. Hagan J, Hardy JD. Lung abscess revisited: a survey of 184 cases. Ann Surg 1983; 197:755.

62. Harber P, Terry PB. Fatal lung abscesses: review of 11 years' experience. South Med J 1981; 74:281.

63. Pohlson EC, McNamara J, Char C, Kurata B. Lung abscess: a changing pattern of the disease. Ann Surg 1985; 150:97.

64. Hirshberg B, Skair-Levi M, Nir-Paz R, et al. Factors predicting mortality of patients with lung abscess. Chest 1999; 115:746.

65. Mori T, Eb T, Takahashi M, et al. Lung abscess: analysis of 66 cases from 1979 to 1991. Intern Med 1993; 32:278.

66. Hammond JM, Potgieter PD, Hanslo D, et al. The etiology and antimicrobial susceptibility patterns of microorganisms in acute community-acquired lung abscess. Chest 1995; 108:937.

67. Bartlett JG. The role of anaerobic bacteria in lung abscess. Clin Infect Dis 2005; 40:923–925.

68. Landay MJ, Christensen EE, Bynum LJ, et al. Anaerobic pleural and pulmonary infections. AJR 1980; 134:233.

69. Stark DD, Federle MP, Goodman PC, et al. Differentiating lung abscess and empyema: radiography and computed tomography. AJR 1983; 141:163.

70. Bartlett JG. Diagnostic accuracy of transtracheal aspiration bacteriology. Am Rev Respir Dis 1977; 115:777.

71. Bartlett JG. The technique of transtracheal aspiration. J Crit Illness 1986; 1:43.

72. Wimberley NW, Bass JB, Boyd BW, et al. Use of a bronchoscopic protected catheter brush for the diagnosis of pulmonary infections. Chest 1982; 81:556.

73. Henriquez AH, Mendoza J, Gonzalez PC. Quantitative culture of bronchoalveolar lavage from patients with anaerobic lung abscesses. J Infect Dis 1991; 164:414.

74. Verma P. Laboratory diagnosis of anaerobic pleuropulmonary infections. Semin Respir Infect 2000; 15:114.

75. Sosenko A, Glassroth J. Fiberoptic bronchoscopy in the evaluation of lung abscesses. Chest 1985; 87:489.

76. Finegold FM, George WL, Mulligan ME. Anaerobic infections. Dis Mon 1985; 31:8.

77. Civen R, Jousimies-Somer H, Marina M, et al. A retrospective review of cases of anaerobic empyema and update of bacteriology. Clin Infect Dis 1995; 20:S224.

78. Wollenman OJ, Finland M. Pathology of staphylococcal pneumonia complicating clinical influenza. Am J Pathol 1943; 19:23.

79. Fisher Am, Trever RW, Curtin JA, et al. Staphylococcal pneumonia: a review of 21 cases in adults. N Engl J Med 1958; 258:919.

80. Francis JS, Doherty MC, Lopatin U, et al. Severe community-onset pneumonia in healthy adults caused by methicillin-resistant *Staphylococcus aureus* carrying the Panton-Valentine Leukocidin genes. Clin Infect Dis 2005; 40:1376–1378.

81. Micek ST, Dunne M, Kollef MH. Pleuropulmonary complications of Panton-Valentine leukocidin-positive community-acquired methicillin-resistant *Staphylococcus aureus*: importance of treatment with antimicrobials inhibiting exotoxin production. Chest 2005; 128:2732–2738.

82. Gillet Y, Issartel B, Vanhems P, et al. Association between *Staphylococcus aureus* strains carrying gene for Panton-vantine Leukocidin and highly lethal necrotizing pneumonia in young immunocompetent patients. Lancet 2002; 359:753–762.

83. Gonzalez BE, Hulten KG, Dishop MK, et al. Pulmonary manifestations in children with invasive community-acquired *Staphylococcus aureus* infection. Clin Infect Dis 2005; 41:583–590.

84. Lina G, Piemont Y, Godail-Gamot F, et al. Involvement of Panton-Valentine Leukocidin-producing *Staphylococcus aureus* in primary skin infections and pneumonia. Clin Infect Dis 1999; 29:1128–1132.

85. Finck-Barbancon V, Duportail G, Meunier O, Colin DA. Pore formation by a two-component leukocidin from *Staphylococcus aureus* within the membrane of human polymorphonuclear leukocytes. Biochim Biophys Acta 1993; 1182:275–282.

86. Bullowa JGM, Chess J, Friedman NJ. Pneumonia due to Bacillus friedlanderi. Arch Intern Med 1937; 60:735.

87. Wang JL, Chen KY, Fang CT, Hseuh PR, Yang PC, Chang SC. Changing bacteriology of adult community-acquired lung abscess in Taiwan: *Klebsiella pneumoniae* versus anaerobes. Clin Infect Dis 2005; 40:915–922.

88. Stack WA, Richardson PD, Logan RO, et al. *Nocardia asteroids* lung abscess in acute ulcerative colitis treated with cyclosporine. Am J Gastroenterol 2001; 96:225.

89. vanBurik JA, Hackman RC, Nadeem SO, et al. Nocardiosis after bone marrow transplantation: a retrospective study. Clin Infect Dis 1997; 24:1154.

90. Ernst A, Gordon FD, Hayek J, et al. Lung abscess complicates *Legionella micdadei* pneumonia in a liver transplant recipient: a case report and review. Transplantation 1998; 65:130.

91. Johnson KM, Huseby JS. Lung abscess caused by *Legionella micdadei*. Chest 1997; 111:252.

92. Senecal JL, St-Antoine R, Beliveau C. *Legionella pneumophilia* lung abscess in a patient with systemic lupus erythematosus. Am J Med Sci 1987; 293:309.

93. Kobayashi K. *Streptococcus milleri* as a cause of pulmonary abscess. Acta Paediatr 2001; 90:233.

94. Jerng JS, Hsueh PR, Teng LJ, et al. Empyema thoracic and lung abscess caused by viridians streptococci. Am Respir Crit Care 1997; 156:1508.

95. Frieden TR, Biebuyck J, Hierholzer WJ Jr. Lung abscess with group beta-hemolytic streptococcus. Case report and review. Arch Intern Med 1991; 151:1655.

96. Roy S, Kaplan EL, Rodriguez B, et al. A family of five cases of group A streptococcal pneumonia. Pediatrics 2003; 112:e61–e65.

97. Harvey RI, Sunstrum JC. *Rhodococcus equi* infection in patients with and without human immunodeficiency virus infection. Rev Infect Dis 1991; 13:139.

98. Verville TD, Huycke MM, Greenfield RA, et al. *Rhodococcus equi* infections of humans. 12 cases and a review of the literature. Medicine (Baltimore) 1994; 73:119.

99. Shapiro JM, Romney BM, Weiden MD, et al. *Rhodococcus equi* endobronchial mass with lung abscess in a patient with AIDS. Thorax 1992; 47:62.

100. Torres-Tortosa M, Arrizabalaga J, Villaneuva JL, et al. Prognosis and clinical evaluation of infection caused by *Rhodococcus equi* in HIV-infected patients: a multicenter study of 67 cases. Chest 2003; 123:1970–1976.

101. Chirinos JA, Lichtstein DM, Garcia J, Tamariz LJ. The evolution of Lemierre syndrome: report of 2 cases and review of the literature. Medicine (Baltimore) 2002; 81:458–465.

102. Lemierre A. On certain septicaemias due to anaerobic organisms. Lancet 1936; 1:701.

103. Cook RJ, Ashton RW, Aughenbaugh GL, Ryu JH. Septic pulmonary embolism: presenting features and clinical course of 14 patients. Chest 2005; 128:162–166.

104. Veld DH, Wuthiekanun V, Cheng AC, et al. The role and significance of sputum cultures in the diagnosis of melioidosis. Am J Trop Med Hyg 2005; 73:657–661.

105. Aaron SD, Vandemheen KL, Ferris W, et al. Combinations antibiotic susceptibility testing to treat exacerbations of cystic fibrosis associated with multiresistant bacteria: a randomized, double-blind, controlled clinical trial. Lancet 2005; 366:433–435.

106. Canton R, Cobos N, de Gracia J, et al., On Behalf of the Spanish Consensus Group for Antimicrobial Therapy in the Cystic Fibrosis Patient. Antimicrobial therapy for pulmonary pathogenic colonization and infection by *Pseudomonas aeruginosa* in cystic fibrosis patients. Clin Microbiol Infect 2005; 11:690–703.

107. Levision ME, Mangura CT, Lober B, et al. Clindamycin compared with penicillin for the treatment of anaerobic lung abscess. Ann Intern Med 1983; 98:466.

108. Gudiol F, Manressa F, Pallares R, et al. Clindamycin vs. penicillin for anaerobic lung infections. Arch Intern Med 1990; 158:2525.

109. Germaud P, Poirier J, Jacqueme P, et al. Monotherapy using amoxicillin/clavulanic acid as treatment of first choice in community-acquired lung abscess during chest physical therapy: a case report. Phys Ther 1988; 68:371.

110. Allewelt M, Schuler P, Bolcskei PL, Mauch H, Lode H. Study Group on Aspiration Pneumonia. Clin Microbiol Infect 2004; 10:163–170.

111. Eykyn SJ. The therapeutic use of metronidazole in anaerobic infection: six years' experience in a London hospital. Surgery 1983; 93:209.

112. Perlino CA. Metronidazole vs. clindamycin treatment of anaerobic pulmonary infection. Arch Intern Med 1981; 141:1424.

113. Sanders CV, Hanna BJ, Lewis AC. Metronidazole in the treatment of anaerobic infections. Am Rev Respir Dis 1979; 120:337.

114. Smith DT. Medical treatment of acute and chronic pulmonary abscesses. J Thorac Surg 1948; 17:72.

115. Cordice JW Jr., Chitkara RK. The role of surgery in treating pleuropulmonary suppurative disease—review of 77 cases managed at Queens Hospital Center between 1986 and 1989. J Natl Med Assoc 1992; 84:145.

116. Pfitzner J, Peacock JM, Tsirgiotis E, et al. Lobectomy for cavitating lung abscess with haemoptysis: strategy for protecting the contralateral lung and also the non-involved lobe of the ipsilateral lung. Br J Anaesth 2000; 85:791.

117. Tseng YL, Wu MH, Lin MY, et al. Surgery for lung abscess in immunocompetent and immunocompromised children. J Pediatr Surg 2001; 36:470.

11

Infective Endocarditis and Its Mimics in the Critical Care Unit

John L. Brusch

Department of Medicine, Harvard Medical School, Cambridge, Massachusetts, U.S.A.

OVERVIEW

Since Osler's comprehensive description of infective endocarditis (IE) in the 1880s, this disease has continuously evolved in respect to its epidemiology, clinical presentations, and therapy.

Over the last 30 years, greater numbers of patients with IE are being cared for in critical care units (CrCU) mainly because of the increased incidence of acute staphylococcal IE. In recent series, approximately 60% of cases of IE are caused by *Staphylococcus aureus* (1). By prolonging the lives of those with acute IE, antibiotics are contributing to the increasing number of cardiac and extracardiac complications of this type of valvular infection. Even in subacute IE, antibiotics have failed to lessen the frequency of embolic complications including mycotic aneurysms (2). This is due to the delay in diagnosis that has not lessened over the last 30 years. The average interval between the onset of valvular infections and diagnosis remains six weeks (3). Although complications of IE affect the heart most frequently, neurological events and sepsis are the most frequent causes of death.

Increasingly, patients being cared for in CrCU are developing IE that is a consequence of the increased reliance on various types of intravascular devices in the care of the critically ill. Even the surgical procedures meant to repair the damage of cardiac infections pose their own unique risks to the patient.

This chapter will focus on the epidemiology, pathogenesis presentation, diagnosis, treatment prevention of the bacteria, and the types of IE that will most likely be encountered in CrCU. Among these are native valve IE (NVE), prosthetic valve endocarditis (PVE), and health-care associated IE (HCIE). The organisms that will be discussed include the various streptococcal species: *Streptococcus viridans*, the nutritionally variant streptococci (NVS) and group B streptococci, gram-negative aerobes, and fungi and of course *S. aureus*. Many infectious and noninfectious disease processes share important clinical features with IE. The most effective of these mimics will also be highlighted.

Epidemiology

IE is usually an infection of the valvular endocardium, rarely of the mural endocardium. Because it can present with noncardiac signs and symptoms, especially subacute disease, the diagnosis of IE may be particularly challenging. Additionally 5% to 10% of cases may be blood culture negative. Histological exam of the involved valvular tissue remains the gold standard for diagnosing IE (4). Because it is uncommon to obtain premortem valvular tissue, Von Reyn et al. developed strict case definitions for the diagnosis of IE (5). By these criteria, only 20% of clinically diagnosed cases could be considered as definite examples of IE. In order to increase this system's sensitivity, The Duke Endocarditis Service in 1994 combined echocardiographic findings with a set of clinical measures (6). These Duke Criteria have far greater positive predictive value and negative predictive value of at least 92% (6). These criteria were further modified in 2000 (see Section on diagnosis).

The incidence of IE has not changed over the last 50 years (approximately 4/100,000 person-years) (7). Those institutions that serve large numbers of intravenous drug abusers (IVDA) and those that perform large numbers of intravascular procedures will generate many more cases than will a community hospital. The incidence of IE is at least two times more common in men than in women. In those greater than 50 years of age, the male incidence is six times that of the female (1,7,8). The risk of developing HCIE is equal among men and women (9). The term HCIE is preferable to that of nosocomial IE because it recognizes the fact that a growing amount of medical care, such as hemodialysis, is provided outside of the hospital proper.

IE has become a disease of the older population. In a series collected in the 1990s (1), the mean age was 50 with 35% greater than 60 years of age and 15% greater than 70 years of age. The major exception to this "graying" trend is IE among IVDA of which 85% are complicated with HIV infection. Several factors have contributed to this rise of IE among elderly (10,11). Among these are:

1. The aging-related atherosclerotic changes to the circulatory system (i.e., calcific valvular disease).
2. The proliferation of cardiac surgery and placement of intravascular devices in older individuals (the majority of patients with hospital acquired staphylococcal bacteremia are in this age group).
3. Those with congenital heart disease are living longer.
4. The age associated dysfunction of the immune system.

There has been a marked increase in cases of HCIE, IVDA IE, and PVE accounting for 22%, 36%, and 16%, respectively, of all cases (1).

Perhaps the most striking change is the rise in cases of acute IE. Currently these account to for more than 50% of cases and growing (1). This reflects the rise of staphylococcal/health-care associated bloodstream infections (HCBSI) (12) coupled with a significant decrease in disease caused by *S. viridans* (13).

Predisposing Cardiac Lesions

Acquired and Congenital Cardiac Abnormalities

The frequency of underlying cardiac lesions in IE of native tissue is dependent on the prevalence of acute IE in the studied population. More than 50% of cases of acute IE have no definable underlying cardiac pathology (14). Congenital heart disease is found in 15% of cases. Congenital bicuspid aortic valve is the most common example found in older patients (20% of cases) (15). A somewhat neglected predisposing condition is asymmetric septal hypertrophy. This accounts for 5% of cases of IE (16). The greater the degree of obstruction the greater is the chance of valvular infection. The mitral valve is the most frequently affected (17). Other contributory congenital conditions are ventricular septal defect, patent ductus arteriosus, and tetralogy of Fallot (18).

In the developed world, rheumatic heart disease (RHD) accounts for <20% of NVE (19). The lifelong risk of individuals with RHD developing IE is approximately 6%, usually of the mitral valve.

Mitral valve prolapse (MVP) accounts for 30% of cases of NVE in younger adults. This rate is most likely related to its prevalence in the general population (5% overall and 20% among females) (18,19). It appears that those who have a pre-existing systolic ejection murmur associated with thickening and redundancy of the valvular leaflets are at a 10- to 100-fold increased risk of developing IE (20).

Degenerative cardiac disease underlies 20% of all cases and 50% of cases of IE in patients >60 years of age (21). These lesions include calcified valvular leaflets, calcified mitral rings, and postmyocardial infarction thrombi. Calcified aortic stenosis may result from calcium deposition either on a congenital bicuspid valve or on a previously normal valve damaged by hemodynamic stress over the years (22). Because of the prevalence of associated illnesses, such as diabetes or renal failure, IE in this group of patients has a poorer than average outcome. The degree of stenosis is often not hemodynamically significant and so is frequently overlooked as a candidate for antibiotic prophylaxis (23).

Forty percent of NVE, excluding IVDA IE, infect only the mitral valve and 40% the aortic solely. The right side of a heart is rarely involved except in cases of IVDA IE (24).

Overall, PVE accounts for 10% to 20% of all cases of IE and 26% in those >60 years of age (25). The 10-year risk of infection of both mechanical and bioprosthetic valves is approximately 5% (26). During the first three months after implantation, mechanical valves are more at risk. However, after one year, bioprosthetic valves exhibit a greater chance of IE due to the ongoing calcification of the leaflets associated with degeneration of the valvular tissue.

Infection of implanted pacemakers (PMs) and cardioverter-defibrillator is becoming more frequent (27). These devices most often become infected within a few months of placement. Infection of PMs may involve the generator pocket (the most common type): there may be infection of proximate leads and those portions of the leads that are in direct contact with the endocardium. The last type is synonymous with true Pacemaker IE (PMIE) (0.5% of all PMs) (28). Seventy five percent of all types of PM infections are caused by staphylococci.

It is important to note that the true risk for development of IE for most underlying cardiac abnormalities has not been accurately quantified for many cardiac conditions (29). Patients with MVP and associated regurgitation have a three- to eightfold increase in risk. Those with a history of prior IE or with prosthetic valves in place have a 60- to 185-fold increased risk.

Extracardiac Predisposing Factors

The incidence of IE among IVDA lies between 1% and 5% per year. IVDA IE causes up to 20% of hospital admissions and 5% to 10% of deaths among narcotics abusers. It appears that IVDA IE is decreasing due to safer injection practices, such as the use of sterile needles and syringes brought about to combat the spread of the HIV virus among this population. Eighty percent of patients are male, probably due to their longer usage of illicit drugs. The tricuspid valve is infected in about 70% of cases with the mitral and aortic valves involved in 20% to 30% of patients. The pulmonic valve is rarely infected. In some series, up to 75% of IVDA IE occurs in the absence of any preexisting valvular abnormalities. Forty three percent of recurrent valvular infections are seen in illicit drug users. Interestingly 7% had prosthetic valves in place. A history of IVDA IE has become the most significant risk factor for recurrent NVE (30–35).

HCIE has been defined as a valvular infection that presents either 48 hours after the patient has been hospitalized or that is associated with a health-care facility-based procedure that has been performed within four weeks of presentation (36,37). Patients with HCIE are older and have a higher rate of underlying valvular disorders and develop bacteremias that are related to a variety of invasive vascular procedures. The incidence of HCIE accounts for approximately 20% of IE overall (1,12) and appears to be ever increasing. Much of this is due to the rise in staphylococcal bacteremia associated with intravascular line infection (12,38,39). HCIE often involves normal valves. Type 1 HCIE results from endocardial trauma to the right ventricular wall produced by an intravascular catheter. Type 2 HCIE occurs in patients who develop left-sided IE due to bacteremias originating from the skin, urinary tract or intravenous lines, or other invasive procedures. In this situation, the left side predominates because of the greater proportion of structural abnormalities on that side (i.e., degenerative valvular disease, MVP). In addition to *S. aureus* and coagulase-negative staphylococci (CONS), gram-negative organisms and fungi are frequently involved. HCIE may be fatal in up to 50% of cases as compared to an overall mortality rate of 11% of IE acquired in the community. This increase in mortality is attributable in part to the older age of the patients with HCIE (64% of patients >60 years of age) (40). An exception to this is that community-acquired cases of *S. aureus* IE have a higher mortality rate than *S. aureus* HCIE. This may be due in part to the higher rate of metastatic complications arising from the prolonged bacteremia prior to the correct diagnosis being made (41).

The major reason for focusing on HCIE has been well expressed by Friedland et al. (9), "nosocomial endocarditis occurs in a definable subpopulation of hospitalized patients and is potentially preventable."

Various types of primary immunodeficiencies as well as diseases that lower the patient's resistance to infection by a variety of mechanisms have been cited as predisposing risk factors for developing IE (42). Among them are a variety of neoplasms, diabetes mellitus, renal failure, liver disease, and the use of corticosteroids. All of these disease states are associated with an increased frequency of bacteremias (43).

The role of dental procedures as a risk factor for developing IE is currently in question (44) and will not be further discussed, especially because most of the patients who develop the IE due to bacteremias secondary to dental work do not require care in CrCU. Suffice it to say that the vast majority of dental associated IE are secondary to an increase in transit bacteremias that arise from poor dental hygiene and are not due to any one specific procedure.

Table 1 presents the recent changes in the characteristics of IE.

MICROBIOLOGY

The exact profile of causative organisms of a given hospital is dependent on the population it serves. The pathogens causing NVE are somewhat different than those that produce PVE or IVDA IE (Table 2). Overall, *S. aureus* produces about 30%

Table 1 Changing Patterns of Infective Endocarditis Since 1966

Marked increase in the incidence of acute IE

Rise of nosocomial, IVDA and prosthetic valve IE
   Change in the underlying valvular pathology: RHD <20% of cases
   Mitral valve prolapse 30% of cases
   Prosthetic valve endocarditis 10–20% of cases
   50% of elderly patients have calcific aortic stenosis
These changes are due to:
   The "graying" of patients (excluding cases of IVDA IE,
     55% of patients >60 yrs of age)
   The increased numbers of vascular procedures

Abbreviations: IE, infective endocarditis; IVDA, intravenous drug abusers; RHD, rheumatic heart disease.

of cases, CONS 16%, *S. viridans* 23%, *S. bovis* 5%, *Enterococcus faecalis* 4%, gram-negative organisms 2%, no growth <5%, and other (including fungi) 17% (45).

    S. viridans has decreased by 35% in frequency while *S. aureus* has increased by 50%. Non–*S. viridans* streptococci have also become more frequent (46). The incidence of culture negative endocarditis has drastically decreased because of markedly improved culture and serologic techniques.

    Overall, *S. viridans* cause <50% of all types of endocarditis. This is a term of classification that has been applied to all nonpneumococcal streptococci excluding groups A, D, and E. The use of this terminology will be continued in this chapter. Members this group include are *Streptococcus salivarius*, *S. sanguis* I and II, *S. mitis*, *S. intermedius*, *S. milleri*, and *S. mutans*. These are generally commensals of the respiratory and gastrointestinal tracts that posses little invasive capacity. They are the classic organisms of subacute IE. Because of their high rate of retrieval from cases of MVP IE, *S. viridans* is increasingly associated with IE occurring in a younger age group (47).

    NVS, although currently classified as Abiotrophia, will be still considered members of the *S. viridans* family. They require the presence of cystine or pyridoxine for growth. These pathogens bind specifically to the extracellular matrix of fibroblasts and endothelial cells. They produce luxuriant valvular vegetations that frequently embolize (48). They may be relatively resistant to penicillin (see Section on therapy) and typically produce subacute disease. The intermedius group (*S. milleri*, *S. anginosus*, and Streptococcal MG (S.MG)) is suppurative and locally

Table 2 Microbiology of Infective Endocarditis in Different Risk Groups

Microorganism recovered (% of cases)	Native valve endocarditis	Intravenous drug users	Prosthetic valve endocarditis	
			Early	Late
Viridans-group streptococci	50	20	7	30
Staphylococcus aureus	19	67	17	12
Coagulase-negative staphylococci	4	9	33	26
Enterococci	8	7	2	6
Miscellaneous	19	7	44	26

invasive. These properties may be related to its polysaccharide capsule. They can produce myocardial abscesses as well as valvular infection. These organisms are capable of producing either acute or subacute IE.

Group D streptococci (*S. faecalis*, *S. faecium*, and the nonenterococcal species *S. bovis* and *S. equinis*) usually produce subacute disease. *S. faecalis* is the most common example. The rise in cases of enterococcal IE appears due to both the increase in third generation cephalosporin use and intravascular invasive procedures. These organisms collectively comprise the third most common cause of IE. They are residents of the gastrointestinal and genitourinary tracts. Enterococcal resistance patterns pose major challenges to the clinician.

S. bovis typically produces subacute IE. Bacteremia/IE with this group often reflects underlying bowel disease ranging from ulcerative colitis to colonic cancer. They are uniformly sensitive to the penicillins.

Group B streptococci produce acute IE not only in the pregnant but in older patients afflicted with a variety of underlying diseases. Their mortality rate is 40% due to the high rate of complications including metastatic infection, arterial thrombi, and congestive heart failure (49). Often valvular replacement is necessary for cure.

Group A streptococcal IE causes acute disease quite similar to that of *S. aureus*. There is up to a 70% mortality rate due to their high rate of suppurative complications. These organisms respond well to penicillin G. Group C and group G streptococci have similar clinical presentation to that of group A IE, but require a synergistic combination of antibiotics for cure.

S. aureus is overall the most common cause of IE and predominates especially in PVE, acute IE, and IVDA IE (50). Approximately 30% of staphylococcal BSIs are complicated by IE; 50% of these are associated with previously abnormal valves. The mortality rate ranges up to 50%. There has been a marked increase in the amount of methicillin-resistant *S. aureus* (MRSA) involved in IE both hospital and community-acquired strains (38,51). Sixty percent of individuals are intermittent carriers of methicillin-sensitive *S. aureus* (MSSA) and MRSA. *S. aureus* is secondary only to CONS as a cause of HCBSI. Fifty percent of the 200,000/yr *S. aureus* bacteremias arise from infected vascular catheters (11). Other risk factors include neoplasms, corticosteroid use, diabetes, IVDA, renal failure, and alcoholism.

CONS is the most common cause of PVE (52). Subacute PVE typically results from this type of infection. NVE is rare but has been reported in previously abnormal valves, usually MVP (53).

Gram-negative rods account for approximately 5% of cases of IE (54). Their inability to adhere efficiently to the valvular endothelium, as compared to the gram-positive cocci, is the major reason for this low rate. Cirrhotics have a risk of developing gram-negative IE with a risk three times that of individuals with healthy livers (55). Of all the gram-negatives, *Pseudomonas aeruginosa* adheres efficiently to the endocardium and accounts for approximately 4% of IVDA IE (33). The *Haemophilus, A. actinomycetemcomitans, C. bacterium hominis, E. corrodens, and Kingella* (HACEK) group are gram-negative bacilli/coccobacilli that reside in the oropharynx. They are the most common cause of gram-negative IE, usually subacute (56) in nature. Complications of this type of IE include massive arterial emboli and congestive heart failure. Combined medical and surgical treatment is usually required for cure.

Polymicrobial IE is most often seen in IVDA and in patients who have undergone cardiac surgery (57). The most frequently isolated organisms are *P. aeruginosa, S. faecalis, S. aureus*, and *S. epidermidis*. The most common combination is that of *S. faecalis* and *P. aeruginosa*. Twenty-eight percent of enterococcal bacteremias have been documented to be polymicrobial. The mortality rate of patients with multiorganism IE is twice that of those infected with a single agent.

Fungal IE has increased by 270% in the last 25 years. Most of this rise in cases is accounted for by infections of patients cared for in CrCU and in those who have undergone cardiac surgery (58). Overall, fungi account for approximately 1% of IE; 5% of IVDA IE, and 13% and 5% early and late PVE, respectively. The risk factors include broad-spectrum antibiotic usage and administration of cytotoxic agents (59).

Candida species are the most common fungi isolated from cases of IE. Two-thirds of these are *C. albicans* (60). *C. albicans* is also the most frequent organism recovered from fungal IE that is associated with infections of all types of intravascular catheters, especially those used for hyperalimentation. The remainder of cases of fungal IE usually involve *aspergillus* isolates most commonly *A. fumigatus* (61). In cases of IVDA fungal IE, *C. albicans*, *C. parapsilosis*, or *C. tropicalis* invade the bloodstream from the skin or from drug paraphernalia (62). In non-IVDA IE, the gastrointestinal tract or the vascular catheter is the most common portal of entry (see Section on clinicopathologic correlations). Contaminated operating room air is usually the source of the *aspergillus* that infects prosthetic valves.

Less than 5% of patients with IE have persistently negative blood cultures. The causes for this are (63) (i) fastidious organisms that are difficult to grow in culture, such as NVS, members of the HACEK group, and Legionella; (ii) recent antimicrobial therapy; (iii) right-sided endocarditis; and (iv) PVE and cultures obtained three months into the valvular infection. Antigen–antibody complexes that develop well into the course of subacute IE inhibit the recovery of organisms from the blood cultures. Recent antibiotic exposure is the most common cause of this (67% of such patients). In the author's experience, the injudicious use of broad-spectrum antibiotics in CrCU can suppress bacterial growth within the valvular thrombus but do not sterilize it. This delay in both diagnosis and initiation of appropriate treatment contributes to the high rate of mortality and morbidity of HCIE.

Table 3 summarizes the properties of the organisms most commonly encountered in cases of IE managed in CrCU.

MICROBIAL PATHOGENICITY

There is clinical significance in classifying IE as subacute or acute. The former is an indolent process lasting as long as 12 months if untreated. It presents with signs and symptoms that are often extracardiac. The latter is a rapidly progressive disease that can kill the victim within a few days with signs of cardiac involvement from beginning of its course (48). This section will examine the specific pathogenic properties of *S. viridans* and *S. aureus*, which enable these organisms to produce respectively the subacute and acute forms of the disease. We will focus on the essential event to the development of IE, the adherence of the pathogen to the endocardium (64). There is a direct correlation between an organism's in vitro adherence capability and its association with human cases of IE (65).

S. viridans has little intrinsic pathogenic potential with the exception of the *S. intermedius* group. They cannot attach directly to normal endothelium but must rely on the presence of a preformed platelet fibrin thrombus, nonbacterial thrombotic endocarditis (NBTE) for adherence to cardiac tissue. This sterile vegetation is the result of abnormal hemodynamic flow or prior damage to the endothelialium (see Section on clinicopathological correlations). Circulating *S. viridans* attach by means

Table 3 Causative Organisms of Infective Endocarditis

Organism	Comments
Staphylococcus aureus	The most common causes of acute IE include PVE, IVDA, and IE related to intravascular infections. Approximately 35% of cases of *S. aureus* bacteremia complicated by IE
Streptococcus viridans (*S. mitior, S. sanguis, S. mutans, S. salivarius*)	70% of cases of subacute IE. Signs and symptoms are immunologically mediated with a very low rate of suppurative complications. Penicillin resistance is a growing problem, especially in patients receiving chemotherapy or bone marrow transplants
Streptococcus milleri group (*S. anginosus, S. intermedius, S. constellatus*)	Up to 20% of streptococcal IE. Unlike other streptococci they can invade tissue and produce suppurative complications
Nutritionally Variant Streptoccoci	5% of subacute IE. Examples require nutritionally variant streptococci active forms of vitamin B6 for growth. Characteristically they produce large valvular vegetations with a high rate of embolization and relapse
Group D streptococci	Third most common cause of IE. They may produce alpha, beta, or gamma hemolysis. Source is GI or GU tracts; associated with a high rate of relapse. Growing problem of antimicrobial resistance. Most cases are subacute
Nonenterococcal group D streptococci (*S. bovis*)	50% of group D IE; associated with lesions of large bowel
Group B *streptococci*	Increasing cause of acute IE in alcoholics, cancer patients, and diabetics as well as in pregnancy. 40% mortality rate. Complications include CHF, thrombi, and metastatic infection. Surgery often required for cure
Groups A, C, and G *streptococci*	More frequently seen in the elderly (nursing homes) and diabetics. 30–70% death rate. Commonly cause myocardial abscesses
Streptococcus pneumoniae	Currently cause <5% of cases; follows acute course. Usually a complication of pneumoniae (1% of cases complicated by IE)
Coagulase negative Staphylococcus aureus	30% of PVE; <5% of IE of native valves; subacute course that is more indolent than that of *Streptococcus viridans*
Pseudomonas aeruginosa	Most commonly acutely seen in IVDA IE (right-sided disease is subacute) and in PVE
Serratia marcescens	NIE (acute IE), often requires surgery for cure
Fungal IE	An increasing problem in the ICU (NIE) and among IVDA. *Candida albicans* as most common example (especially in PVE) as compared to IVDA IE, in which *C. parapsilosis* or *C. tropicalis* predominate. *Aspergillus* species recovered in 33% of fungal IE. Most cases of fungal IE follow a subacute course
Polymicrobial IE	Most common organisms are Pseudomonas and enterococci. It occurs frequently in IVDA and cardiac surgery. It may present acutely or subacutely. Mortality is greater than that of single-agent IE

Abbreviations: IE, infective endocarditis; IVDA, intravenous drug abusers; PVE, prosthetic valve endocarditis; GI, gastrointestinal; GU, genitourinary; CHF, congestive heart failure; NIE, nasocomul infective endocardin.

of molecules on their surfaces that recognize and interact with the extracellular matrix molecules of the NBTE in a "Velcro-like" fashion. These bacterial attachment sites are called microbial surface components recognizing adhesive matrix molecules (MSCRAMMs). The principal MSCRAMM of *S. viridans* is its extracellular production of dextran, which promotes its attachment to the fibrin platelet clot (66). Other MSCRAMMs include those that interact with fibronectin and platelets. After the attachment phase, *S. viridans* promotes the growth of the vegetation by its ability to stimulate local production of tissue factor by monocytes and platelet aggregation. However, the aggregation of platelets does have a negative effect on the bacteria by releasing various antimicrobial peptides and mediators of inflammation (67).

S. aureus possesses a large repertoire of pathogenic mechanisms that have contributed to it becoming the premier bacterial pathogen of this era. The teichoic acid component of its cell wall facilitates its attachment to the nasal mucosa from which it sets up a "beachhead" on the patient's skin (68). Any break in the dermis, accidental or planned (i.e., insertion of intravascular catheter or injection of a recreational drug) promotes entry of the staphylococcus into the microcirculation. Prostatitis and pneumonia are other portals of entry. The organisms then travel to the venules by the lymphatic route. They then infect the venous endothelium (endotheliosis) without the need of a preformed thrombus. They attach to the endothelial cells by means of their MSCRAMM's most notably fibronectin binding proteins and various clumping factors (69). Triggered by the staphylococcal fibro-nectin binding proteins, the venular endandothelium ingests the invaders. *S. aureus* induces the production of tissue factor by both monocytes and endothelial cells. This promotes further thrombosis by means of the extrinsic clotting system. The staphylococci may remain dormant within the endothelial cells for a time but are eventually released back into the circulation. Fibronectin also promotes binding of *S. aureus* to the fibrin sheath that forms in and around the lumen of a vascular catheter (70). Less frequently, the sheath is infected by organisms originating from a distant site (71).

S. aureus has several defenses that shield it from the host's phagocytic system. Among these are proteins A; catalase; alpha, beta, and gamma toxins; and leukoci-dins and its capsule (72). After phagocytosis, 5% of coagulase positive *S. aureus* remain viable for at least several minutes within the leukocyte. The organisms then make use of these cells to travel throughout the patient. Upon the death of the white cell, the still viable staphylococci are deposited into the surrounding tissue or slip back into the intravascular space. The high degree of antibiotic resistance of *S. aureus* must be considered another one of its pathogenic properties.

The chief pathogenic mechanism of CONS is their ability to adhere to implanted foreign bodies. The development of prosthetic materials has transformed an organism that has very limited ability to infect native tissue to one that can pro-duce significant degrees of morbidity and mortality (73). Only 5% of NVE is caused by CONS as compared to 30% of PVE. Binding of CONS to prosthetic material is dependent both on nonspecific factors and production of a glycocalyx by the organ-isms (74). Glycocalyx is an extracellular, slime-like compound that acts to protect the pathogen from phagocytosis but does not block its access to nutritional substances. It also inhibits local immunoglobulin synthesis (75).

S. faecalis also induces the production of fibronectin by endothelial cells (76). This results in a more rapidly proliferating vegetation that then acts as a shield to protect the organisms from administered antibiotics.

Those bacteria that have a prolonged generation time are relatively resistant to those antibiotics which are most effective during the organism's replicative stage. For example, antimicrobial therapy may fail to cure 41% of cases of NVS IE (77).

P. aeruginosa, the most common gram-negative involved in IVDA IE, elaborates many virulence factors including extracellular proteases, elastase, and alkaline proteases (78). These substances produce necrosis in a wide range of tissues, especially the elastic layer of the lamina propria of all calibers of blood vessels. Ecthyma gangrenosum is the classical dermatological manifestation of this process. These toxins also interfere with the function of polymorphonuclear leukocytes, K and T cells, as well as the structure of complement and immunoglobulins. Exotoxin A disrupts protein synthesis and is the factor that is best correlated with systemic toxicity and mortality (79). Many isolates of *P. aeruginosa* are resistant to the bactericidal activity of human serum. Its polysaccharide capsule interferes with phagocytosis and the action of the aminoglycosides.

CLINICAL PRESENTATION AND CLINICOPATHOLOGICAL CORRELATIONS

Clinicopathological Correlations

There are three essential steps in the development of IE: bacteremia with an organism with the ability to infect the endocardium; adherence of that organism to the valvular surface and subsequent invasion of the underlying tissue (64). In all cases of subacute disease, NBTE is the point of attachment for the circulating bacteria. As discussed earlier (see Section "Microbial Pathogenicity"), its presence is not essential for those organisms that are capable of producing acute IE.

In the CrCU, NBTE develops from one of three major processes:

1. Blood loses its laminar characteristics as it flows over valves distorted by atherosclerosis or by rheumatic carditis. These changes in the rheology of blood affect the function and the alignment of the endocardium (80). Leukocytes adhere more readily to this altered surface, and platelets become more reactive in contact with it and become coated with fibrin. Small vegetations develop and in turn increase the degree of turbulence and so accelerate the formation of NBTE.

2. Garrison and Freedman developed a model of IE in which the endocardium of the right side of a rabbit's heart was scarred by a catheter inserted from the femoral vein. This produced a sterile fibrin platelet thrombus, which was subsequently infected by *S. aureus* injected through the catheter (81). This model produces lesions that closely resemble those of early human IE (82). As the infection progresses, the adherent bacteria are covered by successive layers of deposited fibrin. The more superficial organisms are more metabolically active while those deeper into the NBTE were quite indolent. Sequestered within this vegetation, the organisms grew to an impressive concentration (10^9 colony-forming units per gram of tissue) (83). Their ability to reenter the bloodstream produces the continuous bacteremia of IE.

    The use of Swan-Ganz catheters in CrCU re-creates this experimental system. The incidence of IE associated with these catheters ranges from 2.4% to 10% (84). The valvular infection is the consequence of the catheter-induced endothelial damage, which may be seeded by bacteria originating from the catheter itself or from another site. Most of these type 1 HCIE cases were not suspected during the patient's lifetime. Central venous catheters pose a much lower risk (85).

3. In addition to those processes that directly injure endothelium, the jet and Venturi effects play an important role in both the development of NBTE and its location. Rodbard aerosolized bacteria into an agar tube that was constricted in the middle (86). The organisms were deposited on the side of the low pressure sink that lay just beyond the narrowing (the Venturi effect). The particular distribution of thrombi is explained by this model. In mitral insufficiency, NBTE is found on the atrial surface of the valve (the low pressure side); in aortic insufficiency on the ventricular side. In the case of ventricular septal defect, the low pressure side is the right ventricle and the thrombus is located around the orifice of the defect on that side. The endocardium of the right ventricle opposite the septal defect is roughened by the jet of blood (MacCallum's patch), another site that promotes the formation of NBTE (64).

The bacteremias associated with IE occur either spontaneously or are secondary to a variety of invasive procedures (87). For example, transient bacteremia occurs in 10% of patients with severe gingival disease (88). Two percent of patients with burns >60% of their body surface area develop right-sided IE secondary to the bacteremias complicating septic thrombophlebitis. *S. aureus* is the usual organism retrieved (89). Of course, the bacteremias of pneumonia and pyelonephritis play an important role (43).

Table 4 presents the degree of risk of developing bacteremias secondary to certain planned invasive procedures. However the premier source of bacteremias in the CrCU is the noncuffed central venous catheter (Table 5) (90). They account for at least 120,000 cases of bacteremia per year in the United States. These catheters are the major causes of HCBSI due to CONS, *S. aureus*, and Candida species. Seventy-eight percent of *S. aureus* bacteremia (200,000 cases premier) are associated with intravascular catheters (39).

Infection of intravascular catheters arises from four possible sources (91): the site of insertion, the catheter's hub, bacteremic seeding of the catheter, and contamination of the infusate solution. For short-term catheters (mean duration, 7.2–9 days), contamination of the intracutaneous tract by skin flora is the most common type of infection (92). For longer-term devices, infection of the catheter's hub is the major source of catheter-related bloodstream infections. These pathogens reside on the hands of health-care workers who contaminate the hub as they manipulate it for various reasons, such as connecting infusate solutions or various types of measuring devices (93). The microbes then migrate down the luminal wall of the catheter into the bloodstream.

Bacterial adherence to an intravascular catheter is dependent on the host's response to the presence of a foreign body, the pathogenic properties of the organisms, and the location of the catheter (90). A few days after insertion, a sleeve of fibrin/fibronectin is deposited on the device. *S. aureus* and Candida species stick to the fibrin components and not to the fibronectin; the opposite is true for CONS. *S. aureus* and Candida isolates adhere better to polyvinyl chloride catheters than to those made of Teflon (94). In the case of longer-term catheters (mean duration of 109 days) the amount of colonization and biofilm formation found on the luminal side is twice that of the external surface (95).

Table 4 Risk of Bacteremia Associated with Various Procedures

Low (0–20%)	Moderate (20–40%)	High (40–100%)	Organism
	Tonsillectomy		
Bronchoscopy (rigid)			
Bronchoscopy (flexible)			Streptococcal sp. or *S. epidermidis*
Endoscopy			*S. epidermidis*, streptococci, and diphtheroids
Colonoscopy			*Escherichia coli* and Bacteroides sp. *S. epidermidis*
Barium enema			Enterococci; and aerobic gram-negative rods
	Transurethral resection of the prostate		Coliforms, enterococci, *Staphylococcus aureus*
Cystoscopy			Coliforms and gram-negative rods
		Traumatic dental procedures	*Streptococcus viridans*
Liver biopsy (in setting of cholangitis)			Coliforms and enterococci
Sclerotherapy of esophageal varices			*S. viridans*, gram-negative rods, *S. aureus*
Esophageal dilatation			*S. aureus*, *S. viridans*
	Suction abortion		*S. viridans* and anaerobes
Transesophageal echocardiography			Streptococcal sp.

Table 5 Estimated Risk of Catheter Associated Bloodstream Infection for Different Types of Vascular Access

Catheter type	Bloodstream infections 1000 device days
Short plastic peripheral	<2
Arterial	10
Central venous	
Multilumen	30
Swan-Ganz	10
Hemodialysis	50
Long term	
Peripherally inserted central catheters	2
Cuffed central catheters (Hickman, Broviac)	2
Subcutaneous central venous ports (Infusaport, Port-A-Cath)	<1

The infusate itself may be the source of the bacteremia. Contamination of infused solutions is most commonly caused by gram-negative aerobes (i.e., Enterobacter, Pseudomonas, and Serratia species). All of these are able to grow rapidly at room temperature in a variety of solutions. The hypertonic solutions of total parenteral nutrition are bactericidal to most potential pathogens. A notable exception is Candida species (96), which thrive in this medium but are suppressed in normal saline.

All types of products that can be administered intravenously may be tainted during manufacture (intrinsic contamination). Among these are blood products (platelets, albumin, and plasma proteins), intravenous drugs, Vacutainer tubes, and even povidone-iodine (92). Infused solutions may be contaminated after their manufacture (extrinsic contamination) principally by health-care workers' hand carriage of bacteria (97). All of the following have been documented to be so contaminated: hemodialysis-related material, crystalloid solutions, lipid motions, hyperalimentation solutions, multidose vials, and all types of blood-derived products. The sterility of 1% to 2% of all parenterally administered solutions is compromised during administration. Usually the organisms are part of the normal flora of the skin and have little ability to grow in the infusate (98). When the right gram-negative is present, it can multiply to a concentration of 10^3. The risk of fluid contamination is related to the duration of time the infusion apparatus is in place. A more important factor is the degree of manipulation of the system, such as by blood drawing. Contaminated organisms persist in the system until the entire set is changed.

Of particular note is the frequency of HCBSI that are due to infected arterial catheters. Approximately 1% of all these catheters are complicated by bacteremia. Half of these are related to contamination of the infusate (99).

Native Valve Infective Endocarditis

Table 6 presents the clinical presentations of NVE. It is not the intention of this chapter to present a comprehensive review of all the clinical manifestations of IE but to specifically focus on those cases that are found within the CrCU. There are excellent reviews available for the reader (48). Because of the low-grade virulence of the organisms that are involved, the clinical signs and symptoms of subacute IE reflect its immunological origins, such as renal failure due to interstitial nephritis

Table 6 The Early Nonspecific Signs and Symptoms of Subacute Infective Endocarditis[a]

Low-grade fever (absent in 3–15% of patients)
Anorexia
Weight loss
Influenza-like syndromes
Polymyalgia-like syndromes with arthralgias, dull sensorium,
  and headaches resembling typhoid fever
Pleuritic pain
Right upper quadrant pain and right lower quadrant pain
85% of patients present with a detectable murmur;
  all will eventually develop one

[a]The manifestations of subacute bacterial endocarditis (SDE) are caused by emboli
 and/or progressive valvular destruction and/or immunologic phenomena.

or proliferative glomerulonephritis. Arthralgias and arthritis are due to the deposition of immune complexes in the synovia. Lumbosacral spine pain is a classic finding of subacute disease. Its dermal, mucocutaneous, musculoskeletal, central nervous system, and renal presentations are produced by embolization occurring later in the disease. Progressive valvular destruction eventually will result in heart failure. Truly subacute IE can be a mimic of many infectious and noninfectious diseases (see Section on differential diagnostic considerations).

The acute form of the disease heralds itself abruptly and overwhelmingly with suppurative complications both extra and intracardiac. It is the type of NVE that will likely be cared for in the CrCU. The leaflets of the infected valve are rapidly destroyed as bacteria multiply within the ever-growing friable vegetations. The dyspnea and fatigue of severe congestive heart failure, brought about by valvular destruction, appear within a week. These symptoms are often concurrent with a wide range of neuropsychiatric complications.

Arterial embolization causes most of the extracardiac complications of acute IE. Septic emboli are the second most common complication of IE ($115 = 159°C$) (50–35% of cases). They occur more frequently in younger patients, in left-sided disease, and in PVE. IE that is caused by Candida species, *S. aureus*, *H. parainfluenzae*, Aspergillus species, group B streptococci, and NVS is characterized by large friable vegetations that produce macroemboli. The emboli of acute IE produce metastatic infection. A classic example of this process is the right-sided septic emboli of *S. aureus* IVDA that produce small pulmonary abscesses and infarctions. Emboli may occur even 12 months after the microbiological cure of IE. Left-sided emboli most commonly travel to the spleen, brain, kidneys, coronary arteries, and meninges. Cerebral emboli occur in 30% of cases of acute IE. They most frequently involve the middle cerebral artery. Coronary artery emboli produce myocardial infarction in 40% to 60% of cases. They usually do so without producing any significant changes to the patient's electrocardiogram.

Splenic abscesses that are the result of septic emboli may present as persistent bacteremia in the face of successful treatment of the valvular infection itself (100).

In acute IE, life-threatening mycotic aneurysms occur in 2.5% of all patients (101). They result from invasion of arterial walls by septic microemboli. The most common locations are the brain, sinus of Valsalva, abdominal aorta and its branches, spleen, heart, and lungs. There is rarely any warning prior their rupture.

The most frequent major complication of acute IE is congestive heart failure (15–65% of all patients) that is usually due to valvular destruction (102). An infected valve may suffer from any of the following: tearing and fenestration of the leaflets, detachment from the annulus, and rupture of chordae tendinae and/or papillary muscles (103). The jet stream of the incompetent aortic valve may impact the mitral valve and produce erosion or perforation of the leaflets of its chordae tendineae. This is additive to the strain already placed on the left ventricle by the insufficiency itself (104). Congestive heart failure may result unusually from valvular stenosis caused by a large vegetations of fungal or *S. aureus* IE (105). Myocarditis may also lead to congestive heart failure with typical pathological findings of Bracht-Wacther bodies.

Other intracardiac complications of acute IE include aortocardiac fistulas, aneurysms of the sinus of Valsalva, and intraventricular abscesses that may perforate or involve the conduction system of the heart. *S. aureus* may produce multiple myocardial abscesses (20% fatal cases) that may erode into the pericardial sac and produce rapid death by cardiac tamponade (106). These abscesses can rapidly destroy the intraventricular septum and lead to a left to right shunt.

The pericarditis of acute IE is usually due to erosion of a myocardial or ring abscess in the pericardial space or by direct deposition of organisms during the course of the bacteremia. Uncommonly, it may be due to septic coronary artery emboli or rupture of a mycotic aneurysm.

The distinction between the two polar types of IE has become blurred by the use of antibiotics that are given to treat infections that are really undiagnosed endocarditis. This suppresses the growth of bacteria within the thrombus and produces what it is described as "Muted Endocarditis."

Table 7 summarizes involvement of the major organ systems by NVE.

Prosthetic Valve Endocarditis

Early PVE is defined as infection occurring within 60 days of valve implantation. In the case of CONS PVE, this time frame should be extended to 12 months (107). The source of the pathogens of early PVE is chiefly the surgical environment (i.e., operating room and its equipment) that lead to infection with diphtheroids, *S. aureus*, and fungi. These same organisms are involved in the immediate postoperative period due to contamination of infusate, pacing wires, or endotracheal intubation. The profile of pathogens that produce late PVE resembles those found in NVE. The clinical features of PVE are similar to those of NVE. The congestive heart failure of PVE is more severe and develops earlier than that of NVE probably due to the fact that ventricular function is usually already compromised (108). In 10% of patients with mechanical PVE, a large enough thrombus develops to interfere with left ventricular emptying.

The risk of PVE is five times greater when the valve is implanted because of underlying NVE.

PMIE

Clinical presentations of PM infections and PMIE depend on the site of infection (e.g., generator pocket vs. intravascular or epicardial leads, the organism, and the point of origin of the infection (infection of the pocket or bacteremia) (109). Early infections (within a few months of implantation) are usually either acute or subacute infections of the pulse-generator pocket. There may be associated bacteremia. Fever occurs in 33% of patients.

Late infections of the pocket are due to erosion of the overlying skin and always indicate infection of the generator and possibly of the leads themselves. The most significant late infections are those of the transvenous or epicardial leads. With epicardial lead infection, there may be signs and symptoms of pericarditis of mediastinitis as well as bacteremia. Infection of the transvenous electrode produces right-sided IE similar in presentation to that of IVDA IE (pneumonia, septic emboli in 50% of patients). Fever is a universal finding in PMIE.

Intravenous Drug Abusers IE

Fifty-three percent of cases of IVDA IE present with pulmonary manifestations (pneumonia and/or empyema) due to right-sided *S. aureus* septic emboli (110). Occasionally, other sites are infected by septic emboli, such as the meninges, brain, joints, or bones, which may be the heralding event.

Table 7 Organ Involvement in Native Valve Infective Endocarditis

Peripheral stigmata (20% of patients)	Musculoskeletal (40–50% of patients)	Intracardiac
Janeway lesions	Low back pain (presenting symptom)	Valvular vegetations in 15% of patients
Osler nodes	Diffuse myalgias, especially of legs	CHF
Roth spots	Disc space infection	Myocardial abscess
	Hypertrophic osteoarthropathy	Septal abscess (leading to heart block)
	Splenomegaly	Vascular necrosis
	Arthritis (ankle, knee, wrist)	Aortocardiac fistula
		Suppurative pericarditis
		Rupture of papillary muscles, chordae tendinae
		Annular abscess
		Mycotic aneurysm of sinus of Valsalva
		Destruction of valvular leaflets
		Staphylococcus aureus responsible for 55–70% of congestive heart failure

Neurological system	Renal	Mycotic aneurysms	Metastatic infections
Neurological complications are the presenting symptoms in 50–70% of patients	Congestive heart failure and antibiotic toxicity are currently the most common causes of renal failure	Life threatening in 2.5% of patients	Metastatic infections are produced by septic emboli (usually in acute IE) to liver, spleen, gallbladder, coronary arteries (myocardial infarction occurs in 50% of patients), myocardium, lung, and retina
Hemorrhage	Renal abscesses due to highly invasive organisms (i.e., *S. aureus*)	Usually produced by organisms of low invasive capacity (i.e., *Streptococcus viridans*)	
Toxic manifestations (headache, irritability)	Renal infarction (cortical necrosis) occurs in two-thirds of infected patients	Silent until they leak; seen most commonly in brain	
Psychiatric effects (neurosis)	Focal glomerulonephritis occurs in 50% of untreated cases and is associated with renal failure and nephrotic syndrome	Sinus of Valsalva, abdominal aorta and its branches, mesenteric, splenic, coronary, and pulmonary arteries	

(Continued)

Table 7 Organ Involvement in Native Valve Infective Endocarditis (*Continued*)

Neurological system	Renal	Mycotic aneurysms	Metastatic infections
Psychoses, disorientation, delirium (hallucinations) Stroke Meningoencephalitis Dyskinesia Spinal cord and small nerves (girdle pain, paraplegia, weakness, myalgias, and peripheral neuropathy)	"Flea bitten" kidney, multiple emboli and hemorrhages		

Abbreviations: IE, infective endocarditis; CHF, congestive heart failure.

Health-Care Associated IE

The signs and symptoms of community-acquired and HCIE are significantly different. IE, contracted in a health-care setting, presents much more frequently as sepsis (hypotension, metabolic acidosis, and multiple organ failure). The clinical features that are dependent on the host's inflammatory response, such as fever and leukocytosis, occur less frequently in HCIE (55% vs. 25% and 82% vs. 61%, respectively) (1,12,111). Hepatosplenomegaly, Osler nodes, and Janeway lesions occur less often in HCIE. These differences may be explained, at least in part, by the preponderance of elderly who have HCIE as well as the fact that there is a greater rate of underlying valvular disease in this type of IE. Forty-five percent of HCIE occurs in patients with prosthetic valves in place (26). This figure does include cases of early PVE.

It is important to emphasize that prosthetic valves are very susceptible to HCBSI's. Sixteen percent of bacteremic individuals with prosthetic valves in place develop PVE (107). Two-thirds of these had early PVE. The most common sources were intravascular catheters (33%) and wound infections (28%). Thirty-four percent were caused by fungi or gram-negative bacteria. Many of these patients had been given appropriate antibiotic therapy for more than two weeks at the onset of the bacteremia.

DIFFERENTIAL DIAGNOSIS CONSIDERATIONS

History

The usual course of subacute IE is quite indolent. Its most common symptoms are low-grade fever, fatigue, anorexia, back pain (15%), and weight loss. Less commonly, it may present with a cerebrovascular event or congestive heart failure. Both of these usually occur later in the disease process (Table 6). When therapy is delayed for several months, symptoms due to embolic and/or immunological processes come to the fore.

Less than 50% of patients have previously recognized valvular disease. Although the majority of cases of subacute IE are associated with dental disease, most arise not because of oral surgical procedures but from the transient bacteremias of gingival disease. The next most common source of infecting organisms is the urinary tract infection (112). The usual interval between initiating bacteremia and symptoms of subacute IE is two weeks, rarely as long as four weeks.

The clinical course of acute IE is much more aggressive, with the acute onset of high-grade fever. Rapidly progressive valvular destruction and burrowing ring abscesses produce congestive heart failure and cardiac block within a week. The patient should be questioned about intravenous drug abuse or any recent staphylococcal infections, however mild.

Selected Physical Findings

Fifteen percent of cases of subacute IE have normal or subnormal temperatures especially among the elderly (113). Acute IE is almost always marked by a hectic febrile course.

Because of its pathogenesis (see above), murmurs are always present, with rare exceptions, in subacute cases. The characteristics of preexisting murmurs usually do not change until late in the course of subacute disease. Murmurs are absent in about one-third of patients with left-sided acute IE and in two-thirds of those with right-sided disease and mural endocarditis (114).

Currently, the dermal stigmata of IE, including Osler nodes, Janeway lesions, and splinter hemorrhages, are present in only about 20% of patients. Approximately 40% of patients develop various musculoskeletal disorders including arthritis and synovitis (115). The skin and joint manifestations are usually seen in subacute disease. Occasionally, typical septic arthritis may develop from the bacteremia of staphylococcal valvular infection. Splenomegaly is found in less than 30% of cases, usually acute. For other physical findings of IE refer to Table 7.

Laboratory/Radiology Tests

Continuous bacteremia is the hallmark of IE. It may be defined with two blood cultures, positive for the same organism, drawn 12 or more hours apart or at least three out of four cultures positive for the same organism, the first and last separated by at least one hour (6). The author prefers the latter definition with the time span shortened to half an hour. This version is applicable to both subacute and acute cases by recognizing the need to rapidly start antibiotic therapy in acute valvular infection. In those patients with culture positive IE, three sets of blood cultures will detect the pathogen in >99% of cases of IE (116). For confirmation of CONS, five sets should be drawn to rule out the possibility of contamination. At least 64% of patients who have received antibiotics have negative blood cultures (117). The longer the duration of antimicrobial therapy, the longer is the length of time that the cultures remain negative. In these situations, blood cultures should be drawn at least 48 hours after the antimicrobial agent has been discontinued in cases of suspected subacute IE. A delay of one or two weeks in starting treatment of subacute disease is acceptable. If these fail to retrieve a pathogen, then a second set of blood cultures should be obtained between 7 and 10 days later. Blood cultures provide not only the most specific means of diagnosing IE but also the extremely important antimicrobial sensitivity data. In patients with possible acute IE, antibiotic therapy needs to be instituted within a few hours of presentation. Therefore additional treatment must be empiric based on several factors (refer to medical management below).

Up to 50% of positive blood cultures represent contamination (118). Drawing one blood culture is worse than drawing none at all from patients. There is no way to rule out contamination in this case. It is difficult to withhold therapy in such patients who are acutely ill. Because the bacteremia of intravascular infection is continuous, blood cultures can be obtained at any time. The blood samples always should be collected under sterile conditions. The recommended skin preparation is 70% isopropyl alcohol followed by application of an iodophor or tincture of iodine. These solutions need to be allowed to dry completely for greatest effectiveness (119). Each venipuncture should be performed at a different site.

Blood cultures should not be obtained through intravascular lines, except in the process of documenting infection of that line (see below), because of the risk of contamination (120). The diagnosis of catheter-related sepsis or line infection may be established by culturing the catheter by the roll-plate technique (either qualitative, semiquantitative, or quantitative methods), even though it has a disadvantage that the catheter must first be removed and only its external surfaces cultured. A less common but more accurate method is paired quantitative blood cultures obtained from the line and a peripheral vein. Intravascular catheters should not be cultured routinely unless a localized or bloodstream infection is suspected (121). A ratio of colony units of the catheter culture to that from the vein of 10:1 is considered diagnostic of catheter infection.

Replacement of the needle before inoculating the specimen into the blood culture bottle is not necessary. Because the concentration of bacteria is low, 10 mL of blood should be added to each bottle. This produces a 1:10 ratio of blood to broth that can inhibit the suppressive effect of many antibiotics and the patient's own antibodies (122).

Two to five percent of cases of IE have falsely negative blood cultures. This is usually due to prior antibiotic therapy (123). In the author's experience, the second most common cause is the situation in which the pathogen is very deep within the vegetation and is not in direct communication with the bloodstream (124). Less likely is the presence of fastidious organisms (such as members of the HACEK group, Brucella, and fungi).

There is no single ideal growth medium for retrieving the pathogens of IE. Generally trypticase soy broth is used to isolate the aerobic pathogens and thioglycolate for the anaerobic and facultatively anaerobic ones, such as NVS. NVS often requires supplementation of the medium with pyridoxine for growth to take place. With development of various automated blood culture systems and improved media, most pathogens, even the fastidious, can be isolated within five days. It is seldom necessary for cultures to be incubated for two to three weeks as formerly recommended. Various approaches for cultivating the other fastidious organisms are well described elsewhere (125).

Only about 50% of blood cultures in those with Candidal IE are positive. Histoplasma and Aspergillus species are rarely recoverable from the blood. One must consider a fungal pathogen when a case of culture negative IE fails to respond to an appropriate choice of antibiotics. Bone marrow cultures may be useful in isolating fungi as well as mycobacteria and Brucella (126).

Broth supplemented with various types of resins (BACTEC resin) is used in those patients who have received antibiotics prior to obtaining blood cultures. This approach is useful especially in cases of *S. aureus* bacteremia and fungemia. However, its success rate is relatively low (127).

A useful set of criteria for assessing the validity of a positive blood culture has been developed (118). There are three characteristics that denote a true positive culture:

1. The type of organism recovered. For example, CONS recovered in blood cultures of a patient without an intravascular catheter or other prosthetic material usually represents a contaminant.
2. Multiple specimens being positive for the same pathogen.
3. The degree of severity of illness of the patient.

One false positive blood culture can result in an extra four days of hospitalization (128).

To diagnose IE, caused by organisms that are difficult to culture in the hospital's microbiology laboratory (e.g., *Coxiella brunetti*, Brucella sp., and Chlamydia and Legionella), the clinician often resorts to standard serological studies and various types of DNA amplification techniques (129). Measurement of teichoic acid antibodies is useful in deciding the significance of a limited number blood cultures positive for *S. aureus* that do not meet the criteria for a continuous bacteremia.

Cardiac conduction abnormalities develop in 9% of patients. They are due to myocarditis or the development of septal abscesses (130). During the first two weeks of treatment of acute IE, electrocardiography should be performed every 48 to 72 hours because of the high rate of development of septal abscesses. Rheumatoid factor is present in 50% of patients with subacute IE and disappears with successful treatment (43). It represents a "poor man's" circulating immune complex.

The nonspecific findings of elevated sedimentation rate, anemia of chronic disease, proteinuria, and hematuria are not helpful in diagnosing IE.

Because of the interference of the growth of pathogens in blood culture by the widespread use of broad-spectrum antibiotics in the critically ill patient, several types of imaging techniques have been used to indirectly diagnose valvular infection. Radionuclide scans, such as gallium-67 and Indium-111 tagged white cells and platelets, have been used in diagnosing myocardial abscesses. These are plagued by poor resolution and false negatives (131). 2-D echocardiography has become the imaging test of choice for both diagnosis and management of IE (132). There is a great deal of confusion regarding the proper use of echocardiography as well as the respective appropriateness of transthoracic echocardiography (TTE) versus transesophageal echocardiography (TEE). Neither type of echocardiography should be performed in patients with a low pretest clinical probability of IE. Up to 50% of vegetations are sterile (133). There are no echocardiographic criteria that differentiate noninfective findings from infective. Fifteen percent of echocardiographic-defined thrombi are really just valve thickening (134). Additionally, there is a large degree of interobserver variability in reading either type of echocardiography (135). Fifteen percent of cases of IE have no detectable vegetations at any given time.

TTEs can define features down to 5 mm in diameter, TEEs down to 1 mm in diameter (161 = 335 IDC and a 11). Sensitivity of TEE for diagnosing NVE ranges from 48% to 100%; TTE ranges from 18% to 63%. TTE is ineffective in 15% of patients because of their "barrel chests" of chronic pulmonary disease. Because of the attenuation of its beam by the implanted material, TTE has only a 35% sensitivity for detecting PVE as compared to >75% for TEE. TEE is also superior for detecting right-sided vegetations. The sensitivity of TEE is such that it has 100% negative predictive value for IE.

A TTE should be ordered initially in establishing the diagnosis of IE unless there is the possibility of PVE, abnormal body habitus, known valvular abnormality, or *S. aureus* bacteremia (see below medical management). If the TTE is completely normal, the likelihood of valvular infection is very low, and a TEE should not be performed unless there are consistently positive blood cultures without a definable source or the study is technically unsatisfactory.

Table 8 presents the indications for performing echocardiography in NVE and PVE (137,138).

The characteristics of a vegetation can be useful in predicting the risk of embolization and abscess formation. Vegetations >10 mL, which exhibit significant mobility, are three times more likely to embolize than those thrombi without these features (139). Vegetations on the mitral valve, especially the anterior leaflet, were more likely to embolize than those located at other locations (140). Myocardial abscess formation was positively correlated with two factors: aortic valve infection and intravenous drug abuse (141).

All individuals with proven IE should undergo an echocardiographic study in order to provide a baseline so as to monitor response to therapy and to detect the onset of complications, such as aortic regurgitation.

Computed tomography and magnetic resonance imaging currently have almost no role at all in managing cases of IE. The relative "slowness" of the current technology is a major limiting factor (142).

Table 8 American College of Cardiology/American Heart Association Guidelines for Echocardiography in Native Valve and Prosthetic Valve Endocarditis

Indication	Class[a] (native/prosthetic valve)
Detection and characterization of valvular lesions and their hemodynamic severity or degree of ventricular decompensation[b]	I/I
Detection of associated abnormalities (e.g., abscesses, shunts etc.)[b]	I/I
Reevaluation[b] studies in complicated endocarditis (e.g., virulent organisms, severe hemodynamic lesion, aortic valve involvement, persistent fever or bacteremia clinical change, or deterioration)	I/I
Evaluation of patients with high clinical suspicion of culture-negative endocarditis[b]	I/I
Evaluation of persistent bacteremia or fungemia without a known source[b]	Ia/I
Risk stratification in established endocarditis[b]	IIa/-
Routine reevaluation in uncomplicated endocarditis during antibiotic therapy	IIb/IIb
Evaluation of fever and nonpathological murmur without evidence of bacteremia[c]	III/IIa

[a]Class I: evidence and/or general agreement that an echocardiography is useful; IIa: conflicting evidence or divergence of opinion about usefulness, but weight of evidence/opinion favor it; IIb: usefulness is less well established; III: evidence or general opinion that echocardiography is not useful.
[b]Transesophageal echocardiography (TEE) may provide incremental value in addition to information obtained by transthoracic echocardiography. The role of TEE in first-line examination awaits further study.
[c]Prosthetic valves-IIa: for persistent bacteremia; III: for transient bacteremia.
Source: From Ref. 136.

DIAGNOSIS

Presumptive Clinical Diagnosis

Whenever there is a bacteremia with a pathogen capable of infecting a native or prosthetic valve, the possibility of IE must be actively ruled out. It is a "cannot miss" diagnosis. The presence of a continuous bacteremia, by itself, is adequate for the diagnosis of IE because no other infection is capable of producing such. The real challenge comes when the patient clinical signs and symptoms are consistent with endocarditis, but the cultures remain negative (see above).

A definitive pathological diagnosis of IE is achieved by culturing the pathogen from an endocardial vegetation, embolized thrombus, or myocardial abscess. Alternatively, histological examination can confirm active IE. Standard tissue stains have been supplemented by DNA amplification techniques (143).

In 1994, Durack et al. developed criteria that combined the clinical, microbiological, and echocardiographic findings to facilitate diagnosis of IE in a given patient (6).

Major criteria include

- The presence of a continuous bacteremia (see above) with organisms typically involved in IE.
- Specific echocardiographic findings of IE.
  a. Oscillating intracardiac mass on valve or supporting structures or in the path of regurgitant jets or on an iatrogenic device.
  b. Myocardial abscess.
  c. New dehiscence of a prosthetic valve.
  d. New valvular regurgitation.

Minor criteria include

- Predisposing cardiac conditions or intravenous drug use.
- Fever $\leq 38°C$ ($\leq 100.4°F$).
- Vascular phenomena (arterial emboli, septic pulmonary infarcts, mycotic aneurysms, intracranial hemorrhages, and Janeway lesions).
- Immunological phenomena (glomerulonephritis, Osler nodes, Roth spots, and rheumatoid factor).
- Echocardiographic findings not meeting above major echocardiographic criteria.
- Positive blood cultures not meeting above major criteria or serological evidence of the presence of an organism typically involved in IE.

The definitive clinical diagnosis is met by the existence of two major criteria or one major and three minor criteria or five minor criteria.

The diagnosis of IE is rejected when

1. There is a definitive alternative diagnosis.
2. The clinical manifestations of IE resolve after four or less days of antimicrobial therapy.
3. There is no pathological evidence of IE after four or fewer days of antimicrobial therapy.

The modified Duke criteria of 2000 (144) include a category of possible IE. This represents findings that are consistent with IE but neither fulfill the definite criteria nor fit the rejected category.

Table 9 Differential Diagnoses

Noninfectious entities
Antiphospholipid syndrome
Atrial myxoma
Cardiac neoplasms
Polymyalgia rheumatica
Reactive arthritis and Reiter's syndrome
Systemic lupus erythematosus
Thrombotic nonbacterial endocarditis
Temporal arteritis and other forms vasculitis
Cholesterol emboli syndrome
Infectious entities
Lyme disease
Viral hepatitis
Disseminated gonococcal infection/gonococcal arthritis

Note: The presence of a continuous bacteremia differentiates infective endocarditis from its infectious and noninfectious mimics.

The Duke criteria have provided a very useful guideline for the diagnosis of IE. However, they are more suited to diagnose subacute disease than acute because of the preponderance of immunological phenomena in the former. The term possible IE contributes little to the diagnostic process.

Table 9 presents the differential diagnosis of IE.

MIMICS OF ENDOCARDITIS

Many diseases, both infectious and noninfectious, mimic the nonspecific symptoms of IE especially the subacute variety (145). In the era of echocardiography, the absence of valvular vegetations readily excludes many of these entities. For the purpose of this discussion, the mimics of IE are those diseases that damage cardiac valves, induce valvular vegetations, and produce many of the signs and symptoms of IE (i.e., immunological phenomena, embolic events, and musculoskeletal complaints). Of course, in this situation the blood cultures are negative unless the thrombus becomes secondarily infected. Most of these are autoimmune diseases that produce friable vegetations with a high rate of embolization (146). By a variety of mechanisms, these diseases produce endothelial damage that leads to the development of sterile fibrin platelet thrombi. The onset of endocarditis in these diseases may suddenly worsen the degree of the patient's valvular dysfunction. IE, complicating rheumatoid arthritis, are and SLE, is much more common in renal failure and in patients who are receiving prednisone or cyclophosphamide (147). Indeed, penicillin and sulfonamides may promote flare-ups of SLE. Many autoimmune disorders such as scleroderma and systemic vasculitis produce valvular distortion. However, they usually are not associated with thromboembolic disease and should not pose much of a diagnostic challenge.

The major exception to the predominance of autoimmune diseases and probably the most effective mimic of all is atrial myxoma (148). Up to 50% of left atrial myxomas embolize most frequently to the central nervous system. Fifty percent of

Table 10 Mimics of Infective Endocarditis

Disease	Type of valvular involvement	Comments
Antiphospholipid syndrome	Stenosis or regurgitation	Patients have thrombotic events and/or recurrent spontaneous abortions. Antibody titers have no direct correlation with disease activity
Systemic lupus erythematosus	Stenosis or regurgitation occurs in 46% of patients (usually of the mitral valve)	4% of cases of Libman-Sacks endocarditis become secondarily infected usually early in the course of the disease
Rheumatoid arthritis	Regurgitation occurs in 2% of patients	Valvular infection usually occurs later in the course of the disease
Atrial myxoma	Primarily obstruction of the mitral valve due to its "ball valve" effect	It is the most effective mimic due to its valvular involvement, embolic events and constitutional signs and symptoms

cases are marked by significant elevations in temperature. Often the only way to distinguish atrial myxoma from IE is by pathological examination of myxoma tissue retrieved from a peripheral artery or from cardiac surgery. Table 10 presents the most diagnostically challenging mimics of endocarditis.

THERAPY

Nonantibiotic Therapy

Surgery is required eventually in 25% of cases of IE; a great deal of which is performed after bacteriological cure has been achieved. Twenty-five percent of the surgeries are performed during the early phases of the disease, the rest during later stages of IE. Surgery has improved the outcomes of IE. However, due to the increase in IE produced by more virulent pathogens (e.g., *S. aureus*, gram-negatives, and fungi) in impaired hosts, these outcomes have not improved over the last 30 years.

In both NVE and PVE, the most common indication for surgical intervention is congestive heart failure that is refractory to standard medical therapy (149). The other major indications are (i) fungal IE (excluding that produced by Histoplasma capsulatum); (ii) bacteremia that persists after at least seven days of appropriate antibiotic treatment, which is not caused by an extracardiac source (149); (iii) recurrent septic emboli occurring after two weeks of appropriate antibiotic treatment; (iv) rupture of an aneurysm of the sinus of Valsalva; (v) conduction disturbances secondary to a septal abscess; and (vi)"kissing" infection of the anterior mitral valve leaflet in cases of aortic valve IE.

Indications for surgery in PVE are the same with the addition of the presence of prosthetic valve dehiscence and in cases of early PVE. Because of the difficulty in eradicating organisms from prosthetic devices, surgery plays a more immediate role in PVE than in NVE. Not all cases of PVE require surgery. Factors associated with a good outcome with medical therapy alone include (i) infection due to susceptible organisms; (ii) late PVE; (iii) mitral valve infection; and (iv) prompt initiation of antibiotic treatment of bioprosthetic valve PVE (150).

Certain echocardiographic features have been recognized as being positively associated with the need for surgery in IE (151). However, they have not received complete clinical validation. Among these are (i) detectable vegetations following a large embolus; (ii) anterior mitral valve vegetations and >1 cm in diameter; (iii) continued growth of vegetations after four weeks of antibiotic therapy; (iv) development of acute mitral insufficiency; (v) rupture or perforation of a valve; and (vi) periannular extension of infection.

There is no set time for the patient who requires surgery to be on preoperative antibiotics (152). The primary goal of perioperative antibiotics is to prevent bacteremias during the cardiac procedure. It is extremely important to rule out a splenic abscess before cardiac surgery is performed for "refractory IE." These are often clinically occult and can cause a continuous bacteremia that can be misdiagnosed as persistent valvular infection (153). Surgery is frequently required to eradicate a variety of metastatic infections including aneurysms and cerebral abscesses.

Debridement and antibiotic administration often may cure an uncomplicated PM pocket infection. In cases of PMIE, the entire system should be removed for cure. If it has been in place for more than 18 months, extraction of the electrodes can be difficult. Excimer laser sheaths, which have the ability to dissolve the fibrotic attachment bands of the electrodes, can produce complete extraction >90% of cases (154).

An increasingly common problem in CrCU is the management of *S. aureus* bacteremia in the presence of an intravascular catheter. Approximately 25% of these cases represent IE. Separating *S. aureus* IE from cases of uncomplicated staphylococcal bacteremia is essential for determining the length of therapy after removal of short-term lines and determining whether long-term lines need to be removed at all. Hematuria, associated with *S. aureus* bacteriuria, is a useful indicator of sustained *S. aureus* bacteremia. Hematuria is the result of embolic renal infarction or immunologically mediated glomerulonephritis (155). The presence of intracellular bacteria on smears of blood drawn through intravascular catheters is specific for infected devices (156). TEE provides the most specific means of distinguishing uncomplicated *S. aureus* bacteremia from valvular infection. Twenty-three percent of catheter associated staphylococcal bacteremia have evidence of IE on TEE even in the absence of clinical or positive TTE findings. Table 11 presents an approach to management of short-term intravascular catheter associated *S. aureus* bacteremia (157).

Persistent bacteremia after three days of appropriate antibiotic therapy is an independent risk factor for endocarditis as well as death (158).

Surgically implanted long-term catheters (Broviac or Hickman) do not need to be automatically removed except in the presence of IE, infection of the vascular tunnel, suppurative thrombophlebitis or pathogens such as Corynebacterium JK, Pseudomonas species, fungi, *S. aureus*, or mycobacteria (159). Intraluminal infusions of appropriate antibiotics have at least 30% to 50% greater success against sensitive organisms. The use of thrombolytic agents to dissolve the fibrin sheath of the catheter appears to improve the efficacy of the infused antibiotic (137).

Antibiotic Therapy

There are many more challenges to sterilizing an infected thrombus with antibiotic therapy than to sterilizing a large infected vegetation. Among these factors are (i) the density of organisms (10–100 billion bacteria/g of tissue) and (ii) the decreased metabolic and replicative activity of the intrathrombus organisms that make the bacteria less sensitive to the action of most antibiotics (160). In addition, the mobility and phagocytic function of white cells is impaired in the fibrin-rich vegetation.

Table 11 Management of *Staphylococcus aureus* Bacteremia in the
Presence of an Intravascular Catheter

Prompt removal of the catheter
Institution of appropriate antibiotic therapy
Follow-up blood cultures within 24–48 hrs
    If follow-up blood cultures are negative and
        The TEE shows no signs of IE
        There is no evidence of metastatic infection
Then 2 wks of antibiotic therapy would be appropriate
    If follow-up blood cultures are positive and
        The TEE shows signs of IE
Then 4 wks of intravenous therapy is appropriate
    If follow-up blood cultures are positive and
        The TEE shows no signs of IE
Further imaging studies should be performed to rule out other sources of
    bacteremia (osteomyelitis, mediastinitis, splenic abscess)

Abbreviations: TEE, transesophageal echocardiography; IE, infective endocarditis.

The basic principles of antibiotic therapy of IE include:

1. The necessity to employ bactericidal antibiotics because of the "hostile" environment of the thrombus.
2. The minimal inhibitory concentration (MIC) and the minimal bacteriostatic concentration (MBC) of the pathogen need to be determined to insure adequate overkill. It is estimated that in the case of *Escherichia coli* IE, 220 times the MBC of ceftriaxone is required to sterilize the vegetation (161). Determining the bactericidal titer should be limited to those patients who are not responding well to therapy or who are infected by an unusual organism.
3. In general, intermittent dosing of an antibiotic provides superior penetration of tissue as compared to continuous infusion. Its penetration into tissue is directly related to its peak level in serum (162).
4. All patients should be initially treated in a health-care facility for one to two weeks to monitor for hemodynamic stability.
5. In the case of acute IE, antibiotic therapy should be started after three to five sets of blood cultures are drawn within 60 to 90 minutes so as to minimize valvular damage. The selection of the antibiotic regimen is based on the clinical history and physical examination.
6. For cases of subacute IE, treatment may be delayed until the final culture and sensitivity results are available because a delay of one to two weeks does not adversely affect the final outcome.
7. Usually duration of therapy ranges from four to six weeks. A four-week course is quite appropriate for uncomplicated NVE (for sensitive *S. viridans* this sometimes can be decreased to two weeks—see below). Six weeks are required for the treatment of PVE and in those infections with large vegetations such as caused by the HACEK family (117).

A daily temperature maximum of >37°C for 10 days into treatment merits concern. This situation may represent a relatively resistant pathogen, extracardiac infection, pulmonary or systemic emboli, drug fever, *Clostridium difficile* colitis or an infected intravenous site (163). If the pathogen is not sensitive to the administered antibiotic, a thorough search for the cause should be conducted. Mycotic aneurysms are the most difficult to detect. A TTE should be performed. If that is not helpful, then a TEE should be performed (164). Complications, produced by embolic immunological events, are not necessarily related to the failure of treatment for valvular infection itself (165).

Relapse of IE usually occurs within two months of cessation of treatment (166). The risk of relapse is greatly dependent on the infecting organisms. Appropriately treated NVE, caused by *S. viridans*, rarely relapses. Four percent of *S. aureus* IE and 30% of enterococcal IE relapse. Gram-negative organisms, especially *P. aeruginosa*, have higher rates of relapse (167). IE of >3 months duration prior to antibiotic treatment also has a high rate of relapse.

The greatest risk factor for recurrence of IE is a prior case of IE (168). The second most common factor is a past history of IVDA IE. Forty percent of cases of IVDA IE are recurrent.

Isolates of *S. viridans* classically have been quite sensitive to the beta-lactam antibiotics, the aminoglycosides (gentamicin and streptomycin), and vancomycin. Valvular infection caused by these organisms may be cured by a two-week course of a beta-lactam antibiotic combined with gentamicin (169). To undertake a short course approach, the following conditions must exist: a sensitive *S. viridans* (MIC < 0.1 mcg/ml), NVE of < 3 months duration, vegetation size < 10 mm in diameter, no cardiac or extracardiac complications, a low risk for developing aminoglycoside nephrotoxicity, and good clinical response within the first week of therapy.

There is a growing amount of *S. viridans* isolates that are resistant to penicillin (MIC > 0.1 mg/mL). Highly resistant isolates have a MIC that is >1 mg/mL. Thirteen percent of *S. viridans* isolates in this country are highly resistant to penicillin, with 70% being resistant to ceftriaxone (170).

All NVS are resistant to penicillin, many being highly resistant. Many penicillin-sensitive strains are tolerant to the beta-lactam drugs. Tolerance is a phenomenon in which the MBC of antibiotic exceeds its MIC by a factor of 10 (171). Against these isolates, the penicillins behave practically as bacteriostatic compounds.

Although penicillin by itself can cure most cases of *S. viridans*, the third generation cephalosporin, ceftriaxone because of its pharmacokinetics, is the antibiotic of choice because of its twice a day dosing regimen. The combined use of penicillin or glycopeptide with gentamicin is needed to eradicate resistant streptococci. Tolerant streptococci are best managed by a combination of penicillin and gentamicin. Table 12 summarizes the recommendations for treatment of nonenterococcal streptococci.

Since the advent of antibiotics, enterococci have posed major resistance problems due to their ability to develop multiple resistance mechanisms. They are resistant to all the cephalosporins and to the penicillinase-resistant penicillins such as nafcillin and oxacillin. Penicillin and ampicillin are ineffective when used singly against serious enterococcal infection. Aminoglycosides because of their failure to penetrate the bacterial cell wall are ineffective when used alone (172). The success of the serendipitously recognized combination of penicillin and streptomycin opened up the whole field of synergy. The cell wall active antibiotic allows penetration of the aminoglycosides into the bacterial anterior and reach its target, the ribosome. A serum concentration of 3 mg/mL of gentamicin is necessary for synergism. If the isolate is resistant to ampicillin or penicillin synergism is not possible.

Currently, 5% of *E. faecalis* and 40% of *E. faecium* possess high-grade resistance to gentamicin (>2000 mg/mL) (173). Resistance to streptomycin has been

Table 12 Guidelines for Antimicrobial Therapy of Nonenterococcal Streptococcal Infective Endocarditis[a]

Antibiotic	Dosage regimen
Penicillin-sensitive Streptococcus viridans	
Penicillin G[b]	Penicillin G 20,000,000 U IV in four divided doses for 4 wks
Penicillin G[b] and gentamicin[c]	Penicillin 20,000,000 U IV in four divided doses for 2 wks gentamicin 3 mg/kg given q24hrs as a single dose or in divided doses q8hrs for 2 wks (ceftriaxone 2 g IV/1 M for 4 wks may be used in patients with mild reactions to penicillin)
Or ceftriaxone	Ceftriaxone 2 g IV/1 M for 4 wks (may be used in patients with mild reactions to penicillin)
Penicillin-resistant or -tolerant S. viridans	
Penicillin G[b]	Penicillin G 20,000,000 U IV in four divided doses for 4 wks
Gentamicin	Gentamicin 3 mg/kg given q24hrs as a single dose or in divided doses q8hrs for 2 wks
NVS and group B streptococci	
Penicillin G[b]	Penicillin G 20,000,000 U IV in four divided doses for 6 wks
Gentamicin	Gentamicin 3 mg/kg given q24hrs as a single dose or in divided doses q8hrs for 2 wks

Note: Drug dosages:
[a]For patients with normal renal function.
[b]Vancomycin 30 mg/kg IV q12hrs in patients highly allergic to penicillin.
[c]Short course therapy (see text).
Abbreviation: NVS, nutritionally variant streptococci.

prevalent for a long time. Some gentamicin-resistant isolates remain sensitive to streptomycin and vice versa.

Ampicillin resistance, due to beta-lactamase production, has been recognized since the 1980s. This may not be detectable by routine sensitivity testing.

In the absence of ampicillin/penicillin, vancomycin, and aminoglycoside resistance, the combination of a cell wall active antibiotic and an aminoglycoside remains the preferred therapeutic approach. In the setting of normal renal function, the daily dose of ampicillin is 4 g given IV every eight hours. Gentamicin (1.5 mg/kg) is to be given every 12 hours (174).

Vancomycin (1 g IV every 12 hours) is substituted for ampicillin in those allergic to penicillin or for isolates resistant to ampicillin.

When resistance to both gentamicin and streptomycin is present, continuously infused ampicillin, to achieve a serum level of 60 mg/mL, appears to be the best option (175). Quinupristin/dalfoprastin and linezolid should be considered as alternatives. They have the disadvantage of being bacteriostatic antibiotics against the enterococcus (176). In addition, Quinupristin/dalfoprastin is active only against *E. faecium* and not against *E. faecalis*, the most common enterococcal species.

Daptomycin appears to be bactericidal against these organisms, but experience is quite limited in treating IE with this drug (177) (see table for dosages of these antibiotics).

It is extremely important to emphasize the need to obtain MICs and MBCs for ampicillin, the aminoglycosides and vancomycin in all cases of enterococcal IE to arrive at the best therapeutic approach.

Staphylococcus aureus

The penicillinase-resistant penicillins are the drugs of choice in treating MSSA IE; vancomycin is significantly less effective than these compounds against MSSA. It should be used only in valvular infections caused by MRSA or for patients who

Table 13 Antibiotic Therapy of *Staphylococcus aureus* Infective Endocarditis[a]

Valve type (IE type)	Antibiotic	Dosage
Native (MSSA)	Oxacillin +/− gentamicin	Oxacillin 2 g IV q4hrs for 4–6 wks +/− gentamicin 2 mg/kg q24hrs as a single dose or in divided doses q8hrs for 5 days
	or Vancomycin[b,c] +/− gentamicin	Vancomycin 15 mg/kg IV q12hrs for 4–6 wks ± gentamicin 3 mg/kg q24hrs as a single dose or in divided doses q8hrs for 5 days
	or Cefazolin +/− gentamicin	Cefazolin 1.5 g IV q8hrs for 4–6 wks (in patients with mild allergies to penicillin) ± gentamicin 3 mg/kg q24 hrs as a single dose or in divided doses q8hrs for 5 days
Prosthetic (MSSA)	Oxacillin or vancomycin or cefazolin and	Oxacillin 2 g IV q4hrs for 4–6 wks or vancomycin 15 mg/kg IV q12hrs for 4–6 wks or cefazolin 1.5g IV q8hrs for 4–6 wks in patients with mild allergies to penicillin
	Rifampin and Gentamicin	Rifampin 300 mg PO q8hrs for 6 wks Gentamicin 3 mg/kg q24hrs as a single dose or in divided doses q8hrs for 2 wks
Native (MRSA)	Vancomycin[c]	Vancomycin 15 mg/kg IV q12hrs for 4–6 wks
Prosthetic (MRSA)	Vancomycin[c] and	Vancomycin 15 mg/kg IV q12hrs for 4–6 wks
	Rifampin and Gentamicin	Rifampin 300 mg PO q8hrs for 6 wks Gentamicin 3 mg/kg q24hrs as a single dose or in divided doses q8h for 2 wks

[a]For patients with normal renal function.
[b]For patients with severe penicillin allergy.
[c]Substitute linezolid in critically ill patients or those with significant renal failure (refer to discussion in text).
Abbreviations: IE, infective endocarditis; MSSA, methicillin-sensitive *S. aureus*; MRSA, methicillin-resistant *S. aureus.*

Table 14 Therapy for Coagulase-Negative Staphylococcal
Prosthetic Valve Endocarditis[a]

Antibiotic	Dosage regimen
Vancomycin	15 mg/kg q12hrs for 6 wks
Rifampin	300 mg PO q8hrs for 6 wks
Gentamicin	3 mg/kg q24hrs IV as a single dose or in divided doses q12hrs for 2 wks

[a]80% of isolates recovered within the first year after valve replacement are resistant to the beta-lactam antibiotics. After this period, 30% are resistant. Sensitivity to the penicillins must be confirmed because standard sensitivity testing may not detect resistance. If the isolate is sensitive, oxacillin or cefazolin may be substituted.

are significantly allergic to penicillin. Vancomycin has a failure rate of 35% in MSSA IE (178). Although cefazolin is used in treating MSSA IE, especially in patients with mild allergic reactions to penicillins, it should be administered with realization that there have been failures with this drug. This is probably due to production of type A beta-lactamase by the pathogen (179). For the first three to five days of treatment of MSSA or MRSA IE, the addition of gentamicin to the penicillin or vancomycin should be strongly considered in patients who are not at increased risk of aminoglycoside nephrotoxicity. This combination has not been proven to decrease overall mortality. In decreasing the duration of bacteremia and fever, it may minimize the intra- and extra-cardiac complications of *S. aureus* IE (180).

Right-sided IVDA IE, caused by MSSA, has been successfully treated in two weeks of intravenous therapy with a combination of nafcillin/oxacillin and gentamicin (181). This may be due to the fact that in right-sided endocarditis, antibiotic penetration of the vegetation is greater, and there is a lower concentration of bacteria than in left-sided disease due to the lower oxygen tension in the right ventricle. Those cases of IVDA IE in which the patient is HIV positive or there is evidence of left-sided disease or of lung abscess or of other metastatic sites of infection are not suitable for a short course of antibiotic therapy.

To achieve best outcomes for staphylococcal PVE due to MSSA, MRSA, or CONS, a triple drug approach is advised. Rifampin is the key component. Rifampin has the distinctive ability to kill staphylococci adherent to prosthetic material as well as being able to penetrate phagocytes (182). The other two agents are chosen because of their activity against the target isolate with the aim of preventing the development

Table 15 Antibiotic Treatment Options for Treatment of Endocarditis
Due to Highly Resistant Gram-Positive Organisms[a]

Antibiotic dosage
Linezolid 600 mg q24hrs (either PO or IV)[b]
Quinpristin/dalfopristin 7.5 mg/kg q8hrs
Daptomycin 6 mg/kg q24hrs[c]

[a]See text for indications.
[b]Effectiveness of the PO route may approximate that of the IV route (see text).
[c]This higher dose (usual dose = 4 mg/kg q24h) is probably required to treat infective endocarditis due to *Staphylococcus aureus* and enterococci.
Source: From Ref. 188.

Table 16 Therapy of Various Types of Infective Endocarditis[a]

Organism	Antibiotic regimen	Alternative regimen
Culture negative	Ampicillin 2 g IV q4hrs for 4 wks[b] Gentamicin 5 mg/kg q24hrs IV given in a single dose or in divided doses q8hrs for the first 2 wks Oxacillin 2 g IV q4hrs for 4 wks Or if MRSA is suspected or prosthetic material is present, vancomycin 30 mg/kg q 12hrs for 4 wks	Culture negative
Pseudomonas aeruginosa	Ticarcillin 3 g IV q4hrs for 6 wks[b] Tobramycin 5 mg/kg q24hrs IV given in a single dose or in divided doses q8hrs	Ceftazidime[c] 2 g IV q8hrs for 6 wks Aztreonam[d] 2 g IV q6hrs for 6 wks Tobramycin 5 mg/kg IV q24hrs given in a single dose or in divided doses q8hrs
HACEK group	Ampicillin 2 g IV q4hrs for 4–6 wks[b] Gentamicin 5 mg/kg q24hrs as a single dose or in divided doses q8hrs	Cefotaxime[c] 2 g IV q8hrs for 4–6 wks Gentamicin 5 mg/kg q24hrs given in a single dose or in divided doses

[a]For patients with normal renal function.
[b]Preferred regimen (see text).
[c]In patients with mild penicillin allergy.
[d]In patients with severe penicillin allergy.
Abbreviations: MRSA, methicillin-resistant *S. aureus*; HACEK, *Haemophilus, A. actinomycetemcomitans, C. hominis, and Kingella.*

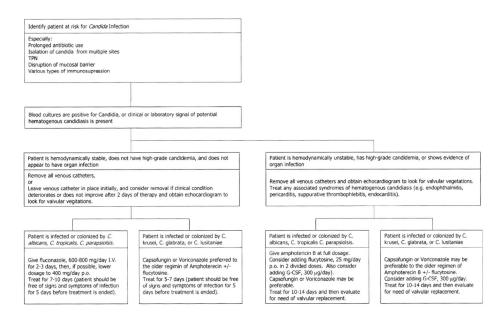

Figure 1 Approach to the patient at risk for candidal endocarditis. *Source*: From Ref. 192.

Table 17 Recommendations for the Prevention of Intravascular Catheter-Related Infections

General

Not recommended
  Preventive strategies incorporating therapeutic antimicrobial agents

During catheter insertion
Strongly recommended
  Full-barrier precautions during central venous catheter insertion
  Subcutaneous tunneling short-term catheters inserted in the internal jugular or femoral
    veins when catheters are not used for blood drawing
  Contamination shield for pulmonary artery catheters.
  Insertion-site preparation with chlorhexidine-containing antiseptics
  Prophylaxis with vancomycin and other therapeutic agents
Recommended
  Subclavian vein, rather than jugular or femoral vein, catheter insertion
Consider
  Insertion-site preparation with tincture of iodine
  Full-barrier precautions during insertion of midline, peripheral artery, and pulmonary
    artery catheters
Not recommended
  Femoral vein catheter insertion

Catheter maintenance
Strongly recommended
  Provide-iodine ointment applied to hemodialysis catheter-insertion sites
  Specialized nursing teams caring for short-term peripheral venous catheters at institutions
    with a high incidence of infection
  Chlorhexidine-silver sulfadiazine-impregnated short-term central venous catheters
  Minocycline-rifampin-impregnated short-term central venous catheters
  Antiseptic chamber-filled hub or hub-protective antiseptic sponge for central venous
    catheters with an expected duration of approximately 2 wk
  Povidone-iodine-saturated sponge enclosed in plastic casing fitted around the central
    venous catheter hubs
  Assess need for intravascular catheters on a daily basis; remove catheters as soon as
    possible after intended use
  Adequate nurse-to-patient ratio in ICUs
  Change needleless system, the device and endcap if present on a regular basis in accordance
    with manufacturers' guidelines and reduce contact with nonsterile water
  Continuing quality-improvement programs to improve compliance with catheter
    care guidelines
  Disinfect catheter hubs and sampling ports before accessing
  Low-dose heparin for patients with short-term central venous catheters
  Low-dose warfarin for patients with long-term central venous catheters
  Pulmonary artery catheters heparin-bonded with benzalkonium chloride.
  Povidone-iodine ointment applied to nontunneled, long-term central venous
    or midline catheter-insertion sites of immunocompromised patients with heavy
    Staphylococcus aureus carriage (i.e., patients with AIDS and cirrhosis)
  Specialized nursing teams caring for catheters used for Total parenteral nutrition (TPN)
Recommended
  Gauze dressings preferred if excessive oozing of blood from insertion site
Consider
  Antiseptic chamber-filled hub or hub-protective antiseptic sponge for central venous
    catheters in ICUs

(Continued)

Table 17 Recommendations for the Prevention of Intravascular Catheter-Related
Infections (*Continued*)

Not recommended
   Routine replacement of central venous catheters
   Mupirocin ointment applied to the insertion site
   Triple antibiotic ointments applied to the insertion sites
   Silver-impregnated, subcutaneous collagen cuffed central venous catheters
   Inline filters for prevention of catheter infection

Abbreviation: TPN, total parenteral nutrition.
Source: From Ref. 194.

of rifampin-resistant organisms. For staphylococci resistant to gentamicin, a fluoroquinolone may be effective (183).

   Linezolid appears to have superior outcomes to vancomycin for many types of
MRSA infections (184). Several studies indicate that this is the case for MRSA IE
(185,186). In seriously ill patients, strong consideration should be given to substituting linezolid for vancomycin. Some studies indicate that there is an advantage to
combining linezolid with gentamicin or imipenem. However in average doses linezolid is a bacteriostatic drug with case reports of failure to cure MRSA IE (187).
Because of its bactericidal properties, daptomycin is quite promising for the treatment of MRSA IE (188). More experience must be gained with this antibiotic and
special attention paid to the myositis associated with its use. Tables 13 and 14 summarize the antibiotic treatment of MSSA, MRSA, and CONS infections of both
native and prosthetic valves. Table 15 presents therapeutic options for treating
highly resistant gram-positive organisms.

   Table 16 summarizes the antibiotic approach to other types of IE that may be
encountered in the CrCU.

Fungal Endocarditis

Combined medical and surgical therapy is necessary for cure of most cases of fungal
IE. Amphotericin B has been the mainstay of medical therapy (189). However the
newer antifungals, caspofungin and voriconazole, hold promise as less toxic and
more effective alternatives to the older compound (190,191). Figure 1 presents the
approach to the patient at risk for candidal endocarditis.

Prophylaxis of IE in the CrCU

Prophylaxis of CrCU IE should be focused on limiting the rate of line related bacteremia in addition to the more traditional methods (193). Table 17 summarizes the
CDC's recommendations to prevent this type of infection (194).

REFERENCES

1. Bouza E, Menasalvas A, Munoz P, et al. Infective endocarditis–A prospective study at
   the end of the twentieth century. Medicine 2001; 80:298–307.
2. Mansur A, Grinberg M, Da Luz P, et al. The complications of infective endocarditis:
   a reappraisal in the 1980s. Arch Intern Med 1992; 152:2428–2432.
3. Starkebaum M, Durack D, Beeson P. The "incubation period" of subacute bacterial
   endocarditis. Yale J Biol Med 1977; 50:49–60.

4. Cunha BA, Gill V, lazar IM. Acute infective endocarditis. Diagnostic and therapeutic approach. Infect Dis Emerg 1996; 10:811–834.

5. Von Reyn CF, Levy BS, Arbeit RD, et al. Infective endocarditis: an analysis based on strict case definitions. Ann Intern Med 1981; 94(Part 1):505–518.

6. Durack DT, Lukes BS, Bright DK. Duke Endocarditis Service. New criteria for diagnosis of infective endocarditis: utilization of specific echocardiographic findings. Am J Med 1994; 96:200–209.

7. Berlin JA, Abrutyn E, Strom BL, et al. Incidence of infective endocarditis in the Delaware Valley, 1988–1990. Am J Cardiol 1995; 76(9):33–36.

8. King H, Harkness JL. Infective endocarditis in the 1980s. Part 1. Aetiology and diagnosis. Med J Aust 1984; 144:536–540.

9. Friedland G, Von Reyn CF, Levy BS, et al. Nosocomial endocarditis. Infect Control 1984; 5:284–288.

10. Terpenning MS, Buggy BP, Kauffman CA. Infective endocarditis: Clinical features in young and elderly patients. Am J Med 1987; 83:626–634.

11. Gladstone JL, Rocco R. Host factor and infectious diseases in the elderly. Med Clinic North Am 1976; 60:1225–1246.

12. Gaynes R. Health care-associated bloodstream infections: a change in thinking. Editorial. Ann Intern Med 2003; 137:850–851.

13. Cabell CH, Jollis JG, Peterson GE, et al. Changing patient characteristics and the effect on mortality in endocarditis. Arch Intern Med 2002; 162:90–95.

14. Kaye D. Changing patterns of infective endocarditis. Am J Med 1985; 78(suppl 6b): 157–162.

15. Delahaye JP, Loire R, Milton H, et al. Infective endocarditis on stenotic aortic valves. Eur Heart J 1988; 9(suppl E):S43–S49.

16. Chagnac A, Rudinki C, Loebel H, et al. Infectious endocarditis in idiopathic hypertrophic subaortic stenosis: report of three cases and review of the literature. Chest 1982; 81:346–361.

17. Hickey AJ, McMahon SW, Wilcken D. Arch without prolapse and bacterial endocarditis: when is antibiotic prophylaxis necessary? Am Heart J 1985; 109:431–435.

18. McKinsey DS, Ratts TE, Bisno Al. Underlying cardiac lesions in adults with infective endocarditis. The changing spectrum. Am J Med 1987; 82:681–688.

19. Starke J. Infections of the heart: infective endocarditis in children. In: Feigin R, Cherry J, eds. Pediatric Infectious Disease. 3rd ed. Philadelphia: WB Saunders, 1992:326–346.

20. Zuppiroli A, Rinaldi M, Kramer-Fox R, et al. Natural history of mitral valve prolapse. Am J Med 1995; 75:1028–1032.

21. Sandre RM, Shafran SD. Infective endocarditis: review of 135 cases over 9 years. Clin Infect Dis 1996; 22:276–286.

22. Selzer A. Changing aspects of the natural history of valvular aortic stenosis. N Engl J Med 1987; 217:91–98.

23. Bansal RC. Infective endocarditis. Medicine 1995; 79:1205–1246.

24. Nager F. Changing clinical spectrum of infective endocarditis. In: Horstkotte D, Bodnar E, eds. Infective Endocarditis. London: ICR Publishers, 1991:25–29.

25. Rutledge RR, Leim BJ, Applebaumb RE. Actuarial analysis of the risk of prosthetic valve endocarditis in 1598 patients with mechanical and bioprosthetic valves. Arch Surg 1985; 120:469–472.

26. Calderwood SB, Swinski LA, Waternaux CM, et al. Risk factors for the development of prosthetic valve endocarditis. Circulation 1985; 72:31–37.

27. Eggimann P, Waldvogel FA. Pacemaker and defibrillator infections. In: Waldvogel FA, Bisno AL, eds. Infections Associated with Indwelling Medical Devices. Washington, D.C.: American Society for Microbiology Press, 2000:247–264.

28. Duval X, Selton-Suty C, Alla F, et al. Endocarditis in patients with a permanent pacemakers: a 1-year epidemiological survey of infective endocarditis due to valvular and/or pacemaker infection. Clin Infect Dis 2004; 39:68.

29. Steckelberg JM, Melton LJ III, Ilstrup DM, et al. Influence of referral bias on the apparent clinical spectrum of infective endocarditis. Am J Med 1990; 88:582–588.
30. Spijerkerman IJ, van Ameidjen EJ, Mientjes GH, et al. Human immunodeficiency virus infection and other risk factors for skin apices and endocarditis among injection drug users. J Clin Epidemiol 1996; 49:1149–1154.
31. Torres-Torotsa M, Rivera A, deAlarcon A, et al. Decrease in the annual frequency of infectious endocarditis among intravenous drug users in southern Spain. Enferm Infecc Microbiol 2000; 18:293–294.
32. Simberkoff MS. Narcotic-associated infective endocarditis. In: Kaplan EL, Taranta AV, eds. Infectious Endocarditis. Dallas: American Heart Association, 1977:46–58.
33. Levine DP. Infectious endocarditis in intravenous drug abusers. In: Levine DP, Sobel JD, eds. Infections in Intravenous Drug Abusers. New York: Oxford University Press, 1991:251–285.
34. Baddour LM. Twelve year review of recurrent native infective endocarditis: disease of the modern antibiotic era. Rev Infect Dis 1988; 10:1163–1170.
35. Hubbell G, Cheitlin MD, Rappaport E. Presentation, management and follow-up evaluation of infective endocarditis in drug addicts. Am Heart J 1981; 102:85–94.
36. Gouello JP, Asfar P, Brenet O, et al. Nosocomial endocarditis in the intensive care unit: an analysis of 22 cases. Crit Care Med 2000; 28:377–382.
37. Fernandez-Guerrero ML, Verdejo C, Azofra J, et al. Hospital-acquired infectious endocarditis not associated with cardiac surgery: an emerging problem. Clin Infect Dis 1995; 20:16–23.
38. Fowler VG Jr., Sanders LL, Kong LK. Infective endocarditis due to *Staphylococcus aureus*: 59 prospectively identify cases with follow-up. Clin Infect Dis 1999; 28:106–114.
39. Safar N, Kluger D, Maki D. A review of risk factors for catheter related bloodstream infection caused by percutaneously inserted noncuffed central venous catheters. Medicine 2002; 81:466–474.
40. Terpenning MS. Infective endocarditis. Geriatr Med 1992; 8:903–912.
41. Wilcox PA, Rayner BL, Whitelaw DA. Community-acquired *Staphylococcus aureus* bacteremia in patients who do not abuse intravenous drugs. Q J Med 1990; 91:41–47.
42. Garvey GJ, Neu HC. Infective endocarditis-an evolving disease. Medicine (Baltimore) 1978; 57:105–127.
43. Weinstein L, Schlesinger JJ. Pathanatomic, pathophysiologic and clinical correlations in endocarditis. N Engl J Med 1974; 29:832–837, 1122–1126.
44. Weinstein L, Brusch JL. Prophylaxis. In: Weinstein L, Brusch JL, eds. Infective Endocarditis. New York: Oxford University Press, 1995:322–337.
45. Watanakunakorn C, Burkert T. Infective endocarditis in a large community teaching hospital, 1980–1990. A review of 210 episodes. Medicine 1993; 72:90–102.
46. Weinstein L, Brusch JL. Microbiology of infective endocarditis and clinical correlates: gram-positive organisms. In: Weinstein L, Brusch JL, eds. Infective Endocarditis. New York: Oxford University Press, 1995:35–72.
47. Baddour LM, Bisno AL. Infective endocarditis complicating mitral valve prolapse: epidemiologic, clinical and microbiologic aspects. Rev Infect Dis 1986; 8:117–137.
48. Weinstein L, Brusch JL. Clinical manifestations of native valve endocarditis. In: Weinstein L, Brusch JL, eds. Infective Endocarditis. New York: Oxford University Press, 1996:165–193.
49. Gallagher P, Natanakunakora C. Group B streptococcal endocarditis: report of seven cases and review of the literature 1962–1985. Rev Infect Dis 1986; 8:175.
50. Petti CA, Fowler VG. *Staphylococcus aureus* bacteremia and endocarditis. In: Durack DT, ed. Infective Endocarditis. Philadelphia: WB Saunders, 2002:413–435.
51. Chambers HF. The changing epidemiology of *Staphylococcus aureus*. Emerg Infect Dis 2001; 7:178–182.
52. Rupp ME, Archer GL. Coagulase-negative Staphylococcus: pathogens associated with medical progress. Clin Infect Dis 1994; 19:231–245.

53. Baddour LM, Phillips TN, Bisno AL. Coagulase-negative staphylococcal endocarditis: occurrence in patients with mitral valve prolapse. Arch Intern Med 1986; 146:119–121.
54. Cohen PS, Maguire JH, Weinstein L. Infective endocarditis caused by gram-negative bacteria: a review of the literature, 1945–1977. Prog Cardiovasc Dis 1980; 22:205–242.
55. Snyder N, Atterbury CE, Correia JP, et al. Increased concurrence of cirrhosis and bacterial endocarditis. Gastroenterology 1977; 33:1107–1112.
56. Ellner JJ, Rosenthal MS, Lerner PI, et al. Infective endocarditis and slow-growing fastidious gram negative bacteria. Medicine 1979; 58:145–158.
57. Baddour G, Mayer J, Henry B. Polymicrobial endocarditis in the 1980s. Rev Infect Dis 1991; 13:963–970.
58. Martin GS, Maninno DM, Eaton S, et al. The epidemiology of sepsis in the United States from 1979 through 2000. N Engl J Med 2003; 348:1546–1554.
59. Leaf H, Simberkoff MS. Fungal endocarditis. In: Horstkotte D, Bodnar E, eds. Infective Endocarditis. London: ICR Publishers, 1991:118–134.
60. McLeod R, Remington JS. Fungal endocarditis. In: Rahimtoola SH, ed. Infective Endocarditis. New York: Grune and Stratton, 1978:211–290.
61. Drexler L, Rytel M, Keelan M, et al. *Aspergillus terreus* infective endocarditis on a porcine heterograft valve. Thorac Cardiovasc Surg 1980; 79:269–274.
62. Mayer AR, Brown A, Weintraub RA, et al. Successful medical therapy for endocarditis due to *Candida parapsilosis*: a clinical and epidemiologic study. Chest 1978:546–549.
63. Pesanti EL, Smith IM. Infective endocarditis with negative blood cultures: an analysis of 52 cases. Am J Med 1979; 66:43–46.
64. Weinstein L, Brusch JL. Pathoanatomical, pathophysiological and clinical correlations. In: Weinstein L, Brusch JL, eds. Infective Endocarditis. New York: Oxford University Press, 1996:138–164.
65. Moreillon P, Overholser CD, Malinverni R, et al. Predictors of endocarditis in isolates from cultures of blood following dental extractions in rats with periodontal disease. J Infect Dis 1980; 157:990–995.
66. Scheld WM, Valone JA, Sande MA. Bacterial adherence in the pathogenesis of endocarditis. J Clin Invest 1978; 61:1394–1404.
67. Yeaman MR. The role of platelets in antimicrobial host defense. Clin Infect Dis 1997; 25:951–958.
68. Aly R, Shinefield H. Role of teichoic acid in the binding of *Staphylococcus aureus* to normal epithelial cells. J Infect Dis 1980; 157:141–144.
69. Tompkins DC, Blackwell LJ, Hatcher VB, et al. *Staphylococcus aureus* proteins that bind to human endothelial cells. Infect Immun 1992; 60:965–969.
70. Hammill RJ. Role of fibronectin in infective endocarditis. Rev Infect Dis 1987; 9(suppl 4): S360–S371.
71. Drake T. *Staphylococcus aureus* induced tissue factor expression in cultured valve endothelium. J Infect Dis 1980; a57:749–753.
72. Sheagren J. *Staphylococcus aureus*, the persistent pathogen. N Engl J Med 1984; 310: 1368–1574.
73. Christensen GD, Bisno AL, Parisi B, et al. Nosocomial septicemia due to multiply antibiotic-resistant *Staphylococcus epidermidis*. Ann Intern Med 1982; 96:1–10.
74. Cristina AB. Biomaterial-centered infection: microbial adhesions versus tissue integration. Science 1987; 37:1588–1595.
75. Gotz F, Georg P. Colonization of medical devices by coagulase-negative staphylococci. In: Waldvogel FA, Bisno AL, eds. Infections Associated with Indwelling Medical Devices. Washington, D.C.: ASM Press, 2000:55–88.
76. Drake TA, Rodgers GM, Sande MH. Tissue factor is a major stimulus of vegetation formation in enterococcal endocarditis in rabbits. J Clin Invest 1984; 70:1750–1753.
77. Stein DS, Nelson KE. Endocarditis due to nutritionally deficient streptococci: therapeutic dilemma 1987; 9:908–916.

78. Doring J, Maier M, Mueller E. Virulence factors of *Pseudomonas aeruginosa*. Antimicrob Agents Chemother 1987; 39:136–148.

79. Young F. Human immunity in *Pseudomonas aeruginosa*: in-vitro interaction of bacteria, polymorphonuclear leukocytes and serum factors. J Infect Dis 1972; 26:257–263.

80. Burrig KL, Schute Terhau, Sen J, et al. Special role of the endocardium in the pathogenesis of endocarditis. In: Horskotte D, Bodnar E, eds. Infective Endocarditis. London: ICR Publishers, 1991:3–9.

81. Garrison PK, Freedman LR. Experimental endocarditis. I. Staphylococcal endocarditis in rabbits resulting from placement of a polyethylene catheter in right side of the heart. J Biol Med 1978; 22:394–410.

82. Freedman LR, Valone J Jr. Experimental infective endocarditis. Prog Cardiovasc Dis 1979; 22:169–180.

83. Durack DT, Beeson PM, Petersdorf RG. Experimental bacterial endocarditis. III. Production and progress of the disease in rabbits. Br J Exp Pathol 1972; 50:50–53.

84. Rowley KM, Cluff KS, Smith GJW. Right-sided infective endocarditis as a consequence of a flow directed pulmonary artery catheterization. N Engl J Med 1984; 311: 1152–1156.

85. Greene JF, Fitzwater JE, Clemmer TP. Septic endocarditis and indwelling pulmonary artery catheters. JAMA 1975; 33:891–897.

86. Rodbard S. Blood velocity and endocarditis. Circulation 1963; 27:18–28.

87. Everett ED, Hirschmann JV. Transient bacteremia and endocarditis prophylaxis. A review. Medicine (Baltimore) 1977; 56:61–77.

88. Loesche WJ. Indigenous human flora and bacteremia. In: Kaplan EL, Taranta AV, eds. Infective Endocarditis. Dallas: American Heart Association, 1977:40–45.

89. Baskin RW, Rosenthal A, Bruitt BA. Acute bacterial endocarditis, a silent source of sepsis in the burn patient. Ann Surg 1976; 184:618–625.

90. Raad H, Bodey GP. Infectious complications of indwelling vascular catheters. Clin Infect Dis 1992; 15:197–210.

91. Durack DT. Prevention of infective endocarditis. N Engl J Med 1995; 332:38–44.

92. Sheretz RJ. Pathogenesis of vascular catheter infection. In: Infections Associated with Indwelling Medical Devices. Washington, D.C.: ASM Press, 2000:111–125.

93. Sitges-Serra A, Linares J, Garau J. Catheter sepsis: the clue is the hub. Surgery 1985; 97:355–357.

94. Sheth NK, Franson TR, Rose HD. Colonization of bacteria on polyvinylchloride Teflon intravascular catheter in hospitalized patients. J Clin Microbiol 1983; 18:1061–1063.

95. Raad I, Costerton JW, Sabharwar U, et al. Central venous catheters (CVC) studied by quantitative cultures and scanning electron microscopy (SEM): the importance of luminal colonization. Program and Abstracts of the 31st Interscience Conference on Antimicrobial Agents and Chemotherapy. Abstract 450 1991. Washington, D.C.: American Society of Microbiology, 1991.

96. Jarvis WR. Nosocomial outbreaks: The Center for Disease Control's hospital infections program experience. 1980–1991. Am J Med 1991; 91(suppl B):101S–106S.

97. Finland M, Barnes MW. Changing etiology of bacterial endocarditis in the antibacterial era: experiences in The Boston City Hospital 1933–1955. Ann Intern Med 1970; 72: 341–348.

98. Snydman DR, Reidy MD, Perry LK, et al. Safety of changing intravenous (IV) administration sets containing burettes at longer than 48 hour intervals. Infect Control 1987; 8:113–116.

99. Maki DG, Rhame FS, Mackel DC, et al. Nationwide epidemic of septicemia caused by contaminated intravenous products. Am J Med 1976; 60:471–485.

100. Johnson JD, Raff MJ, Barnwell PA. Splenic abscess complicating infectious endocarditis. Arch Int Med 1983; 143:906–912.

101. Wilson WR, Lie JT, Houser OW, et al. The management of patients with mycotic aneurysm. Curr Clin Topics Infect Dis 1981; 2:151–181.

102. Lerner PI, Weinstein L. Infective endocarditis in the antibiotic era. N Engl J Med 1966; 274:199–206, 259–266, 323–331, 388–393.

103. Weinstein L. Life-threatening complications of infective endocarditis and their management. Arch Int Med 1988; 146:953–957.

104. Roberts WC, Buchbinder NA. Healed left-sided infective endocarditis: a clinicopathological study of 59 patients. Am J Cardiol 1976; 40:876–883.

105. Ghosh PK, Miller HJ, Vidne BA. Mitral obstruction in bacterial endocarditis. Br Heart J 1985; 53:340–344.

106. Crawford HH, Badke FR, Amon KW. Effectively undisturbed pericardium on left ventricular size and performance during acute volume loading. Am Heart J 1983; 105: 267–270.

107. Fang G, Keys T, Gentry L. Prosthetic valve endocarditis resulting from nosocomial bacteremia. Ann Intern Med 1993; 119:560–567.

108. Horskotte D. Prosthetic valve endocarditis. In: Horskotte D, Bodnar E, eds. Infective Endocarditis. London: ICR Publishers, 1991:233–261.

109. Arber, Pras E, Coopperman Y, et al. Pacemaker endocarditis. Report of 44 cases and review of the literature. Medicine (Baltimore) 1994; 73:299–315.

110. Cherubin CE, Sapira JD. The medical complications of drug addiction and medical assessment of intravenous drug users: 25 years later. Ann Intern Med 1993; 119: 1017–1028.

111. Werner BS, Schulz R, Fuchs JB, et al. Infective endocarditis in the elderly in the era of transesophageal echocardiography: clinical features and prognosis compared with younger patients. Am J Med 1976; 100:90–97.

112. Weinstein L, Rubin R. Infective endocarditis-1973. Prog Cardiovasc Dis 1973; 16:239–274.

113. Libman E, Friedberg CK. Subacute Bacterial Endocarditis. Oxford: Oxford University Press, 1948.

114. Weinstein L. Infective endocarditis: past, present and future. J R Coll Phys Lond 1972; 6:161–163.

115. Churchill M, Geraci J, Hunder G. Musculoskeletal manifestations of bacterial endocarditis. Ann Intern Med 1977; 87:755–762.

116. Weinstein MP, Towns ML, Quartey SM, et al. The clinical significance of positive blood cultures in the 1990s: a prospective comprehensive evaluation of the microbiology, epidemiology, and outcome of bacteremia and fungemia in adults. Clin Infect Dis 1997; 24:584–602.

117. Weinstein L. Infective endocarditis. In: Braunwald E, ed. Heart Disease: A Textbook of Cardiovascular Medicine. 3rd ed. Philadelphia: WB Saunders, 1988:113.

118. Bates D, Lee TH. Rapid classification of positive blood cultures; prospective validation of a multivariate algorithm. JAMA 1992; 267:1962–1966.

119. Weinstein MP. Current blood culture methods in systems: clinical concepts, technology and interpretation of results. Clin Infect Disease 1996; 23:40–46.

120. Miller M, Casey J. Infective endocarditis: new diagnostic techniques. Am Heart J 1978; 96:123–130.

121. Safar N, Fine JP, Maki D. Meta-analysis: evidence for diagnosing intravascular device-related bloodstream infection. Ann Intern Med 2005; 142:451–466.

122. Murray PR, Traynor P, Hopson D. Critical assessment of blood culture techniques: analysis of recovery of complicated facultative anaerobes, strict anaerobic bacteria and fungi in aerobic and anaerobic blood culture bottles. J Clin Microbiol 1992; 30:1462–1468.

123. Von Scoy RE. Culture-negative endocarditis. Mayo Clin Proc 1982; 57:149–154.

124. Keefer CS. Subacute bacterial endocarditis: active cases without bacteremia. Ann Intern Med 1937; 11:714–734.

125. Barbari EF, Cockerill FR, Steckelburg JM. Infective endocarditis due to unusual or fastidious microorganisms. Mayo Clin Proc 1997; 72(6):532–542.

126. Vansdoy RE. Culture negative endocarditis. Mayo Clin Proc 1982; 57:149–156.

127. Lichtlen P. General principles of conservative treatment of infective endocarditis. In: Horstkotte D, Bodnar E, eds. Infective Endocarditis. London: ICR Publishers, 1991: 85–92.

128. Bates D, Goldmann L, Lee TH. Contaminant blood cultures and resource utilization. JAMA 1991; 265:365–369.

129. Hoen B, Selton-Suty C, Lacassin F, et al. Infective endocarditis in patients with negative blood culture: analysis of 8 cases in a one year nationwide survey in France. Clin Infect Dis 1995; 20:501–506.

130. Arnette N, Roberts SI. Valve ring abscesses in active infective endocarditis. Circulation 1976; 54:140–145.

131. Oates E, Sarno RC. Detection of bacterial endocarditis with indium-III labeled leukocytes. Clin Nucl Med 1988; 13:691–693.

132. Lindner JR, Case RA, Dent JM, et al. Diagnostic value of echocardiography in suspected endocarditis. An evaluation based upon the pretest probability of disease. Circulation 1996; 93:730–740.

133. Lowry RW, Zogbhi WA, Baker WB, et al. Clinical impact of transesophageal echocardiography in the diagnosis and management of infective endocarditis. Am J Cardiol 1994; 73:1089–1091.

134. Chirillo F, Bruni A, Giujusa T, et al. Echocardiography in infective endocarditis: reassessment of the diagnostic criteria of vegetation as evaluated from the precordial and transesophageal approach. Am J Card Imaging 1995; 9:174–179.

135. Roe MT, Abramson MA, Li J, et al. Clinical information determines the impact of transesophageal echocardiography on the diagnosis of infective endocarditis by the Duke criteria. Am Heart J 2000; 139:945–953.

136. Cheitlin MD, Armstrong WF, Aurigemma GP, et al. ACC/AHA/ASE 2003 guideline update for the clinical application of echocardiography: summary article. A report of the American College of Cardiology/American Heart Association task force on practice guidelines. Circulation 2003; 108:1146–1153.

137. Ascher DP, Shoupe BA, Maybee D, et al. Persistent catheter-related bacteremia: clearance with antibiotics and urokinase. J Pediatr Surg 1993; 28:628–635.

138. Durack DT, Beeson PB. Experimental bacterial endocarditis. Part II. Survival of bacteria in the endocarditis vegetation. Br J Exp Pathol 1972; 53:50–53.

139. Sanfillipo AJ, Picard MH, Newell JB, et al. Echocardiographic assessment of patients with infectious endocarditis: prediction of risk for complications. J Am Coll Cardiol 1991; 18:1191–1199.

140. Rohmann S, Erbel R, Gorge T, et al. Clinical relevance of vegetation localization by transesophageal echocardiography in infective endocarditis. Eur Heart J 1992; 12:446–452.

141. Omari B, Shapiro S, Gintzon L, et al. Predictive risk factors for perivalvular extension of native valve endocarditis. Clinical and echocardiographic analyses. Chest 1989; 96(6): 1273–1279.

142. Jeang M, Fuenfes F, Gately A, et al. Aortic root abscess: initial experience using magnetic resonance imaging. Chest 1986; 89(4):613–615.

143. Goldenberger D, Kunzli A, Vogt P, et al. Molecular diagnosis of bacterial endocarditis by broad-range PCR amplification and direct sequencing. J Clin Microbiol 1997; 35:2733–2739.

144. Li JS, Sexton DJ, Mick N, et al. Proposed modifications to the Duke criteria for diagnosis of infective endocarditis. Clinic Infect Dis 2000; 30:633–644.

145. Rosenblum G, Carsons S. Mimics of endocarditis. In: Cunha B, ed. Infectious Diseases in Critical Care Medicine. New York: Marcel Dekker, 1998:435–434.

146. Maksimowicz-McKinnon K, Mandell BF. Understanding valvular heart disease in patients with systemic autoimmune diseases. Cleveland Clinic J Med 2004; 11:881–885.

147. Brusch JL. Cardiac infections in the immunosuppressed patient. In: Cunha B, ed. Infections in the Compromised Host Infectious Disease Clinics of North America. Philadelphia: WB Saunders Co, 2001:613–638.

148. Fisher J. Cardiac myxoma. Cardiovasc Rev Rep 1983; 9:1195–2001.

149. Bauernschmitt R, Jakob HG, Vahl C-F, et al. Operation for infective endocarditis: results after implementation of mechanical valves. Ann Thorac Surg 1998; 65:359–364.

150. Truninger K, Attenhofer Jost CH, Seifert B, et al. Long-term follow-up of prosthetic valve endocarditis: What characteristics identify patients who were treated successfully with antibiotics alone? Heart 1999; 82:714–720.

151. Bayer AS, Bolger AF, Taubert KA, et al. Diagnosis and management of infective endocarditis and its complications. Circulation 1998; 25:2936–2948.

152. Olaison L, Hogevik H, Myken P, et al. Early surgery in infective endocarditis. Q J Med 1996; 89:267–278.

153. Magilligan D. Cardiac surgery in infective endocarditis. In: Horstkotte D, Bodnar E, eds. Infective Endocarditis. London: ICR Publishers, 1991:210.

154. Wilkoff BL, Byrd CL, Love CJ, et al. Pacemaker lead extraction with the laser sheath: results of the patient lead extraction with the excimer sheath (Plexes) trial. J Am Coll Cardiol 1999; 33:1671–1685.

155. Lee BK, Crossley K, Gerding DN. The association between *Staphylococcus aureus* bacteremia and bacteruria. Am J Med 1978; 65:303–310.

156. Torlakovic E, Hibbs JR, Miller JS, et al. Intracellular bacteria in blood smears in patients with central venous catheters. Arch Int Med 1995; 155:1547–1553.

157. Fowler V, Li J, Core GR, et al. Role of echocardiography in evaluation of patients with *Staphylococcus aureus* bacteremia in 107 patients. J Am Coll 1997; 30:107–218.

158. Chang FY. A prospective multicenter study of *Staphylococcus aureus* bacteremia: incidence of endocarditis, risk factors for mortality and clinical impact of methicillin-resistant. Medicine (Baltimore) 2003; 82:322–332.

159. Press OW, Ramsey PV, Larson EB, et al. Hickman catheter infections in patients with malignancies medicine 1984; 63:189–200.

160. Joly V, Pangon B, Vallois JM, et al. Value of antibiotic levels in serum and cardiac vegetations for predicting antibacterial effect of ceftriaxone in experimental *E. coli* endocarditis. Antimicrob Agents Chemother 1987; 31:1632–1635.

161. Gengo F, Schentag J. Rate of methicillin penetration into normal heart valves and experimental endocarditis lesions. Antimicrob Agents Chemother 1982; 21:456–459.

162. Fraimow HJ, Abrutyn E. Pathogens resistant to antimicrobial agents: epidemiology, molecular mechanisms and clinical management. Infect Dis Clin North Am 1995:497–530.

163. Douglas A, Moore-Gillon J, Eykyn J. Fever during treatment of infective endocarditis. Lancet 1986; 1:1341–1343.

164. Blumberg E, Robbins SN, Adimora A, et al. Persistent fever in association with infective endocarditis. Clin Infect Dis 1992; 15:980–996.

165. Sexton DJ, Spelman D. Current best practices and guidelines: assessment and management of complications in infective endocarditis. In: Durack DT, ed. Infectious Disease Clinics of North America. Philadelphia: WB Saunders Company, 2002:16507–16521.

166. Wilson W, Giuliani E, Danielson G, et al. Management of complications of infective endocarditis. Mayo Clin Proc 1982; 57:162–169.

167. Weinstein L, Brusch JL. In: Weinstein L, Brusch JL, eds. Medical Management. New York: Oxford University Press, 1996:256–304.

168. Welton DE, Young JB, Gentry WO, et al. Recurrent infective endocarditis: analysis of predisposing factors and clinical features. Am J Med 1979; 66:932–939.

169. Francioli P, Ruch W, Stamboulian D. Treatment of streptococcal endocarditis with a single daily dose of ceftriaxone and netilmicin for 14 days: a prospective multicenter study. Clin Infect Dis 1995; 21:1406–1410.

170. Doern GV, Ferraro MJ, Bruggermann AB, et al. Emergence of high rates of antimicrobial resistance among viridans streptococci in the United States. Antimicrob Agents Chemother 1995; 39:2243–2247.

171. Pulliam L, Inokuchi S, Hadley WK, et al. Penicillin tolerance in experimental streptococcal endocarditis. Lancet 1979; 2:957–961.

172. Eliopoulos GM. Antibiotic resistance in enterococcus species: an update. In: Remington J, Schwarz M, eds. Current Clinical Topics in Infectious Diseases. Cambridge, MA: Blackwell Scientific, 1996:21–51.

173. Eliopoulos GM. Aminoglycoside resistant enterococcal endocarditis. Med Clin North Am 1993; 17:117–172.

174. Fantin B, Carbon C. Importance of the aminoglycoside dosing regimen in the penicillin-netilmicin combination for treatment of *Enterococcus faecalis*-induced experimental endocarditis. Antimicrob Agents Chemother 1990; 34:2387–2391.

175. Wilson WR, Karchmer AW, Dsajani AS, et al. Antibiotic treatment of adults with infective endocarditis due to streptococci, enterococci, staphylococci and HACEK microorganisms. JAMA 1995; 274:1705–1714.

176. Thompson RL, Lavin B, Talbot GH. Endocarditis due to vancomycin-resistant *Enterococcus faecium* in an immunocompromised patients: cure by administering combination therapy with Quinpristin/dalfopristin and high dose ampicillin. South Med J 2003; 96:818–820.

177. Eliopoulos GM, Thavin-Eliopoulos C, Moellering RC Jr. Contribution of animal models in the search for effective therapy for endocarditis due to enterococci with high-level resistance to gentamicin. Clin Infect Dis 1992; 15:58–62.

178. Karchmer AW. *Staphylococcus aureus* and vancomycin: the sequel. Ann Intern Med 1991; 115:739–741.

179. Nannini EC, et al. Relapse of type A beta-lactamase-producing *Staphylococcus aureus* native valve endocarditis cefazolin therapy: revisiting the issue. Clin Infect Dis 2003; 37:1194–1198.

180. Korzeniowski O, Sande MH. The national collaborative endocarditis study group combination antimicrobial therapy for *Staphylococcus aureus* endocarditis in patients addicted to parenteral drugs and in non-addicts: a prospective study. Ann Intern Med 1982; 92:619–624.

181. Chambers HF. Short-course combination and oral therapies of *Staphylococcus aureus* endocarditis. Med Clin North Am 1993; 7:69–80.

182. Karchmer AW. Infections of prosthetic heart valves. In: Waldvogel F, Bisno Al, eds. Infections Associated with Indwelling Medical Devices. Washington, D.C.: American Society for Microbiology, 2000:145–172.

183. Chuard C, Herrmann M, Roehner P, et al. Treatment of experimental foreign body infections caused by methicillin-resistant *Staphylococcus aureus*. Antimicrob Agents Chemother 1990; 34:2312–2317.

184. Stevens DL, Herr D, Lampiris H, et al. Linezolid versus vancomycin for the treatment of methicillin-resistant *Staphylococcus aureus* infections. Clin Infect Dis 2002; 34:1481–1490.

185. Howden BP, Ward PB, Charles PG, et al. Treatment outcomes for serious infections caused by methicillin-resistant *Staphylococcus aureus* with reduced vancomycin susceptibility. Clin Infect Dis 2004; 38:521–528.

186. Jacquiline C, Batard E, Perez L, et al. In vivo efficacy of continuous infusion versus intermittent dosing of linezolid compared to vancomycin in a methicillin-resistant *Staphylococcus aureus* rabbit endocarditis model. Antimicrob Agents Chemother 2002; 46:3706–3711.

187. Sperber SJ, Levine JF, Gross PA. Persistent MRSA bacteremia in a patient with low Linezolid levels. Clin Infect Dis 2003; 36:675–676.

188. Sakoulas G, Eliopoulos GM, Alder J, et al. Efficacy of daptomycin in experimental endocarditis due to methicillin-resistant *Staphylococcus aureus*. Antimicrob Agents Chemother 2003; 47:1714–1718.

189. Ellis ME, Al Abdely H, Sandridge A, et al. Fungal endocarditis: evidence in the world literature 1965–1995. Clin Infect Dis 2001; 32:50–62.

190. Walsh T, Pappas P, Winston DJ, et al. Voriconazole versus liposomal amphotericin B for empirical antifungal therapy. N Engl J Med 2002; 366:1745–1747.

191. Mora-Duarte J, Betts R, Rotstein C, et al. Comparison of caspofungin amphotericin B for invasive candidiasis. N Engl J Med 2002; 347:2020–2029.
192. Anaisse EJ, Bishara AB, Solomkin JS. Fungal infection. In: Souba WW, Fink MP, Jurkovich GJ, et al eds. New York: Web Professional Publishing 2005:1486–1487.
193. Dajani AS, Taubert KA, Wilson W, et al. Prevention of bacterial endocarditis: recommendations by the American Heart Association. Circulation 1997; 96:358–366.
194. Centers for Disease Control and Prevention. Guidelines for the prevention of intravascular catheter-related infections. Morb Mortal Wkly Report 2002; 51:1–29.

12

Acute Myocarditis and Acute Pericarditis in the Critical Care Unit

Jason M. Lazar
Department of Cardiology, State University of New York Downstate Medical Center, Brooklyn, New York, U.S.A.

Diane H. Johnson and Burke A. Cunha
Infectious Disease Division, Winthrop-University Hospital, Mineola, and State University of New York School of Medicine, Stony Brook, New York, U.S.A.

ACUTE MYOCARDITIS

Introduction

Acute myocarditis is a common sequelae of systemic infection by many organisms. It is estimated to occur in 5% to 15% of common infections. Acute myocarditis develops from direct infection or after infection with the heart as a target of immune injury (1). Most cases are subclinical, but acute myocarditis can progress to congestive heart failure and death. It may also preset with ventricular arrhythmias or resemble acute myocardial infarction (MI). Myocarditis can become a chronic progressive disease and is estimated to account for 10% to 20% of cases of dilated cardiomyopathy (2). This chapter provides an overview of the clinical course of acute infectious myocarditis.

Infectious Causes

The clinical syndrome of myocarditis was first described in the mid-1800s in patients with mumps and epidemic pleurodynia. Myocarditis was encountered during the influenza A pandemic during the first part of the century. Although the causative agent of myocarditis is not always identified, most cases of infectious myocarditis in the United States and Europe are viral in origin (3–5).

The group B coxsackieviruses are responsible for most cases of documented human disease. Other enteroviruses, including the coxsackie A and echoviruses, are important causes of myocarditis as well (4). Historically, poliovirus was a cause of myocarditis; however, its incidence has markedly declined due to widespread vaccination efforts. These enteroviruses are RNA viruses that attach to receptors on the cardiac myocyte and cause cell destruction and the subsequent initiation of a host immune response. Other commonly encountered viruses that may result in myocarditis clinically include: varicella, cytomegalovirus (CMV), Epstein-Barr virus (EBV), rubeola, rubella, hepatitis B, and adenovirus (6). Arboviruses, such as dengue and the rabies virus, are also causes of myocarditis (5,7). Currently, HIV infection is often associated with cardiomyopathy.

Bacterial pathogens are responsible for some cases of myocarditis and reach the myocardium by direct hematogenous spread of microorganisms or from contiguous spread from an infected heart valve. *Gonococci, Meningococci, Brucella, Salmonella, Staphylococci*, and *Streptococci* have all been reported to cause bacterial myocarditis (5). Bacteria such as *Corynebacterium diphtheriae* and *Clostridium perfringens* elaborate toxins that can damage the myocardial tissue (8,9). Some organisms causing atypical pneumonias, such as *Mycoplasma pneumoniae, Legionella pneumophila, Chlamydia pneumoniae*, and *Chlamydia psittaci*, are unusual but are known causes of myocarditis.

Lyme disease, which is caused by the spirochete *Borrelia burgdorferi*, is known to cause myocarditis, which usually manifests as conduction disturbances. Infections with rickettsia commonly cause myocarditis as well, e.g., Rocky Mountain spotted fever and scrub typhus (10). In South America, myocarditis secondary to Chagas disease caused by *Trypanosoma cruzzi* is fairly common. The other trypanosome species, *T. gambiense* and *T. rhodesiense*, that cause African sleeping sickness can infect the heart as well. *Trichinella spiralis, Toxoplasma gondii*, and *Echinococcus* are causes of myocarditis in developing nations (11).

Disseminated fungal infections such as aspergillosis, cryptococcosis, and candidiasis have all been reported to result in myocarditis, with the majority occurring in immunocompromised individuals (12). The infectious causes of myocarditis and the associated clinical and laboratory features are listed in Table 1.

Clinical Presentation

The majority of cases of acute infectious myocarditis are presumed to be asymptomatic, leaving its incidence and course ill defined. Alternatively, acute myocarditis may result in congestive heart failure, chest pain mimicking acute MI, and/or arrhythmias. Because these conditions are more commonly associated with primary myocardial disease, the diagnosis of acute myocarditis poses a challenge.

Congestive Heart Failure

The overall incidence of myocarditis in acute heart failure is unknown. It has been reported to accompany between 4% and 80% of cases of acute and chronic cardiomyopathy collectively (13), but occurs more frequently in patients with symptoms of shorter duration. In patients presenting with signs and symptoms of congestive heart failure, active myocarditis should be considered when there is a young patient age, absence of cardiac history, and the onset of symptoms during or immediately following a systemic or viral illness. The illness may present with flu-like symptoms of respiratory or gastrointestinal nature including fever, chills, cough, coryza, myalgia, pharyngitis, anorexia, and diarrhea. Of note, cardiac involvement is more likely to occur in patients reporting myalgias during the prodromal illness (14).

The signs and symptoms of heart failure due to myocarditis are similar to other causes. Dyspnea, orthopnea, paroxysmal nocturnal dyspnea, and fatigue are manifestations of left ventricular (LV) dysfunction. Abdominal discomfort related to hepatomegaly and peripheral edema result from right ventricular failure. The duration of symptoms is brief (less than three months) in over two-thirds of patients with biopsy-proven myocarditis (13). In addition, substernal or precordial chest pain

(*Text continued on page 274*)

Table 1 Causes of Myocarditis and Pericarditis, Clinical Features, and Diagnostic Tests

Causes	Associated clinical features	Diagnostic tests
Myocarditis		
Viral Group B	Fever	Isolation of virus from throat or stool
Coxsackieviruses	Upper respiratory tract symptoms Chest pain (pleurodynia) Skin rash	↑ Titer IgM coxsackie B antibody or ≥4× rise in IgG antibody titer (CF) between acute and convalescent sera Isolation of virus or viral proteins from myocardial biopsy
Echoviruses	Fever Upper respiratory tract symptoms Loose stool or diarrhea Skin rash	↑ Titer IgG echovirus antibody or four fold rise in IgG antibody titer (CF) between acute and convalescent sera Isolation of influenza virus from nasopharynx, throat or sputum
Influenza A	Fever	Isolation of influenza virus from nasopharynx, throat, or sputum
Influenza B	Headache Myalgias Eye pain Nonproductive cough Sore throat	Four-fold rise in IgG antibody titer between acute and convalescent sera (EIA, IFA, CF, HIA) Isolation of virus or viral proteins from myocardium
Adenovirus	Rhinorrhea Pharyngitis Tracheitis Pneumonia Conjunctivitis Cervical adenitis	Culture of adenovirus from pharynx sputum, conjunctiva, urine Four-fold rise in IgG adenovirus antibody titer between acute and convalescent sera (EIA, IFA)
Measles (rubella)	Fever Cough Coryza Conjunctivitis Koplik spots Descending blotchy maculo-papular rash that becomes confluent	In early phase, multinucleated giant cells seen in stained nasal secretions, sputum Leukopenia Measles-specific IgM antibody (HIA, EIA, IFA, CF) or Four-fold rise in IgG titer between acute and convalescent sera
Rubella	Fever Mild conjunctivitis Posterior cervical/occipital adenopathy Arthralgia Pink, macular/papular rash beginning on face spreading downward Palatal petechias (Forscheimer spots)	Isolation of virus from nasopharynx Rubella specific IgM antibody (EIA or HAI or four fold rise in titer between rubella-specific IgG antibodies (EIA, HAI)

(Continued)

Table 1   Causes of Myocarditis and Pericarditis, Clinical Features, and Diagnostic Tests (*Continued*)

Causes	Associated clinical features	Diagnostic tests
Varicella	Prodromal flu-like symptoms Rash initially macular, becomes, vesicular, then pustular Rash erupts in crops	Tzanck prep of lesions-multinucleated giant cells Basophilia Demonstration of virus by IFA from material from a lesion Varicella specific IgG antibodies between acute and Convalescent sera (EIA, CF)
Mumps	Parotitis mostly bilateral, but can be unilateral (25%) Fever Epididymo-orchitis in men (-30%)	↑ Amylase Isolation of virus from blood, nasopharynx, secretions from Stensen's duct, cerebrospinal fluid (CSF), urine ↑ Mumps specific IgM, or four-fold rise in IgG, IFA mumps antibody between acute and convalescent sera
Polio	Fever Aseptic meningitis Muscle pain, cramps, twitching Asymmetric paralysis Sensation remains intact	Mild CSF pleocytosis (predominantly lymphs), slightly elevated protein Isolation of virus from throat, stool Four-fold rise in CF antibody, EIA, or IFA titer or polio antibody
Epstein-Barr virus	Fever Fatigue Periorbital edema Pharyngitis (may be exudative) Posterior cervical or generalized lymphadenopathy Splenomegaly	Mildly ↑ LFTs Lymphocytosis with atypical lymphocytes Positive heterophile antibody monospot test Positive IgM viral capsid antigen high titers present serum 1–6 wks after onset of illness ↑ ESR
Myocarditis *Viral* Cytomegalovirus	Fever Malaise, fatigue Myalgia, headache Splenomegaly Pharyngitis and cervical adenopathy are uncommon Prodromal symptoms: anorexia, nausea vomiting, fatigue arthralgia, myalgia, pharyngitis, cough, possible rash Distortion of taste Icterus Tender hepatomegaly	Mildly ↑ LFTs Lymphocytosis with atypical lymphocytes Latex agglutination test for CMV antibody Four fold rise in CMV IgG antibody titer PCR evaluation of blood Markedly elevated LFSs Initial lymphopenia followed by lymphocytosis with atypical lymphocytes
Dengue	Saddle-back fever curve Mild conjunctivitis Severe headache	Leukopenia Virus may be isolated from blood

Table 1   Causes of Myocarditis and Pericarditis, Clinical Features, and Diagnostic Tests (*Continued*)

Causes	Associated clinical features	Diagnostic tests
	Myalgias, especially back, lower extremities	Presence of dengue specific IgM antibody (EIA, CF, IFA)
	Pain with eye movement	Four-fold rise in titer between acute and convalescent IgG antibody (EIA, CF, IFA)
	Pinpoint vesicles on posterior soft palate	
	Skin rash initially erythema, becoming morbiliform on thorax, inner arms, followed by appearance of pruritic maculopapular desquamating rash	
Lymphocytic choriomeningitis	Initial nonspecific illness–occasional	
	lymphadenopathy or maculopapular rash resolves in 2–4 days	Leukopenia, thrombocytopenia
		CSF: lymphocyte predominance, usually elevated CSF pressure
	Illness recurs with severe headache, meningitis	Isolates of virus in blood (early), and CSF (late)
		↑LCM IgM titer or four-fold rise LCM IgG titer titers (CF, IFA) between acute and convalescent sera
Rabies	Prodromal-flu–like illness	No test available for diagnosis prior to onset of clinical disease
	Hyperactivity, hallucinations, bizarre	
	Hypertension	Microscopic examination of brain tissue for Negri bodies from rabid animals
	Salivation	
	Paralysis	Positive CF or ELISA antibody from CSF (not detected until after onset of clinical illness)
Yellow fever	Early	Serum is positive by mouse intracerebral inoculation in less than 5 days
	Fever, relative bradycardia, myalgia	
	Severe headache	Postmortem pathological examination of liver
	Lumbosacral pain	
	Conjunctival ejection	
	Coated tongue with red edges	
	Later	
Bacterial Neisseria gonorrhoeae	Jaundice, delirium, acidosis, shock	
	Urethritis-usually purulent discharge, dysuria	
	Mucopurulent cervicitis in females	Intracellular gram-negative diplococci on Gram stain of urethral, cervical secretions, synovial fluid
	Arthritis	
	Pustular skin rash on distal extremities	Blood cultures in disseminated disease

(*Continued*)

Table 1 Causes of Myocarditis and Pericarditis, Clinical Features, and Diagnostic Tests
(*Continued*)

Causes	Associated clinical features	Diagnostic tests
Neisseria meningitidis	Fever	Elevated PMNs in CSF
	Macular or petechial skin rash-most commonly found on axillae, flanks, wrists, ankles	Cultures of blood, CSF, nasopharynx
		Aspirate from skin lesion
	Meningitis	
Brucella	Fever	Blood cultures
	Arthralgia, myalgia	Acute and convalescent serological titers
	Anorexia, weight loss	
	Splenomegaly on 20%	
Salmonella	Fever with relative bradycardia	Blood cultures
	Constipation or diarrhea	Isolation of organism from stool
	Abdominal tenderness	Acute and convalescent serological titers
	Mild hepatosplenomegaly	
	Gastroenteritis	
Myocarditis		
Bacterial Staphylococcus aureus	Fever	Blood cultures
		Organism cultures from infected site
		Elevated teichoic acid antibody
Streptococcus pyogenes	Fever	Blood cultures
	Sandpaper-like rash	Throat culture
	Erythema marginatum	Elevated ASO, anti-DNAase B, antihyaluronidase
	Arthritis	Elevated ESR
	Pharyngitis	
	Subcutaneous modules	
Corynebacterium diphtheriae	Sore throat	"Chinese letter" arrangement on Gram stain of membrane
	Tonsillar membrane-dirty gray, may be green or necrotic-may extend over soft palate	Culture of membrane (if diphtheria is suspected, alert lab to use selective media)
	Hoarseness, dyspnea, stridor	
	Neuropathy with severe disease	
Legionella pneumophila	Pneumonia	Fluorescent antibody staining of sputum
	Relative bradycardia	Isolation of organism of sputum
	Abdominal pain, diarrhea	Four-fold rise in titer between acute and convalescent sera
	Mental confusion	Elevated serum *Legionella* antibody titer
		Legionella urinary antigen
Mycoplasma pneumoniae	Cough, usually nonproductive, may be accompanied by wheezing	Elevated cold agglutinin titer Mycoplasma IgM, IgG serology
	Headache	Detection of *M. pneumoniae* antigen in sputum
	Pharyngitis	
	Minority have myringitis	Sputum cultures require special media
	Erythema multiforme	
	Other skin rashes	

Table 1 Causes of Myocarditis and Pericarditis, Clinical Features, and Diagnostic Tests (*Continued*)

Causes	Associated clinical features	Diagnostic tests
Chlamydia pneumoniae	Fever Pharyngitis with hoarseness Sinusitis	Culture of pharyngeal swab *C. pneumoniae* IgM, IgG serology
Chlamydia psittaci	History of bird exposure Fever Pharyngitis with hoarseness Splenomegaly Hepatomegaly Relative bradycardia Epistaxis	Four-fold rise in serological titer
Borellia burgdorferi	History of tick exposure Bull's-eye rash Headache Meningismus Arthralgias	Serological testing including Western blot
Rickettsia rickettsii	Often history of tick exposure Fever Headache Myalgia Nausea, vomiting, abdominal pain Rash-initially maculopapular around wrists, ankles, becomes petechial	Isolation of organism from blood Demonstration of organism from biopsy of skin lesion Serological testing
Rickettsia tisutsugamushi	Papule, which ulcerates to form an eschar at site of chigger bite High temperature Severe headache Myalgias Tender lymphadenopathy in region of bite Conjunctival injection Ocular pain	Weil-Felix–antibodies to OX-K in 50% Four-fold rise in ~50% serological titer
Mycarditis *Parasitic*		
Trypanosoma orazii	Chagoma—indurated, crythematous area on skin if parasite enters there Romana sign—periorbital/palpebral edema Fever Malaise Hepatosplenomegaly Generalized lymphadenopathy	Detection of parasites in buffy coat/blood Detection of parasites in lymph nodes, bone marrow aspirate, pericardial fluid Serological testing for *T. cructi* IgG, IgM
Trichinella spirulis	Most infections asymptomatic Diarrhea, nausca, vomiting, abdominal pain	Eosinophilia Low ESR (approx. 0)

(*Continued*)

Table 1 Causes of Myocarditis and Pericarditis, Clinical Features, and Diagnostic Tests
(*Continued*)

Causes	Associated clinical features	Diagnostic tests
	Periorbital edema, subconjunctival hemorrhage	Four-fold rise between acute and convalescent serology
	Fever	Trichinella cysts seen on muscle biopsy
	Myositis	
Toxoplasma gondii	Asymptomatic cervical lymphadenopathy	*T. gondii* IgM/IgG serology
	Occasionally mononucleosis-like illness	Toxoplasma cysts in tissue from biopsy specimen
Fungal (Note: most common in immunocompromized biosis as a result of disseminated infection)		
Cryptococcus neoformans	Headache, dizziness, somnolence, impaired memory, judgement with CNS disease	Culture of organism from CSF, sputum, urine, blood
	Dull chest pain, cough, dyspnea with pulmonary disease	India ink preparation of CSF may assist in presemptive diagnosis
	Skin lesions—popular, pastular, or nodular	Visualization of organism in histological specimen
		Detection of cryptococcal polysaccharide antigen from serum and/or CSF
Aspergillus species	High fever	Isolation of organism from blood, CSF, bone marrow (rarely positive)
	Consolidation on chest X-ray	
	Rarely cerebral infarct due to CNS invasion	Isolation from sputum in appropriate clinical sening
	Necrotizing skin lesions	Visualization of organism in histological specimen
Candida species	Fever	Isolation of organism from blood
	Fluffy infiltrates on retina eye examination	Visualization of organism in histological specimen
	Nodular skin lesions	
Pericarditis *Viral Group B* Coxsackieviruses	Fever	Isolation of virus from throat, stool ↑ Coxsackie B IgM titer or four-fold rise in antibody titer between acute and convalescent sera
	Upper respiratory tract symptoms	
	Chest pain (pleurodynia)	
	Skin rash	

(*Continued*)

Table 1   Causes of Myocarditis and Pericarditis, Clinical Features, and Diagnostic Tests (*Continued*)

Causes	Associated clinical features	Diagnostic tests

Echoviruses	Fever
	Upper respiratory tract
	  symptoms
		Isolation of virus or viral proteins
		  from pericardium
		  ↑ Echovirus IgM titer or four-
		  fold rise in IgG antibody titer
		  (CF) between acute and
		  convalescent sera

	Diarrhea Skin rash	Isolation of virus or viral proteins from pericardium

Influenza A	Fever	Isolation of influenza virus
		  from nasopharynx, throat, or
		  sputum

Influenza B	Headache
	  Myalgia
	  Eye pain
	  Nonproductive cough
	  Sore throat
		Four-fold rise in IgG antibody
		  titer between acute and
		  convalescent sera (EIA, IFA,
		  CF, HIA)
		  Isolation of virus or viral
		  proteins from pericardium

Adenovirus	Rhinorrhea
	  Pharyngitis
	  Tracheitis
	  Pneumonia
	  Conjunctivitis
	  Cervical adenitis
		Culture of adenovirus from
		  pharynx sputum, conjunctive,
		  urine
		  Four-fold rise in adenovirus IgG
		  antibody titer between acute
		  and convalescent sera

Mumps	Parotitis, mostly bilateral,
	  but can be
	  unilateral (25%)
	Fever
	  Epididymo-orchitis in men
	  (30%)
		↑ amylase
		  Isolation of virus from blood,
		  nasopharynx, secretions from
		  Stensen's duct, CSF, urine
		  ↑ mumps-specific IgM or four-
		  fold rise in IgG, IFA, mumps
		  antibody between acute and
		  convalescent sera

Pericarditis *Viral*		

Epstein-Barr virus	Fever
	Periorbital edema
	Pharyngitis (may be exudative)
	Posterior cervical or generalized
	Lymphadenopathy
	Splenomegaly
		Mildly ↑ LFTs
		Lymphocytosis with atypical
		  lymphocytes
		Positive monospot antibody test
		Positive IgM viral capsid antigen
		  high titers present in serum
		  1–6 wks after onset of illness,
		  ↑ ESR

Cytomegalovirus	Fever
	  Melaise, fatigue
	  Myalgia, headache
	  Splenomegaly
	  Pharyngitis and cervical
		Mildly ↑ LFTs
		  Lymphocytosis with atypical
		  lymphocytes
		  Latex agglutination test for
		  CMV antibody

(*Continued*)

Table 1 Causes of Myocarditis and Pericarditis, Clinical Features, and Diagnostic Tests (*Continued*)

Causes	Associated clinical features	Diagnostic tests
	adenopathy are uncommon	Four-fold rise in IgG antibody titer, PCR of blood
Hepatitis B	Prodromal symptoms: anorexia nausea, vomiting, fatigue, arthralgia, myalgia, pharyngitis, cough, possible rash	Markedly elevated LFTs Initial lymphopenia followed by lymphocytosis with atypical lymphocytes
	Distortion of taste Iaterus Tender hepatomegaly	Detection of HBsAg in serum
Varicella zoster virus	Prodromal flu-like symptoms Rash initially macular, becomes vesicular, then pustular Rash erupts in crops	Tzanck prep of lesions shows multinucleated giant cells Basophilia Demonstration of virus by DFA from material from a lesion Varicella specific IgM antibody (EIA) Four-fold rise in varicella-specific IgG antibodies between acute and convalescent sera (EIA, CF)
Bacterial		
Mycoplosma pneumoniae	Cough, usually nonproductive, may be accompanied by wheezing Headache Pharyngitis Minority have myringitis Erythema multiforme Other skin rashes	Elevated cold agglutinin titers ($>1{:}64$) Mycoplasma IgM titers Sputum culture viral require special media
Legionella pneumophila	Pneumonia Relative bradycardia Abdominal pain, diarrhea Mental confusion	DFA staining of sputum Isolation of organism from sputum $>4\times$ rise in titer between acute and convalescent sera Initial serum Legionella antibody titer ($>1{:}256$) Legionella urinary antigen
Chlamydia pneumoniae	Fever Pharyngitis with hoarseness Sinusitis	Culture of pharyngeal swab *C. pneumoniae* IgM titer
Borella burgdorferi	History of tick exposure Bulls eye rash Headache Meningismus Arthralgias	Serologic testing (western blot)
Actinomyces spp.	Pericarditis, usually a result of thoracic disease	Presence of sulfur granules in specimen taken from sterile site

(*Continued*)

Table 1   Causes of Myocarditis and Pericarditis, Clinical Features, and Diagnostic Tests (*Continued*)

Causes	Associated clinical features	Diagnostic tests
	Chest pain Fever Weight loss Mass lesion or multiple small Cavities on chest X-ray Spontaneous drainage of empyema through chest wall	Organism cultured from tissue or pus Isolation of organism from pericardial fluid
Nocardio spp.	Anorexia, weight loss Cough Dyspnea Hemoptysis Chest X-ray findings heterogeneous	Isolation of organism from blood, pus or sputum Isolation of organism from pericardium
Myocabacterium *tuberculosis*	Often contiguous infection from lung Chest pain Weight loss Night sweats Dyspnea Cough Echocardiography may show multiple loculations of pericardial fluid	Pericardial fluid usually shows lymphocytic predominance with elevated protein and moderately decreased glucose; pH usually 7.0–7.3 AFB smear of pericardial fluid rarely positive AFB culture of pericardial fluid
Pericarditis *Fungal* *Histoplasm* *capsulatum*	Fever Weight loss Nonproductive cough Hilar adenopathy Patchy infiltrates on chest X-ray Pericarditis may result as an inflammatory response to inflamed mediastinal lymph nodes	Blood pericardial fluid in acute primary pulmonary histoplasmosis Isolation of organism from sputum, blood cultures from pericardial fluid rarely positive
Coccidioides immitis	Fever Cough Night sweats Erythema nodosum Cardiac involvement rare	Isolation of organism from sputum (hazardous) Coccidioides immities IgM antibody from serum (high serum titers in disseminated disease)
Cryptococcus *neoformans*	Headache, dizziness, somnolence, impaired memory, judgment with CNS disease Dull chest pain, cough, dyspnea with pulmonary disease Skin lesions-papular, pustular, or nodular	Culture of organism from CSF, sputum, urine, blood India ink preparation of CSP may assist in presumptive diagnosis Visualization of organism in histological specimen Detection of cryptococcal antigen from serum and/or CSF

(*Continued*)

Table 1 Causes of Myocarditis and Pericarditis, Clinical Features, and Diagnostic Tests (*Continued*)

Causes	Associated clinical features	Diagnostic tests
Aspergillus spp.	High fever Consolidation on chest X-ray Rarely cerebral infarction due to CNS invasion Necrotizing skin lesions	Isolation of organism from blood, CSF, bone marrow (rarely positive) Isolation from sputum in appropriate clinical setting Visualization of organism in histological specimen
Candida spp.	Fever Fluffy infiltrates in retina Nodular skin lesions	Isolation of organism from blood Visualization of organism in histological specimen
Parasites *Entamoeba* *histolytica*	Pericarditis occurs as a complication of liver abscess Fever Weight loss Abdominal pain Hepatic tenderness Diarrhea Chest pain	Isolation of organism from stool Isolation of organism from liver abscesses Isolation of organism from pericordial fluid Elevated serum antiamebic (HI) antibody test
Toxoplasma gondii	Asymtomatic cervical lymphadenopathy	*T. gondii* IgM titer
Occasionally	mononucleosis-like illness	Toxoplasma cysts in tissue from biopsy specimen.

Abbreviations: CMV, cytomegalovirus; CNS, central nervous system, ELISA, enzyme-linked immunosorbent assay; IgG, immunoglobulinG; PCR, polymerase chain reaction; ESR, erythrocyte sedimentation rate; CSF, cerebrospinal fluid; PMN, polymorphonuclear leukocytes; AFB, acid-fast bacilli; CF, complement filtration; EIA, enzyme immunoassay; IFA, immunofluorescence assay; HIA, hemagglutination inhibition assay; LFT, liver function test; CSF, cerebrospinal fluid; LCM, lymphocytic choriomeningitis; ASO, antistreptolysin O.

occurs in approximately one-third of patients and is likely related to contiguous involvement of the pericardium (myopericarditis). Other physical findings include tachycardia disproportionate to the degree of fever, tachypnea, and narrowed pulse pressure from low cardiac output. LV failure results in leftward displacement of the apical impulse, the presence of a third and/or fourth heart sound, a systolic murmur of mitral regurgitation, and rales on pulmonary auscultation. Elevation of jugular venous pressure and peripheral edema arise from right-sided failure. The presence of a pericardial rub indicates contiguous pericarditis. This finding along with chest pain is important as pericardial involvement is predictive of future recurrences of myocarditis (15).

Nonspecific markers of inflammation, including erythrocyte sedimentation rate and white blood cell count, are neither sensitive nor specific for myocarditis. In the Myocarditis Treatment Trial for acute and subacute forms of myocarditis, leukocytosis was present in one of five patients, and about half had elevated erythrocyte sedimentation rates (16). Increased white blood cell count and other markers of stronger immune response were associated with more profound cardiac dysfunction presentation. CPK-MB isoenzyme, a more specific marker of myocyte injury, is quite insensitive in active myocarditis, as only 6% of patients have elevated serum levels (17).

However, the frequency of CPK-MB elevation is higher (approximately 75%) in patients with ST segment elevation on electrocardiogram (EKG). By comparison, one-third of patients had elevated serum levels of Troponin I, another biochemical marker of myocardial injury (17). Troponin I did not correlate with the histological severity of myocarditis, but elevated serum levels were associated with symptoms of less than one-month duration. Serum brain natriuretic peptide levels, which provide diagnostic and prognostic value in patients with congestive heart failure, are likely nonspecific in myocarditis, but have not been well studied.

The EKG is almost always abnormal in active myocarditis (14,18). ST-segment and T-wave changes are most common and may be diffuse or focal. The ST segments may be depressed or elevated. ST elevations are associated with elevation of CPK levels thereby prompting suspicion of recent MI. The presence of ST elevation without reciprocal ST depression has been proposed to be useful in differentiating myocarditis (19). The presence of pathological Q waves may further mimic MI. Other EKG findings include conduction abnormalities such as atrioventricular block and bundle branch block. Overall, EKG findings are rather nonspecific in suspected myocarditis. The chest X-ray may reveal cardiomegaly and pulmonary edema, although myocardial dysfunction may not be apparent on portable films that are taken in the critical care setting.

Cardiac imaging modalities such as echocardiography and cardiac blood pool imaging may show both diffuse and regional wall motion abnormalities during active myocarditis. In one study, LV dysfunction was found in 69% of patients with biopsy-proven myocarditis and in 88% of patients presenting with congestive heart failure (20). In most cases of LV dysfunction, the LV was normal in size and not dilated as expected in other types of cardiomyopathy. Failure of the LV to dilate might be related to decreased ventricular compliance associated with LV hypertrophy, a common echocardiographic and pathological finding in myocarditis, Nevertheless, reduced LV systolic function with normal LV chamber size in the setting of congestive heart failure provides another clue as to the possibility of myocarditis (21). LV dysfunction occurs in one-fourth of patients with the right ventricular also normal in size in most cases. Magnetic resonance imaging using T2-weighted images detecting tissue water content as an indicator of inflammation may be useful. The addition of early and late gadolinium enhancement may help distinguish myocarditis from MI (22). Segmental early subendocardial defects with corresponding segmental subendocardial or transmural delayed high enhancement is characteristic of patients with MI, whereas patients with myocarditis exhibit normal first pass perfusion imaging, nonsegmental nonsubendocardial delayed enhancement (focal or diffuse) predominantly in the inferolateral location, and visualization of hyper-enhancing nodules.

Although the diagnosis of myocarditis may be made with reasonable certainty on clinical grounds, endomyocardial biopsy remains the gold standard. The presence of myocyte injury and lymphocytic infiltrate are required for histological criteria. Recently, the role of endomyocardial biopsy has been questioned. In a randomized, placebo-controlled trial of 111 patients with LVEF, less than 45% had histological evidence of myocarditis immunology.

Suppressive therapy consisting of prednisone with either cyclosporine or azathioprine did not affect survival or improve LVEF (16). The low incidence of myocarditis found on biopsy as well as the lack of demonstrable clinical benefit of immunosuppression has resulted in the utility of endomyocardial biopsy being challenged. Therefore, the utility of endomyocardial biopsy remains uncertain and the procedure is not routinely performed.

Noninvasive detection of myocardial inflammation has been attempted with gallium-67 imaging and indium-111 antimyosim antibodies, which bind to areas of myocardial necrosis. However, these techniques have not gained widespread acceptance for use in suspected myocarditis.

Therefore acute myocarditis has a wide spectrum. LV dysfunction is central to the diagnosis but may have other causes such as sepsis-induced cardiac dysfunction. Recently, Tako-tsubo–like LV dysfunction has been described and is being recognized with increasing frequency. It is characterized by transient LV apical ballooning in the absence of coronary disease, associated with chest pain, dyspnea, and syncope. It is more common in females and occurs frequently after emotional or physical stress. The pathophysiology is poorly understood, but myocarditis had been hypothesized.

The course of congestive heart failure related to myocarditis is quite variable. Myocarditis may resolve spontaneously with complete resolution of symptoms. Spontaneous improvement in LVEF is common. LV function returns to normal in about half of the patients, making it difficult to draw meaningful conclusions about the clinical effects of immunosuppression in uncontrolled trials. In the Myocarditis Treatment Trial, the mean LVEF improved from 26% to 34%, but as aforementioned, was unaffected by immunosuppressive agents (16). Higher LVEF and less intensive conventional therapy at baseline were independent predictors of survival. Patients with fulminant lymphocytic myocarditis have a better prognosis than those with acute nonfulminant myocarditis (23). CMV is the most common specific finding in immunocompetent patients with fatal myocarditis (24).

The medical management of myocarditis heart failure includes diuretics and angiotensin-converting inhibitors. Digitalis may be used with caution as patients with myocarditis are particularly sensitive to its effects (2). Intravenous gamma globulin has been advocated to attenuate inflammatory cytokines during the acute treatment of myocarditis. Although a recent review identified three case series having shown gamma globulin to improve LV function, one randomized controlled trial of 62 patients found no benefit with respect to cardiac function, outcome, or event-free survival (25). Additional attempts at suppressing inflammation with aspirin and anti-inflammatory agents have been disappointing. In five animal studies of coxsacchie B3– and B4–induced myocarditis, aspirin, indomethacin, and ibuprofen resulted in a two to threefold increase in inflammation, myocyte necrosis, and mortality when compared to placebo (26). The deleterious effect was more prominent during the acute and subacute phases of myocarditis. The possible contribution of microvascular spasm to the progression of myocarditis toward dilated cardiomyopathy provides a rationale for the use of calcium channel blockers in acute myocarditis (2). However, their use in myocarditis has not been studied and should not be considered as multiple studies have demonstrated clinical deterioration associated with calcium channel blockers in congestive heart failure. Similarly, enhanced nuclear factor-kappaB expression suggests a protective effect of PPAR-gamma activators, which has not yet been studied. Bed rest is generally recommended to patients with active myocarditis as animal studies have shown myocardial necrosis to be enhanced by exercise (15). Critically ill patients often require mechanical circulatory support such as percutaneous. In one study, 71% of patients with fulminant myocarditis supported with percutaneous extracorporeal membrane oxygenation survived with spontaneous improvement of LV function (27). LV assist devices have been implanted in patients with myocarditis as a bridge to cardiac transplantation but has also recently been found to provide a bridge to

LV recovery in 11% of patients. Patients with myocarditis and postpartum cardio-myopathy are most likely to spontaneously recover (28).

Myocardial Infarction

Acute myocarditis should also be considered in suspected acute MI with normal coronary arteries and no other identifiable causes (21). Chest pain, fever, EKG changes, CPK-MB elevation, and regional wall motion abnormalities on cardiac imaging studies are common on both entities. As above, a young patient age, preceding viral syndrome, and ST-segment elevation on EKG in the absence of reciprocal ST depressions suggest acute myocarditis. Nonetheless, most cases of acute coronary syndrome result from atherosclerotic plaque rupture and thrombosis. Myocarditis is usually first suspected when normal coronary arteries are found on cardiac catheterization after patients are treated in a conventional manner with antianginal agents, anticoagulation, and thrombolytic therapy. Active myocarditis was found on biopsy in 33% of such patients up to six years after biopsy (29). Despite the theoretical concerns of myocardial hemorrhage and cardiac tamponade, one study found thrombolytic therapy to be uncomplicated in patients with viral myopericarditis misdiagnoses for acute MI (30). Although small in size, this study also showed a favorable long-term outcome for acute myocarditis mimicking acute MI without recurrent cardiac events.

Arrhythmias

Acute infectious myocarditis may also present with arrhythmias and conduction disturbances. Premature ventricular and supraventricular complexes occur most frequently and have been observed during the first three days of hospitalization in one-third of patients admitted for myocarditis (31). The overall incidence of arrhythmias likely decreases with time after presentation. In one study, complex ventricular ectopy decreased from 28% at one week to 8% at three months (31). Ventricular tachycardia is presumably less common, but may be responsible for 5% to 15% of cases of sudden death in young athletes related to myocarditis. The overall risk of malignant arrhythmias is unknown as its prevalence remains undetermined. One study found myocarditis to be present in four to six young asymptomatic athletes with minor rhythm disturbances and/or echocardiographic abnormalities (32). Ventricular arrhythmias and sudden cardiac death may be the initial manifestation of myocarditis and occur in the absence of LV dysfunction. Surviving patients should be referred for electrophysiological testing.

ACUTE PERICARDITIS

Acute pericarditis is characterized clinically by chest pain, a pericardial friction rub, and serial electrocardiographic findings. The most commonly identified causes are infection, uremia, bacteria, acute MI, and trauma.

Infectious Causes

Many of the same agents that are responsible for the development of acute infectious myocarditis can cause pericarditis as well. In fact, illness most often manifests as a myopericarditis. The enteroviruses, especially Coxsackie group B (which is the agent of epidemic pleurodynia), are again the most commonly implicated pathogens (33).

Other viruses, such as CMV, EBV, mumps, herpes, varicella, and hepatitis B, have all been reported to cause pericarditis, but incidence is low (34).

At one time, bacteria were the major cause of pericarditis, but since the development of antimicrobials, purulent pericarditis is unusual. It is occasionally encountered as a complication of pneumococcal and staphylococcal pneumonia or bacteremia. *Hemophilus influenza* type B was also responsible for the development of pericarditis in children, but the incidence of this is decreasing as well due to the use of the *H. influenzae* type B conjugate vaccine. Streptococcal and meningococcal infections may result in the development of pericardial disease, as can infection with *L. pneumophila* and *M. pneumoniae*. The aerobic gram-negative rods have been reported to cause disease, especially in debilitated or immunocompromised hosts (35,36).

Mycobacterium tuberculosis is a well-known cause of primary pericarditis and results from hematogenous spread or direct extension of the infection to the pericardium. Cases that develop acutely may result in cardiac tamponade. The incidence of tuberculosis pericarditis has been rising, due to the increasing incidence of tuberculosis in the area of HIV infection (35,37).

Pericarditis occurs with some disseminated fungal infections, especially histoplasmosis, aspergillosis, and candidiasis; however, it is unusual with coccidioidomycosis. Pericardial involvement is more commonly seen in immunocompromised individuals. Parasitic disease of the pericardium is rare, but cases of pericarditis secondary to *T. gondii*, *E. histolytica*, and schistosomes have been reported (35). The infectious causes of pericarditis and their associated clinical and laboratory features are listed in Table 1.

Clinical Presentation

The chest pain of pericarditis is classically described as a sharp or stabbing sensation located in the substernal or pericardial areas, with radiation to the left trapezius region (38). It is usually persistent, variable in intensity, and worsened by lying supine and relieved upon sitting up. Pleural-like pain may also be present. A pericardial cause should always be considered in the evaluation of pain in the trapezius ridge. Dyspnea is also a common symptom of acute pericarditis and is likely related to shallow respiration to avoid pleuropericardial discomfort.

On physical examination, the most characteristic sign is a pericardial friction rub. Although the friction rub is pathognomonic for pericarditis, it is appreciated in only two-thirds of patients. Therefore, the absence of a rub does not exclude the diagnosis of pericarditis (38). The rub is a scratchy, superficial sound heard best at the lower left sternal border with the patient leaning forward using the diaphragm of the stethoscope. It often becomes obvious during inspiration. The rub typically has three components representing pericardial–epicardial contact during rapid ventricular filling, atrial systole, and ventricular systole. Although rubs may be confused with murmurs, the left parasternal location and the failure of a sound to radiate to areas expected of murmurs may help to identify a pericardial rub (39). The second diastolic component of atrial contraction is the most specific finding to pericarditis. Other physical findings include fever and tachycardia.

Chest X ray may reveal enlargement of the cardiac silhouette due to pericardial effusion. Pleural effusions are evident in one-fourth of patients with acute pericarditis and are usually left-sided in contradistinction to the right-sided effusion seen in congestive heart failure (40). The presence of a pulmonary infiltrate of pleural effusion favors pleuroperocarditis or pulmonary infarction.

The EKG is abnormal in over 90% of patients (41). The classic evolutionary changes occur in half of the patients. During the first few hours of acute pericarditis, patients develop diffuse ST-segment elevations without reciprocal changes. ST depressions can occur in leads, AVR and V1. Of note, the T waves remain upright. Over weeks, the ST segments return to baseline and depression of the PR segment develops in 80% of patients (42). After the ST segments return to baseline, the T waves become inverted and ultimately normalized. Although both acute pericarditis and MI are associated with ST-segment elevation, several important EKG features may help to differentiate these two entities (41). ST elevations are diffuse in pericarditis and usually localized in acute MI. Pericarditis is more commonly associated with PR-segment depression and less commonly with Q waves than acute MI. In addition, T-wave inversion is present during ST-segment elevation in MI. However, in acute pericarditis, the T waves invert after the ST segments return to baseline. In other words, "the T waves flip after the STs dip." Diffuse ST elevations may be seen in young healthy subjects with "early repolarization." As compared to early repolarization, acute pericarditis is more likely when inspection of level V6 shows the height of the ST segment to exceed one-fourth the amplitude of the T wave (43). Low voltage may also be present in the presence of pericardial effusion. Of note, typical EKG findings occur less commonly in uremic pericarditis.

Nonspecific markers of inflammation, including erythrocyte sedimentation rate and white blood cell count, are neither sensitive nor specific for pericarditis. Serum CPK levels are usually within normal limits but may be mild to moderately elevated with underlying myocarditis. Elevated CPK levels are associated with more prominent EKG changes. Patients clinically suspected of acute pericarditis should undergo echocardiography.

Echocardiography is the most sensitive technique for detecting pericardial effusion. As pericardial fluid appears as an echo-free space, its size, distribution, and hemodynamic significance can be assessed (44). However, the absence of a pericardial effusion does not rule out the diagnosis of pericarditis, although its presence is further suggestive of the diagnosis.

After exclusion of other ominous underlying conditions such as MI, the clinical course of acute pericarditis is usually self-limited. However, 10% to 20% of patients may develop chronic relapsing pericarditis (42). The management of acute pericarditis includes the symptomatic relief of chest pain with nonsteroidal anti-inflammatory agents and analgesics. Most patients should be admitted to the hospital for observation of complications including cardiac tamponade and arrhythmias. Aspirin and indomethacin are the initial agents used. The use of glucocorticoids is controversial as recurrences are common when therapy is discontinued.

The complications of acute infectious pericarditis include cardiac tamponade and cardiac arrhythmias. Cardiac tamponade is the most frequent and often life-threatening complication of acute pericarditis. Pericardial inflammation results in an effusion within the pericardial space that is detectable in half of the patients with pericarditis. Cardiac tamponade develops in 15% of patients with pericarditis and effusion. The hemodynamic significance of a pericardial effusion is more closely related to its rapidity of accumulation than to its volume. Rapid accumulation of an effusion does not allow for stretching of the pericardium. Consequently, tamponade may develop even in the presence of a small effusion, and large chronic effusions may not cause tamponade. Cardiac tamponade is not an all-or-none phenomenon, but is a spectrum of compressive physiology (45). Pericardial fluid restricts diastolic filling of the right ventricle and then the left ventricle, resulting in low cardiac output.

On physical examination, there is tachycardia, hypotension, and narrowed plus pressure reflecting decreased stroke volume. Pulsus paradoxus, an inspiratory decrease of >10 mmHg in systolic blood pressure during quiet respiration, is a late finding. In the absence of dehydration, there should be elevation of jugular venous pressure as systemic venous pressure is increased. On auscultation, the lungs are clear. Pulses alternans in which the amplitude of QRS complexes alternate from beat to beat is present. Echocardiographic findings include right atrial and right ventricular chamber collapse, inferior vena cava distension, and variation of mitral and tricuspid flow velocity with respiration on Doppler examination. Pericardiocentesis or open surgical drainage of the effusion is indicated for signs of cardiac tamponade. Although needle pericardiocentesis can usually be performed earlier, surgical drainage is considered safer. In the absence of tamponade, pericardiocentesis for laboratory evaluation of pericardial fluid carries a low diagnostic yield of 14% and is generally not recommended (46). Therapeutic pericardiocentesis provides a diagnostic etiology in about a third of cases.

Summary

In summary, acute infectious myocarditis has a variable clinical course and a wide clinical spectrum ranging from asymptomatic EKG changes to progressive heart failure and death. It may also present with arrhythmia and/or sudden cardiac death or can mimic MI. The clinical factors that should raise suspicion of active myocarditis include young patient age, absence of cardiac history, recent or present viral syndrome, a brief duration of symptoms, coexisting pericarditis, and the absence of reciprocal ST depressions in suspected MI. Laboratory markers of active inflammation are generally not helpful. Cardiac imaging studies often reveal regional and diffuse wall motion abnormalities without chamber enlargement. Endomyocardial biopsy is required for definitive diagnosis; however, a strong presumptive diagnosis can be made clinically.

In the appropriate clinical setting, a fourfold rise in acute and convalescent antibody titers, IgM-specific antibodies, isolation of virus from another site such as the throat or stool, or positive blood culture would strongly suggest the etiological agent of infection. Treatment of acute myocarditis is generally supportive.

Acute pericarditis is characterized clinically by chest pain, a pericardial friction rub, and serial electrocardiographic changes. Although the presence of a pericardial friction rub is path gnomonic of pericarditis, its absence does not exclude the diagnosis. Differentiating electrocardiographic features from acute MI includes ST segment of diffuse nature, resolution of ST elevation prior to T-wave inversion, and PR-segment depression. Laboratory markers of active inflammation are generally not helpful. All patients suspected of pericarditis should be referred for echocardiography. Further management includes the treatment of chest pain with anti-inflammatory agents and analgesics as well as observation for complications, including cardiac tamponade and arrhythmias.

REFERENCES

1. Mason JW. Distinct forms of myocarditis. Circulation 1991; 83:1110–1111.
2. Sole MJ, Liu P. Viral myocarditis: a paradigm for understanding the pathogenesis and treatment of dilated cardiomyopathy. J Am Cull Cardiol 1993; 22:A99–A105.

3. Woodruff JF. Viral myocarditis: a review. Am J Pathol 1980; 101:427–478.

4. See DM, Tilles JG. Viral myocarditis. Rev Infec Dis 1991; 13:951–956.

5. Savoia MC, Oxman MN. Myocarditis, pericarditis. In: Mandell GL, Bennett JE, Dolin R, eds. Principles and Practice of Infectious Diseases, 4th ed. New York: Churchill Livingstone, 1995:799–813.

6. Maje SS, Adolph RJ. Myocarditis; unresolved issues in diagnosis and treatment. Clin Cardiol 1990; 13:69–79.

7. Obeyeshere I, Hermon Y. Myocarditis and cardiomyopathy after arbovirus infections. Br Heart J 1972; 34:821–827.

8. Gore J. Myocardial changes in fatal diphtheria: summary of observations in 221 cases. Am J Med Sci 1948; 215:257–266.

9. Smith RH, Lazar JM. Myocarditis. Infect Dis Prac 1996; 20:94–95.

10. Nontrowitz NE, Smith RH. Myocarditis update. Emerg Med 1993; 25:69–74.

11. Lerner AM. Pericarditis-myocarditis. In: Gorbach SL, Bartlett JG, Blacklow NR, eds. Infectious Diseases. Philadelphia: WS Saunders, 1992:565–572.

12. Atkinson JB, Connor DH, Robinowitz M, et al. Cardiac fungal infections. Review of autopsy findings in 60 patients. Hum Pathol 1984; 15:935–942.

13. Chow LC, Dittrich HC, Shabetai R. Endocardial biopsy in patients with unexplained congestive heart failure. Ann Intern Med 1988; 109:535–539.

14. Lewes D, Rainford DJ, Lane WF. Symptomless myocarditis and myalgia in viral and mycoplasma pneumonia infections. Br Heart J 1974; 36:924–932.

15. Johnson RA, Palacios I. Dilated cardiomyopathies of the adult. N Engl J Med 1982; 307:1119–1126.

16. Mason JW, O'Connell JB, Hershkowitz A, et al. A clinical trial of immunosuppressive therapy for myocarditis. N Eng J Med 1995; 333:269–275.

17. Smith SC, Ladenson JH, Mason JW, et al. Elevations of cardiac troponin I associated with myocarditis. Circulation 1997; 95:163–168.

18. Karjalainen J, Heikkila J. "Acute pericarditis": myocardial enzyme release as evidence for myocarditis. Am Heart J 1986; 111:546–552.

19. Nakashima H, Honda Y, Katayama T. Serial electrocardiographic findings in acute myocarditis. Intern Med 1994; 33:659–666.

20. Pinamonti B, Albert E, Cigalotto A, et al. Echocardiographic findings in myocarditis. Am Coll Cardiol 1992; 20:85–89.

21. Laissey JP, Hyafil F, Juliard JM, et al. Differentiating acute myocardial infarction from myocarditis: diagnostic value of early-and delayed-perfusion cardiac MR imaging. Radiology 2005; 237:75–82.

22. Dec GW Jr, Waldman H, Fallon JT, et al. Viral myocarditis mimicking acute myocardial infraction. J Am Coll Cardiol 1992; 20:85–89.

23. McCarthy RE III, Boehmer JP, Hruban RH, et al. Long-term outcome of fulminant myocarditis as compared with acute (non-fulminant) myocarditis. N Eng J Med 2000; 342:690–695.

24. Kyto V, Vuorinen, Saukko P, Lautenschlager I, et al. Cytomegalovirus infection of the heart is common in patients with fatal myocarditis. Clin Infect Dis 2005; 40:683–688.

25. Robinson JL, Hartling L, Crumley E, et al. A systematic review of intravenous gamma globulin for therapy of acute myocarditis. BMC Cardiovasc Disord 2005; 5:12–17.

26. Meune C, Spaulding C, Mahe I, et al. Risks versus benefits of NSAIDS including aspirin in myocarditis: a review of the evidence from animal studies. Drug Safety 2003; 26(13):975–981.

27. Asaumi Y, Yasuda S, Morii I, et al. Favourable clinical outcome in patients with cardiogenic shock due to fulminant myocarditis supported by percutaneous extracorporeal membrane oxygenation. Eur Heart J 2005; 26:2185–2192.

28. Simon MA, Kormos R, Murali S, et al. Myocardial recovery using ventricular assist devices. Circ 2005; 112(SI):I32–I36.

29. Dec GW, Palacios IF, Fallon JT, et al. Active myocarditis in the spectrum of acute dilated cardiomyopathies. N Eng J Med 1985; 312:885–890.

30. Millaire A, de Groote P, Decoulx E, et al. Outcome after thrombolytic therapy of nine cases of myopericarditis misdiagnosed as myocardial infarction. Eur Heart J 1995; 16:333–338.
31. Vikerfors T, Stjema A, Olcen P, et al. Acute myocarditis. Acute Med Scand 1988; 223:45–52.
32. Zeppolli P, Santini C, Palmieri V, et al. Role of myocarditis in athletes with minor arrhythmias and/or echocardiographic abnormalities. Chest 1994; 106:373–380.
33. Smith WG. Coxsakie B myopericarditis in adults. Am Heart J 1970; 80:34–36.
34. Fowler No, Manitas GT. Infectious pericarditis. In: Mandell GL, Bennett JE, Dolin R, eds. Principles and Practice of Infectious Diseases. 4th ed. New York: Churchill Livingstone, 1955:799–815.
35. Savoia MC, Oxman MV. Myocarditis and pericarditis. In: Mandell GL, Bennett JE, Dolin R, eds. Principles and Practice of Infectious Diseases. 4th ed. New York: Churchill Livingstone, 1995:799–815.
36. Maisch B. Pericardial diseases with a focus on etiology. Curr Opin Cardiol 1994; 9: 379–388.
37. Ortbals DW, Avioli LV. Tuberculous pericarditis. Arch Intern Med 1979; 139:231–234.
38. Shabetai R. Acute pericarditis. Cardiol Clin 1990; 8:639–671.
39. Spodick DH. Diagnostic electrocardiographic sequences in acute pericarditis: significance of PR segment and PR vector changes. Circulation 1973; 48:575.
40. Weiss JM, Spodick DH. Association of left pleural effusion with pericardial disease. N Engl J Med 1983; 308:696.
41. Spodick DH. Differential diagnosis of acute pericarditis. Prog Cardiovasc Dis 1971; 14:192.
42. Spodick DH. Diagnostic electrocardiogram in acute pericarditis: distributions of morphologic and axial changes by stages. Am J Cardiol 1974; 33:470.
43. Ginzton LE, Laks MM. The differential diagnosis of acute pericarditis from the normal variant: new electrocardiographic criteria. Circulation 1982; 65:1004.
44. Kronzon I, Cohen ML, Winer HE. Contribution of echocardiography to the understanding of the pathophysiology of cardiac tamponade. J Am Coll Cardiol 1983; 1:1180–1182.
45. Reddy PS, Curtiss EI. Cardiac tamponade. Cardiol Clin 1990; 8:627–633.
46. Permanyer-Miralda G, Sagrista-Sauleda J, Soler-Soler J. Primary acute pericardial disease. A prospective series of 231 consecutive patients. Am J Cardiol 1985; 56:623.

13

Central Intravenous Line Infections in the Critical Care Unit

Burke A. Cunha

*Infectious Disease Division, Winthrop-University Hospital, Mineola, and
State University of New York School of Medicine, Stony Brook,
New York, U.S.A.*

INTRODUCTION

Intravenous (IV) central venous catheters (CVC) are used in critical care units (CCU) for medication, fluid, or nutritional access. IV CVCs may be inserted peripherally, i.e., peripherally inserted central catheters in central veins. Complications of CVCs may be mechanical/infectious. The three most common infectious complications of CVC include bacteremia, septic thrombophlebitis, and acute bacterial endocarditis (ABE). The most common organisms associated with CVC infection are methicillin-sensitive *Staphylococcus aureus* (MSSA)/methicillin-resistant *S. aureus* (MRSA), *S. epidermitis*, also known as coagulase-negative staphylococci (CoNS), and less commonly aerobic gram-negative bacilli. Fungal IV CVC infections may occur in any patient with CVCs in place for an extended period of time or receiving total parental nutrition. Enterococci are uncommon causes of CVC, excluding femoral lines. Because most patients in CCUs have one or more CVCs, clinicians caring for patients in the CCU should be familiar with the infectious complications of CVC. Physicians consulting in the CCU should be familiar with the differential diagnosis therapy of CVC infections (1–10).

OVERVIEW OF CVC INFECTIONS

There are several factors that predisposed to CVC infections. After aseptic insertion technique, the most important factors predisposing to infection are duration and location of insertion of CVCs. IV CVC line infections are a function of time. CVC-related line infection is rare before seven days; or after seven days, there is a gradual increase over time in the incidence of IV CVC line infections. The number of lumens may increase the potential for IV CVC infection. In a patient with otherwise unexplained fever in the CCU, the longer a CVC is in place the more likely the CVC is the likely cause of fever. Other important determinants of IV CVC line

Table 1 Pathogens Associated with Intravenous-Line Infections

Most common pathogen*s*
  Staphylococcus aureus (MSSA/MRSA)
  Staphylococcus epidermidis/CoNS
  Enterobacter agglomerans
  Enterobacter cloacae
Less common microorganisms
  Enterococci (VSE/VRE; vancomysin-sensitive enterococci/
    vancomycin-resistant enterococci)
  Burkholderia (*Pseudomonas*) *cepacia*
  Stenotrophomonas (*Xanthomonas*) *maltophilia*
  Citrobacter freundii

Abbreviations: MSSA, methicillin-sensitive *S. aureus*; MRSA, methicillin-resistant *S. aureus*; CoNS, coagulase-negative staphylococci.
Source: From Ref. 1.

infections are the anatomical location of CVC. The best anatomical location with the lowest potential for infection is the subclavian vein. The next best location is the internal jugular vein, and the least desirable location from an infectious perspective is the femoral location. It should be appreciated that peripheral IV lines rarely result in IV line infections. Even if phlebitis and bacteremia develops from a peripheral IV line, the discontinuous/low-grade bacteremia does not result in endocarditis. The reticuloendothelial system rapidly eliminates microorganisms introduced in the blood stream via peripheral IV lines. If peripheral IV lines are associated with a intermittent/low-grade *S. aureus* bacteremia, *S. aureus* ABE is not a complication, (Tables 1 and 2) (1–5,11–18).

IV LINE INFECTIONS

The main diagnostic difficulty with CVC infections is that only 50% of CVCs that are infected have any indicators of infection present locally. CVC IV line infection is straightforward when the insertion site is red and painful. But half of the time there are no superficial signs of IV line infection. It is usually straightforward to differentiate chemical phlebitis or IV line infiltration from cellulitis at the CVC insertion site.

Table 2 Risk Factors Associated with Central Intravenous-Line Infections

Important risk factors for central IV line infections
  Aseptic insertion technique
  Duration of catheterization (catheter days)
  Location of catheter placement
  Multiple lines
Less important factors in central IV line infections
  Contaminated infusate
  Number of catheter lumens (single vs. triple lumen)
  Secondary bacteremias
  Host defense status

Abbreviation: IV, intravenous.
Source: From Refs. 1, 3, 4.

The skin at the IV insertion site in IV phlebitis or with IV infiltration is swollen and painful but is not erythematous and the patient does not have otherwise unexplained fever. IV line infections secondary to CVC must be suspected in CCU patients with fever where the other causes of fever in the CCU have been ruled out. Then the diagnosis of CVC-related infection should be entertained. The likelihood of CVC-related infection is more likely the longer the CVC has been in place and, as mentioned, is also related to the anatomical location of the insertion, i.e., femoral lines are much more likely to become infected than subclavian lines (1–8).

IV line infection in the absence of local manifestations may be diagnosed by blood cultures and semiquantitative catheter tip cultures. If IV line infection is suspected from a CVC, the catheter should be removed and the tip sent for a semi-quantitative culture. Simultaneously, the patient should have blood cultures drawn, but not drawn through the removed or other CVCs unless there is no venous access. IV line infection is diagnosed if the blood culture isolate, excluding skin contaminants acquired during venipuncture, is the same organism recovered from the removed CVC tip culture. For the CVC tip culture to be considered positive, ≥ 15 colonies should be present. Positive tip cultures without bacteremia indicate the catheter colonization of noninfection. Bacteremia without a positive CVC tip culture indicates bacteremia unrelated to the line. IV line infection is only diagnosed if there are ≥ 15 or greater colonies, from culturing the removed catheter tip, and they are the same species as the blood culture isolates (1,3,15–19).

The therapy of uncomplicated IV line infections is for two weeks with anti-MSSA/MSRA antibiotics. Near the end of the therapy, MSSA/MRSA ABE should be ruled out by transthoracic echocardiography (TTE)/transesophageal echocardiography (TEE). Elevated teichoic acid antibody titers/otherwise unexplained elevated erythrocytes sedimentation rate (ESR) is a clue to the possibility of ABE following MSSA/MRSA bacteremia. Cardiac echocardiography should be done in a patient with a high-grade/persistent *S. aureus* bacteremia following an IV CVC infection, particularly with an otherwise unexplained elevated ESR or teichoic acid antibody level. In patients without prosthetic valves. TTE is sufficient; TEE is a low-yield procedure. For prosthetic valves, TEE is preferred. Antimicrobial coated CVCs have not been shown to decrease IV line infection greater than seven days after placement (20–35).

SEPTIC THROMBOPHLEBITIS

Simple uncomplicated phlebitis may be associated with low-grade fevers $\geq 102°F$ and is not associated with bacteremia. If bacteremia complicates phlebitis, it is due to skin organisms, usually *S. aureus* or CoNS, and the bacteremia is intermittent and is of low intensity. Typically, if blood cultures are positive, they are present in a 1/2, 2/0, 2/2, 0/4, etc., indicative of blood culture contaminants. Septic thrombophlebitis is an IV septic process within the vein. The clinical findings resemble phlebitis except that the patient usually has fevers of $\geq 102°F$ and is often accompanied by rigors. Blood culture positivity may be continuous or discontinuous and is usually of a high-grade 3/4 or 4/4 positive blood cultures. The diagnosis of septic thrombophlebitis may be suspected clinically and confirmed by removal of the central IV line, and pus emanating from the catheter wound and palpable cord is usually present. Therapy for septic thrombophlebitis is venotomy, with appropriate anti MSSA/MRSA therapy for four weeks.

S. AUREUS ACUTE BACTERIAL ENDOCARDITIS

S. aureus is the commonest cause of ABE at the present time. *S. aureus*, either MSSA/MRSA, is capable of attacking normal and abnormal heart valves. This is in contrast to SBE due to avirulent pathogens, e.g., *Staphylococcus veridans* group that requires pre-existing valvular damage and capsular production to cause SBE. The factors that predispose to MSSA/MRSA ABE include high-grade/continuous MSSA/MRSA bacteremia from a CVC, invasive cardiac procedure, e.g., radio-frequency ablation or a distant protected focus, e.g., abscess. ABE is not a complication of peripheral IV line infection.

The clinical diagnosis of *S. aureus* ABE demonstrates two diagnostic features. First, the patient must have a high-grade/continuous *S. aureus* bacteremia, i.e., 3/4 or 4/4 positive blood cultures. The second criterion is the demonstration of vegetation by TTE/TEE. *S. aureus* bacteremia that is not high grade/prolonged indicates a transient staphylococcal bacteremia and is not indicative of endocarditis per se. In *S. aureus* endocarditis, the bacteremia characteristically is of high grade and prolonged. High-grade prolonged *S. aureus* bacteremia without a vegetation demonstrated by TTE/TEE should suggest an extracardiac focus or abscess. Patients with ABE may or may not have a new/rapidly changing cardiac murmur. If the endo-carditis is recent, there may have been sufficient valvular damage to result in a cardiac murmur. There is no indication to get a TTE/TEE to rule out endocarditis in patients without bacteremia. If a cardiac vegetation is demonstrated and no concomitant bacteremia is present from an organism that is a known endocarditis pathogen, then the vegetation is an incidental finding and not indicative of ABE. Sterile vegetations, also known as marantic endocarditis, may occur in association with malignancy as well as nonmalignant disorders, e.g., Liebman–Saks endocarditis. Therefore the diagnosis of *S. aureus* ABE rests on demonstrating a high-grade continuous bacteremia that is persistent in a patient with demonstrable vegetation by cardiac EKG, murmur may or may not be present. In non-IVDAs, the fever in ABE is usually $\geq 102°F$ (Table 3).

The treatment of MSSA/MRSA ABE is for four to six weeks of anti-staphy-lococcal therapy. For MSSA ABE, treatment is usually with oxacillin, nafcillin, and first-generation cephalosporins, e.g., cephazolin. In penicillin-allergic patients with MSSA/MRSA ABE, vancomycin quinupristin/dalfopristin, minocycline, linezolid, and daptomycin have been used. All of the drugs used to treat MRSA are also effec-tive against MSSA, but the reverse is not true. Because the therapy of MRSA/MSSA is prolonged, i.e., four to six weeks, oral therapy for all or part of the therapy is desirable. The only two antibiotics available to treat MRSA ABE orally are minocy-cline and linezolid. If fever/bacteremia persists after a week of appropriate therapy then the clinician should re-evaluate drug treatment to be sure that the drug is being dosed optimally, as well as the nonantibiotic causes of apparent antibiotic failure, i.e., myocardial abscess and noncardiac septic foci. If the problem is drug-related, daptomy-cin offers the best option for terminating the bacteremia/curing the endocarditis. Daptomycin is concentration-dependent on the killing kinetics and is the most potent anti-staphylococcal antibiotic available against MSSA/MRSA. Although the usual dose of daptomycin for bacteremia/ABE is 6 mg/kg (IV) q24 hours (with normal renal function), the dose of daptomycin may be increased if the patient is not responding to daptomycin or other anti-staphylococcal antibiotics. Daptomycin given at a dose of 12 mg/kg (IV) q24 hours (with normal renal function) has been used safely without side effects for over four weeks (36–44). If the problem is not drug-related and is related to a

Table 3 Infectious Complications of Central Venous Catheters

Intravenous line–related bacteremias
   Diagnostic features
      Low grade/short duration/discontinuous MSSA/MRSA bacteremias
      Temperatures usually ≤102°F
   Therapy
      Remove CVC
      Antibiotic therapy × 2 wks
Septic thrombophlebitis
   Diagnostic features
      IV line infection
      Usually high grade/continuous bacteremias
      Pus from CVC site when removed
      ± Palpable venous cord
      Temperatures usually ≥102°F
      TTE/TEE negative if no ABE
   Therapy
      Remove CVC
      Empiric antibiotic therapy × 2–4 wks
      ±Venotomy
MSSA/MRSA ABE
   Diagnostic features
      High grade/continuous bacteremia
      Cardiac vegetation by TTE/TEE
      Cardiac murmur may not be present early
      ESR ↑ usually 30–50 mm/hr range
      Teichoic acid antibody titers usually elevated (>1:4)
   Therapy
      Antibiotic treatment directed against MRSA until susceptibility
        to methicillin known. Treat MSSA or MRSA, ABE for 4–6 wks

Abbreviations: CVC, central venous catheters; IV, intravenous; TTE, transthoracic echocardiography; TEE, transesophageal echocardiography; MRSA, methicillin-resistant *S. aureus*; MSSA, methicillin-sensitive *S. aureus*; ESR, erythrocytes sedimentation rate; ABE, acute bacterial endocarditis.
Source: From Refs. 1, 39, 42.

protected focus, e.g., abscess myocardial, *S. aureus*, acute bacteremia meningitis, or extra cardiac septic complications, then surgical drainage may be needed to eradicate the infection.

REFERENCES

1. Cunha BA. Intravenous line infections. Crit Care Clin 1998; 8:339–346.
2. Sherertz RJ. Update on vascular catheter infections. Curr Opin Infect Dis 2004; 17: 303–307.
3. Seifert H, Jansen B, Farr BM. Catheter-related infections. 2d ed. New York: Marcel Dekker, 2004.
4. Maki DG. Infections caused by intravascular devices used for infusion therapy: pathogenesis, prevention, and management. In: Infections Associated with Indwelling Medical Devices. 2d ed. Washington: American Society for Microbiology, 1994.
5. Norwood S, Ruby A, Civetta J, Cortes V. Catheter-related infections and associated septicemia. Chest 1991; 99:968–975.

6. Johnson A, Oppenheim BA. Vascular catheter-related sepsis: diagnosis and prevention. J Hosp Infect 1992; 20:67–78.

7. Toltzis P, Goldman DA. Current issues in central venous catheter infection. Annu Rev Med 1990; 41:169–176.

8. Corona ML, Peters SG, Narr BJ, Thompson RL. Infections related to central venous catheters. Mayo Clin Proc 1990; 65:979–986.

9. Arnow PM, Quimosing EM, Beach M. Consequences of intravascular catheter sepsis. Clin Infect Dis 1993; 16:778–784.

10. Farr BM, Hanna H, Raad I. Nosocomial infections related to use of intravascular devices inserted for long term vascular access. In: Mayhall G, ed. Hospital Epidemiology and Infection Control. 3rd ed. Baltimore: Lippincott Williams & Wilkins, 2004.

11. Raad I, Bodey GP. Infectious complications of indwelling long-term central venous catheters. Infect Dis 1992; 15:197–210.

12. Clarke DE, Raffin. Infectious complications of indwelling long-term central venous catheters. Chest 1990; 97:966–972.

13. Sitges-Serra A, Pi-Suner T, Garces JM, Segura M. Pathogenesis and prevention of catheter-related septicemia. Am J Infect Control 1995; 23:310–316.

14. Read II, Hohn DC, Gilbreath J, et al. Prevention of central venous catheter-related infections by using maximal sterile barrier precautions during insertion. Infect Control Hosp Epidemol 1994; 15:231–238.

15. Early TF, Gregory RT, Wheeler JR, Snyder SO, Gayle RG. Increased infection rate in double lumen versus single lumen Hickman catheters in cancer patients. S Med J 1990; 83:34–36.

16. Moro ML, Vigano EF, Lepri AC. The Central Venous Catheter-Related Infections Study Group. Risk factors for central venous catheter-related infections in surgical and intensive care units. Infect Control Hosp Epidemiol 1994; 15:253–264.

17. Ullman RF, Gurevich I, Schoch PE, Cunha BA. Colonization and bacteremia related to duration of triple-lumen intravascular catheter placement. Am J Infect Control 1990; 18: 201–207.

18. Raad I, Costerton W, Sabharwal U, Sacilowski M, Anaissie E, Bodey GP. Ultrastructural analysis of indwelling vascular catheters: a quantitative relationship between luminal colonization and duration of placement. J Infect Dis 1993; 168:400–407.

19. Maki DG, Weise CE, Sarafin HW. A semiquantitative culture method for identifying intravenous-catheter-related infection. N Engl J Med 1977; 296:1305–1309.

20. Hill PC, Birch M, Chambers S, et al. Prospective study of 424 cases of Staphylococcus aureus bacteremia: determination of factors affecting incidence and mortality. Intern Med J 2001; 31:97–107.

21. Fatkenheuer G, Preuss M, Salzberger B, et al. Long term outcome and quality of care patients with Staphylococcus aureus bacteremia. Eur J Clin Microbiol Infect Dis 2004; 23:157–162.

22. Kim SH, Park WB, Lee KD, et al. Outcome of Staphylococcus aureus bacteremia in patients with eradicable foci versus noneradicable foci. Clin Infect Dis 2003; 37:794–797.

23. Mylotte JM, McDermott C. Staphylococcus aureus bacteremia caused by infected intravenous catheters. Am J Infect Control 1987; 15:1–6.

24. Malanoski GJ, Samore MH, Pefanis A, Karchmer AW. Staphylococcus aureus catheter-associated bacteremia. Arch Intern Med 1995; 155:1161–1166.

25. Jensen AG. Importance of focus identification in the treatment of Staphylococcus aureus bacteremia. J Hosp Infect 2002; 52:29–36.

26. Finkelstein R, Sobel JD, Nagler A, Merzbach D. Staphylococcus aureus bacteremia endocarditis: comparison of nosocomial community-acquired infection. J Med 1984; 15: 193–211.

27. Lesens O, Hansmann Y, Storck D, Christmann D. Risk factors for metastatic infection in patients with Staphylococcus aureus bacteremia with and without endocarditis. Eur J Intern Med 2003; 14:227–231.

28. Espersen F, Frimodt-Moller N. *Staphylococcus aureus* endocarditis: a review of 119 cases. Arch Intern Med 1986; 146:1118–1121.

29. Chang FY, MacDonald BB, Peacock JE, et al. A prospective multicenter study of *Staphylococcus aureus* bacteremia. Incidence of endocarditis, risk factors for mortality, and clinical impact of methicillin resistance. Medicine 2003; 82:322–332.

30. Bayer AS, Lam K, Ginzton L, Norman DC, Chiu CY, Ward JL. *Staphylococcus aureus* bacteremia: clinical serological echocardiographic findings in patients with and without endocarditis. Arch Intern Med 1987; 147:457–462.

31. Mirimanoff RO, Glauser MP. Endocarditis during *Staphylococcus aureus* septicemia in a population of non-drug addicts. Arch Intern Med 1982; 142:1311–1313.

32. Kaech C, Elzi L, Sendi P, et al. Course and outcome of *Staphylococcus aureus* bacterae-mia: a retrospective analysis of 308 episodes in a Swiss tertiary-care centre. Clin Microbio Infect 2006; 12:345–352.

33. Fowler VG Jr., Olsen MK, Corey GR, et al. Clinical identifiers of complicated *Staphylococcus aureus* bacteremia. Arch Intern Med 2003; 163:2066–2072.

34. Raad II, Sabbagh MF. Optimal duration of therapy for catheter-related *Staphylococcus aureus* bacteremia: a study of 55 cases and review. Clin Infect Dis 1992; 14:75–82.

35. Rupp ME, Lisco SJ, Lipsett PA, et al. Effect of a second-generation venous catheter impregnated with chlorhexidine and silver sulfadiazine on central catheter-related infections—a randomized, controlled trial. Ann Inter Med 2005; 143:570–580.

36. Sacks-Berg A, Strampfer MJ, Cunha BA. Intravenous line sepsis due to suppurative thrombophlebitis. Heart Lung 1987; 16:318–320.

37. Mayhall CG. Diagnosis and management of infections of implantable devices used for prolonged venous access. Curr Clin Top Infect Dis 1992; 12:83–110.

38. Cunha BA. Clinical usefulness of highly elevated teichoic acid antibody (TAA) titers. Infect Disease Pract 2005; 29:378–380.

39. Cunha BA. Persistent *S. aureus* bacteremia: a clinical approach. Infect Disease Pract 2005; 29:444–446.

40. Cunha BA, Hamid N, Kessler, Parchuri S. Daptomycin cure after cefazolin treatment fail-ure of Methicillin-sensitive *Staphylococcus aureus* (MSSA) tricuspid valve acute bacterial endocarditis from a peripherally inserted central catheter (PICC) line. Heart Lung 2005; 34:442–447.

41. Cunha BA, Eisenstein L, Hamid N. Pacemaker induced *S. aureus* mitral valve acute bacterial endocartitis complicated by persistent bacteremia from an infection coronary stent: cure with prolonged/high dose daptomycin without toxicity. Heart & Lung 2006; 35:217–222.

42. Cunha BA. Clinical manifestations and antimicrobial therapy of methicillin resistant *Staphylococcus aureus* (MRSA). Clinical Microbiology & Infection 2005; 11:33–42.

43. Cunha BA, ed. Antibiotic Essentials. 5th ed. Royal Oak, Michigan: Physicians Press, 2006.

14

Intra-Abdominal Surgical Infections and Their Mimics in the Critical Care Unit

Meghann L. Kaiser and Samuel E. Wilson
Department of Surgery, University of California, Irvine School of Medicine, Orange, California, U.S.A.

INTRODUCTION

Postsurgical patients in the intensive care unit (ICU) often confront a myriad of medical and new surgical complications. Among these, intra-abdominal infections remain the most formidable adversary, affecting an estimated 6% of all critically ill surgical patients. Organ dysfunction continues to be a major manifestation of these infections, resulting in a high mortality of 23% (1).

Intra-abdominal infection in the surgical ICU (SICU) patient may occur as a complication of a previous condition or arise de novo. In either event, it is evident that the critically ill patient is predisposed to a different set of disease states and pathogens than the clinician might routinely encounter. Moreover, given the complex background of concomitant illnesses in these individuals, physicians must be prepared to interpret a variety of atypical presentations. The burden of the diagnostician in the care of the ICU patient, however, remains not only of sensitivity but also of specificity; accordingly, the physician must be alert to a variety of clinical pictures that may masquerade as abdominal infection in the SICU patient. In this chapter, we will review the unique characteristics of intra-abdominal infections in critically ill patients, as well as the challenges faced in their diagnosis and treatment.

TERTIARY PERITONITIS

With a startling mortality of 20% to 50%, the diagnosis and treatment of tertiary peritonitis has remained a source of intense research for some time (2). Tertiary peritonitis, or intra-abdominal infection persisting beyond a failed surgical attempt to eradicate secondary peritonitis, represents a blurring of the clinical continuum, often characterized by the lack of typically presenting signs and symptoms. Nevertheless, prompt diagnosis is essential for cure, and given the grim propensity of this complication to strike already critically ill patients—rapidly devolving into multi-organ system failure—the intensivist should be equipped with the necessary knowledge to suspect, confirm, and treat this serious illness.

Early Recognition

The gradual postoperative transitional period between a diagnosis of secondary and tertiary peritonitis causes the clinical presentation of tertiary peritonitis to be quite subtle. Moreover, because patients are frequently sedated, intubated, or otherwise incapacitated, history and physical exam in the early stages of disease are often an insensitive means to a diagnosis. Therefore, the physician must pay particular attention to those secondary peritonitis patients whose conditions place them at risk, including malnutrition and the several variables detailed under the acute physiological and chronic health evaluation score (APACHE) II scoring system such as age, chronic health conditions, and certain physiologic abnormalities while in the ICU (3). In these individuals, fever, elevated C reactive protein (CRP), and leukocytosis—although admittedly nonspecific in the postsurgical patient—should be addressed quickly and assertively, even when lacking other evidence of infection, such as abdominal tenderness and absent bowel sounds (3). As one might reasonably predict, clinical evidence of tertiary peritonitis becomes increasingly more obvious the farther the disease has progressed, eventually leading to multi-organ system failure. To this end, further scoring systems have been developed to determine the probability that tertiary peritonitis is in fact present postsurgically. Two such systems, the Sepsis-related Organ Failure Assessment and the Goris scores, attempt to objectively sum the failure of the respiratory, cardiovascular, nervous, renal, hepatic and coagulation systems. Even though first postoperative day scores are elevated in patients both with and without tertiary peritonitis, subsequent second and third day scores are seen to fall in those without the disease, whereas remaining steady in patients later diagnosed by re-operation with tertiary peritonitis (4). Although these findings may be interesting and statistically significant, their clinical application—in overall terms of mortality avoided—remains to be proven. By pausing for evidence of changing widespread system failure over time, the clinician risks losing the opportunity to avoid medical catastrophe.

Radiologic tools, then, become a mainstay of the physician's investigation. Two such studies, gallium-67 scintigraphy and computed tomography (CT) scan, are commonly used for the detection of intra-abdominal infection. On the whole, CT is generally the preferred choice. At 97.1% accuracy, it is the more accurate of the two, with an enviable specificity of 100%. Isotope scans suffer in terms of accuracy for the postoperative patient because of false-positive uptake in areas of surgical injury. Moreover, CT has the potential to contribute both diagnostically and therapeutically in the care of patients, as will be discussed later. Finally, CT may be done on demand, whereas Ga-67 requires one to two days for concentration of the isotope at the site of infection. Scintigraphy, however, is not entirely without its own merits. With a sensitivity of 100% relative to 93.7% for CT, it is superior for uncovering early infection prior to the development of discreet fluid collections. Also, it is worth considering that in centers where indium-111 and technetium-99m exametazine-labeled leukocyte scans are available, a higher level of scintigraphy accuracy may be attained, albeit at greater expense. Furthermore, as an incidental advantage, nucleotide scanning has been known to reveal extra-abdominal infections such as pneumonia and cellulitis that might imitate tertiary peritonitis (5). Therefore, one might consider this as a second option for the relatively stable patient, in which CT has failed to provide a definitive answer but signs and symptoms persist. Other studies, such as plain film and ultrasound, are impaired by the nonspecific finding of intra-peritoneal free air and other features that might normally be expected in the postoperative patient (6).

Microbiology and Pathogenesis

The flora of tertiary peritonitis is different from that of secondary peritonitis. Whereas a culture of secondary peritonitis might produce a predominance of *Escherichia coli*, *Streptococci*, and *Bacteroides*—all normal gut flora—tertiary peritonitis is more apt to culture *Pseudomonas*, coagulase-negative *Staphylococcus*, *Enterococci*, and *Candida* (7,8). The obvious explanation for these differences is the mode of infection: secondary peritonitis is typically community acquired, but tertiary peritonitis occurs in an ICU setting. Time spent in the ICU necessarily implies that the patients affected are critically ill and likely already treated with antimicrobials. Some theorize that disease begins when the gut is weakened by surgical manipulation, hypoperfusion, antibiotic elimination of normal gut flora, and a lack of enteral feeding, thereby creating an opportunity for selected resistant native bacteria to translocate across the mucosal border (9). In fact, independent risk factors for postsurgical enterococcal infection include APACHE II scores greater than 12 and inadequate antibiotic coverage (8). Therefore, empiric antibiotic therapy should be broadly launched to cover the wide range of likely organisms, and later targeted to the specific determined pathogen and sensitivity. Appropriate first agents include, among others, carbapenems or the anti-pseudomonal penicillins, or a regimen of aminoglycosides with either clindamycin or metronidazole for the penicillin-allergic patient (6).

Treatment

When possible in selected patients, the treatment of tertiary peritonitis may be accomplished by image-guided percutaneous drainage of intra-abdominal abscesses, generally using CT. Percutaneous drainage is not without its inconveniences: complications such as fistulas, cellulitis, and obstructed, displaced, or prematurely removed drains occur in 20% to 40% of patients (10,11). Nevertheless, the efficacy of this technique is real: Cinat et al. found this method to be 90% successful in postoperative abscess. Abscesses involving the appendix, liver or biliary tract, and colon or rectum were also found to be particularly responsive at rates of 95%, 85% and 78%, respectively, although pancreatic abscesses and those involving yeast were correlated with poor outcomes by this treatment method (10). Khurrum Baig et al. echoed the success of percutaneous drainage in treating abscesses secondary to colorectal surgery, but questioned the applicability of these findings to patients with other than well-defined intra-abdominal abscesses (11).

Other considerations include planned relaparotomy and open management. Data is far from optimal, as these critically ill patients cannot ethically be randomized to different treatment groups. However, it would appear at this time that these strategies still result in an unacceptably high mortality of around 42% (12,13). A study by Schein found a particularly high mortality of 55% in the specific subgroup of diffuse postoperative peritonitis treated by planned relaparotomy, with or without open management. Furthermore, Schein went on to state that open management was associated with over twice the mortality of closed: 58% versus 24% (14). Although necessary flaws in study design make it difficult to say whether these approaches offer an advantage over the more traditional ones, it is nevertheless clear that they are far from ideal.

The hurdles in addressing the challenge of tertiary peritonitis have led to exploration of potential future therapies. Some are in keeping with traditional surgical/mechanical means: case studies have surfaced detailing the success of laparoscopy, even in the face of diffuse peritonitis and multiple abscesses (15). Other concepts favor a medicine-based approach, rooted in emerging ideas on the disease's basic pathology. As it is believed that bacteria migrate out of the intestines secondary to mucosal weakening, strategies that strengthen the mucosa, such as early postoperative enteral feeding or selective elimination of endogenous pathogenic bacteria, have each been tried with mixed results. Likewise, it has been argued that the progression from secondary to tertiary peritonitis represents a crippling of the body's immune system; in support of this belief, granulocyte colony stimulating factor and interferon-γ have each produced limited success in small patient groups, and successfully treated individuals all demonstrated some recovery of immune cell functioning. Another idea has been postulated that a relative lack of corticosteroid exists to fulfill the demands of extreme stress, and it has been seen that supplying patients with stress doses of hydrocortisone can dramatically improve the vascular effects of septic shock. Finally, some researchers have investigated the possibility that alleviating the hyper-catabolic state of patients with tertiary peritonitis might decrease mortality. Growth hormone and insulin-like growth factor-1 have both been tried with intermittent positive and negative outcomes (9).

NEW ONSET PERITONITIS

Antibiotic-associated *Clostridium difficile* Diarrhea in the ICU Patient

Epidemiology, Pathogenesis, and Risk Factors

The anaerobe *Clostridium difficile* causes twice as many cases of diarrhea as all other bacterial and protozoal causes combined. In hospitalized patients, *C. difficile* is responsible for 30% of diarrhea cases, and in hospitalized patients receiving antibiotic therapy—as is the case for many postsurgical patients—this number rises to an impressive 50% to 70%. *C. difficile*–associated diarrhea (CDAD), is theorized to arise in patients colonized by the pathogen when protective normal gut flora is simultaneously suppressed by broad-coverage antibiotic exposure. Although clindamycin, ampicillin, and the third-generation cephalosporins such as ceftazidime, ceftriaxone and cefotaxime are the most commonly associated antimicrobials, the newer, broader-spectrum quinolones such as gatifloxacin and moxifloxacin can also increase risk, and in fact any antibiotic, including, surprisingly, metronidazole and vancomycin, may rarely predispose patients to the disease. Other risk factors for CDAD include age, >60 years, the winter season, antineoplastic agents (especially methotrexate), recent gastrointestinal surgery, enemas, stool softeners, postpyloric enteric tube feedings (e.g., J-tubes), and even use of proton-pump inhibitors in hospitalized patients (16,17).

Diagnosis

A CDAD diagnosis is reached based on a number of clinical and laboratory findings such as low-grade fever, median leukocytosis of around 16,000 WBCs/mm^3, occasional hypoalbuminemia secondary to a protein-losing enteropathy, and, in 5% of patients, even the dramatic presentation of acute abdomen. Sigmoidoscopy, when performed in equivocal cases, will show whitish or yellowish pseudomembranes over-lying the mucosa in 41% of cases, and radiologic studies, although nonspecific, will often show signs of inflammation such as cecal dilatation, air–fluid levels, and mucosal thumbprinting. Even though diagnosis is often confirmed using the enzyme-linked immunoassay, it is worth bearing in mind that these tests are only about 85% sensitive. Even polymerase chain reaction (PCR), culture, and the cytotoxicity assay—considered to be the gold-standard in terms of specificity—are likewise imper-fect; therefore, a negative test result should not undermine the weight of sound clinical judgment when other likely causes of nosocomial diarrhea have been ruled out (16,17).

Treatment and Prevention

Therapy for mild cases may consist only of discontinuing the offending antibiotics, or switching to antibiotics less likely to perpetuate CDAD, such as aminoglycosides, macrolides, sulfonamides, or tetracyclines: up to a quarter of cases will resolve fol-lowing this step alone. For moderate-to-severe cases, metronidazole, either orally or intravenously, is the first line of therapy. In the 20% to 30% of patients who will relapse, a second course of metronidazole is recommended, followed by vancomycin enema for persistent symptomatic infection. Other treatments, such as intravenous immunoglobulin, cholestyramine which binds the bacterial toxin, and probiotics such as *Lactobacillus*, the yeast *Saccharomyces boulardii*, and even donor feces or "stool transplantations" to seed the re-growth of normal gut flora, have all been tried with success but as yet are not commonly done. Of course, prevention remains the most effective means of addressing the *C. difficile* dilemma, and precautions such as contact isolations for known carriers, conscientious hand-washing, gloves, and bleach disinfection of hospital surfaces, endoscopes and other equipment should never be overlooked (16,17).

Acalculous Cholecystitis

Acalculous cholecystitis, with its difficulty in diagnosis and attendant high mortality, should be a consideration in jaundiced postoperative patients. Although this disease occurs in only about 0.19% of SICU patients, it nevertheless accounts for around 14% of all acute cholecystitis patients, and the mortality ranges from 15% to 41% (18,19). With this in mind, physicians caring for high-risk populations should care-fully evaluate the signs and symptoms of this disease, and even a low level of clinical suspicion should prompt more thorough investigation.

Risk Factors and Pathophysiology

Although the pathogenesis of acalculous cholecystitis has not been entirely elucidated, it is apparent that the critically ill patient is particularly prone. Risk factors include recent trauma, burn injury, or nonbiliary tract operations, atherosclerosis, diabetes, hypertension, chronic renal failure, hemodynamic instability such as congestive heart failure or shock, and use of total parenteral nutrition (TPN) (18–21). One patient has been reported in the literature with acalculous cholecystitis secondary to a diaphrag-matic hernia mechanically obstructing the cystic duct (19). Only about 13% have a history indicative of gallbladder disease (21). Given these associations, it is likely that there are multiple triggering factors contributing to a common disease state. An experimental form of the disease is produced by a combination of decreased blood flow to the gallbladder, cystic duct obstruction, and bile concentration (21). It can be conjectured that a partially ischemic state, together with the effects of stasis, creates a favorable environment for the growth of enteric bacteria, ultimately leading to inflammation, often with accompanying gangrene, empyema, perforation, and abscess at rates much higher than those seen with calculous cholecystitis (18,20,21). *E. coli* is the organism most commonly isolated (19).

Presentation and Diagnosis

In addition to having one or more of the above risk factors, acalculous cholecystitis patients frequently present with the classical signs and symptoms of the calculous form, such as right upper quadrant pain, Murphy's sign, nausea and vomiting, abdominal distention, decreased bowel sounds, fever, jaundice, and abdominal mass (19,21); although patients with mental status changes often lack pain and other symptoms, absence of any one clue should not exclude such a serious possibility (18,22). Laboratory values suggesting the diagnosis include leukocytosis, hyperamylasemia, and elevated aminotransferases (22). Nevertheless, these findings are nonspecific, and given the likelihood of atypical presentation, the equivocal patient generally warrants radiologic and/or nucleotide (isotope) tests including ultrasound, CT scan, and cholescintigraphy such as hepatobiliary iminodiacetic acid (HIDA) scan. Of these, cholescintigraphy demonstrating an abnormal gallbladder ejection fraction of <40% in 45 minutes has been found most accurate, with a sensitivity of 90% to 100%, and a specificity of 88% (18,23); however, patients receiving TPN for a prolonged period may exhibit delayed gallbladder emptying, producing a false-positive result. CT detects roughly two-thirds of cases (18). Ultrasound, by contrast, when searching for the typical signs of thickened gallbladder wall, sludge, pericholecystic fluid, emphysematous change, and hydrops has recently been shown just 30% sensitive in critically ill trauma patients (23). Finally, diagnostic laparoscopy, although invasive, is nevertheless acceptably safe and allows direct visualization of the organ. In many cases, a combination of studies will be necessary to secure a diagnosis (24).

Treatment

Cholecystectomy, together with antibiotics, is the definitive treatment for acalculous cholecystitis. Laparoscopic surgery may be possible, and this being minimally invasive might be considered an attractive option in the critically ill patient. Surgeons, however, must be prepared to encounter many possible complications, including the increased likelihood of gangrene and empyema, both of which are difficult to manage laparoscopically, as well as the tendency to encounter adhesions in any postoperative patient. For poor surgical candidates, another treatment option is laparoscopic cholecystotomy. This procedure is safe and effective in relieving sepsis, but is contraindicated in the cases of gangrene and perforation, and of course, subject to all the limitations of laparoscopy (25). Appropriate antibiotic treatment would center on coverage of gut flora, such as a beta-lactamase inhibitor penicillin along with an anti-anaerobic agent.

Colorectal Anastomotic Leakage

Risk Factors, Prevalence, and Long-term Sequelae

Approximately 3% to 6% of large bowel surgical anastomoses constructed by experienced surgeons may leak. Anastomotic breakdown is the most common cause of stricture formation and also predisposes to increased local recurrence of cancer, a lower cancer specific survival, and poor colorectal function. Risk factors for anastomotic leakage include male gender, obesity, malnutrition, cardiovascular disease and other underlying chronic disease states, steroid use, alcohol abuse, smoking, inflammatory bowel disease, and preoperative pelvic irradiation. Specific operations that predispose to the development of a leak include emergency indications for surgery, low anterior resection, colorectal anastomoses, particularly difficult or long surgeries lasting over two hours, intraoperative septic conditions, and perioperative blood transfusions (26).

Diagnosis

The diagnosis of an anastomotic leak in the postoperative patient is relatively straightforward. A typical triad indicative of infection includes fever, leukocytosis, and pelvic pain. Given these signs and symptoms, together with the appropriate surgical history, anastomotic leakage should be high on the differential diagnosis. Other clues that might prompt clinical suspicion include absence of bowel sounds on postoperative day 4 or diarrhea before day 7, greater than 400 mL of fluid from an abdominal drain by day 3, and renal failure by day 3. Further evidence can be gleaned from CT scan with rectal contrast, which will reveal leakage of contrast with a sensitivity of 98%, as well as any abscesses that may be present as a result. CT is reported to be a superior modality to plain film with contrast enema, which in one review was positive in only 54% of patients who were later determined to have anastomotic breakdown (26).

Treatment

Following intravenous fluid resuscitation and antibiotic therapy to cover gut flora, laparotomy to lavage the abdominal cavity and either place a protecting stoma or an end colostomy is generally indicated for the more severe anastomotic leak. In less severe cases, where rectal contrast is seen to be contained by CT imaging, further surgery is not always necessary. In either event, any abscess formed must be drained, preferably percutaneously with CT guidance when possible (26).

Perforated Gastroduodenal Ulcer

Although markedly decreased in incidence by improved critical care management, gastroduodenal ulceration leading to perforation and peritonitis may complicate the course of ICU stays.

Risk Factors

Perforated ulcer represents yet another potential source of abdominal infection in the postoperative patient. Nonsurgical patients in the ICU are also predisposed to the development of ulcers. Curling's ulcers, or stress ulcers, affect in particular burn patients with septic complications; Cushing's ulcers develop in patients with central nervous system pathology involving midbrain damage, such as occurs after head trauma. In addition, many patients will be treated with nonsteroidal antiinflammatory drugs and exogenous steroids during their ICU stay, which may contribute to mucosal barrier breakdown and delay recognition of ensuing infection. Risk factors predicting ulcer perforation include smoking, exposure to nonsteroidal anti-inflammatory drugs, cocaine abuse, and *Helicobacter pylori* infection (27,28). Effective as they are, acid-suppressing drugs do not eliminate the risk entirely (29), and thus the possibility of ulcer perforation should be considered as an explanation of intra-abdominal infection in the ICU patient.

Presentation and Diagnosis

Perforation most typically presents as an acute abdomen with sudden onset of pain, occasionally accompanied by nausea and vomiting, diffuse abdominal tenderness, rigidity of the abdominal wall, and ileus. As with other illnesses, perforation in the ICU patient may manifest in less obvious ways. Plain abdominal and upright chest films exhibiting signs of free air may detect 85% of free perforations (30) and is often the radiologic modality of first choice. CT scan, although frequently rendered unnecessary in the face of a positive plain film, may nevertheless disclose a remaining few diagnoses: Chen et al. found pneumoperitoneum on CT to be 100% sensitive (31). Moreover, other signs such as fluid collections and soft tissue inflammation also demonstrated by CT may be of further help.

Treatment

Although there has been debate in recent years with regard to a 12-hour period of observation and supportive treatment before proceeding to surgical intervention for perforation, the poor prognosis associated with delay in definitive treatment and the relatively straightforward surgical procedure has persuaded many surgeons against this approach (28). Currently, direct suture repair, often with omental patch reinforcement, is the usual treatment of choice. Subsequent eradication of *H. pylori*—for example, using ampicillin, metronidazole, and a proton pump inhibitor, otherwise known as "triple therapy"—has been shown to decrease the recurrence of ulcers at one year from 38% to 5% (27).

Spontaneous Bacterial Peritonitis

Spontaneous bacterial peritonitis (SBP), is a bacterial infection of intraperitoneal ascitic fluid and resulting peritoneal inflammation that occurs in the absence of other inciting factors, e.g., a perforated viscus. With a 10% to 30% incidence of SBP among random hospital admissions of cirrhotic patients with ascites, and a mortality of 20% to 40% equivalent to that of an esophageal variceal bleed, SBP is a formidable threat to the cirrhotic ICU patient (32,33).

Risk Factors and Pathogenesis

SBP occurs when enteric bacteria, most commonly *E. coli*, *Klebsiella pneumoniae*, and *pneumococcus*, translocate across the gut mucosa to mesenteric lymph nodes. From there, impaired opsonization and phagocytosis in these patients allows bacteria to colonize the ascitic fluid and generate an inflammatory reaction. Hematogenous spread is the possible explanation for gram-positive monoisolates. Complications develop secondary to this inflammation, as intravascular blood volume drops and hepatorenal failure predictably ensues. Renal failure is, in fact, the most sensitive predictor of in-hospital mortality (33).

Although cirrhotic individuals comprise the vast majority of SBP patients, ascites from other etiologies may also become infected, including ascites secondary to fulminant hepatic failure, cardiac etiologies, nephrotic syndrome, and even

Budd-Chiari syndrome (33–36). Among patients with ascites, major additional independent risk factors include ongoing gastrointestinal hemorrhage, a previous episode of SBP, high serum bilirubin, and probably ascites protein <10 g/L (32).

Presentation, Diagnosis, and Differential Diagnosis

SBP generally presents with symptoms typical of peritonitis—e.g., fever, abdominal pain, ileus, diarrhea, vomiting, leukocytosis, and rarely, shock (32). Atypical presentations may consist of acute prerenal renal failure or sudden onset new hepatic encephalopathy with rapidly declining hepatic function. Given this wide range of potential signs and symptoms, SBP is no longer considered to be a purely clinical diagnosis, but is based principally on laboratory findings. The primary sensitive indicator of SBP is a polymorphonuclear (PMN) count of $>250/mm^3$ (in traumatic bloody taps, the total PMN count is corrected by subtracting one PMN per 250 red blood cells) (32). The high incidence of SBP warrants diagnostic paracentesis in cirrhotic patients with ascites and fever or abdominal findings immediately upon hospital admission, and additional paracenteses in any of these patients subsequently developing the signs and symptoms of peritonitis or gastrointestinal bleeding (32). Although a PMN count $>250/mm^3$ may be further supported by positive single organism ascites fluid cultures, this test is only about 60% sensitive even under optimal conditions—bedside aerobic and anaerobic cultures of 10 mL each into blood culture bottles—and moreover requires unacceptable delay as a practical indication of treatment (32). Although recent studies have shown promising results of 100% sensitivity in the diagnosis of SBP using certain urine reagent strips, these findings are not yet supported by sufficient experience to advocate their routine clinical use (37).

Secondary peritonitis is bacterial peritonitis secondary to a viscus perforation, surgery, abdominal wall infection, or any other acute inflammation of intra-abdominal organs. In the postsurgical ICU patient, differentiating SBP from secondary peritonitis is particularly challenging, yet nonetheless pivotal in determining appropriate management. Secondary peritonitis often occurs in the wake of obvious causes, but in settings where underlying issues are subtle, a diagnosis of SBP may be mistakenly seized and acted upon. Thus, a diagnosis of secondary peritonitis should generally be considered when patients fail antibiotic therapy for SBP. Characteristics of ascites fluid strongly favoring secondary peritonitis over SBP include isolation of multiple organisms, isolation of anaerobic or fungal organisms, or an ascites glucose level <50 mg/dL with a protein concentration of >10 g/L and lactic dehydrogenase concentration greater than that of normal serum. These indicators are all very sensitive but nonspecific for a diagnosis of secondary peritonitis, and their presence must be weighed against the remaining clinical picture before any firm diagnoses are reached (32).

Treatment and Prognosis

Initial empiric treatment for SBP must cover gram-negative aerobic bacteria from the family of *Enterobacteriacae* as well as nonenterococcal *Streptococcal* species, and must adequately penetrate into the peritoneal fluid. Low dose, short course cefotaxime—2 g twice a day for five days—is generally considered the first line therapy, but other cephalosporins such as cefonicid, ceftriaxone, ceftizoxime, and ceftazidime are equally effective, and even oral, lower cost antibiotics such as amoxicillin with clavulanic acid will achieve similar results. For patients with penicillin allergy, oral fluoroquinolones such as ofloxacin are yet another suitable option, except in those with a history of failed quinolone prophylaxis implying probable resistance.

Follow-up paracentesis is recommended after 48 hours of antibiotic therapy to assess response: a fall >25% in the number of ascites PMN cells is considered a success (32).

However, antimicrobials are not the only means of management: because renal impairment secondary to decreased intravascular volume is a major cause of mortality in SBP, further management may be aimed at preventing this fluid shift. The addition of albumin to an antibiotic regimen has been shown to decrease in-hospital mortality almost two-thirds from 28% to 10%. It is considered especially beneficial for patients with already impaired renal function and a creatinine >91 µmol/L, or advanced liver disease as evidenced by serum bilirubin >68 µmol/L (33). Nevertheless, the future outlook for patients with SBP is bleak: of those that survive the initial episode 30% to 50% will survive one year further, and only 25% to 30% will live a second year. Given these odds, patients with a history of SBP should be considered for liver transplantation, as well as long-term antibiotic prophylaxis in the interim (33).

Prophylaxis

On weighing the cost of antimicrobials and the threat of inducing antibiotic resistance against the gravity of SBP, prophylaxis is indicated only for patients with the highest risk, namely, those with a previous episode of SBP, ongoing gastrointestinal bleeding, or an ascitic fluid protein <10 g/L. Fluoroquinolones, such as norfloxacin and ciprofloxacin, are the antimicrobials recommended for prophylactic purposes (33). In cirrhotic patients with ascites lacking these risk factors, the one- and three-year incidences of SBP are 0% and 3% respectively, and do not justify regular long-term prophylaxis (32).

INFECTIOUS COMPLICATIONS OF PANCREATITIS

Pancreatitis is a serious but generally self-limited disorder, which spontaneously resolves in 48 to 72 hours for the great majority of patients; however, 20% will develop severe acute pancreatitis as defined by the presence of three or more Ranson criteria (38). Among this subset, infected pancreatic necrosis is the leading cause of death (39).

Presentation and Diagnosis

In addition to the typical signs and symptoms of pancreatitis such as moderate epigastric pain radiating to the back, vomiting, tachycardia, fever, leukocytosis, and elevated amylase and lipase, patients with severe acute pancreatitis present with relatively greater abdominal tenderness, distension, and even symptoms of accompanying multiorgan failure (38). In these patients, the intensivist must maintain a high level of clinical suspicion for necrosis and possibly infection as well. CT scan with intravenous contrast is 80% to 90% sensitive for the detection of necrotic areas as a focal lack of enhancement (40). Infection is estimated to develop in 30% to 70% of patients with necrotic pancreatitis (40). However, necrosis both with and without infection often manifest with similar clinical presentations because necrosis alone causes a systemic inflammatory response, and additional diagnostic data is generally needed to differentiate these (41). Although CT only rarely shows gas bubbles as evidence of necrotic infection, CT-guided percutaneous aspiration of necrotic areas is 90% sensitive in yielding a diagnosis of this complication, and by sampling multiple necrotic areas in a diffusely necrotic pancreas, detection may be higher still (40).

Enterococcus species are the organisms most frequently isolated, although many different pathogens including *Candida* species and *Pseudomonas aeruginosa* are frequently seen (38,42).

Treatment and Prophylaxis

The distinction between sterile and infected necrotic pancreatitis is crucial, as the former may be handled medically when necrosis affects less than 30% of the organ, whereas the latter often demands surgical debridement (38). Patients with infected necrotic pancreatitis will return to the operating room for an average of two to three operations as determined necessary by recurrence of clinical signs and symptoms combined with evidence from follow-up postoperative CT scans (41). Recently, several studies have explored the potential of laparoscopy for infectious pancreatic necrosis, but this approach is rarely feasible in instances of extensive necrosis, and data is not yet sufficient to compare the safety and efficacy of laparoscopic surgery versus laparotomy for this indication (43). Percutaneous drainage has a low success rate of just 32% and is generally insufficient management except in the case of a well-defined abscess, or one remote from the pancreas (41). Runzi et al., recently published a small study in which antimicrobial therapy alone resulted in similar outcomes to antimicrobials combined with surgery (42); however, nonsurgical management is not currently common practice for infectious necrotic pancreatitis.

An appropriate antibiotic regimen is the second arm of a successful treatment plan: given the wide range of possible offending organisms, a gram stain is recommended to tailor specific initial therapies prior to culture results. For gram-negative organisms, a single agent quinolone or carbapenen is effective; for gram-positives β-lactamase–resistant drugs, vancomycin, and even linezolid must considered. When yeast are identified, high dose fluconazole or caspofungin should be sufficient. In any case, if infection develops despite antibiotic prophylaxis, a different class of drugs must be administered for treatment than was given for prophylaxis (43).

A meta-analysis by Bassi et al. found that antimicrobial prophylaxis for patients with necrotic pancreatitis successfully decreases the incidence of infection by half and triples overall survival (44). Although current literature does not specifically favor any specific antibiotic as prophylaxis, it is nonetheless clear that microbial coverage must be broadly targeted. One to two week courses of cefuroxime, imipenem with cilastin, and ofloxacin with metronidazole have each been tried with success (42).

MIMICS OF ABDOMINAL INFECTION

Multiple conditions may mimic a postsurgical abdominal infection and must be considered when searching for diagnosis. An exhaustive list of these is beyond on the scope of this chapter; however, the reader should be aware of the general possibilities. Fever, for instance, in the postoperative patient, is not always secondary to infection. Particularly relevant to the postsurgical patient are events such as atelectasis, myocardial infarction, stroke, hematoma formation and even pulmonary embolism that may occasionally present with a fever component. Other causes that warrant deliberation include drug or transfusion reaction, malignancy, collagen vascular disease, endocrine causes such as hyperthyroidism, and less common etiologies such as disordered heat homeostasis secondary to an ischemic hypothalamic injury or even familial malignant hyperthermia. Pain is yet another symptom that may be misleading: Abadir et al. published a study in which patients with segmental infarction of the omentum or epiploic appendages presented with localized peritonitis, mimicking appendicitis, diverticulitis, and cholecystitis (45). Furthermore, it is important to interpret radiological findings with an open mind. A fluid collection on CT does not necessarily represent an abscess. Again, high on the differential that must be considered is hematoma, and one may explore other diagnoses given the individual patient history. For example, Yu et al. found that the fundus of the excluded stomach following gastric bypass surgery may fill with air, fluid, and contrast material, thus closely resembling a loculated fluid collection (46). Finally, entertain where appropriate the idea of extra-abdominal infections. A myocardial infarction involving the inferior wall of the heart and lower lobe pneumonias, for instance, may present with abdominal pain and fever despite extra-abdominal origins.

DE NOVO COINCIDENTAL INTRA-ABDOMINAL INFECTION

When presenting an overview on the topic of postoperative abdominal infection, it is worth mentioning for completeness' sake the possibility of coincidental infection. A patient status post-aneurysm repair has the same likelihood of developing appendicitis, for example, as any member of the general population in the same age group. Therefore, the conscientious physician considers all possibilities appropriate for the patient's complete history—not surgical history only—when constructing a thorough differential.

REFERENCES

1. Barie PS, Hydo LJ, Eachempati SR. Longitudinal outcomes of intra-abdominal infection complicated by critical illness. Surg Infect (Larchmt) 2004; 5(4):365–373.
2. Evans HL, Raymond DP, Pelletier SJ, et al. Diagnosis of intra-abdominal infection in the critically ill patient. Curr Opin Crit Care 2001; 7(2):117–121.
3. Malangoni MA. Evaluation and management of tertiary peritonitis. Am Surg 2000; 66(2): 157–161.
4. Paugam-Burtz C, Dupont H, Marmuse JP, et al. Daily organ-system failure for diagnosis of persistent intra-abdominal sepsis after postoperative peritonitis. Intensive Care Med 2002; 28(5):594–598.
5. Tsai SC, Chao TH, Lin WY, et al. Abdominal abscesses in patients having surgery: an application of Ga-67 scintigraphic and computed tomographic scanning. Clin Nucl Med 2001; 26(9):761–764.
6. Marshall JC. Intra-abdominal infections. Microbes Infect 2004; 6(11):1015–1025.
7. Marshall JC, Innes M. Intensive care unit management of intra-abdominal infection. Crit Care Med 2003; 31(8):2228–2237.
8. Sitges-Serra A, Lopez MJ, Girvent M, et al. Postoperative enterococcal infection after treatment of complicated intra-abdominal sepsis. Br J Surg 2002; 89(3):361–367.
9. Buijk SE, Bruining HA. Future directions in the management of tertiary peritonitis. Intensive Care Med 2002; 28(8):1024–1029.
10. Cinat ME, Wilson SE, Din AM. Determinants for successful percutaneous image-guided drainage of intra-abdominal abscess. Arch Surg 2002; 137(7):845–849.
11. Khurrum Baig M, Hua Zhao R, Batista O, et al. Percutaneous postoperative intra-abdominal abscess drainage after elective colorectal surgery. Tech Coloproctol 2002; 6(3): 159–164.

12. Christou NV, Barie PS, Dellinger EP, et al. Surgical Infection Society intra-abdominal infection study. Prospective evaluation of management techniques and outcome. Arch Surg 1993;128(2):193–198.
13. Bosscha K, Hulstaert PF, Visser MR, et al. Open management of the abdomen and planned reoperations in severe bacterial peritonitis. Eur J Surg 2000; 166(1):44–49.
14. Schein M. Planned reoperations and open management in critical intra-abdominal infections: prospective experience in 52 cases. World J Surg 1991; 15(4):537–545.
15. Hakimi AA, White NB, Hodgson WJ. Laparoscopic repair of intraabdominal abscesses in a septic patient. Surg Rounds 2005; 123–127.
16. Oldfield EC. *Clostridium difficile*-associated diarrhea: risk factors, diagnostic methods, and treatment. Rev Gastroenterol Disord 2004; 4(4):186–195.
17. Riley TV. Nosocomial diarrhoea due to *Clostridium difficile*. Curr Opin Infect Dis 2004; 17(4):323–327.
18. Kalliafas S, Ziegler DW, Flancbaum L, et al. Acute acalculous cholecystitis: incidence, risk factors, diagnosis, and outcome. Am Surg 1998; 64(5):471–475.
19. Coelho JC, Campos AC, Moreira M, et al. Acute acalculous cholecystitis. Int Surg 1991; 76(3):146–148.
20. Ryu JK, Ryu KH, Kim KH. Clinical features of acute acalculous cholecystitis. J Clin Gastroenterol 2003; 36(2):166–169.
21. Howard RJ. Acute acalculous cholecystitis. Am J Surg 1981; 141(2):194–198.
22. Owen CC, Jain R. Acute acalculous cholecystitis. Curr Treat Options Gastroenterol 2005; 8(2):99–104.
23. Puc MM, Tran HS, Wry PW, et al. Ultrasound is not a useful screening tool for acute acalculous cholecystitis in critically ill trauma patients. Am Surg 2002; 68(1):65–69.
24. Brandt CP, Priebe PP, Jacobs DG. Value of laparoscopy in trauma ICU patients with suspected acute acalculous cholecystitis. Surg Endosc 1994; 8(5):361–364.
25. Yang HK, Hodgson WJ. Laparoscopic cholecystostomy for acute acalculous cholecystitis. Surg Endosc 1996; 10(6):673–675.
26. Chambers WM, Mortensen NJ. Postoperative leakage and abscess formation after colorectal surgery. Best Pract Res Clin Gastroenterol 2004; 18(5):865–880.
27. Behrman SW. Management of complicated peptic ulcer disease. Arch Surg 2005; 140(2): 201–208.
28. Svanes C. Trends in perforated peptic ulcer: incidence, etiology, treatment, and prognosis. World J Surg 2000; 24(3):277–283.
29. Gunshefski L, Flancbaum L, Brolin RE, et al. Changing patterns in perforated peptic ulcer disease. Am Surg 1990; 56(4):270–274.
30. Grassi R, Romano S, Pinto A, et al. Gastro-duodenal perforations: conventional plain film, US and CT findings in 166 consecutive patients. Eur J Radiol 2004; 50(1):30–36.
31. Chen CH, Huang HS, Yang CC, et al. The features of perforated peptic ulcers in conventional computed tomography. Hepatogastroenterology 2001; 48(41):1393–1396.
32. Rimola A, Garcia-Tsao G, Navasa M, et al. Diagnosis, treatment and prophylaxis of spontaneous bacterial peritonitis: a consensus document. International Ascites Club J Hepatol 2000; 32(1):142–153.
33. Mowat C, Stanley AJ. Review article: spontaneous bacterial peritonitis—diagnosis, treatment and prevention. Aliment Pharmacol Ther 2001; 15(12):1851–1859.
34. Shaked Y, Samra Y. Primary pneumococcal peritonitis in patients with cardiac ascites: report of 2 cases. Cardiology 1988; 75(5):372–374.
35. Ackerman Z. Ascites in Nephrotic syndrome. Incidence, patients' characteristics, and complications. J Clin Gastroenterol 1996; 22(1):31–34.
36. Barrio J, Castiella A, Gil I, et al. Spontaneous bacterial peritonitis by campylobacter fetus in Budd-Chiari syndrome without liver cirrhosis. Liver 1999; 19(1):69–70.
37. Kramer L, Druml W. Ascites and intraabdominal infection. Curr Opin Crit Care 2004; 10(2):146–151.

38. Malangoni MA, Martin AS. Outcome of severe acute pancreatitis. Am J Surg 2005; 189(3):273–277.
39. Mishra G, Pineau BC. Infectious complications of pancreatitis: diagnosis and management. Curr Gastroenterol Rep 2004; 6(4):280–286.
40. Choe KA. Imaging in pancreatic infection. J Hepatobiliary Pancreat Surg 2003; 10(6): 401–405.
41. Lee MJ, Wittich GR, Mueller PR. Percutaneous intervention in acute pancreatitis. Radiographics 1998; 18(3):711–724.
42. Runzi M, Niebel W, Goebell H, et al. Severe acute pancreatitis: nonsurgical treatment of infected necroses. Pancreas 2005; 30(3):195–199.
43. Solomkin JS, Umanskiy K. Intraabdominal sepsis: newer interventional and antimicrobial therapies for infected necrotizing pancreatitis. Curr Opin Crit Care 2003; 9(5):424–427.
44. Bassi C, Lavin M, Villatoro E. Antibiotic therapy for prophylaxis against infection of pancreatic necrosis in acute pacreatitis. Conchrane Database Syst Rev 2003; CD002941.
45. Abadir JS, Cohen AJ, Wilson SE. Accurate diagnosis of infarction of omentum and appendices epiploicae by computed tomography. Am Surg 2004; 70(10):854–857.
46. Yu J, Turner MA, Cho SR, et al. Normal anatomy and complications after gastric bypass surgery: helical CT findings. Radiology 2004; 231(3):753–760.

15

Clostridium difficile–associated Diarrhea and Colitis in the Critical Care Unit

Marci Drees
Department of Geographic Medicine and Infectious Diseases,
Tufts-New England Medical Center, Boston, Massachusetts, U.S.A.

Sherwood L. Gorbach
Nutrition/Infection Unit, Department of Public Health and Family Medicine,
Tufts University School of Medicine, Boston, Massachusetts, U.S.A.

OVERVIEW

History

Pseudomembranous colitis (PMC) was first recognized by J.M. Finney and William Osler in 1893. Rare in the pre-antibiotic era, PMC was primarily associated with colonic, pelvic, or gastric surgery (1). In the 1950s, PMC was linked to antibiotic use; *Staphylococcus aureus* was frequently isolated from stool cultures in patients with PMC and was its presumed etiology. In the early 1970s, the disease became known as "clindamycin colitis" because of strong linkage to that particular antibiotic. Later in that decade *Clostridium difficile* proved to be the cause. Since that time, *C. difficile* infection has been nearly exclusively associated with use of various types of antibiotics and has become a major and growing problem in hospitals worldwide.

Definitions

Antibiotic-associated diarrhea (AAD) is defined as otherwise unexplained diarrhea associated with antibiotic use. Only 10% to 30% of AAD is attributable to *C. difficile* (2–5), and is known as *C. difficile*–associated diarrhea (CDAD). However, *C. difficile* causes the majority (60–75%) of the more severe form, antibiotic-associated colitis, and 96 to 100% of PMC (3).

Epidemiology

The overall attack rate of AAD in hospitals is 3.2% to 29% (5). Over 300,000 cases of CDAD occur annually in the United States alone, with an incidence among hospitalized and long-term care patients of 25 to 60 cases per 100,000 bed-days (6).

In acute care hospital patients, incidence ranges from 1 to 10 cases per 1000 discharges, but can vary significantly even within a single hospital (5). The risk of acquiring *C. difficile* while hospitalized directly relates to length of hospital stay, with 13% colonization after two weeks and 50% at greater than four weeks of hospitalization (1,7). Overall, approximately 20% of hospitalized patients become colonized, whereas 8% develop diarrhea (8). Incidence is higher during winter, which may reflect increased patient census, severity of illness, and antibiotic use due to high rates of respiratory infections (7). Outpatient cases are much less common, accounting for around 20,000 cases per year in the United States (7.7 cases per 100,000 person-years) (6). A retrospective cohort study of 265,000 health maintenance organization members found the overall risk of CDAD at less than one case per 10,000 antibiotic prescriptions (5).

Even though *C. difficile* is not nationally notifiable in the United States, data from the National Nosocomial Infections Surveillance System indicates that the incidence of *C. difficile* disease increased significantly during 1987–2001 (7). Several studies have reported recent increases in both incidence and severity of CDAD in the United States, Canada, and the United Kingdom (9). In Oregon, a 1994 to 2000 cohort of patients with CDAD had a 15.3% mortality rate, compared with 3.5% mortality during the previous 10 years (10). In Quebec, annual incidence increased from 35.6 cases per 100,000 population in 1991 to 156.3 cases per 100,000 in 2003. Among patients ≥65 years, incidence increased from 867 to 1681 cases per 100,000. Disturbingly, the case-fatality rate also increased from 4.7% in 1991 to 13.8% in 2003 (11). Seventy-nine deaths have been reported during 2003 and early 2004 (12). The reasons behind this increase in incidence and severity of disease may include increasing illness severity, changes in antimicrobial and other medication [such as proton pump inhibitor (PPI)] use, and diminished resources for housekeeping and infection control; it has also been suggested that there has been introduction of new strains of *C. difficile* with increased virulence and transmissibility (13).

C. difficile infection has significant economic ramifications. CDAD can add up to two weeks of hospitalization, at a cost of $6000 to $10,000 per case (4). On average, each case of CDAD adds $2000 to $5000 to the cost of health care (5,14). The mean lifetime cost for recurrent CDAD has been estimated at nearly $11,000 per case (5). Overall, *C. difficile* incurs an estimated $1 billion in health care costs in the United States annually (15).

Transmission

C. difficile is ubiquitous, persisting as a highly resistant spore that may survive for months in the environment. The gastrointestinal tracts of young mammals, including humans, appear to be a reservoir. It has been cultured from soil, swimming pools, and salt, fresh, and tap water (5). In the hospital setting, it has been cultured from telephones, call buttons, shoes of health care workers, fingernails, and numerous other objects (1). *C. difficile* is transmitted via the fecal-oral route, either directly (hand carriage by health care workers and patient-to-patient contact) or indirectly (from contaminated environments) (7). *C. difficile* has been found in infected patients' rooms up to 40 days after discharge (1). Fecal carriage among health care workers is rare. Most cases of disease appear to be caused by acquisition of the organism from an exogenous source, rather than from endogenous colonization; in fact, colonization with either toxigenic or nontoxigenic strains appears to protect from clinical disease (5).

Risk Factors

Antibiotic use is clearly the major risk factor for CDAD. Normal intestinal flora consists of 10^{11} to 10^{12} bacteria per gram of feces, with over 100 distinct, primarily anaerobic, species. Together these bacteria exert a protective effect, known as "colonization resistance" (16), against *C. difficile* by depleting carbon sources required for *C. difficile* growth (5), prevention of access to adherence sites, and production of inhibitory substances (16). Antibiotics alter this normal gut flora, allowing overgrowth of *C. difficile*. Although longer duration of antibiotic use confers greater risk of CDAD, cases following a single dose, such as for perioperative prophylaxis, have been reported (4). Parenteral and oral antibiotics bestow similar levels of risk (4). Some hospitalized patients develop CDAD without any antibiotic exposure. One study found that 18 (11%) of 157 hospitalized patients with CDAD had no prior antibiotic exposure; 12 such patients were immunocompromised (10).

Although initially attributed to clindamycin use, CDAD can be caused by any antibiotic, including metronidazole, antifungal, and antiviral medications. However, certain antibiotics have clearly stronger association with CDAD (Table 1). Antibiotics with significant antianaerobic activity, and to which *C. difficile* has either innate or acquired resistance, pose the highest risk. Clindamycin, penicillins, and cephalosporins are most commonly associated with CDAD. Clindamycin-resistant strains have been responsible for large outbreaks in multiple hospitals (14,17). In this setting, clindamycin use is significantly associated with disease caused by the epidemic strain, whereas the use of other antibiotics is not (17). Cephalosporins have higher attributable risk for CDAD given their higher usage rates compared to clindamycin (18). Among cephalosporins, ceftriaxone in particular has been implicated due to extensive biliary excretion resulting in high fecal concentrations (19). Recent studies have also linked CDAD to fluoroquinolones (18,20), particularly the newer quinolones, such as gatifloxacin, with expanded anti-anaerobic spectrum (21). Odds ratios (OR)

Table 1 Levels of Risk of *Clostridium difficile*–associated Diarrhea Among Various Antimicrobial Agents

High risk
  Clindamycin
  Second and third generation cephalosporins, particularly ceftriaxone
  Ampicillin, amoxicillin, and extended-spectrum penicillins
Medium risk
  Quinolones, particularly newer generation
  First-generation cephalosporins
  Narrow-spectrum penicillins (aside from amoxicillin and ampicillin)
  Carbapenems
  Ureidopenicillins (piperacillin, ticarcillin)
  Tetracycline
  Macrolides
  Trimethoprim
  Sulfonamides
Low risk
  Aminoglycosides
  Vancomycin
  Metronidazole
  Bacitracin

for acquiring CDAD range from 15.6 to 42 for clindamycin, 1.4 to 28.6 for cephalosporins, 3.4 to 4.9 for penicillins, and 3.1 for vancomycin. Use of multiple antibiotics is associated with an OR of 1.6 to 22.6 (22). Anticancer drugs, such as cisplatin and the antimetabolite methotrexate, inhibit mitosis of intestinal epithelial cells and may create an environment suitable for *C. difficile* proliferation (23). These drugs as well as paclitaxel have been associated with CDAD (24).

Host factors play an essential role in determining outcome after exposure to antibiotics and to *C. difficile*. Intrinsic predisposing host factors include advanced age, severity of underlying disease, bedridden status, documented underlying infection (8,14), renal failure (22), hematologic malignancy, transplantation (particularly lung) (9), burns, and gastrointestinal disease, including functional or structural bowel obstruction (25). The risk for CDAD was found to be eight times greater for patients with severe underlying disease compared to those with mild/moderate disease (8). HIV per se is not a risk factor for CDAD, and data is conflicting whether HIV-positive patients develop more severe disease (5). Iatrogenic predisposing factors include use of any agent, such as laxatives or narcotics, that alters gastrointestinal motility (5), gastrointestinal surgery, tube feeding, PPI use, and use of medical devices (7). Regarding tube feeding, *C. difficile* is often not actively investigated because nearly 60% of tube-fed patients develop diarrhea, which is frequently attributed to tube feeding formulas. However, one case–control study of 76 tube-fed patients found a ninefold risk of developing CDAD (11-fold among those with postpyloric tips) (26). This may be due to direct inoculation during feeding tube manipulation, lack of protective dietary fiber in the formulations, or bypassing of the acidic stomach pH. Even though spores are not affected, stomach acid kills vegetative cells, decreasing the inoculum by 99% (16,26). Similarly, potent acid suppression may facilitate survival of *C. difficile*, as well as alter the gastrointestinal flora (27). A multivariate analysis found that among 81 patients who developed CDAD, use of PPI, but not H2 blockers, was significantly associated with CDAD (OR 2.1, 95% CI 1.2–3.5) (27). Among 21 patients with relapsing disease, 19 (90%) were receiving PPIs, compared to 35 (65%) of those without relapses (OR 5.2, 95% CI 1.1–24.6) (27).

Host immune response plays a particularly vital role in determining whether patients become colonized or develop clinical disease. The majority (>60%) of older children and adults have detectable antibodies against *C. difficile* toxins (6), and serum levels of antitoxin A IgG rise rapidly after colonization, indicating a systemic amnestic response to the toxin (8). Serum IgG and IgA and mucosal IgA all appear to be involved in protection (6). Serum antitoxin A IgG and fecal antitoxin A IgA levels are higher in patients who develop mild CDAD than in those with prolonged, severe diarrhea (8). For patients with severe underlying disease, 88% of those with IgG levels ≤3.0 enzyme linked immunosorbent assay (ELISA) units developed CDAD, compared to 20% with higher levels; among patients with mild to moderate underlying disease, 43% with low IgG levels developed CDAD, versus none with higher levels. Using multiple logistic regression analysis, the odds of developing CDAD for patients with serum IgG levels ≤3.0 ELISA units were 48 times greater than for those with IgG levels > 3.0 units, after adjustment for age, sex, and severity of disease (8).

Another study found fewer macrophages and IgA-producing cells in patients with CDAD, particularly in those with PMC, compared to controls with non–*C. difficile* diarrhea (28). Immune response also appears important in relapsing disease; children with recurrent CDAD had lower serum IgG against toxin A than controls (6). There is no evidence that serum antibodies are protective against colonization (8).

MICROBIOLOGY

C. difficile is a gram-positive, large (2–17 μm), spore-forming anaerobic bacillus. It is closely related to *C. sordellii* but not to other toxigenic Clostridia, such as *C. perfringens*, *C. botulinum*, and *C. tetani*. Difficult to isolate in the laboratory (hence its name), *C. difficile* can be grown on highly selective cefoxitin, cycloserine, and fructose agar media (5). *C. difficile* colonizes the luminal surface of the colon but is generally noninvasive. Outside of the gastrointestinal tract, *C. difficile* demonstrates low pathogenicity, although it may enhance that of other bacteria in mixed infections (29).

C. difficile produces two heat-labile protein exotoxins (toxins A and B), the largest known bacterial toxins (30). These toxins are optimally expressed at body temperature (5). Purified toxins are capable of causing the full spectrum of disease (15). Although most strains produce both toxins, some produce toxin B only but can be equally pathogenic. Nontoxigenic *C. difficile* strains are not believed to cause human disease, although rare cases of CDAD caused by strains producing neither toxin A nor B have been reported (6). Toxigenic strains are not equally virulent; some strains that clearly possess toxin genes demonstrate low levels of gene transcription, resulting in minimal toxin production (31).

Toxin A is a 308-kDa enterotoxin that produces acute inflammation, induces fluid secretion, and causes necrosis of the epithelium in the rabbit ileal loop model (30). Toxin B is a 270-kDa cytotoxin that is more potent than toxin A in tissue culture (6). The toxins appear to act synergistically (15). Both toxins are internalized and inactivate proteins in the Rho subfamily, which regulate the F-actin cytoskeleton. This results in disaggregation of actin, opening the tight junctions between cells, and resulting in characteristic cell rounding and cell death (6,15). Both toxins are also pro-inflammatory, inducing release of cytokines, phospholipase A2, platelet-activating factor (30), tumor necrosis factor–α, and substance P (9). This results in activation of the enteric nervous system, leading to neutrophil chemotaxis and fluid secretion. *C. difficile* also produces tissue degradation enzymes, such as collagenase and hyaluronidase (1). Some strains also produce an actin-specific binary toxin, which is encoded by the *cdtA* and *cdtB* genes and is cytotoxic to Vero cells in culture. Binary toxin has been associated with more severe *C. difficile* disease, but whether strains possessing binary toxin are truly more pathogenic requires further study (32). One study found that 10.3% (22/214) of toxigenic strains harbored this binary toxin (33), but 65.3% (32/49) of strains in a recent hospital outbreak demonstrated *cdtA* and *cdtB* genes (8).

AAD can be caused by other enteric pathogens. Although generally recognized as a cause of food poisoning, several studies have found evidence of enterotoxigenic strains of *C. perfringens* type A in patients with AAD but not in controls. Elderly hospitalized patients seem to be at particular risk (34). As mentioned above, *S. aureus* was routinely found in cases of PMC prior to the discovery of *C. difficile*; although it is felt that this largely represents misdiagnosis, as *S. aureus* may have the potential to cause a similar syndrome. *Candida albicans* has been found in large quantities (>100,000 organisms/g stool) in patients with AAD who subsequently improved after receiving antifungal therapy, but it remains unclear whether this represents true infection. *Salmonella* species have also been shown to cause PMC and have been implicated in rare cases of AAD. However, testing for these organisms is not routinely done.

CLINICAL PRESENTATION

Most patients exposed to *C. difficile*, even after antibiotic exposure, become asymptomatically colonized. Colonization rates of 25% to 80% are seen in healthy infants and neonates (1), but clinical illness is rare. For unclear reasons, colonization appears to wane with advancing age, and only 3% of healthy adults are colonized. Colonization increases to 20% to 30% of hospitalized adults (4), but clinical symptoms develop in only one-third of those who become colonized (6). Once colonization is established, the risk of symptomatic CDAD decreases (1).

Symptoms can begin within the first day of antibiotic use, or up to six weeks after completion of the antibiotic course (6). Most commonly, symptoms develop within four to nine days (1). Diarrhea is frequently watery or mucoid and may contain blood or be greenish in color. Mild disease is defined as diarrhea without any systemic symptoms such as fever or hemodynamic changes. Moderate disease may result in profuse diarrhea, abdominal distention or pain, fever, tachycardia, and oliguria, but responds readily to volume resuscitation. Pseudomembranes are seen in more advanced disease and are characterized by raised yellow plaques 2 to 10 mm in diameter, frequently with normal intervening mucosa (Fig. 1) (1,28). Histologically, the membranes are composed of inflammatory cells, fibrin, mucin, and cellular debris (28). PMC primarily affects the large bowel, although the small intestine may rarely be involved. Occasionally patients may present without diarrhea but with marked leukocytosis and abdominal pain, due to primary right-sided involvement (6). In the setting of ileus, CDAD should still be considered in absence of diarrhea.

Severe or fulminant disease may result in hemodynamic instability requiring pressor support and/or mechanical ventilation (9), occult bleeding, and severe oliguria. Fulminant colitis develops in 1% to 3% of cases and can lead to ileus, toxic

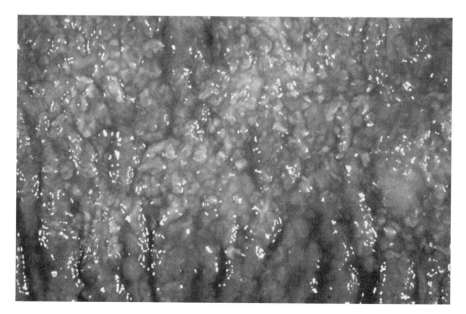

Figure 1 Typical endoscopic findings in *Clostridium difficile*–associated pseudomembranous colitis with widely disseminated, punctate yellow plaques with normal intervening mucosa.

megacolon, intestinal perforation, and death. The first warning sign may be diminishing diarrhea, due to decreased colonic muscle tone. Dallal et al. report that of 44 patients undergoing colectomy for fulminant colitis, five (11%) presented with frank peritonitis, hypotension, or both (9).

With appropriate treatment, the overall mortality for PMC is < 1% in most series (35), but mortality as high as 24% has been reported among critically ill patients (36). Among patients requiring surgery, mortality rates after colectomy have ranged from 38% to 80% in small series (9). In one study of patients with fulminant colitis requiring colectomy, the need for preoperative vasopressor support significantly predicted postoperative mortality (9).

Other complications of CDAD include hyperpyrexia, transverse volvulus (5), and protein-losing enteropathy, resulting in hypoalbuminemia and anasarca. Reactive arthritis, similar to Reiter's syndrome caused by other enteric pathogens, may occur one to four weeks after infection (6,37). Extracolonic *C. difficile* is rare, but case series have described isolation of the organism from pleural fluid, peritoneal fluid, blood, bone, prosthetic joints, wounds (including necrotizing fascitiis), and splenic, vaginal, and perianal abscesses. Generally these infections are polymicrobial, making it difficult to ascertain the contributing pathogenicity of the *C. difficile* itself. However, pure extracolonic cultures of *C. difficile* have been described (29,37).

Unfortunately, relapsing CDAD is common even with appropriate treatment, occurring in 20% to 25% of infections. Relapse generally occurs 3 to 21 days after completion of anticlostridial therapy and is due to recurrence rather than reinfection (36). However, one study did find that 50% of relapses were due to reinfection with a different strain, rather than recrudescence of the original infecting strain (15). Most will respond to a second course of therapy, but those who have had two or more recurrences have a 65% risk of further relapse (15,36), and 3% to 5% will have more than six relapses. Up to 26 relapses have been described in a single patient (36). Patients with chronic renal insufficiency, high leukocyte counts ($\geq 15,000$ cells/mL), multiple previous episodes of CDAD, community-acquired disease, and who require continued antibiotic therapy have higher risk of relapse (6). Patients who develop PMC may also be at greater risk; in 63 patients with CDAD who underwent flexible sigmoidoscopy, 17 (30.4%) of 56 patients with PMC relapsed, compared to zero of seven patients without PMC (38).

DIFFERENTIAL DIAGNOSTIC CONSIDERATIONS

The majority of AAD cases cannot be attributed to any specific microorganism. A number of theories have been advanced to explain the role of antimicrobial drugs in producing diarrhea not associated with *C. difficile*. By disturbing the normal bowel flora, antibiotics destroy organisms responsible for producing short chain fatty acids, resulting in longer nonabsorbable molecules reaching the colon and an osmotic diarrhea (2). Carbohydrate metabolism is also affected, with similar results. The breakdown of primary bile acids, which are potent colonic secretory agents, may also be affected (4). In addition, certain antibiotics have direct effects on the gastrointestinal system. For example, erythromycin increases the gastric emptying rate, clavulanate stimulates bowel motility, and neomycin causes malabsorption (1). Penicillin has rarely been noted to cause segmental colitis (4). Hospitalized patients are frequently subjected to polypharmacy, and medication lists should be carefully examined for other contributing agents, such as laxatives, antacids, electrolyte supplements (particularly magnesium), nonsteroidal antiinflammatory drugs (NSAIDS), contrast, products containing lactose or sorbitol, and antiarrhythmic and cholinergic medications. Ulcerative colitis may present similarly to CDAD, and typhlitis should be considered in neutropenic patients (39). Only 2% to 3% of AAD has been proven to be caused by alternate pathogens, such as *C. perfringens*, *S. aureus*, and *C. albicans* (1); routine testing for these organisms is not recommended. Although PMC is much more specific for *C. difficile*, other potential etiologies include early ischemia, verotoxin-producing organisms such as *Escherichia coli* 0157:H7, and medications (gold, chlorpropanide, or NSAIDS). Hospitalized patients without history of antibiotic use and without significant amounts of diarrhea or abdominal pain are unlikely to have *C. difficile*; 94% to 97% of patients meeting these criteria will have negative cytotoxin assays (5). Testing for *C. difficile* is not recommended in infants under one year, for nondiarrheal stool specimens (except in setting of ileus) or for test of cure (5).

Given the wide spectrum of disease caused by *C. difficile*, there are no pathognomonic findings on history or physical exam. Diarrhea is seen in nearly all cases, but can range from insignificant "nuisance" diarrhea to profuse, cholera-like diarrhea. In more severe disease, abdominal pain, bloating, and tenderness are generally present, and rarely the disease can present as an acute abdomen. One study found that 35% of patients with fulminant colitis caused by *C. difficile* were diagnosed at autopsy (9), suggesting that a significant number of deaths due to "sepsis" in critically ill patients may be related to *C. difficile*.

Although nonspecific, leukocytosis is common in CDAD and can precede the diarrhea and abdominal pain. Band forms are frequently present. One prospective study of 400 inpatients with white blood cell (WBC) counts ≥15,000 cells/mL found *C. difficile* infection in 11% of those with WBC of 15 to 19,900 cells/mL, 15% of those with WBC 20 to 29,000 cells/mL, and 34% of those with WBC ≥30,000 cells/mL. A retrospective analysis found proven *C. difficile* in 25% of patients with WBC ≥30,000 (excluding those with leukemia). Conversely, among 133 outpatients with WBC ≥15,000, only one (1%) was proven to have *C. difficile* (40). Other supporting laboratory findings include hypoalbuminemia and fecal leukocytes. Fecal leukocytes have 28% to 40% sensitivity and 92% specificity (5). Fecal lactoferrin assays have been found to have sensitivity of 75% to 90%, but are nonspecific (46%) (5).

Radiologic studies are also nonspecific but can support the diagnosis. Plain abdominal films may reveal mucosal edema or paralytic ileus and are useful in ruling out free intraabdominal air and toxic megacolon. Computed tomography (CT) may show diffusely thickened colon with edematous mucosa (6). One study of 39 patients with CDAD who underwent CT found that all were diagnostic when combined with the clinical scenario, showing ascites and colonic wall thickening or massive dilatation. Eleven patients had right-sided colitis, whereas nine had left-sided colitis and 19 had pancolitis (9). Barium enemas are not recommended due to the risk of perforation (39).

If endoscopy is performed and pseudomembranes are visualized, the likelihood of *C. difficile* is high. However, mucosa can be normal or can demonstrate minimal erythema (39). One study of 179 patients with undiagnosed diarrhea who underwent flexible sigmoidoscopy found 63 (35.2%) patients with CDAD, of whom 56 (88.9%) had PMC. Twenty-nine (52%) of these patients had negative cytotoxin assays from stool sampled during sigmoidoscopy; nine of these patients had stool samples available for culture, all of which demonstrated toxigenic *C. difficile* (38). Another study of 20 patients who underwent flexible sigmoidoscopy for CDAD found a false negative rate of 10%. Of the two patients not diagnosed, one had strictly right-sided disease and the other had poor bowel preparation (9). Endoscopy should be avoided in patients with severe disease with colonic dilatation.

DIAGNOSIS

The gold standard for diagnosis of *C. difficile* infection is the tissue culture cytotoxin assay for toxin B, which can detect as little as 10 pg of toxin (4). The assay reveals characteristic cytopathic effects on cell culture monolayers; preincubation with neutralizing antibodies demonstrates the specificity of the cytotoxicity (Fig. 2). Sensitivity and specificity are high (94–100% and 99%, respectively) (6). However, this test requires tissue culture capability. It has been supplanted largely by cytotoxin enzyme immunoassay (EIA), which requires 100 to 1000 pg of either toxin A or B, and can provide results within hours. The EIA has high specificity (92–98%); sensitivity can be as low as 71%, but can be increased to 90% with testing of three stool samples. More than one assay for diagnosis is required in 5% to 20% of patients (6). False negative assays may be due to toxin instability, degradation of toxin by proteases derived from other bacteria, or the presence of other bacteria-derived toxin-binding components (38). Assays that test for both toxins are preferred, as 1% to 2% of strains produce only toxin B (4). Fatal PMC was reported in a patient with a *C. difficile* strain that produced nonfunctional toxin A; the

(A)   **(B)**   **(C)**

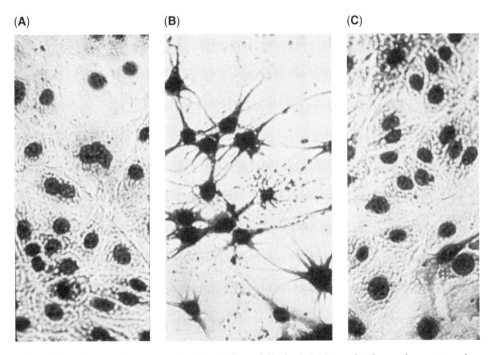

Figure 2 Tissue culture assay for *Clostridium difficile*. (**A**) Normal primary human amnion cells. (**B**) Typical changes (cell rounding) after application *C. difficile* toxin. (**C**) Tissue culture after neutralization with *Clostridium sordelli* antitoxin.

repeated negative cytotoxin A assays resulted in delay of diagnosis and contributed to the patient's death (41).

Stool culture is highly sensitive for *C. difficile* but has several disadvantages. Because nontoxigenic strains are frequently present, culture must be accompanied by toxin-culture assay and broth culture of isolates to identify toxigenic strains. As a result, diagnosis may be delayed by three to four days, and most laboratories no longer perform *C. difficile* cultures (4). Latex agglutination assays lack sensitivity and specificity, as they detect the enzyme glutamate dehydrogenase rather than toxin (1). Polymerase chain reaction (PCR) is very sensitive, but requires significant technical expertise. However, a rapid detection method developed in Spain using nested PCR of the toxin B genes has been found to be 96% sensitive and 100% specific and can be performed in several hours (1). This assay is not yet widely available.

TREATMENT

Whenever possible, the inciting antibiotic should be discontinued or changed. For mild disease, no further treatment may be necessary. Diarrhea may resolve in 25% of patients just with discontinuation of antibiotics (6). Supportive care, such as intravenous fluids and electrolyte replenishment, should be offered if necessary. Antiperistaltic agents, such as narcotics and loperamide, should be avoided as they may promote a dire complication, toxic megacolon (4). Treatment of asymptomatic carriers is ineffective (42), may prolong the carrier state, and is not advised. Asymptomatic carriage usually is transient and resolves spontaneously (39).

Indications for treatment include severe diarrhea, persistent diarrhea despite stopping antibiotics, evidence of systemic toxicity, and the need to continue antibiotics (Table 2) (4). Duration of treatment is usually 10 days, although many experts recommend continuing anticlostridial therapy for one week following discontinuation of the inciting antibiotic. Empiric treatment while awaiting cytotoxin

Table 2 Treatment of *Clostridium difficile*–associated Diarrhea

General supportive measures
Discontinue inciting antibiotic(s) if possible, or change to antibiotic rarely associated with CDAD
Correct fluid and electrolyte imbalances
Avoid use of antiperistaltic agents
Anti-clostridial antibiotics
Metronidazole 500 mg orally three times daily for 10 days
Vancomycin 125 mg orally four times daily for 10 days (first-line therapy in severely ill, pregnant, or lactating patients)
Metronidazole 500 mg intravenously three times daily (in patients with ileus or inability to take oral medications)
Relapsing disease
Repeat 10-day course of metronidazole or vancomycin
Lactobacillus GG: one capsule twice daily for 14 days
Saccharomyces boulardii: 500 mg capsules twice daily for four weeks
IVIG: 400 mg/kg every three weeks
Consider administration of fecal organisms via nasogastric tube or retention enema

Abbreviations: CDAD, *C. difficile*–associated diarrhea; IVIG, intravenous immunoglobulin; GG.

results, or if the first assay is negative, is advisable in severely ill patients with suspected *C. difficile* disease. One study found that patients who died from fulminant colitis were twice as likely as those who survived to have had an initial false-negative toxin (9). Typical response is fairly rapid, with decreased fever within one day and improvement of diarrhea in four to five days. In patients who fail to respond, one should consider lack of compliance, an alternate diagnosis, or the inability of drug to reach the colon, such as with ileus or megacolon (4).

Oral metronidazole and oral vancomycin are the two agents most commonly used for CDAD. Currently published guidelines from the Society for Healthcare Epidemiology of America, the American College of Gastroenterology, and the Hospital Infection Control Practices Advisory Committee all recommend metronidazole as the first-line agent (42). Both have similar response rates (90–97%), but metronidazole has much lower cost and vancomycin has the potential to promote colonization with vancomycin-resistant enterococcus. A 10-day course of high-dose oral vancomycin (500 mg four times daily) costs US $7358 compared to $765 for a 10-day course of oral metronidazole (dosed at 500 mg three times daily) (42).

Metronidazole is typically dosed orally at 500 mg three times daily or 250 mg four times daily. Metronidazole is well absorbed and difficult to detect in healthy volunteers without diarrhea (43), reaching relatively low fecal concentrations (0.4–24.4 µg/g feces after 400 mg orally or 500 mg intravenously) (35). Parenteral therapy may be required in the setting of severe ileus or toxic megacolon. Intravenous metronidazole is primarily excreted in the upper gastrointestinal tract, and approximately 14% of the dose is excreted in feces (3). However, fecal concentrations of the drug have been shown to exceed the minimum inhibitory concentration (MIC) with parenteral therapy (6). Metronidazole treatment failures occur, although documented drug resistance of *C. difficile* is rare. However, *C. difficile* isolates rarely undergo sensitivity testing. One study found no metronidazole resistance even among 10 primary treatment failures (43). Another study found only one isolate with high-level resistance to metronidazole (MIC > 64 µg/mL by agar dilution testing) of 100 tested (35). The mechanism of resistance is not well understood. No antibiotic resistance plasmids have ever been reported in *C. difficile* (17). The rate of treatment failure may be increasing; in Quebec in 2003, 87 of 110 patients with high leukocyte counts, creatinine levels, or both, were treated initially with metronidazole. Complicated CDAD developed in 34 (39.1%), and 20 (23.0%) died (11).

Indications for oral vancomycin therapy include pregnancy, lactation, intolerance of metronidazole, or failure to respond to metronidazole within three to five days of treatment (4). Because of the recent experience with metronidazole-treatment failures, and the low fecal levels achieved with this drug, some experts have moved to treatment of more severely ill patients with vancomycin (39). Parenteral vancomycin is not effective. The typical oral dose is 125 mg four times daily. In the setting of ileus or severe disease, one can increase the dose to 250 to 500 mg four times daily (4). Adjunctive intracolonic vancomycin, administered via retention enema, has been shown to be effective in small, uncontrolled case series of patients with severe or fulminant colitis not responding to standard therapy (3). Vancomycin resistance has not been reported. In the 2003 outbreak in Quebec, initial treatment with vancomycin was associated with a 79% lower risk of complicated CDAD compared with metronidazole, after adjustment for confounding factors (adjusted OR 0.2, 95% CI 0.06–0.8) (11).

Alternate agents for the treatment of CDAD include teicoplanin, fusidic acid, and bacitracin (6). Teicoplanin is available in Europe but not in the United States, and has been touted to be superior to vancomycin in terms of both bacteriologic and symptomatic cure (42). Both fusidic acid and bacitracin have been shown to be less effective than vancomycin (42). Anion exchange resins, such as cholestyramine, bind toxin in the colon but have been associated with treatment failures when used alone. Rifaximin, newly available in the United States for treatment of travelers' diarrhea, has wide antibacterial activity and poor absorption, leading to high intraluminal concentrations. It was compared in vitro with metronidazole and vancomycin against 93 *C. difficile* isolates, and demonstrated superior intrinsic activity (44). In small clinical trials it was as effective as vancomycin (42). It is not Food and Drug Administration–approved for the treatment of CDAD, however.

A minority of patients (0.39–3.6%) with *C. difficile* colitis require surgery (45). Surgery is indicated for patients with peritoneal signs, systemic toxicity, toxic megacolon, perforation, multiorgan failure, or progression of symptoms despite appropriate antimicrobial therapy (39,45). Total colectomy with end ileostomy is the procedure of choice. Select patients with disease clearly limited to the ascending colon have been treated successfully with right hemicolectomy, but intraoperative colonoscopy should be performed to rule out left-sided disease (9).

Treatment of relapsing disease can become problematic. Most authorities recommend repeating a second 10-day course of metronidazole, with 92% response rates (46). For patients with multiple relapses, a variety of options have been tried: long courses of metronidazole, vancomycin, or both; vancomycin plus rifampin; tapered or pulsed dosing of vancomycin; or vancomycin plus cholestyramine (36). Of note, cholestyramine binds vancomycin as well as *C. difficile* toxin, so doses should be separated by several hours (46).

Recovery of normal fecal flora may take days to weeks after the discontinuation of antibiotics (16). Aside from cost, repeated courses of anticlostridial therapy have the disadvantage of perpetuating this disruption in intestinal flora. To break this cycle, alternate treatments have been attempted, including feces or fecal flora via enema or nasogastric tube, nontoxigenic *C. difficile* (46), and probiotics. Stool transplantation was shown effective in one small case series. Filtered stool from patients' family members or healthy volunteers was administered via nasogastric tube to 18 patients with at least two relapses of CDAD. Two patients died from apparently unrelated causes and one patient had one additional relapse, but the remaining patients were cured (overall 94% cure rate). The author notes that the procedure was well tolerated and most patients felt symptomatically better within 24 to 48 hours (36). This study was retrospective and uncontrolled, however.

Probiotics are nonpathogenic microorganisms that, when ingested, may benefit the health or physiology of the host (47). Probiotics have been beneficial in the setting of travelers' diarrhea, rotavirus infection, and AAD (48), but most have only been studied thus far in small, open label, or uncontrolled trials. Organisms include brewers yeast (*Saccharomyces cerevisiae*), *S. boulardii*, *Lactobacillus* GG (LGG), and *L. plantarum* LP299v (47). *S. boulardii* was studied in conjunction with metronidazole or vancomycin in patients with multiple recurrences of CDAD, and decreased relapses compared to placebo (35% vs. 65%, $p = 0.04$) (46). Lactobacilli are a diverse group of lactose-fermenting organisms that have several immune-enhancing effects, including augmentation of phagocyte function and enhancement of humoral and cell-mediated immune responses (48).

LGG is a human isolate resembling *L. casei* subspecies *rhamnosus* that has inhibitory activity against a wide range of bacteria, including *C. difficile*. Unlike some other lactobacilli, it can survive digestion and persist in the colon for at least one week (2). Data regarding its efficacy is conflicting, however. One study of 188 children receiving antibiotics and LGG found a significant decrease in antibiotic-associated diarrhoea (AAD) (24% in placebo group vs. 7% in LGG group), as well as decreased duration of diarrhea and improved stool consistency (48). Similar findings were reported in a study from Finland (49). However, another prospective, randomized, placebo-controlled trial of 267 adults found no difference in the incidence of diarrhea during a 21-day follow-up period (2).

Because the host immune response to *C. difficile* challenge plays a major role, passive immunotherapy with intravenous IgG (IVIG) has been studied in patients with recurrent or refractory CDAD (8). A dose of 400 mg/kg every three weeks was found to produce a marked increase in serum antitoxin A/B levels, and resolution of diarrhea (46). Five children with relapsing disease and low antitoxin A IgG levels responded favorably to IVIG, and several studies in adults have also shown favorable results (15).

PREVENTION

Prevention of *C. difficile* colonization and subsequent infection requires aggressive infection control within hospitals and other institutions (Table 3). Hand washing and use of barrier precautions (gown and gloves) during patient contact requires continual emphasis. Of note, the widely used alcohol-based hand sanitizing solutions do not destroy *C. difficile* spores; this may be contributing to the recent increases in CDAD described above. When CDAD is suspected, patients should be placed in enteric precautions while laboratory testing is ongoing, until the diagnosis can

Table 3   Hospital Infection Control Policies for *Clostridium difficile*–associated Diarrhea

Patient interventions
    Use enteric precautions (gown and gloves upon entering room) for patients with confirmed
       or suspected CDAD
    Place patients with confirmed or suspected CDAD in private rooms and bathrooms
    Consider diagnosis and order cytotoxin assays promptly
    Avoid unnecessary use of acid suppression (i.e., proton pump inhibitors) and
       gastrointestinal motility agents
    Consider prophylactic use of probiotics in patients at particularly high risk of CDAD
Hospital staff interventions
    Improve hand hygiene compliance
    Encourage use of soap and water rather than alcohol-based hand sanitizers after contact
       with *C. difficile*–infected patients
Environmental interventions
    Clean patient rooms with hypochlorite solutions (1 part bleach to 10 parts water, prepared
       daily and allowed to air dry)
    Individually assign thermometers, blood pressure cuffs, and stethoscopes
    Avoid use of rectal thermometers
    Adequately disinfect all equipment used by multiple patients
Hospital policy interventions
    Pursue multidisciplinary interventions to improve appropriate antibiotic use
    May need to restrict high-risk antimicrobials
    Cohort nursing staff
    Cohort patients if necessary in outbreak setting

Abbreviation: CDAD, *Clostridium difficile*–associated diarrhea.

be excluded. Patients should be isolated in private rooms (with private bathrooms) or cohorted with other *C. difficile*–infected patients. Enteric precautions can be removed when diarrhea ceases without test of cure. Patient rooms should be disinfected with freshly prepared hypochlorite solutions (1 part bleach to 10 parts water) and allowed to air dry.

Appropriate antibiotic use is vital; one study found 30% of all antimicrobial-days of therapy in a teaching hospital unnecessary (16). Even a few doses of certain antibiotics can cause prolonged disruption of fecal flora, therefore one should strive to avoid improper initiation of antibiotics. During epidemics, hospital-wide restriction of implicated antibiotics has been effective (4). One epidemic linked to a clonal clindamycin-resistant *C. difficile* isolate responded to restriction of clindamycin; a decrease in the mean number of cases per month from 11.7 to 5.7 was observed within the first six months, with further decline to 3.5 cases per month during the second year of restriction (14). The number of isolates resistant to clindamycin decreased from 91% to 35% (14). The total costs of antibiotics with antianaerobic activity increased, as agents such as imipenem and pipercillin–tazobactam were substituted for clindamycin, but the hospital experienced overall net savings due to decreased number of CDAD cases (14). Even in the absence of an epidemic, restriction of third-generation cephalosporin usage has been associated with decreased rates of *C. difficile* (19).

Vaccination to prevent CDAD has also been studied. Hamster studies have shown protection from lethal ileocecitis with parenteral formalin-inactivated toxins A and B, and full protection from death and diarrhea with a combination of intranasal and intraperitoneal inactivated culture filtrate vaccine plus cholera toxin and Ribi adjuvants. Passive immunization with antitoxin A–neutralizing antibodies protected against lethal disease, whereas full protection against diarrhea required antibodies to both toxins. IgG monoclonal antibodies against the cell-binding domain of toxin A provided complete protection in gnotobiotic mice (15). In humans, an investigational parenteral toxoid vaccine using inactivated toxins A and B was recently tested in healthy volunteers for safety and immunogenicity. The vaccine was well tolerated and all subjected seroconverted (15). Whether the antibody titers elicited are sufficient to protect against disease is unknown. An initial pilot test of three patients with chronic, relapsing CDAD found no recurrent disease during two-month follow-up.

REFERENCES

1. Hurley BW, Nguyen CC. The spectrum of pseudomembranous enterocolitis and antibiotic-associated diarrhea. Arch Intern Med 2002; 162:2177–2184.
2. Thomas MR, Litin SC, Osmon DR, et al. Lack of effect of *Lactobacillus* GG on antibiotic-associated diarrhea: randomized, placebo-controlled trial. Mayo Clin Proc 2001; 76:883–889.
3. Apisarnthanarak A, Razavi B, Mundy LM. Adjunctive intracolonic vancomycin for severe *Clostridium difficile* colitis: case series and review of the literature. Clin Infect Dis 2002; 35:690–696.
4. Bartlett JG. Antibiotic-associated diarrhea. N Engl J Med 2002; 346(5):334–339.
5. Thielman NM, Wilson KH. Antibiotic-associated colitis. In: Mandell GL, Bennett JE, Dolin R, eds. Mandell, Douglas, and Bennett's Principles and Practice of Infectious Diseases. 6th ed. Philadelphia, Pennsylvania: Elsevier Churchill Livingstone Publications, 2005:1249–1263.
6. Mylonakis E, Ryan ET, Calderwood SB. *Clostridium difficile*-associated diarrhea: a review. Arch Intern Med 2001; 161:525–533.

7. Archibald LK, Banerjee SN, Jarvis WR. Secular trends in hospital-acquired *Clostridium difficile* disease in the United States, 1987–2001. J Infect Dis 2004; 189:1585–1589.

8. Kyne L, Warny M, Qamar A, et al. Asymptomatic carriage of *Clostridium difficile* and serum levels of IgG antibody against toxin A. N Engl J Med 2000; 342 (6):390–397.

9. Dallal RM, Harbrecht BG, Boujoukas AJ, et al. Fulminant *Clostridium difficile*: an under appreciated and increasing cause of death and complications. Ann Surg 2002; 235(3):363–372.

10. Morris AM, Jobe BA, Stoney M, et al. *Clostridium difficile* colitis: an increasingly aggressive iatrogenic disease? Arch Surg 2002; 137:1096–1100.

11. Pépin J, Valiquette L, Alary M-E, et al. *Clostridium difficile*-associated diarrhea in a region of Quebec from 1991 to 2003: a changing pattern of disease severity. CMAJ 2004; 171(3):466–472.

12. Pindera L. Quebec to report on *Clostridium difficile* in 2005. CMAJ 2004; 171(7):715.

13. Valiquette L, Low DE, Pépin J, et al. *Clostridium difficile* infection in hospitals: a brewing storm. CMAJ 2004; 171(1):27–29.

14. Climo MW, Israel DS, Wong ES, et al. Hospital-wide restriction of clindamycin: effect on the incidence of *Clostridium difficile*-associated diarrhea and cost. Ann Intern Med 1998; 128:989–995.

15. Giannasca PJ, Warny M. Active and passive immunization against *Clostridium difficile* diarrhea and colitis. Vaccine 2004; 22:848–856.

16. Donskey CJ. The role of the intestinal tract as a reservoir and source for transmission of nosocomial pathogens. Clin Infect Dis 2004; 39:219–226.

17. Johnson S, Samore MH, Farrow KA, et al. Epidemics of diarrhea caused by a clindamycin-resistant strain of *Clostridium difficile* in four hospitals. N Engl J Med 1999; 341(22):1645–1651.

18. Gerding DN. Clindamycin, cephalosporins, fluoroquinolones, and *Clostridium difficile*-associated diarrhea: this is an antimicrobial resistance problem. Clin Infect Dis 2004; 38:646–648.

19. Thomas C, Stevenson M, Williamson J, et al. *Clostridium difficile*-associated diarrhea: epidemiological data from Western Australia associated with a modified antibiotic policy. Clin Infect Dis 2002; 35:1457–1462.

20. McCusker ME, Harris AD, Perencevich E, et al. Fluoroquinolone use and *Clostridium difficile*-associated diarrhea. Emerg Infect Dis 2003; 9(6):730–733.

21. Gaynes R, Rimland D, Killum E, et al. Outbreak of *Clostridium difficile* infection in a long-term care facility: association with gatifloxacin use. Clin Infect Dis 2004; 38:640–645.

22. Safdar N, Maki DG. The commonality of risk factors for nosocomial colonization and infection with antimicrobial-resistant *Staphylococcus aureus*, *Enterococcus*, gram-negative bacilli, *Clostridium difficile*, and *Candida*. Ann Intern Med 2002; 136:834–844.

23. Emoto M, Kawarabayashi T, Hachisuga T, et al. *Clostridium difficile* colitis associated with cisplatin-based chemotherapy in ovarian cancer patients. Gynecol Oncol 1996; 61:369–372.

24. Husain A, Aptaker L, Spriggs DR, et al. Gastrointestinal toxicity and *Clostridium difficile* diarrhea in patients treated with paclitaxel-containing chemotherapy regimens. Gynecol Oncol 1998; 71:104–107.

25. Kent KC, Rubin MS, Wroblewski L, et al. The impact of *Clostridium difficile* on a surgical service: a prospective study of 374 patients. Ann Surg 1998; 227(2):296–301.

26. Zimmaro Bliss D, Johnson S, Savik K, et al. Acquisition of *Clostridium difficile* and *Clostridium difficile*-associated diarrhea in hospitalized patients receiving tube feeding. Ann Intern Med 1998; 129:1012–1019.

27. Dial S, Alrasadi K, Manoukian C, et al. Risk of *Clostridium difficile* diarrhea among hospital inpatients prescribed proton pump inhibitors: cohort and case-control studies. CMAJ 2004; 171(1):33–38.

28. Johal SS, Lambert CP, Hammond J, et al. Colonic IgA producing cells and macrophages are reduced in recurrent and non-recurrent *Clostridium difficile* associated diarrhea. J Clin Pathol 2004; 57:973–979.

29. Wolf LE, Gorbach SL, Granowitz EV. Extraintestinal *Clostridium difficile*: 10 years' experience at a tertiary-care hospital. Mayo Clin Proc 1998; 73:943–947.

30. Guerrant RL, Steiner TS, Lima AAM, et al. How intestinal bacteria cause disease. J Infect Dis 1999; 179(suppl 1):S331–S337.

31. Philips C. Serum antibody responses to *Clostridium difficile* toxin A: predictive and protective? Gut 2001; 49:167–168.

32. McEllistrem MC, Carman RJ, Gerding DN, et al. A hospital outbreak of *Clostridium difficile* disease associated with isolates carrying binary toxin genes. Clin Infect Dis 2005; 40:465–472.

33. Gonçalves C, Decré D, Barbut F, et al. Prevalence and characterization of a binary toxin (actin-specific ADP-ribosyltransferase) from *Clostridium difficile*. J Clin Microbiol 2004; 42(5):1933–1939.

34. Modi N, Wilcox MH. Evidence for antibiotic induced *Clostridium perfringens* diarrhea. J Clin Pathol 2001; 54:748–751.

35. Wong SS-Y, Woo PC-Y, Luk W-K, et al. Susceptibility testing of *Clostridium difficile* against metronidazole and vancomycin by disk diffusion and etest. Diagn Microbiol Infect Dis 1999; 34:1–6.

36. Aas J, Gessert CE, Bakken JS. Recurrent *Clostridium difficile* colitis: case series involving 18 patients treated with donor stool administered via a nasogastric tube. Clin Infect Dis 2003; 36:580–585.

37. Jacobs A, Barnard K, Fishel R, et al. Extracolonic manifestations of *Clostridium difficile* infections: presentation of 2 cases and review of the literature. Medicine 2001; 80(2): 88–101.

38. Johal SS, Hammond J, Solomon K, et al. *Clostridium difficile* associated diarrhea in hospitalized patients: onset in the community and hospital and role of flexible sigmoido-scopy. Gut 2004; 53:673–677.

39. Yassin SF, Young-Fadok TM, Zein NN, et al. *Clostridium difficile*-associated diarrhea and colitis. Mayo Clin Proc 2001; 76:725–730.

40. Wanahita A, Goldsmith EA, Musher DM. Conditions associated with leukocytosis in a tertiary care hospital, with particular attention to the role of infection caused by *Clostridium difficile*. Clin Infect Dis 2002; 34:1585–1592.

41. Johnson S, Kent SA, O'Leary KJ, et al. Fatal pseudomembranous colitis associated with a variant *Clostridium difficile* strain not detected by toxin A immunoassay. Ann Intern Med 2001; 135:434–438.

42. Bricker E, Garg R, Nelson R, et al. Antibiotic treatment for *Clostridium difficile*-associated diarrhea in adults. Cochrane Database Systematic Rev 2004 (most recent update; Accessed Feb 2005).

43. Sanchez JL, Gerding DN, Olson MM, et al. Metronidazole susceptibility in *Clostridium difficile* isolates recovered from cases of *C. difficile*-associated disease treatment failures and successes. Anaerobe 1999; 5:201–204.

44. Marchese A, Salerno A, Pesce A, et al. In vitro activity of rifaximin, metronidazole, and vancomycin against *Clostridium difficile* and the rate of selection of spontaneously resistant mutants against representative anaerobic and aerobic bacteria, including ammonia-producing species. Chemotherapy 2000; 46:253–266.

45. Synnott K, Mealy K, Merry C, et al. Timing of surgery for fulminating pseudomembranous colitis. Br J Surg 1998; 85:229–231.

46. Kyne L, Kelly C. Recurrent *Clostridium difficile* diarrhoea. Gut 2001; 49:152–153.

47. Marteau PR, de Vrese M, Cellier CJ, et al. Protection from gastrointestinal diseases with the use of probiotics. Am J Clin Nutr 2001; 73(suppl):430S–436S.

48. Vanderhoof JA. Probiotics: future directions. Am J Clin Nutr 2001; 73(suppl):1152S–1155S.

49. Arvola T, Laiho K, Torkkeli S, et al. Prophylactic *Lactobacillus* GG reduces antibiotic-associated diarrhoea in children with respiratory infections: a randomized study. Pediatrics 1999; 104(5):e64.

16

Severe Skin and Soft Tissue Infections in the Critical Care Unit

Mamta Sharma and Louis D. Saravolatz
*Division of Infectious Disease, Department of Medicine, St. John Hospital and
Medical Center, and Wayne State University School of Medicine,
Detroit, Michigan, U.S.A.*

INTRODUCTION

Skin and soft tissue infections are common and vary widely in severity from minor pyodermas to severe necrotizing infections. Most of these infections are superficial and treated with regimens of local care and antimicrobial therapy. However, others like necrotizing infections are life threatening and require a combined medical and surgical intervention. Prompt recognition and treatment is paramount in limiting the morbidity and mortality associated with these infections, and thus a thorough understanding of the various etiologies and presentation is essential in the critical care setting. It is also important to discriminate between infectious and noninfectious causes of skin and soft tissue inflammation. A detailed history and examination are necessary to narrow the possible etiologies of infection. In many instances surface cultures are unreliable and misleading because surface colonizing organisms can be mistaken for pathogens. In instances in which the diagnosis is in doubt, aspiration, biopsy, or surgical exploration of the skin can be considered. Here we review causes of severe skin and soft tissue infection, highlighting the clinical presentation, diagnosis, and approach to management in the critical care setting.

MICROBIAL FLORA

Physiological factors that control the bacterial skin flora include humidity, water content, skin lipids, temperature, and rate of desquamation. The pH of the skin is usually around 5.6. Besides containing secretory Immunoglobulin (IgA), sweat also possesses sufficient salt to create a high osmotic pressure, which may be responsible for inhibiting many microbial species. In spite of these barriers to colonization, the skin provides an excellent venue of various microenvironments. Differences in cutaneous microflora may relate to variability in skin surface temperature and moisture content as well as the presence of different concentrations of skin surface lipids that

321

may be inhibitory to various microorganisms. Colonization with organisms sensitive to desiccation, such as gram-negative bacilli, is not favored. The predominant bacterial flora of the skin is the various species of coagulase-negative staphylococci (*S. epidermidis*, *S. capitis*, *S. warneri*, *S. hominis*, *S. haemolyticus*, *S. lugdunensis*, and *S. auricularis*), *Corynebacterium* species (diphtheroids), and *Propionibacterium* species. Humans are a natural reservoir for *Staphylococcus aureus* (*S. aureus*), and asymptomatic colonization is far more common than infection. Colonization of the nasopharynx, perineum, or skin, particularly if the cutaneous barrier has been disrupted or damaged, may occur shortly after birth and may recur anytime thereafter (1–4). The anterior nares are reservoirs for *S. aureus.* Approximately 20% of individuals always carry one type of strain and are called persistent carriers. A large proportion of the population, approximately 60%, harbors *S. aureus* intermittently, and the strains change with varying frequency. Such persons are called intermittent carriers. Finally, approximately 20% almost never carry *S. aureus* and are called non-carriers (5–7). Carriage rates are higher than in the general population for injection drug users, persons with insulin-dependent diabetes, patients with dermatologic conditions, patients with long-term indwelling intravascular catheters, and those with human immunodeficiency virus infection. High nasal carriage rates are found in patients with *S. aureus* skin infections as demonstrated from nasal cultures taken at the time the *S. aureus* infection was present (5). *Micrococcus* spp., *Peptostreptococcus*, *Streptococcus viridans*, and *Enterococcus* spp. can also be isolated. *Acinetobacter* spp. are found on the skin of about 25% of the population in the axillae, toe webs, groin, and antecubital fossa. *Proteus*, *Pseudomonas*, *Enterobacter*, and *Klebsiella* are rarely found. Antibiotics disturb the balance within commensal flora and leave the surface vulnerable to colonization by exogenous gram-negative bacilli and fungi. The principal fungal flora is lipophilic yeasts of the genus *Malassezia*, and nonlipophilic yeasts such as *Candida* spp. are also inhabitants of the skin (1,2,4).

Primary skin infections occur in otherwise normal skin and are usually caused by group A streptococci or *S. aureus*. Secondary infections complicate chronic skin conditions (e.g., eczema or atopic dermatitis). A deficiency in the expression of antimicrobial peptides may account for the susceptibility of patients with atopic dermatitis to skin infection with *S. aureus* (8). These underlying disorders act as a portal of entry for virulent bacteria. Other factors predisposing to skin infections include vascular insufficiency, disrupted venous or lymphatic drainage, sensory neuropathies, diabetes mellitus, previous cellulitis, foreign bodies, accidental or surgical trauma, burns, poor hygiene, obesity, and immunodeficiencies.

CLASSIFICATION OF SKIN AND SOFT TISSUE INFECTIONS

Infections of the skin and soft tissue can be divided based on the depth of penetration and the ability of the organism to produce necrosis. Infection of the outermost layer of skin, the epidermis, is termed impetigo. Extension into the superficial dermis with involvement of lymphatics is typical of erysipelas, whereas cellulitis is an extension into the subcutaneous tissue. In necrotizing fasciitis (NF) there is involvement of fascia, whereas in myonecrosis there is involvement of muscle. A clinically useful distinction with important management implications subdivides soft tissue infections into non-necrotizing and necrotizing processes (9). In some systemic infections, cutaneous manifestations are non-infectious complications of the illness as in purpura fulminans.

Impetigo

Impetigo is the most common, contagious, superficial skin infection produced by *S. aureus* or streptococcus. There are two clinical presentations: bullous impetigo and nonbullous impetigo, and both begin as a vesicle (10). Bullous impetigo, like staphylococcal scalded skin syndrome (SSSS) and the staphylococcal scarlatiniform syndrome, represents a form of cutaneous response to the two extracellular exfoliative toxins produced by *S. aureus* of phage group II (usually type 71). The group A streptococci responsible for impetigo belong to different M serotypes (2,49,52,55,57, 59–61) from those of strains that produce pharyngitis (1,2,4,6,25) (11,12). Crusted impetigo is usually associated with a mixed flora of both *S. aureus* and streptococci. *S. aureus* is known to be the primary pathogen in both bullous and nonbullous impetigo. They are common in exposed areas, such as hands, feet, and legs, and are often associated with traumatic events, such as minor skin injury or insect bite. Predisposing factors include warm ambient temperature, humidity, poor hygiene, and crowded conditions. Systemic complications are very uncommon.

Staphylococcal Scalded Skin Syndrome

SSSS, first described in 1956, is a generic term applied to a group of exfoliative dermopathies caused by an exfoliative (or epidermolytic) exotoxin, produced by various strains of *S. aureus*, mainly of phage group II (usually type 71) (13–15). It primarily affects neonates and young children, although adults with underlying diseases are also susceptible. Two variants of the toxin, the exfoliative toxin A and B, have been described. These exotoxins induce pathological changes in the epidermis that closely resemble a scald caused by boiling water, hence the name SSSS (16–18). Histologically, these toxins cause intraepidermal cleavage through the granular layer without damage or alteration of the keratinocytes, bullae formation, and slippage of the upper epidermal layer with the application of gentle pressure (a positive Nikolsky's sign). *S. aureus* enterotoxin (A through D) and toxic shock syndrome toxin 1 (TSST-1) are frequently associated with staphylococcal scarlet fever. The clinical response to these exotoxins is varied. Thus, the manifestations of SSSS include several primarily age-dependent presentations: (i) a generalized exfoliative syndrome seen in newborns (Ritter's disease or Pemphigus neonatorum) and children, but can rarely develop in adults; (ii) bullous impetigo, a localized pustulosis in children; and (iii) staphylococcal scarlet fever, a form of SSSS that does not progress beyond the initial stage of a generalized erythematous eruption.

SSSS occurs abruptly or few days after a recognized staphylococcal infection with fever, skin tenderness, and scarlatiniform rash. The lesions begin as a vesicle that gradually enlarges into flaccid bullae that rupture, leaving a tender, moist surface that eventually heals. Localized infection occurs, usually in the nasopharynx, umbilicus, or urinary tract. Large flaccid clear bullae form over two to three days, and result in separation of sheets of skin. Exfoliation exposes large areas of bright red skin surface (19,20). Fluid and electrolyte loss can lead to hypovolemia and sepsis syndrome. In adults the mortality rate approaches 60% (21). With appropriate therapy the lesions heal within two weeks. Toxic epidermal necrolysis (TEN) typically occurs as a drug reaction. The lesions are similar to SSSS; however, there is more extensive destruction of the epidermis and the stratum corneum layer, recovery is prolonged, and scarring is more frequent. TEN is often fatal and should be treated like a widespread burn. Most cases of SSSS are diagnosed on clinical grounds and are easily treated with antibiotics, which rapidly eliminate the staphylococci producing the toxin. Laboratory investigations are required only if the clinical findings are equivocal or when outbreaks occur. Because the condition is the result of exotoxins, which may be produced by staphylococci at a distant site, the blister fluid in generalized SSSS tends to be sterile, whereas the fluid in localized bullous impetigo will contain *S. aureus*. Staphylococci producing enterotoxions ET can usually be cultured from the nares, conjunctiva, or nasopharynx. Biopsy of the blister is one of the most definitive diagnostic tests in SSSS. One study revealed a positive blister biopsy result with intraepidermal cleavage in all 30 adults with SSSS (20). Blood cultures are usually negative because the organisms are frequently noninvasive, particularly in children. In one study only 3% of children had a positive blood culture, in contrast to 20 (62.5%) of 32 adults (17,20,22–24).

Treatment: Severe forms require more aggressive treatment with intravenous antistaphylococcal antibiotics and extra care of denuded skin to prevent secondary infection and fluid losses, and to maintain body temperature, especially in neonates. In methicillin sensitive strains, a penicillinase-resistant penicillin nafcillin or oxacillin (2 g IV every four to six hours) is the drug of choice. Cefazolin (1–2 g IV every eight hours) is an alternative treatment that can also be used in patients with histories of delayed type penicillin allergy. In methicillin-resistant strains (MRSA) vancomycin (1 g or 15 mg/kg IV every 12 hours), sulfamethaxole/trimethoprim (1600/320 IV every 12 hours), linezolid (600 mg IV or orally every 12 hours), and other agents such as daptomycin (4 mg/kg/day IV) for skin and soft tissue infections (6 mg/kg/day IV for severe infections) and quinupristin-dalfopristin (7.5 mg/kg IV every eight hours) are treatment options (25,26). Linezolid, daptomycin, and quinupristin-dalfopristin can be used for vancomycin intermediate *S. aureus* and vancomycin-resistant *S. aureus* (VRSA) strains (25). Oritavancin, dalbavancin, tigecyline, and telavancin are newer agents under development for treatment of resistant strains (27).

Toxic Shock Syndrome

Toxic-shock syndrome (TSS) is a rapid-onset illness causing fever, hypotension, rash, multiple organ system dysfunction, and desquamation. Infection with *S. aureus* produces classical TSS, whereas *Streptococcus pyogenes* causes a modified form of TSS known as either streptococcal TSS (STSS), or toxic-shock–like syndrome (TSLS). TSLS displays many of the typical TSS symptoms with the addition of severe soft tissue necrosis (28). Diagnosis of TSLS caused by streptococci is based on a constellation of clinical and laboratory signs as proposed by the Centers for Disease Control and Prevention (Table 1) (29,30).

There are two clinical forms of TSS: menstrual TSS and nonmenstrual TSS. Menstrual TSS starts within three days of the beginning or end of menses and is primarily associated with the use of high absorbency tampons. Clinical signs include high fever, capillary leak syndrome with hypotension and hypoalbunemia, generalized nonpitting edema, and a morbilliform rash, followed by desquamation after a few days. TSST-1 and staphylococcal enterotoxins are the paradigm of a large family of pyrogenic exotoxins called superantigens (SAg). For nonmenstrual TSS, the offending pathogen can virtually colonize any site in the body (31–34). Recurrent menstrual TSS is a well-described phenomenon (35,36). Two conditions are required for recurrence of TSS: persistent colonization with a toxigenic strain of *S. aureus* and persistent absence of neutralizing antibody. Recurrent TSS develops exclusively among patients who fail to develop a humoral immune response to the implicated

Table 1 Streptococcal Toxic-Shock Syndrome: Clinical Case Definition

An illness with the following clinical manifestations occurring within the first 48 hrs of
   hospitalization or, for a nosocomial case, within the first 48 hrs of illness:
   Hypotension defined by a systolic blood pressure less than or equal to 90 mmHg for adults
      or less than the fifth percentile by age for children aged less than 16 yrs. Multiorgan
      involvement characterized by two or more of the following:
      Renal impairment: creatinine greater than or equal to 2 mg/dL (greater than or equal to
         177 μmol/L) for adults or greater than or equal to twice the upper limit normal for
         age. In patients with preexisting renal disease, a greater than twofold elevation over the
         baseline level
      Coagulopathy: platelets less than or equal to 100,000/mm^3 (less than or equal to
         100×10^6/L) or disseminated intravascular coagulation, defined by prolonged clotting
         times, low fibrinogen level, and the presence of fibrin degradation products
      Liver involvement: alanine aminotransferase, aspartate aminotransferase, or total
         bilirubin levels greater than or equal to twice the upper limit of normal for the patient's
         age. In patients with preexisting liver disease, a greater than twofold increase over the
         baseline level
      Acute respiratory distress syndrome defined by acute onset of diffuse pulmonary
         infiltrates and hypoxemia in the absence of cardiac failure or by evidence of diffuse
         capillary leak manifested by acute onset of generalized edema, or pleural or peritoneal
         effusions with hypoalbuminemia
      A generalized erythematous macular rash that may desquamate. Soft tissue necrosis,
         including necrotizing fasciitis or myositis, or gangrene
Laboratory criteria for diagnosis
   Isolation of group A *Streptococcus.*
Case classification
   Probable: a case that meets the clinical case definition in the absence of another identified
      etiology for the illness and with isolation of group A *Streptococcus* from a nonsterile site
   Confirmed: a case that meets the clinical case definition and with isolation of group A
      Streptococcus from a normally sterile site (e.g., blood or cerebrospinal fluid, or less
      commonly, joint, pleural, or pericardial fluid)

staphylococcal toxin (37). Diagnosis of TSS is based on a constellation of clinical
and laboratory signs as proposed by the Centers for Disease Control and Prevention
(Table 2) (28).

   In the late 1980s, a disease similar in appearance to TSS, yet caused by invasive
streptococci, was recognized and referred to as "toxic strep," "streptococcal TSLS,"
or STSS. This condition was found to share many clinical features with TSS. M types
1, 3, 12, and 28 have been the most common isolates from patients with shock and multiorgan failure (38,39). In the majority of cases toxin-producing group A streptococci
have been isolated, with Streptococcal pyrogenic exotoxin-A (Spe-A) production being
most closely linked with invasive disease. However, group A streptococci producing
Streptococcal pyrogenic exotoxin-B (Spe-B), Streptococcal pyrogenic exotoxin-C
(Spe-C), streptococcal SAg, and mitogenic factor, as well as nongroup A streptococci,
have been found to be causative in individual cases of STSS as well. Similar to classic
TSS, the clinical signs of STSS are postulated to be mediated by massive cytokine release
(primarily TNF-alpha, IL-1b, and IL-6) as a result of toxin/SAg activity, in addition,
streptolysin O, produced by 100% of streptococcal strains associated with STSS, has
also been shown to cause TNF-α and IL-1 β production, and has been demonstrated
to act synergistically with Spe-A (40–45). Very young, elderly, diabetic, or immunocompromised persons are more susceptible to the acquisition of invasive streptococcal

Table 2 Toxic Shock Syndrome: Clinical Case Definition

An illness with the following clinical manifestations:
  Fever: temperature greater than or equal to 102.0°F (greater than or equal to 38.9°C)
  Rash: diffuse macular erythroderma
  Desquamation: 1–2 wks after onset of illness, particularly on the palms and soles
  Hypotension: systolic blood pressure less than or equal to 90 mmHg for adults or less than
    fifth percentile by age for children aged less than 16 yrs; orthostatic drop in diastolic
    blood pressure greater than or equal to 15 mmHg from lying to sitting, orthostatic
    syncope, or orthostatic dizziness
  Multisystem involvement (three or more of the following):
    Gastrointestinal: vomiting or diarrhea at onset of illness
    Muscular: severe myalgia or creatine phosphokinase level at least twice the upper
      limit of normal
    Mucous membrane: vaginal, oropharyngeal, or conjunctival hyperemia
    Renal: blood urea nitrogen or creatinine at least twice the upper limit of normal for
      laboratory or urinary sediment with pyuria (greater than or equal to five leukocytes per
      high-power field) in the absence of urinary tract infection
    Hepatic: total bilirubin, alanine aminotransferase enzyme, or aspartate aminotransferase
      enzyme levels at least twice the upper limit of normal for laboratory
    Hematologic: platelets less than 100,000/mm^3
    Central nervous system: disorientation or alterations in consciousness without focal
      neurologic signs when fever and hypotension are absent
Laboratory criteria
  Negative results on the following tests, if obtained:
    Blood, throat, or cerebrospinal fluid cultures (blood culture may be positive for
      Staphylococcus aureus)
    Rise in titer to Rocky Mountain spotted fever, leptospirosis, or measles
Case classification
  Probable: a case which meets the laboratory criteria and in which four of the five clinical
    findings described above are present
  Confirmed: a case which meets the laboratory criteria and in which all five of the clinical
    findings described above are present, including desquamation, unless the patient dies
    before desquamation occurs

infection such as STSS. However, the majority of cases of STSS have occurred in young, otherwise healthy persons between 20 and 50 years of age. An absence of protective immunity is postulated as a potential risk factor in this population. STSS has also been well described as a complication of wounds, varicella, and influenza A. A controversial association of invasive group A streptococcal infections such as STSS with prior non-steroidal anti-inflammatory drug (NSAID) use has been suggested (46). The link has been proposed to be depression of the cellular immune response by NSAIDs.

Clinically, STSS shares many features with TSS. Fever, hypotension, myalgias, liver abnormalities, diarrhea, emesis, renal dysfunction, and hematologic abnormalities may be present in TSS caused by either staphylococci or streptococci. Diffuse macular erythroderma likewise is frequently present in disease caused by both bacteria and is often accompanied by mucous membrane findings, such as conjunctival injection and delayed desquamation of palms and soles.

Nonetheless, certain important differences exist between STSS and TSS. The skin is often the portal of entry in STSS, with soft tissue infections developing in 80% of patients (38). The initial presentation of STSS is often localized pain in an extremity, which rapidly progresses over 48 to 72 hours to manifest both local and systemic signs of STSS. Cutaneous signs may include localized edema and erythema, a bullous and hemorrhagic cellulitis, NF or myositis, and gangrene. Soft tissue involvement of this nature is distinctly uncommon in staphylococcal TSS.

Blood cultures are positive in 60% of patients with STSS (38), as compared with less than 3% in TSS. Mortality in STSS is between 30% and 80%, whereas in staphylococcal TSS ranges from 3% to 5% (47,48).

Treatment: Group A streptococcus is susceptible to penicillin and other β-lactam antibiotics in vitro; however clinical treatment failure occurs when penicillin is used alone in severe group A streptococcus infections (49). This may be attributed to the large inoculum size, the so-called Eagle effect (50,51). These large inoculum reach the stationary growth phase very quickly. Penicillin and other β-lactam antibiotics are ineffective in the stationary growth phase because of reduced expression of penicillin-binding proteins in this phase. Moreover, toxin production is not inhibited by β-lactam antibiotics during the stationary growth phase. The greater efficacy of clindamycin is multifactorial: it inhibits protein synthesis, and its efficacy is unaffected by inoculum size or the stage of bacterial growth. Clindamycin also suppresses synthesis of penicillin-binding proteins, and has a longer post antibiotic effect than β-lactam antibiotics. Lastly clindamycin causes suppression of lipopolysaccharides (LPS)-induced monocyte synthesis of TNF (51–54). Prompt antimicrobial therapy with high dose penicillin and clindamycin should be instituted. Aggressive fluid resuscitation is needed because of intractable hypotension and diffuse capillary leak. Human polyspecific intravenous immunoglobulin (IVIG) has been suggested as a potential adjunctive therapy for invasive group A streptococcus diseases mainly because of its ability to neutralize a wide variety of SAg and to facilitate opsonization of streptococci. An observational cohort study of IVIG in patients with STSS reported decreased mortality rates in patients treated with IVIG compared to controls (67% vs. 34%) (55). A double blind placebo trial was prematurely terminated because of slow recruitment. Analyses of primary end point revealed a reduced mortality in IVIG treated group as compared with placebo (10% vs. 36%), although statistical significance was not reached. A significant increase in plasma neutralizing activity against SAgs expressed by autologous isolates was noted in the IVIG group after treatment (56). If IVIG is to be used, it should be given early and more than one dose should be used, because batches of IVIG have variable neutralizing activity (57). In addition, prompt surgical exploration and debridement of deep seated streptococcal infection should be performed (see discussion of NF).

For management of TSS anti-staphylococcal agents are selected with consideration of susceptibility testing. Supportive care includes aggressive intravenous fluid resuscitation and vasopressors as needed. The suspected focus of infection requires specific attention. Specifically, management includes the removal of any vaginal device in menstrual cases and the removal of packed dressings in conjunction with drainage and debridement in cases associated with postsurgical wounds.

Furuncles and Carbuncles

Furuncle is a deep inflammatory nodule that develops from predisposing folliculitis. A carbuncle is a more extensive process that extends into the subcutaneous fat in areas covered by thick, inelastic skin. Multiple abscesses separated by connective tissue septa develop and drain to the surface along the hair follicle. *S. aureus* is the most common etiological agent. Infections occur in areas that contain hair follicles such as neck, face, axillae, and buttocks, and sites predisposed to friction and perspiration.

Predisposing factors include obesity, defects in neutrophil dysfunction, and diabetes mellitus. Bacteremia can occur and result in osteomyelitis, endocarditis, or other metastatic foci.

Erysipelas

Erysipelas is a distinctive superficial cellulitis of the skin with prominent lymphatic involvement. In typical erysipelas, the area of inflammation is raised above the surrounding skin; there is a distinct demarcation between involved and normal skin, and the affected area has a classic orange peal (peau d'orange) appearance. The induration and sharp margin distinguish it from the deeper tissue infection of cellulitis, in which the margins are not raised and merge smoothly with uninvolved areas of the skin (Fig. 1). Systemic signs of chills and fever are common. Flaccid bullae filled with clear fluid may develop on the second or third day. Occasionally the infection spreads more deeply and causes cellulitis, abscess, and NF. Desquamation may occur in 5 to 10 days, and scarring is very uncommon. Erysipelas is almost always caused by group A streptococcus, though streptococci of groups G, C, and B, and rarely *S. aureus* can also be responsible. Formerly the face was commonly involved but now up to 85% of cases occur on the legs and feet largely due to lymphatic venous disruptions (11,58). Erysipelas can spread rapidly if not treated promptly. Blood cultures are positive in only about 5% of cases (58).

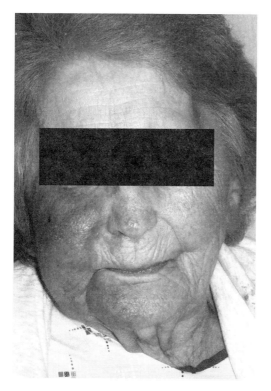

Figure 1   Facial erysipelas involving the right cheek. Sharp demarcation between the erythema and right cheek is evident.

Treatment: There has never been a documented report of group A streptococci resistant to penicillin, and thus penicillin remains the drug of choice, penicillin G 200,000 U every six hours. Other alternative agents include first generation cephalosporins or clindamycin. Agents such as erythromycin and the other macrolides are limited by their rates of resistance, and the fluoroquinolones are generally less active than the β-lactam antibiotics against β-hemolytic streptococci.

Cellulitis

Cellulitis is an acute, spreading pyogenic inflammation of the dermis and subcutaneous tissue (59,60). *S. aureus* and group A β-hemolytic streptococcus species are the common organisms (Fig. 2). Cellulitis commonly begins as erythema, edema, and pain and lacks demarcation. It often occurs in the setting of local skin trauma from skin bite, abrasions, surgical wounds, contusions, or other cutaneous lacerations. Edema also predisposes patients to cellulitis. Specific pathogens are suggested when infections follow exposure to seawater (*Vibrio vulnificus*) (61,62), fresh water (*Aeromonas hydrophila*) (63), or aquacultured fish (*Streptococcus iniae*) (64). Lymphedema may persist after recovery from cellulitis or erysipelas and predisposes patients to recurrences. In addition, spread to adjacent structures may result in osteomyelitis. Cellulitis infrequently occurs as a result of bacteremia. Uncommonly, pneumococcal cellulitis occurs on the face or limbs in patients with diabetes mellitus, alcohol abuse, systemic lupus erythematosus, nephritic syndrome, or a hematological cancer (65). Meningococcal cellulitis occurs rarely, although it may affect both children and adults (66). Bacteremic cellulitis due to *V. vulnificus* with hemorrhagic bullae may follow the ingestion of raw oysters by patients with cirrhosis, hemochromatosis, or thalassemia. Cellulitis caused by gram-negative organisms usually occurs through a cutaneous source in an immunocompromised patient but can also develop through bacteremia. *Cryptococcus neoformans*, *Fusarium*, *Proteus*, and *Pseudomonas* spp have been associated with bloodstream infections. Immunosuppressed patients are particularly susceptible to the progression of cellulitis from regional to systemic infections.

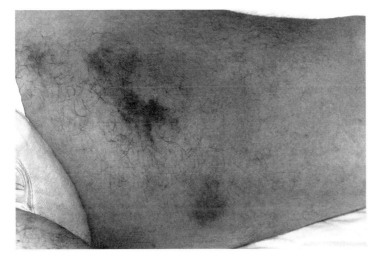

Figure 2 Cellulitis of the left thigh in an alcoholic patient blood; cultures grew group B *streptococcus*.

The distinctive features including the anatomical location and the patient's medical and exposure history should guide appropriate antibiotic therapy. Periorbital cellulitis involves the eyelid and periocular tissue and should be distinguished from orbital cellulitis because of complications of the latter: decreased ocular motility, decreased visual acuity, and cavernous-sinus thrombosis.

Diagnostic studies: Diagnosis is generally based on clinical and morphologic features of the lesion. Culture of a needle aspirate is not generally indicated because of a low yield. Among 284 patients, a likely pathogen was identified in 29%. Of 86 isolates, only three represented mixed culture. Gram-positive organisms (mainly *S. aureus*, group A or B streptococci, and *Enterococcus faecalis*) accounted for 79% of cases; the remainder were caused by gram-negative bacilli (*Enterobacteriaceae*, *H. influenzae*, *P. multocida*, *Pseudomonas aeruginosa*, and *Acinetobacter* spp.) (59). Bacteremia is uncommon in cellulitis with only 2% to 4% yielding a pathogen (59). Blood cultures appear to be positive more frequently with cellulitis superimposed on lymphedema. Radiography and computed tomography are of value when clinical setting suggests a subjective osteomyelitis or there is clinical evidence to suggest adjacent infections such as pyomyositis or deep abscesses. When it is difficult to differentiate cellulitis from NF, a magnetic resonance imaging (MRI) may be helpful, although surgical exploration for a definite diagnosis should not be delayed when the latter condition is suspected.

Treatment: Because most cases are caused by streptococci and *S. aureus*, β-lactam antibiotics with activity against penicillinase-producing *S. aureus* are the usual drugs of choice. Specific treatment for bacterial causes is warranted after an unusual exposure (human or animal bite or exposure to fresh or salt water), in patients with certain underlying conditions (neutropenia, splenectomy, or immunocompromise), or in the presence of bullae and is described in Table 3.

Erysipeloid

The localized cutaneous infection caused by *Erysipelothrix rhusiopathiae* presents as a subacute cellulitis (termed "erysipeloid"). It is usually due to contact with fish, shellfish, or infected animals. Contact with this pathogen may occur in recreational settings, domestic exposures, or after lacerations among abattoirs or chefs (67). Lesions are slightly raised and violaceous. Other organisms that cause skin and skin structure infections following exposure to water and aquatic animals include *Aeromonas*, *Plesiomonas*, *Pseudallescheria boydii*, and *V. vulnificus*. *Mycobacterium marinum* can also cause skin infection, but this infection is characterized by a more indolent course. For *erysipelothrix* bacteremia or endocarditis, penicillin G (12 million–20 million units IV daily) is the drug of choice; alternative antimicrobials include ciprofloxacin, cefotaxime, or imipenem-cilastatin.

Bites

Each year, several million Americans are bitten by animals, resulting in approximately 10,000 hospitalizations. Ninety percent of the bites are from dogs and cats, and 3% to 18% of dog bites and 28% to 80% of cat bites become infected, with occasional sequelae of meningitis, endocarditis, septic arthritis, and septic shock. Animal or human bites can cause cellulitis due to skin flora of the recipient of the bite or the oral flora of the biter. Severe infections develop after bites as a result of hematogenous spread or undetected penetration of deeper structures. In a prospective,

Table 3 Antimicrobiol Therapy and Pathogens Associated with Specific Risk Factors

Risk factor	Pathogen	Recommended therapy	Alternative therapy
Dog and cat bites	*Pastcurella multocida* and other *Pastcurella* spp. *Staphylococcus aureus*, *Capnocytophaga*, *streptococcus* *Neisseria canis*, *H. felix*, *Capnocytophaga canimorsus*, anaerobes	Ampicillin/sulbactam 1.5–3 g IV q.i.d	Ciprofloxacin 500 mg PO or 400 mg IV b.i.d + clindamycin 600–900 mg IV t.i.d
Human bites	*Eikenella corrodens*, anaerobes, *S. aureus*, *Streptococcus viridans*	Ampicillin/sulbactam 1.5–3 g IV q.i.d	Ciprofloxacin 500 mg PO or 400 mg IV b.i.d + clindamycin 600–900 mg IV t.i.d
Salt water	*Vibrio vulnificus*	Doxycycline 200 mg IV followed by 100–200 mg IV b.i.d	Cefotaxime 1–2 g IV b.i.d or ciprofloxacin 500 mg PO or 400 mg IV b.i.d
Fresh water or use of leeches	*Aeromonas* species	Ciprofloxacin 400 mg IV b.i.d	Imipenam/cilastatin 500 mg IV q.i.d
Butcher, fish handler or veterinarian	*Erysipelothrix rhusiopathiae*	Penicillin G 12–20 million units IV every 4 hrs daily	Ciprofloxacin or cefotaxime or imipenam/cilastatin 500 mg IV q.i.d
Intravenous drug users	MRSA, *Pseudomonas aeruginosa*	Vancomycin 1 g IV b.i.d + ceftazidime 1–2 g IV t.i.d or cefepime 1–2 g IV b.i.d	Linezolid 600 mg PO or IV b.i.d + tobramycin 5.0/kg/day[a] or ciprofloxacin

Note: Dose to be adjusted for azotemia except for ceftriaxone, doxycycline, clindamycin, and linezolid.
[a]Based on once a day dose of 5.0 mg/kg, however can be given as 1.7 mg/kg IV t.i.d.
Abbreviation: MRSA, methicillin-resistant *Staphylococcus aureus*.

multicenter study of infected dog and cat bites *Pasteurella* spp. was the most common isolate from both dog bites (50%) and cat bites (75%). *Pasteurella canis* was the most common isolate of dog bites and *P. multocida* subspecies the most common isolate of cat bites. Other common aerobes include *Streptococci*, *Staphylococci*, *Moraxella*, and *Neisseria*. Common anaerobes include *Fusobacterium*, *Bacteroides*, *Porphyromonas*, and *Prevotella*. *Capnocytophaga canimorsus* is an invasive organism usually occurring in immunosuppressed patients after a dog bite (68,69). Human bites are usually associated with mixed aerobic and anaerobic organisms including *S. viridans* and other streptococci, *S. aureus*, *Eikenella corrodens*, *Fusobacterium*, and *Prevotella*. Clenched fist injuries may lead to infection, tendon tear, joint disruption, or fracture (70). For treatment refer to Table 3.

Ecthyma Gangrenosum

Ecthyma gangrenosum is the classic skin lesion associated with *P. aeruginosa* infection in granulocytopenic patients (71–73), and has been reported in 2% to 28% of patients with pseudomonas bacteremia. Rarely this lesion may be caused by other organisms, including *S. aureus*, *Aeromonas*, *Serratia*, *Klebsiella*, *Escherichia coli*, *Capnocytophaga*, *Aspergillus*, and *Candida*. Neutropenic patients with overwhelming septicemia develop a patchy dermal and subcutaneous necrosis. The characteristic skin lesion starts with erythematous macular eruptions that become bullous with central ulceration and necrosis. These are usually multiple, occurring in different stages of development, which may concentrate on the extremities or the head and neck. Diagnosis of the etiologic agent may occur with biopsy of the lesion being cultured or isolated from blood cultures. Treatment is primarily by administration of intravenous antimicrobial therapy and by debridement of multiple lesions, which may lessen the bacterial burden.

Chancriform Lesions: Anthrax

A bioterrorism-associated anthrax outbreak occurred suddenly in the United States in 2001. Out of the 22 cases 11 had the cutaneous form (74). After incubation of one to eight days, a painless, sometime pruritic, papule develops on an exposed area. The lesion enlarges and becomes surrounded by a wide zone of brawny, erythematous, gelatinous, and nonpitting edema. As the lesion evolves it becomes hemorrhagic, necrotic, and covered by an eschar. Frequently lymphadenopathy is present. If untreated bacteremic dissemination can occur. Incision and debridement should be avoided because it increases the likelihood of bacteremia (75). A skin biopsy after the initiation of antibiotics can be done to confirm the diagnosis by culture, polymerase chain reaction, or immunohistochemical testing. With the concern that strains may have been modified to be resistant to penicillin, treatment with ciprofloxacin or doxycycline has been recommended (76).

Purpura Fulminans

Purpura fulminans is an acute illness most commonly associated with meningococcemia but also seen with pneumococcal or staphylococcal disease (77,78). It is typically characterized by disseminated intravascular coagulation (DIC) and purpuric skin lesions. There are four primary features of this syndrome: large purpuric skin lesions, fever, hypotension, and DIC. However, five cases associated with *S. aureus* strains have been reported from the Minneapolis-St. Paul, Minnesota, metropolitan area. These strains produced high levels of TSST-1, staphylococcal enterotoxin serotype B, or staphylococcal enterotoxin serotype C. Only two of the five patients survived (79). Staphylococcal purpura fulminans may be a newly emerging illness associated with SAg production. There are no specific guidelines for the therapeutic management of this serious manifestation other than assuring that anti-staphylococcal agents are selected with consideration of susceptibility testing.

Necrotizing Cellulitis

Infectious gangrene is a cellulitis that rapidly progresses, with extensive necrosis of subcutaneous tissues and the overlying skin. Pathologic changes are those of necrosis and hemorrhage of the skin and subcutaneous tissue. In most instances, necrotizing cellulitis has developed secondary to introduction of the infecting organism at the site of infection. Streptococcal gangrene is a rare form caused by group A streptococci that occurs at the site of trauma but may occur in the absence of an obvious portal of entry. Cases may follow infection at an abdominal operative wound, around an ileostomy or colostomy, at the exit of a fistulous tract, or in proximity to chronic ulceration. The organisms responsible include *Clostridium*, *Bacteroides*, and *Peptostreptococcus*. The diagnosis is suggested when gas is present or when necrosis develops rapidly in an area of cellulitis. Gram stain and culture of skin drainage, aspirate fluid, or surgical specimens should reveal the pathogenic organisms (80–82).

Treatment consists of immediate surgical exploration beyond the involved gangrenous and undermined tissue. Areas of cutaneous necrosis are excised. Repeat exploration is commonly performed within 24 hours. Antibiotic therapy should be guided by Gram-stain results or empirically consist of high dose intravenous penicillin G (3–4 million units every four hours) or ampicillin (2 g every four hours), with the addition of clindamycin.

Necrotizing Fasciitis

NF is a rapidly spreading infection that involves the fascia and subcutaneous tissue with relative sparing of underlying muscle. The mortality of this disease remains alarmingly high ranging from 6% to 76% (83). Delayed diagnosis and delayed debridement have been shown to increase mortality. Type 1 NF is polymicrobial with at least one anaerobic species isolated in combination with one or more facultative anaerobic species such as nontypable streptococci and enterobacteriaceae (Fig. 3). Type 1 NF is common in postoperative infections and includes Fournier's gangrene. Type 2 NF is typically monomicrobial, most often caused by group A streptococcus (84), *Clostridium perfringens*. Other organisms that have rarely been implicated in monobacterial infections include *Serratia marcescens*, *Flavobacterium odoratum*, *Ochrobactrum anthropi*, *V. vulnificus*, and group G streptococcus and *S. aureus* (85). NF presents either as an acute and life-threatening condition usually caused by group A streptococcus or clostridium spp., or as a subacute process, usually caused by mixed aerobic and anaerobic organisms. The primary site is the superficial fascia. Bacteria proliferate within the superficial fascia and elaborate enzymes and toxins. The precise mechanism of spread has not been fully elucidated but has been attributed to the expression of hyaluronidase, which degrades the fascia. The key pathological process resulting from this uncontrolled proliferation of bacteria is angiothrombotic microbial invasion and liquefactive necrosis of the superficial fascia. As this process progresses, occlusion of perforating nutrient vessels to the skin causes progressive skin ischemia. This event is responsible for the cutaneous manifestations. As the condition evolves, ischemic necrosis of the skin ensues with gangrene of subcutaneous fat, dermis and epidermis, manifesting progressively as bullae formation, ulceration, and skin necrosis. In early stages (stage 1 NF) the disease is indistinguishable from severe soft tissue infection such as cellulitis and erysipelas and presents with only pain tenderness and warm skin. Margins of the skin are poorly defined with tenderness extending beyond the apparent area of involvement. Blister or bulla formation is an important diagnostic clue. It signals the onset of skin ischemia (stage 2 NF). The late stage (stage 3 NF) signals the onset of tissue necrosis and is characterized by hemorrhagic bullae, skin anesthesia, and gangrene. Systemic manifestation such as fever, hypotension, and multiorgan failure can occur

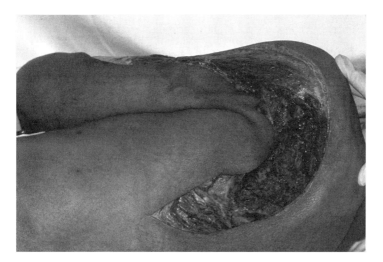

Figure 3 Necrotizing fasciitis of left arm and shoulder in a patient with intravenous drug user (IVDU) who injected in the left arm. Patient underwent disarticulation. One set of blood cultures grew *Gemella morbillorum* and second set grew *Streptococcus constellatus*. Operative cultures obtained from left arm grew *Klabsiella oxytoca*, *Peptostreptococcus micros*, and *P. prevoti.*

(86–89). The effects are classically caused by SAg produced by group A streptococcus. NSAIDs are postulated to potentiate tissue damage by decreasing granulocyte adhesion and phagocytosis and increasing cytokine production.

NF is a clinical diagnosis with corroborative operative findings that include the presence of grayish necrotic fascia, a lack of resistance of normally adherent superficial fascia, a lack of bleeding of the fascia during dissection, and the presence of foul smelling "dishwater pus." Features reported to be indicative of NF on the computed tomography scan include deep fascial thickening, enhancement, and fluid and gas in the soft tissue planes. Negative deep fascial involvement on MRI effectively excludes NF. Fine needle aspiration, frozen section of tissue biopsy, fascial biopsy, and skin biopsy for histopathology are all useful in diagnosis of NF. The lack of bleeding may be seen or murky dishwater pus exudates may ooze from the incision site.

Pathognomonic for NF is a positive "finger" test. The finger test can be used to delineate the extent of infection into the adjacent normal appearing skin. A 2-cm incision down to the deep fascia is made under local anesthesia. Probing of the level of the superficial fascia is then performed. The lack of bleeding, foul smelling dishwater pus, and minimal tissue resistance to finger dissection constitute a positive finger test, which is diagnostic of NF (90). If a diagnosis of NF is made, emergent surgical debridement and/or fasciotomy should be considered. Debridement beyond the visible margin of infection is necessary. Repeated debridements may be required and should continue until the subcutaneous tissue can no longer be separated from the deep fascia. Fasciotomy may be performed at the time of debridement. If infection progresses despite serial debridements and antibiotics, amputation may be life saving. A combination of broad-spectrum antibiotics, such as a penicillin, and an aminoglycoside or a third generation cephalosporin, and clindamycin or metronidazole can be started depending on the clinical presentation. Once the Gram-stain, culture and sensitivity results are obtained, the antibiotic regimen can be altered based on these findings. The use of IVIG as an adjunctive treatment for patients with STSS has been used on the basis of retrospective studies and one small prospective randomized trial, but conclusive evidence supporting its use remains limited. IVIG contains many antibodies, which neutralize the exotoxins/SAgs secreted by the strep-tococcus and are involved in the pathogenesis of STSS. Because STSS and NF are mediated by the streptococcal toxins and inflict their tissue destruction via some of the same cytokines, it was postulated that IVIG would be as effective a treatment in NF as it was in STSS. This has yet to be conclusively demonstrated in a clinical trial. For treatment refer to Table 4.

Fournier's Gangrene

It originates as a necrotic black area on the scrotum. It is a fulminant, rapidly progressive subcutaneous infection of the scrotum and penis, which spreads along fascial planes and may extend to the abdominal wall. More than 60% of the patients have diabetes mellitus. Fournier's gangrene occurs commonly without a predispos-ing event or after uncomplicated hemorrhoidectomy. Less commonly this can occur after urological manipulation or as a late complication of deep anorectal suppuration. Fournier's gangrene is characterized by necrosis of the skin and soft tissues of the scrotum and or perineum that is associated with a fulminant, painful, and severely toxic infection (91,93) (91,92). The infection is usually polymicrobial. Successful treatment is again based on early recognition and vigorous surgical debridement. Empiric antibiotic treatment is appropriate until culture results are available. Infec-tion is often polymicrobial. The therapeutic benefit of hyperbaric oxygen treatment remains controversial in this as well as other forms of NF.

Clostridium Myonecrosis (Gas Gangrene)

C. perfringens type A is the most common organism. Although initial growth of the organism occurs within the devitalized anaerobic milieu, acute invasion and destruc-tion of healthy, living tissue rapidly ensues. Historically, clostridial myonecrosis was a disease associated with battle injuries, but 60% of cases now occur after trauma. It is a destructive infectious process of muscle associated with infections of the skin and soft tissue. It is often associated with local crepitus and systemic signs of toxemia, which are formed by anaerobic, gas forming bacilli of the clostridium species. The infection most often occurs after abdominal operations on the gastrointestinal tract; however, penetrating trauma and frostbite can expose muscle, fascia, and subcuta-neous tissue to these organisms. Common to all these conditions is an environment containing tissue necrosis, low oxygen tension, and sufficient nutrients (amino acids and calcium) to allow germination of clostridial spores. The systemic manifestations of gas gangrene are related to the elaboration of potent extracellular protein toxins, especially the α-toxin, a phospholipase C, and θ-toxin, a thiol-activated cytolysin (94–97). Clostridia are gram-positive, spore forming, obligate anaerobes that are widely found in soil contaminated with animal excreta. They may be isolated from the human gastrointestinal tract and from the skin in the perineal area. *C. perfringens* is the most common isolate (present in 80% of cases) and is among the fastest-growing clostridial species, with a generation time, under ideal conditions, of ~eight minutes. This organism produces collagenases and proteases that cause widespread tissue destruction, as well as α-toxin, which have a role in the high mortality asso-ciated with myonecrosis. The α-toxin causes extensive capillary destruction and hemolysis, leading to necrosis of the muscle and overlying fascia, skin, and subcuta-neous tissues. Patients complain of sudden onset of pain at the site of trauma or

Table 4 Antimicrobiol Therapy and Microbiology Associated with Diabetic Foot Infection
and Necrotizing Fasciitis

Clinical syndrome	Pathogen	Recommended therapy	Alternative therapy
Diabetic foot infection	*Staphylococcus aureus*, *Streptococcus Enterobacteriaceae*, *Pseudomonas aeruginosa* anaerobes (*Bacteroides*, *Peptostreptococcus*)	Ampicillin/sulbactam 1.5–3 g IV q.i.d or piperacillin/ tazobactam 3.375 g IV q.i.d or ceftriaxone 1–2 g IV q.d or ciprofloxacin + metronidazole 500 mg IV or PO t.i.d[a]	Imipenam/cilastatin 500 mg IV q.i.d or clindamycin + ciprofloxacin 500–750 mg PO or 400 mg IV b.i.d or cefepime 2 g IV b.i.d
Type 1 NF	Anarobes (*Bacteroides*, *Peotostreptococcus*) *Escherichia coli*, *Enterobacter*, *Klebseilla*, *Proteus*	Ampicillin 1–2 g IV every 4–6 hr p + gentamicin + metronidazole 0.5 g t.i.d or q.i.d or clindamycin 900 mg t.i.d	Imipenam/cilastatin 500 mg q.i.d or ampicillin/ sulbactam + gentamicin 5.0 mg[b] or pipercillin/ tazobactam 3.375 g IV q.i.d
Type 2 NF	Group A *streptococcus*	Penicillin 2–3 mu IV every 3–4 hr + clindamycin 900 mg IV t.i.d ± IVIG	Cefazolin 1–2 g IV t.i.d or vancomycin + clindamycin 900 mg IV t.i.d

Note: Dose adjusted for azotemia except for ceftriaxone, doxycycline, clindamycin and linezolid.
[a]When methicillin-resistant *Staphylococcus aureus* suspected use vancomycin, linezolid or other active agents.
[b]Based on once a day dose of 5.0 mg/kg/day, however can be given as 1.7 mg/kg IV t.i.d.
Abbreviations: NF, necrotizing fasciitis; IVIG, intravenous immunoglobulins.

surgical wounds, which rapidly increases in severity. The skin becomes edematous
and tense. Hemorrhagic bullae are common, as is a thin watery, foul smelling discharge. Examination of the wound discharge reveals abundant large, box-car shaped
gram-positive rods with a paucity of surrounding leukocytes. The usual incubation
period between injury and the onset of clostridial myonecrosis is two to three days
but may be as short as six hours. A definitive diagnosis is based on the appearance
of the muscle on direct visualization by surgical exposure. Initially, the muscle is pale,
edematous, and unresponsive to stimulation. As the disease process continues, the
muscle becomes frankly gangrenous, black, and extremely friable. This occurs with
septicemia and shock. Nearly 15% of patients have positive blood cultures. Serum
creatinine phosphokinase levels are always elevated with muscle involvement. The
mortality rate associated with gas gangrene approaches 60%. Among the signs that
predict a poor outcome are leukopenia, thrombocytopenia, hemolysis, and severe
renal failure. Myoglobinuria is common and can contribute significantly to worsening
of renal function. Frank hemorrhage may be present and is a harbinger of DIC. Successful treatment of this life-threatening infection depends on early recognition and
debridement of all devitalized and infected tissues. When extremities are involved,
amputation is frequently indicated. The role of hyperbaric oxygen therapy has not
been established (100% oxygen at 3 atm), but it may have a role early in the treatment
of seriously ill patients (98,99). The mainstay of treatment is surgical debridement,

and this should not be delayed. A less life-threatening form of this disease is known as clostridium cellulitis. In this process, the bacterial tissue invasion is primarily superficial to the fascial layer, without muscle involvement. Prompt recognition and treatment as described earlier can reduce the associated morbidity and mortality. High dose penicillin G is the drug of choice. Protein synthesis inhibitors such as combining clindamycin with penicillin have had considerably better efficacy than penicillin alone. *Clostridium septicum* bacteremia is associated with underlying colon cancer or neutropenic enterocolitis (100). *Clostridium sordelli* has been reported to cause rapidly progressive myonecrosis with fulminant shock syndrome, particularly in obstetric patients. Black tar heroin use has resulted in outbreak of *Clostridium botulinism, C. tetani*, and *C. sordelli* in intravenous drug users.

Nonclostridial Myonecrosis

Nonclostridial myonecrosis encompasses at least five relatively distinct entities that differ from gas gangrene in their pathogenesis, clinical features and bacteriology: Streptococcal myositis ± NF type 2 (see earlier discussion under NF), synergistic nonclostridial anaerobic myonecrosis ± NF type 1 (see earlier discussion under NF), anaerobic streptococcal myonecrosis, *A. hydrophila* myonecrosis, and infected vascular gangrene.

Anaerobic streptococcal myonecrosis clinically resembles subacute clostridial gas gangrene. The involved muscles are discolored; in contrast to gas gangrene, early cutaneous erythema is prominent. If not treated, the infection progresses to gangrene and shock. The infection is usually mixed, anaerobic streptococci with group A streptococcus or *S. aureus*. Treatment involves the use of high dose penicillin and antistaphylococcal agent, if indicated, and surgical debridement.

Rapidly progressive myonecrosis resembling clostridial gangrene but caused by *A. hydrophila* may occur after injuries sustained in freshwater, or in conjunction with medicinal leech therapy. Cellulitis often develops within 12 to 24 hours, accompanied by excruciating pain, marked edema, and bullae. Bacteremia is often documented. Treatment requires prompt antimicrobial therapy and wide surgical debridement.

Infected vascular gangrene is a focal, usually indolent, and primarily ischemic process in the small muscles of a distal lower extremity already gangrenous from arterial insufficiency. Diabetic patients are prone to develop this complication, which usually does not extend beyond the area of vascular gangrene to involve viable muscle. Proteus spp., Bacteroides spp., and anaerobic streptococci are among the bacteria found in such lesions (101,102).

DIABETIC FOOT INFECTION

This term defines any inframalleolar infection in a person with diabetes mellitus. These include paronychia, cellulitis, myositis, abscesses, NF, septic arthritis, tendonitis, and osteomyelitis. The most common lesion requiring hospitalization is the infected diabetic foot ulcer (Fig. 4). Neuropathy plays a central role, with disturbances of sensory, motor, and autonomic functions leading to ulcerations due to trauma or excessive pressure on a deformed foot. This wound may progress to become actively infected, and by contiguous extension the infection can involve deeper tissues. This sequence can be rapid, especially in an ischemic limb. Various immunologic disturbances, especially involving the polymorphonuclear leukocytes, may affect some

(A)

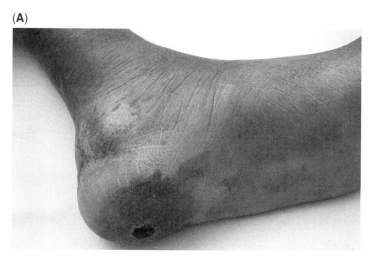

(B)

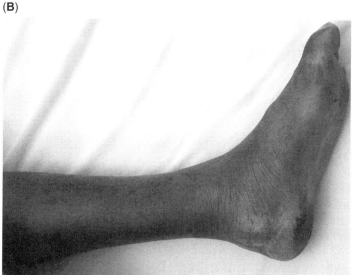

Figure 4 (**A**) Limb threatening left diabetic foot ulcer. (**B**) Rapid progression to gas gangrene. Patient underwent below knee amputation. Operative cultures grew group G *streptococcus*, methicillin-resistant *Staphylococcus aureus*, *Streptococcus viridans*, *Enterococcus* spp., and *Bacteroides fragilis.*

diabetic patients. *S. aureus* and the β-hemolytic streptococci (groups A, C, G, and especially group B) are the most commonly isolated pathogens. Chronic wounds develop a more complex colonizing flora, including enterococci, enterobacteriaceae, obligate anaerobes, *P. aeruginosa*, and other nonfermentative gram-negative rods. Hospitalization, surgical procedures, and prolonged antibiotics predispose patients to colonization and infection with MRSA or vancomycin-resistant enterococcus. Community-acquired cases of MRSA are becoming more common. Finally, the two reported cases of VRSA involved a diabetic patient with a foot infection (103–105).

Therapy: Initial therapy is empirical and should be based on severity of infection and available microbiological data, such as recent culture results or current smear findings from adequately obtained specimens. The microbiology can be identified by culture only if specimens are collected and processed properly. Deep tissue specimens, obtained aseptically at surgery, contain the true pathogens more often than do samples obtained from superficial lesions. A curettage, or tissue scraping with a scalpel, from the base of a debrided ulcer provides more accurate results. An antibiotic regimen should always include an agent active against staphylococci and streptococci. Previously treated or severe cases may need extended coverage that also includes commonly isolated gram-negative bacilli and *Enterococcus* spp. Necrotic, gangrenous, or foul smelling wounds usually require antianaerobic therapy. For moderate to severe infection ampicillin/sulbactam or piperacillin/tazobactam can be used. For life-threatening infections imipenam/cilastin may be a consideration. A high prevalence of MRSA may require use of vancomycin, or other appropriate agents against these organisms. The duration of treatment for life-threatening infection may be two weeks or longer. Many infections require surgical procedures that range from drainage and excision of infected and necrotic tissues to revascularization or amputation. For treatment refer to Table 4.

SKIN AND SOFT TISSUE INFECTIONS IN INJECTION DRUG USERS

The mechanism by which infection is established probably relates to tissue trauma, direct effects of drugs, tissue ischemia, and inoculation of bacteria. As a result of repeated injections into a single site, skin and surrounding tissue are damaged, develop local ischemia and necrosis, and become susceptible to infection. Opiates suppress T-cell functions and also inhibit phagocytosis, chemotaxis, and killing by neutrophils and macrophages. Infection ranges from cellulitis to skin and soft tissue abscesses, and occasionally fasciitis and pyomyositis. The most common sites of involvement correspond to injection sites: the upper and lower extremities, the groin and antecubital fossa, with the microbiology being monomicrobial or polymicrobial involving *S. aureus*, *S. viridans*, *S. pyogenes*, *Streptococcus anginosus group*, *E. corrodens*, anaerobic organisms like clostridium spp. and *Prevotella*, and gram-negative enteric organisms including *E. coli*, *Klebsiella*, *Proteus mirabilis*, *Pseudomonas*, and *Enterobacter* (106–108). Black tar heroin use has resulted in outbreaks of *C. botulinism*, *C. tetani*, and *C. sordelli* in intravenous drug users. For treatment refer to Table 3.

PYOMYOSITIS

Pyomyositis is an infection of the skeletal muscle predominantly caused by *S. aureus* and *Streptococcus* spp. (109,110). Other rare organisms include enterobacteriaceae and anaerobic bacteria. Case reports of *Aspergillus fumigatus*, *C. neoformans*, *Mycobacterium tuberculosis*, and *M. avium-intracellulare* have been reported (111,112). It was originally recognized in patients who acquired the disease in the tropics. Predisposing conditions include diabetes mellitus, cirrhosis, immunosuppressive illness, and HIV, and has been reported in intravenous drug abusers. Presumed pathogenesis involves a prior bacteremia, commonly transient. Bacterial infection of the muscle usually occurs after a penetrating wound, vascular insufficiency, or a contiguous spread. Common muscle involvement includes deltoid, psoas, biceps, gastrocnemius, gluteal, and quadriceps, though any muscle group can be involved. Patients will typically present with fever, pain, tenderness, and swel-

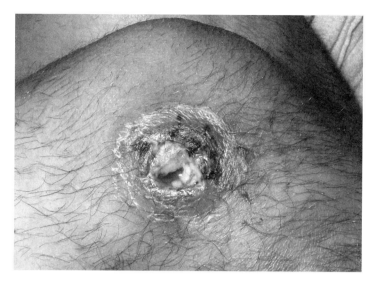

Figure 5 Right leg abscess, cultures grew methicillin-resistant *Staphylococcus aureus* (community acquired).

ling of the involved muscle. Bacteremia is present in 5% to 35% of cases. The diagnosis is best established by computed tomography scan or MRI.

Treatment consists of drainage (percutaneous or open-incision). Initial antibiotics should consist of intravenous administration of a β-lactamase–resistant penicillin. Initial vancomycin therapy should be considered if MRSA is suspected. Early modification of initial antimicrobial therapy is based on Gram-stain and culture results.

COMMUNITY-ACQUIRED METHICILLIN-RESISTANT *S. AUREUS*

Community-acquired MRSA has become increasingly endemic in many parts of the world (113,114). The most common clinical syndrome has been skin and soft tissue infections (Fig. 5). *S. aureus* has been a very uncommon cause of NF, but in a recent study 14 patients were identified as community-acquired MRSA with clinical and intraoperative findings of NF, necrotizing myositis, or both (115). Unfortunately, there are no obvious epidemiologic clues to this etiologic agent, and one sees patients with no prior antimicrobial therapy developing this infection. The organism appears somewhat unique in its characteristics by possessing the staphylococcal cassette chromosome Mec IV gene for methicillin resistance and the Panton Valentine Leukocidin genes encoding for a toxin presumably responsible for necrosis in soft tissue sites as well as the lungs. This organism has prompted many clinicians to add vancomycin, sulfamethoxazole/trimethoprim, linezolid, daptomycin, or other agents effective against MRSA in the empiric treatment of skin and soft tissue infections.

SUMMARY

A wide variety of skin and soft tissue infections can occur in the critical care settings. The rise in immunocompromised patients such as those with AIDS, transplant recipients, and those receiving chemotherapy or prolonged corticosteroid therapy have led to diverse etiologies, clinical manifestations, and severity. *S. aureus* remains the most common pathogen causing infections from minor skin lesions to severe life-threatening illness such as purpura fulminans. However a variety of other pathogens may be identified and need to be considered with certain epidemiologic clues. Community-acquired MRSA has become increasingly prevalent in many parts of the world. The most common clinical syndrome has been skin and soft tissue infection, but in a recent study 14 patients were identified as community-acquired MRSA with clinical and intraoperative findings of NF, necrotizing myositis, or both.

Important considerations when evaluating patients include underlying medical conditions; exposure history; and presenting signs, symptoms, and radiographic patterns. The key to treating serious skin and soft tissue infections successfully is prompt recognition, followed by appropriate antibiotic and surgical intervention as needed to decrease the morbidity and mortality.

REFERENCES

1. Roth RR, James WD. Microbiology of the skin: resident flora, ecology, infection. J Am Acad Dermatol 1989; 20:367–390.
2. Roth RR, James WD. Microbiol ecology of the skin. Annu Rev Microbiol 1988; 42:441–464.
3. Greene JN. The microbiology of colonization, including techniques for assessing and measuring colonization. Infect Control Hosp Epidemiol 1996; 17:114–118.
4. Granto PA. Pathogenesis and indigenous microorganisms of humans. In: Murray PR, Banon EJ, Jorgersas JH, Pyaller MA, Yolken RH, eds. Manual of Clinical Microbiology. 8th ed. Washington, DC: ASM Press, 2003; 1:44–54.
5. Kluytmans J, Belkun AV, Verbrugh H. Nasal carriage of *Staphylococcus aureus*: epidemiology, underlying mechanisms, and associated risks. Clin Microbiol Rev 1997: 505–520.
6. Eiff CV, Becker K, Machka K, et al. Nasal carriage as a source of *Staphylococcus aureus* bacteremia. N Engl J Med 2001; 344:11–16.
7. Williams REO. Healthy carriage of *Staphylococcus aureus*: its prevalence and importance. Bacteriol Rev 1963; 27:56–71.
8. Ong PY, Ohtake T, Brandt C, et al. Endogenous antimicrobial peptides and skin infections in atopic dermatitis. N Engl J Med 2002; 347:1151–1160.
9. Lewis RT. Soft tissue infections. World J Surg 1998; 22:146–151.
10. Dajani AS, Ferrieri P, Wannamaker LW. Natural history of impetigo. II. Etiologic agents and bacterial interactions. J Clin Invest 1972; 51:2863.
11. Bisno AL, Stevens DL. Streptococcal infections of skin and soft tissues. N Engl J Med 1996; 334:240–245.
12. Scales J, Fleischer A, Krowchuk D. Bullous impetigo. Arch Pediatr Adolesc Med 1997; 151:1168–1169.
13. Melish ME, Glasgow LA. The staphylococcal scalded-skin syndrome. N Engl J Med 1970; 282:1114–1119.
14. Dajani AS. The scalded skin syndrome: relation to phage group II staphylococci. J Infect Dis 1972; 125:548–551.
15. Kondo IS, Sakuri S, Sarai Y, et al. Two serotypes of exfoliatin and their distribution in Staphylococcal strain isolated from patients with scalded skin syndrome. J Clin Microbiol 1975; 5:397–400.
16. Yamasaki O, Yamguchi T, Sugai M, et al. Clinical manifestations of staphylococcal scalded-skin syndrome depend on serotypes of exfoliative toxins. J Clin Microbiol 2005; 43:1890–1893.

17. Ladhani S, Joannou CL, Lochrie DP, et al. Clinical, microbial, and biochemical aspects of the exfoliative toxins causing staphylococcal scalded-skin syndrome. Clin Microbiol Rev 1999; 12:224–242.
18. Lina G, Gillet Y, Vandenesch F, et al. Toxin involvement in staphylococcal scalded skin syndrome. Clin Infect Dis 1997; 25:1369–1373.
19. Elias, PM, Fritsch P, Epstein EH Jr. Staphylococcal scalded skin syndrome. Arch Dermatol 1997; 113:207–219.
20. Ladhani S, Evans, RW. Staphylococcal scalded skin syndrome. Arch Dis Child 1998; 78: 85–88.
21. Gemmell CG. Staphylococcal scalded skin syndrome. J Med Microbiol 1995; 43:318–327.
22. Cribier B, Piemont Y, Grosshans E. Staphylococcal scalded skin syndrome in adults: a clinical review illustrated with a case. J Am Acad Dermatol 1984; 30:319–324.
23. Brochers SL, Gomez EC, Isseroff RR. Generalized staphylococcal scalded skin syndrome in an anephric boy undergoing hemodialysis. Arch Dermatol 1984; 120:912–918.
24. Goldberg NS, Ahmed T, Robinson B, et al. Staphylococcal scalded skin syndrome mimicking acute graft-versus-host disease in a bone marrow transplant recipient. Arch Dermatol 1989; 125:85–87.
25. Lowy FD. Staphylococcus aureus infections. N Engl J Med 1998:520–532.
26. Markowitz N, Quinn EL, Saravolatz LD. Trimethoprim-sulfamethoxazole compared with vancomycin for the treatment of *Staphylococcus aureus* bacteremia. Ann Intern Med 1992; 117(5):390–398.
27. Anstead GM, Owens AD. Recent advances in the treatment of infections due to resistant *Staphylococcus aureus*. Curr Opin Infect Dis 2004; 17:549–555.
28. Manders SM. Toxin-mediated streptococcal and staphylococcal disease. J Am Acad Dermatol 1998; 39(3):383–398.
29. Centers for Disease Control and Prevention. Epidemiology Program Office, Division of Public Health surveillance and Informatics. Case definitions for infectious conditions under public health surveillance. Part 1. Case definitions for nationally notifiable infectious disease. Available at http://www.cdc.gov/epo/dphsi/casedef/notiable.htm (accessed June 11, 2005).
30. The Working Group on Severe Streptococcal Infections. Defining the group A streptococcal toxic shock syndrome: rationale and consensus definition. JAMA 1993; 269:390–391.
31. Chesney PJ, Davis JP, Purdy WK, et al. Clinical manifestation of toxic shock syndrome. JAMA 1981; 246:741–748.
32. Shands KN, Schmid GP, Dan BB, et al. Toxic shock syndrome in menstruating women. Association with tampon use and *Staphylococcus aureus* and clinical features in 52 cases. N Engl J Med 1980; 303:1436–1442.
33. Parsonnet J. Non menstrual toxic shock syndrome: new insights into diagnosis, pathogenesis, and treatment. Curr Clin Top Infect Dis 1996; 16:1–20.
34. Kain KC, Schulzer M, Chow AW. Clinical spectrum of nonmenstrual toxic shock syndrome (TSS): comparison with menstrual TSS by multivariate analyses. Clin Infect Dis 1993; 16:100–106.
35. Davis JP, Osterholm MT, Helms CM, et al. Tri-state toxic shock syndrome study. II. Clinical and laboratory findings. J Infect Dis 1982; 145:441–448.
36. Davis JP, Chesney PJ, Wand PJ, et al. Toxic-shock syndrome: epidemiologic features, recurrence, risk factors, and prevention. N Engl J Med 1980; 303:1429–1435.
37. Stolz SJ, Davis JP, Vergeront JM, et al. Development of serum antibody to toxic shock toxin among individuals with toxic shock syndrome in Wisconsin. J Infect Dis 1985; 151:883–889.
38. Stevens DL. Invasive group A streptococcus infections. Clin Infect Dis 1992; 14:2–13.
39. Johnson Dr, Stevens DL, Kaplan EL. Epidemiologic analysis of group A streptococcus serotypes associated with severe systemic infections, rheumatic fever, or uncomplicated pharyngitis. J Infect Dis 1992; 166:374–382.
40. Teglund AN, Thulin P, Gan BS. Evidence for superantigen involvement in severe group A streptococcal tissue infections. J Infect Dis 2001; 184:853–860.

41. Hackett SP, Stevens DL. Streptococcal toxic shock syndrome: synthesis of tumor necrosis factor and interleukin-1 by monocytes stimulated with pyrogenic exotoxin A and streptolysin O. J Infect Dis 1992; 165:879–885.

42. Fast DJ, Schlievert PM, Nelson RD. Toxin shock syndrome-associated staphylococcal and streptococcal pyrogenic toxins are potent inducers of tumor necrosis factor production. Infect Immun 1989; 57:291–294.

43. Saouda M, Wu W, Conran P, et al. Streptococcal pyrogenic exotoxin B enhances tissue damage initiated by other *Streptococcus pyogenes* products. J Infect Dis 2001; 184: 723–731.

44. Proft T, Sriskandan S, Yang L. Superantigens and streptococcal toxic shock syndrome. Emerg Infect Dis 2003; 9:1211–1218.

45. Forni AL, Kaplan EL, Schlievert PM, Roberts RB. Clinical and microbiological characteristics of severe group A streptococcus infections and streptococcal toxic shock syndrome. Clin Infect Dis 1995; 21(2):333–340.

46. Factor SH, Levine OS, Schwartz B, et al. Invasive group A streptococcal disease: risk factors for adults. Emerg Infect Dis 2003; 8:970–977.

47. McCormick JK, Yarwood JM, Schlievert PM. Toxic shock syndrome and bacterial superantigens: an update. Annu Rev Microbiol 2001; 55:77–104.

48. Darenberg J, Söderquist B, Normark BH. Differences in potency of intravenous polyspecific immunoglobulin G against streptococcal and staphylococcal superantigens: implications for therapy of toxic shock syndrome. Clin Infect Dis 2004; 38:836–842.

49. Stevens DL. Dilemmas in the treatment of invasive streptococcus pyogenes infections. Clin Infect Dis 2003; 37:341–343.

50. Eagle H. Experimental approach to the problem of treatment failure with penicillin. I. Group A streptococcal infection in mice. Am J Med 1952; 13:389.

51. Stevens DL, Gibbons AE, Bergstrom R, et al. The Eagle effect revisited: efficacy of clindamycin, erythromycin, and penicillin in the treatment of streptococcal myositis. J Infect Dis 1988; 158:23–28.

52. Stevens DL, Yan S, Bryant AE. Penicillin-binding protein expression at different growth stages determines penicillin efficacy in vitro and in vivo: an explanation for the inoculum effect. J Infect Dis 1993; 167:1401–1405.

53. Stevens DL, Bryant AE, Yan S. Invasive group A streptococcal infection: new concepts in antibiotic treatment. Int J Antimicrob Agents 1994; 4:297–301.

54. Gemmell CG, Peterson PK, Schmeling D, et al. Potentiation of opsonization and phagocytosis of *Streptococcus pyogenes* following growth in the presence of clindamycin. J Clin Invest 1981; 67:1249–1256.

55. Kaul R, McGeer A, Norrby-Teglund A, et al. Intravenous immunoglobulin therapy for streptococcal toxic shock syndrome—a comparative observational study. Canadian Streptococcal study group. Clin Infect Dis 1999; 28:800–807.

56. Darenberg J, Ihendyane N, Sjolin J, et al. Intravenous immunoglobulin G therapy in streptococcal toxic shock syndrome: a European randomized, double blind, placebo controlled trial. Clin Infect Dis 2003; 37:333–340.

57. Norrby-Telgund A, Basma H, Anderson J, et al. Varying titres of neutralizing antibodies to streptococcal superantigens in different preparations of normal polyspecific immunoglobulin G (IVIG): implications for therapeutic efficacy. Clin Infect Dis 1998; 26: 631–638.

58. Jorup-Ronstrom C. Epidemiological and complicating features of erysipelas. Scand J Infect Dis 1986; 18:519–524.

59. Swartz MN. Cellulitis. N Engl J Med 2005; 350:904–912.

60. Swartz MN, Pasternack MS. Cellulitis and subcutaneous tissue infections. In: Mandell GL, Bennett JE, Dolin R, eds. Principles and Practices of Infectious Disease. 6th ed. Philadelphia: Elsevier, Churchill Livingstone, 2005; 1:1172–1194.

61. Bisharat N, Agmon V, Finkelstein R, et al. Clinical, epidemiological, and microbiological features of *Vibrio vulnificus* biogroup 3 causing outbreaks of wound infection and bacteraemia in Israel. Israel Vibrio Study Group. Lancet 1999; 354:1421–1424.

62. Bonner JR, Coker AS, Berryman CR, et al. Spectrum of vibrio infections in a gulf coast community. Ann Intern Med 1983; 99:464–469.

63. Gold WL, Salit IE. Aeromonas hydrophilia infections of the skin and soft tissue: report of 11 cases and review. Clin Infect Dis 1993; 16:69–74.

64. Weinstein MR, Litt M, Kertesz Da, et al. Invasive infections due to a fish pathogen, *Streptococcus iniae*. *S. iniae* Study Group. N Engl J Med 1997; 337(9):589–594.

65. Capdevila O, Grau I, Vadillo M, et al. Bacteremic pneumococcal cellulitis compared with bacteremic cellulitis caused by *Staphylococcus aureus* and *Streptococcus pyogenes*. Eur J Clin Microbiol Infect Dis 2003; 22(6):337–341.

66. Porras MC, Martinez VC, Ruiz IM, et al. Acute cellulitis: an unusual manifestation of meningococcal disease. Scand J Infect Dis 2001; 33(1):56–59.

67. Brooke CJ, Riley TV. *Erysipelothrix rhusiopathiae*: bacteriology, epidemiology and clinical manifestations of an occupational pathogen. J Med Microbiol 1999; 48(9):789–799.

68. Talan DA, Citron DM, Abrahamian FM, et al. Bacteriologic analysis of infected dog and cat bites. N Engl J Med 1999; 340:85–92.

69. Moal GL, Landron C, Grollier G, et al. Meningitis due to *Capnocytophaga canimorsus* after receipt of a dog bite: case report and review of the literature. Clin Infect Dis 2003; 36:e42–e46.

70. Talan DA, Abrahamian FM, Moran GJ, et al. Clinical presentation and bacteriologic analysis of infected human bites in patients presenting to emergency departments. Clin Infect Dis 2003; 37:1481–1489.

71. Greene SL, Su WP, Muller SA. Ecthyma gangrenosum: report of clinical, histopathologic, and bacteriologic aspects of eight cases. J Am Acad Dermatol 1984; 11:781–787.

72. Huminer D, Siegman-Igra Y, Morduchowicz G, et al. Ecthyma gangrenosum without bacteremia. Report of six cases and review of the literature. Arch Intern Med 1987; 147(2): 299–301.

73. Sevinsky LD, Viecens C, Ballesteros DO, et al. Ecthyma gangrenosum: a cutaneous manifestation of Pseudomonas aeruginosa sepsis. J Am Acad Dermatol 1993; 29(1):104–106.

74. Inglesby TV, O'Toole, Henderson DA, et al. Anthrax as a biological weapon 2002: updated recommendation for management. JAMA 2002; 287:2236–2252.

75. Swartz MN. Recognition and treatment of Anthrax: an update. N Engl J Med 2001; 345:1621–1626.

76. Centers for Disease Control and Prevention update: investigation of bioterrorism resulted anthrax and interim guidelines for exposure management and antimicrobial therapy. Mor Mortal Wkly Rep 2001; 50:909–919.

77. Harrison OB, Robertson BD, Faust SN, et al. Analysis of pathogen host cell interactions in purpura fulminans: expression of capsule, type IV pilli, and Por A by *Neisseria meningitides* in vivo. Infect Immun 2002; 70:193–201.

78. Carpenter CT, Kaiser AB. Purpura fulminans in pneumococcal sepsis: case report and review. Scand J Infect Dis 1997; 29(5):479–483.

79. Kravitz GR, Dries DJ, Peterson ML, et al. Purpura fulminans due to Staphylococcus aureus. Clin Infect Dis 2005; 40:941–947.

80. Seal DV. Necrotizing fasciitis. Curr Opin Infect Dis 2001; 14:127–132.

81. Kuncir EJ, Tillou A, St. Hill CR, et al. Necrotizing soft tissue infections. Emerg Med Clin N Am 2003; 21:1075–1087.

82. Nicholas RL, Florman S. Clinical presentations of soft-tissue infections and surgical site infections. Clin Infect Dis 2001; 33:S84–S93.

83. McHenry CR, Pitrowski JJ, Petrinic D, et al. Determinants of mortality in necrotizing soft tissue infections. Ann Surg 1995; 221:558–563.

84. Giuliano A, Lewis F Jr., Hardy K, et al. Bacteriology of necrotizing fasciitis. Am J Surg 1977; 134:52–57.

85. Sharma M, Khatib R, Fakih M. Clinical characteristics of necrotizing fasciitis caused by Group G streptococcus: case report and review of the literature. Scand J Infect Dis 2002; 34(6):468–471.

86. Patino JF, Castro D. Necrotizing lesions of the soft tissue: a review. World J Surg 1991; 15:235–239.

87. Chapnik EK, Abter EI. Necrotizing soft tissue infections. Infect Dis Clin North Am 1996; 10:835–855.

88. Cunningham JD, Silver L, Rudikoff D. Necrotizing fasciitis. A plea for early diagnosis and treatment. Mt Sinai J Med 2001; 68:253–261.

89. Wong CH, Wang YS. The diagnosis of necrotizing fasciitis. Curr Opin Infect Dis 2005; 18:101–106.

90. Kaul R, McGeer A, Low DE, Green K, Schwartz B. Population-based surveillance for group A streptococcal necrotizing fasciitis: clinical features, prognostic indicators, and microbiologic analysis of seventy-seven cases. Ontario Group A Streptococcal Study. Am J Med 1997; 103(1):18–24.

91. Anderson TJ, Green SD, Childers BJ. Massive soft tissue injury: diagnosis and management of necrotizing fasciitis and purpura fulminans. Plast Reconstr Surg 2001; 107: 1025–1035.

92. Jones RB, Hirschmann JV, Brown GS, et al. Fournier's syndrome: necrotizing subcutaneous infection of the male genitalia. J Urol 1979; 122; 279–282.

93. Nickels JC, Morales A. Necrotizing fasciitis of the male genitalia (Fournier's gangrene). Can Med Assoc J 1983; 129:445–448.

94. Cline KA, Turnbull TL. Clostridial myonecrosis. Ann Emerg Med 1985; 14:459–466.

95. Gorbach SL, Thadepalli H. Isolation of clostridium in human infections: evaluation of 114 cases. J Infect Dis 1975; 131:S81–S85.

96. Bryant AE, Chen RYZ, Nagata Y. Clostridial gas gangrene. I. Cellular and molecular mechanisms of microvascular dysfunction induced by exotoxins of *Clostridium perfringens*. J Infect Dis 2000; 182:799–780.

97. Stevens DL, Bryant AE. The role of clostridial toxins in the pathogenesis of gas gangrene. Clin Infect Dis 2002; 35:S93–S100.

98. Stephans MB. Gas gangrene. Potential for hyperbaric oxygen therapy. Postgrad Med 1996; 99:217–220.

99. Tibbles PM, Edelsberg JS. Hyperbaric-oxygen therapy. N Engl J Med 1996; 334: 1642–1648.

100. Stevens DL, Musher DM, Watson DA, et al. Spontaneous nontraumatic gangrene due to *Clostridium septicum*. Rev Infect Dis 1990; 12:286–296.

101. DiNubile MJ, Lipsky BA. Complicated infections of skin and skin structures: when the infection is more than skin deep. J Antimicrob Chemother 2004; 53(S2):ii37–ii50.

102. Pasternack MS, Swartz MN. Myositis. In: Mandell GL, Bennett JE, Dolin R, eds. Principles and Practices of Infectious Disease. 6th ed. Philadelphia: Elsevier, Churchill Livingstone, 2005; 1:1194–1204.

103. Lipsky BA, Pecoraro RE, Wheat JL. The diabetic foot: soft tissue and bone infection. Infect Dis Clin North Am 1990; 4:409–432.

104. Wheat LJ, Allen SD, Henry M, et al. Diabetic foot infections: bacteriologic analysis. Arch Intern Med 1986; 146:1935:40.

105. Sapico FL, Witte JL, Canawati HN, et al. The infected foot of the diabetic patient: quantitative microbiology and analysis of clinical features. Rev Infect Dis 1984; 6(suppl 1): 171–176.

106. Murphy EL, DeVita D, Liu H, et al. Risk factors for skin and soft-tissue abscesses among Injection drug users: a case control study. Clin Infect Dis 2001; 33:35–40.

107. Chen JL, Fullerton KE, Flynn NM. Necrotizing fasciitis associated with injection drug usc. Clin Infect Dis 2001; 33:6–15.

108. Ebright JR, Pieper B. Skin and soft tissue infections in injection drug users. Infect Dis Clin North Am 2002; 16:697–712.

109. Levin MJ, Gardner P, Waldvogel FA. Tropical pyomyositis: an unusual infection due to *Staphylococcus aureus*. N Engl J Med 1971; 284:196–198.
110. Crum NF. Bacterial pyomyositis in the United States. Am J Med 2004; 117:420–428.
111. Miralles GD, Bregman Z. Necrotizing pyomyositis caused by *Mycobacterium avium* complex in a patient with AIDS. Clin Infect Dis 1994; 18:833–834.
112. Sharma M, Khatib R, Fakih M. *Cryptococcus neoformans* myositis without dissemination. Scand J Infect Dis 2002; 34(11):858–859.
113. Fridkin SK, Hageman JC, Morrison M, et al. Methicillin resistant *staphylococcus aureus* disease in three communities. N Engl J Med 2005; 352:1436–1444.
114. Johnson LB, Saravolatz LD. Community-acquired MRSA: current epidemiology and management issues. Infect Med 2005; 22:16–20.
115. Miller LG, Perdeau-Remington, Reig Gunter, et al. Necrotizing fasciitis caused by community associated methicillin resistant *Staphylococcus aureus* in Los Angeles. N Engl J Med 2005; 352:1445–1453.

17

Infections in Patients on Steroids in the Critical Care Unit

John N. Sheagren
Department of Internal Medicine, Advocate Illinois Masonic Medical Center, Chicago, Illinois, U.S.A.

INTRODUCTION

For over half a century, steroids (corticosteroids and glucocorticoids) have been used to suppress inflammatory, autoimmune, and other immunologic processes (1–3). Their benefits are unquestioned; however, their costs are high. When needed, their multifactorial enhancing and suppressing molecular and cellular effects on metabolic systems lead to hypertension, electrolyte abnormalities, and mineral disorders, especially osteoporosis (1–3). Their impacts on inflammatory systems impair tissue integrity and repair and result in a variety of infectious complications (4), the focus of this chapter.

While steroids still need to be used in nearly every specialty of medicine, clinicians are constantly searching for "steroid sparing," immunosuppressive/anti-inflammatory treatments for the multitudes of inflammatory and autoimmune disorders suffered by their patients. This chapter will provide an historical overview of the relationship between steroids and infections, how the host's defense system is organized to defend against microbial invasion by specific organisms, how steroids alter each aspect of the inflammatory system generally to increase the likelihood of each such infection, and, paradoxically, how steroids can actually be used to treat some specific infectious diseases. Several years ago, all these topics were reviewed in great detail (5); and most of the data and concepts provided in that review are still relevant today.

HISTORICAL ASPECTS OF STEROIDS AND INFECTIONS

The historical relationships between the function of the adrenal gland and infection were masterfully summarized in a review article in 1953 by Kass and Finland (6). They pointed out that Dr. Harvey Cushing in the early 1900s noted that adrenalectomy (hypoadrenalism) was associated with increased susceptibility to and mortality from infection. Physiologic replacement doses of an adrenal extract, containing the adrenal cortical hormones, corrected the problem of increased mortality from infection in experimental animals.

The evolution through the late 1800s and early 1900s of the understanding of the adrenal cortex as compared to the adrenal medulla lead to the observation that the life of experimental animals could be prolonged by the administration of adrenal cortical but not adrenal medullary (epinephrine hormone) administration. Not only was the life of the adrenalectomized animal extended with adrenal cortical extracts, but such extracts also corrected the increased susceptibility to infection as well as the other metabolic and hemodynamic abnormalities which they had described.

In 1912, Dr. Harvey Cushing was the first to define the disease produced by adrenal cortical steroid excess. It was not for another 20 years, however, that he wrote the definitive paper on the syndrome, which subsequently came to be called "Cushing's Syndrome." While such patients were hypertensive and experienced a variety of fluid and electrolyte abnormalities, Dr. Cushing noted that infection was the primary cause of death in about half (6).

In the late 1940s, Hench et al. (7) at the Mayo Clinic described the first clinical uses of supraphysiologic doses of cortisone on a variety of systemic inflammatory diseases, especially rheumatoid arthritis. Not long afterward, case reports appeared describing a wide variety of infectious complications occurring in patients on such doses of steroids. Kass went on to perform a series of elegant laboratory studies confirming that steroid therapy produced a dose-related increase in susceptibility to a variety of infectious agents in experimental animals (8).

HOST DEFENSES/IMMUNITY AGAINST INFECTIONS

An excellent review of the actions of steroids on immunity has recently been published (9). That review noted and summarized a variety of studies over the past half century that at least have partially clarified the multiple actions of steroids on the immune system. The complexity of such effects is enormous: In some situations, steroids up regulate and enhance immunologic functions, while in others, they down regulate and/or suppress immunity. Franchimont (9) outlines in some detail the molecular, cellular, and pharmacologic properties of steroids and pointed out that steroids exert both negative and positive effects on various limbs and components of the immune response. While modulating genes involved in the priming of the innate (nonspecific) immune response, they suppress cellular [T helper-1 (Th-1)] immunity and promote humoral [T helper 2 (Th-2)] immunity in the adaptive (specific or acquired) immune response. Franchimont goes on to suggest the ex vivo therapeutic use of steroids might represent a way positively to modulate cellular responses in autoimmune diseases while avoiding long-term systemic steroid side effects.

In my earlier review of this topic (5), I proposed a simple organization of the immune system in order to permit a better understanding of how each component functions to defend the host against microbial invaders, as well as in a more focused fashion to help explain how steroids affect each limb of immunity. Table 1 outlines an organizational structure of the immune system, useful in understanding the host defense systems against infections. Briefly, the immune system is broken down into the nonspecific (innate) and the specific (acquired or adaptive) immune systems.

Table 1 A Simplified Organization of the Host Defense System

Nonspecific (innate) immunity
Barrier systems: skin, mucous membranes, cilia, and mucus
Complement system (via the alternative pathway)
WBCs: neutrophils, macrophages, and eosinophils
Specific (acquired or adaptive) immunity
Macrophages, including dendritic (antigen processing) cells
Cellular immune response: mediated by Th-1 lymphocytes, which release cytokines to activate surrounding macrophages which then become more efficient microbial killers
Humoral immune response: mediated by Th-2 lymphocytes, which subsequently activate surrounding B lymphocytes to evolve into plasma cells which produce the various classes of immunoglobulins/antibodies. Antibodies either opsonize bacteria to permit phagocytosis or directly lyse and kill bacteria with the help of the complement system (this time via the "classical" pathway)

Abbreviations: Th-1, T helper 1; Th-2, T helper 2; WBCs, white blood cells.

The Nonspecific (Innate) Immune System

The first lines of defense against microbial invaders are the skin and mucous membranes, breaks in which, for example, create entry points for colonizing acute invasive bacteria, mostly *staphylococci* and *streptococci*, to enter the body. Once in the subcutaneous or submucosal tissues, these microbes replicate and initiate activation (via a variety of their cell materials, toxins, and enzymes) of the complement system, at this initial point through its "alternative" pathway (10). Complement components not only enhance local vasoactive and mediator contributions to the local inflammatory response, but generate chemotactic fragments which draw in surrounding leukocytes.

The white blood cells (WBCs) are the most important nonspecific participants in this initial phase of host defense, for complement's alternative pathway does not itself directly participate in bacterial killing. Because all organisms, whether opsonized or not, activate the alternative limb of the compliment pathway, it is the response of WBCs, predominantly the neutrophils and macrophages, which are the most important host defense elements in this initial, nonspecific phase of the host defenses. The vast majority of microbial invaders are stopped in their tracks by the combination of the barrier systems and the complement assembled WBCs.

The Specific (Acquired or Adaptive) Immune System

Macrophages (including dendritic cells) are crucial to antigen processing and initiate both the cellular (Th-1) lymphocyte activation and response and the humoral (Th-2) immune response. Further, macrophages are also *effector* cells in the fully developed cellular immune response, responsible, when activated, for intracellular killing of a variety of important pathogens. Th-1 lymphocytes reacting to specific antigen stimulation release cytokines, which subsequently assemble and activate available surrounding macrophages to become highly efficient killers of facultative intracellular microbes; such organisms can survive ingestion in unactivated macrophages and go on to cause further tissue damage (11).

The humoral immune response has as its primary role the production of immunoglobulins, most importantly antibodies of the immunoglobulin M (IgM) and immunoglobulin G (IgG) classes (12). These antibodies are either directly bactericidal [along with complement (10), this time via the "classical" pathway] or important opsonins leading to more efficient phagocytosis and cellular killing, especially of a variety of encapsulated microbes (the prototypic organism being *Streptococcus pneumoniae*). Opsonins probably also help in the defense against a variety of gram-negative organisms, especially neisseria and certain other gram-negative rods.

MICROBIAL DEFENSE BY THE VARIOUS COMPONENTS OF THE IMMUNE SYSTEMS

While the preceding paragraphs have discussed the components of the host defense/ immune systems and alluded to some of the microbes dealt with by each component of immunity, the next few paragraphs will focus on the specific microbes expected when there are deficiencies in those host defense systems (Table 2).

Infections Expected in Deficiencies of the Nonspecific/Innate Immune System

The barrier systems are most important in protecting against invasion by the acute pyogenic bacteria such as the beta-hemolytic streptococci and *Staphylococcus aureus*. The classic example of such defects is the patient with exfoliative types of dermatitis (such as an exfoliating drug eruption or Stevens/Johnson Syndrome) or the extensively burned patient (13). The sequence of events in such patients is usually the following: first occurs colonization and then infection with gram-positive cocci (*streptococci* and *staphylococci*), which are generally antibiotic susceptible and therefore treatable. Next come the colonization and then infection with gram-negative bacilli such as the coliform bacteria, Klebsiella, and *Pseudomonas aeruginosa*. Intense antibacterial antibiotic therapy may again stabilize such patients for a while, but then overgrowth with a variety of yeasts, such as *Candida albicans*, or the other candida species creates an extremely difficult clinical situation. Also, burn wound colonization and infection with a variety of viruses sometimes occur (such as the herpes viruses or other DNA viruses). Deficiencies in the complement system may

Table 2 Microbes Defended Against by the Various Components of the Host Defense/ Immune Systems

Immune system component	Defends against
Nonspecific/innate immune system (barrier systems, complement via the "alternative" pathway, and leukocytes, mainly the neutrophil)	Acute pyogenic bacteria (streptococci, staphylococci, some gram negatives such as neisseria, etc.)
Specific (acquired or adaptive) immunity:	
Cellular immunity (Th-1, lymphocytes, and macrophages)	The group of microbes collectively known "facultative intracellular pathogens" (see text)
Humoral immunity (Th-2 lymphocytes, plasma cells, and complement via the "classical" pathway)	IgM and IgG antibodies protect primarily encapsulated, pyogenic bacteria (classically, *Streptococcus pneumoniae*, *Hemophilus influenzae*, and *Neisseria*; may also help against some other gram negative rods

Abbreviations: Th-1, T helper 1; Th-2, T helper 2; IgM, immunoglobulin M; IgG, immunoglobulin G.

lead also to infections with acute pyogenes and seem particularly to increase susceptibility to neisseria (14). Finally, defects in numbers or function of neutrophils classically lead to infections with *streptococci* and *staphylococci* and, after repeated courses of antibiotics, to a variety of gram-negative bacilli, and then yeasts.

Specific (Acquired or Adaptive) Immunity

Cellular Immunity

As noted earlier, the cellular immune system is composed of Th-1 lymphocytes, the cytokines they produce, and the macrophages which on the afferent side process antigen to initiate the cellular immune response and on the efferent side become activated by the Th-1 lymphocytokines to become the ultimate killer cells of cellular immunity. As shown in Table 2, the cellular immune system defends against the group of organisms collectively known as the "facultative intracellular pathogens" (FIPs), microorganisms that generally survive inside nonimmune host macrophages (15). These types of microbes may be effectively dealt with when they are ingested by cytokine "activated" macrophages, i.e., those whose microbicidal systems have been turned on by cytokines released by specifically sensitized Th-1 lymphocytes (11,16). Thus, in nonimmune hosts, FIPs may live symbiotically within macrophages, deriving, in fact, some of their metabolic needs from the host cells themselves. However, once the immune response has been generated by antigen processing cells, which program subsets of Th-1 lymphocytes against antigens peculiar to each specific invading FIP, such organisms are either killed, or at least held in check, for prolonged periods of time. Those organisms, lying dormant but still alive within host tissues, mostly within activated macrophages (which pathologically are recognized as epitheloid cells or giant cells combining to form granulomas), may, when the cellular immune responses have become suppressed, begin to grow and cause a "reactivated" infection, proceeding on to cause local and/or systemic host damage. The major causes of the suppression of the cellular immune system are prolonged periods of exogenous stress, usually accompanied by malnutrition, certain specific viral infections, especially the human immunodeficiency virus, and systemic immunosuppressive agents, particularly steroids.

The types of microbes known as FIPs contained by cellular immunity and which are most important in infecting humans (as noted in Table 2) are several types of bacteria (listeria, salmonellae, mycobacteria, and nocardia) and fungi (cryptococcus, histoplasmosis, coccidioidomycosis, and the yeasts, especially candida species). Several parasites are also primarily controlled by the cellular immune system (toxoplasmosis, *Pneumocystis carinii*, leishmania, cryptosporidium, and strongyloids).

Humoral Immunity

The humoral immune system consists of Th-2 lymphocytes and the B cells, which are activated and programmed to evolve into plasma cells producing the various classes of immunoglobulins. These immunoglobulins/antibodies are important in defending against a variety of pathogens. As noted earlier, the humoral/antibody mediated immune system also is aided by the complement system, now via the "classical" pathway, and is important in both opsonization and direct bactericidal activity (10,12). Particularly important in host defense are the IgM and IgG antibody classes. Such antibodies help protect the host primarily against the encapsulated, pyogenic bacteria, the classical organisms being *S. pneumoniae*, *Hemophilus influenzae*, and *Neisseria* (12).

Antibody mediated defenses may also help against some other gram-negative rods such as the coliform bacteria and klebsiella (Table 2).

MAJOR EFFECTS OF STEROIDS ON IMMUNITY

It is important for the reader to be aware that different doses of steroids (glucocorticoids) are used to achieve different therapeutic results in patients; further, different steroid doses have quite different effects on host inflammation and immunity (Table 3). I have arbitrarily classified these dose effects into the following ranges: physiologic, pharmacologic, and suprapharmacologic doses of steroids.

Physiologic Doses of Steroids

Physiologic doses of steroids are those in the daily range from 20 to 30 mg of hydrocortisone, the amount that the unstressed adrenal cortex produces over 24 hours (15). Thus, if a patient is on from 5 to 10 mg of prednisone for an underlying inflammatory disease, such a dose range (equivalent to 20–40 mg of hydrocortisone) represents essentially physiologic replacement of adrenal cortical function. Individuals on such doses have a relatively intact immune system, although a variety of long-term metabolic effects do occur (especially bone loss and osteoporosis). Such patients are not at a substantially increased risk of infectious complications. One needs to be aware, however, that should such a patient encounter the increased stress of trauma or infection, they then need to be treated with increased stress doses of hydrocortisone, in the range from 100 to 200 mg (20–40 mg of prednisone) daily. Again, patients treated properly during such periods of stress seem to be at no increased risk of infection, unless the period of stress and the administration of the aforementioned doses of glucocorticoids are prolonged beyond a few days (15).

Pharmacologic Doses of Steroids

These doses of prednisone (hydrocortisone is rarely used in such situations) are in the range of 1 mg/kg (40–100 mg) per day, doses typically used to treat a variety of acute inflammatory/autoimmune conditions. Such doses of prednisone are equivalent to 200 to 500 mg of hydrocortisone daily and when continued for more than four to six weeks, begin to produce the classical changes of Cushing's Syndrome with fat redistribution (moon facies, buffalo hump, and truncal obesity) and thinning of the skin, including the presence of striae and increasing bruisability. Further, these doses of steroids effectively block the access of acute inflammatory cells, especially neutrophils and macrophages, to foci of inflammation and infection, resulting in both reduced symptoms of the underlying inflammatory disease and reduced evidence of an infection as it progresses (16,17). Infections expected under such conditions are those caused by the acute pyogenic bacteria (again, streptococci and staphylococci). Also, rapid colonization and usually only superficial invasion occur with yeasts (*C. albicans* and other candida species), resulting in oral, pharyngeal, vaginal, and intertriginous infections (16).

The cellular (Th-1) immune system becomes suppressed after two to four weeks of such doses of steroids, resulting in impaired access of macrophages to inflammatory and infectious sites and decreased cytokine activation of macrophages by already programmed Th-1 lymphocytes (18). In such patients, positive delayed type

Table 3 Approximate Dose-Response Effects of Steroids on Host Defense/Immune Systems

Steroid doses/day	Effect on immunity	Infections expected
Physiologic: Nonstressed dose range state: 20–30 mg of hydrocortisone (5–7.5 mg of prednisone or equivalent)	None	None
Stressed state[a]: 100–200 mg of hydrocortisone (20–40 mg of prednisone) per day	None (unless prolonged)	None (unless prolonged)
Pharmacologic dose range: 200–500 mg of hydrocortisone (40–100 mg of prednisone or equivalent)	*Nonspecific/innate immunity* impairs inflammatory cell (esp. neutrophil) access to inflammatory/infections foci; increases fragility and therefore likelihood of breaks in the barrier systems (skin/mucous membranes)	Acute pyogenic bacteria (*staphylococci, streptococci,* superficial yeast infections)
	Cellular (Th-1) immunity becomes markedly suppressed within 14–28 days; results in impaired access of macrophages (MP) to inflammatory/ infectious sites and deceases MP activation; converts positive delayed type skin tests (e.g., tuberculin) to negative	Facultative intracellular pathogens (e.g., mycobacteria, systemic mycoses, listeria, salmonella, chlamydia, rickettsia, trypanosoma, leishmania, and strongyloids)
	Humoral (Th-2) immunity: These doses of steroids produce little effect; may even enhance some antibody responses	None in particular; however, note that even opsonized bacteria require the neutrophil for killing!
"Suprapharmacologic" dose range: 5000–10,000 mg of hydrocortisone (1–2 g of prednisone or equivalent) per day	Massive suppression of nonspecific/innate, cellular and even humoral immunity; effects present within 48 hrs; these negative immune effects reverse quickly when such doses are discontinued	Mostly infections with acute pyogenes, then (if such doses are continued) with gram-negative rods, then with facultative intracellular pathogens
Usually given in "pulse" doses over a 3 to 5 to 7-day period	Effects on the immune systems of pulse doses not well studied; probably minimal at 3–5 days; some effects probable at 7 days and beyond	None or acute pyogenic bacterial infection (at 5–7 days)

[a]Trauma, infection, metabolic hyper- or hypoactivity (e.g., hypo- or hyperthyroidism, pregnancy, severe fluid/electrolyte abnormalities, etc.).
Abbreviations: MP, macrophages; Th-1, T helper 1; Th-2, T helper 2.

hypersensitivity skin tests turn negative (19,20), and latent infections with FIP may become reactivated (21) and disseminate (e.g., those caused by tuberculosis, histoplasmosis, leishmania, strongyloidiasis, etc.).

The humoral (Th-2) immune system is not substantially affected even by these pharmacologic doses of steroids (22,23). It is important to realize, of course, that even though *S. pneumoniae* may be effectively opsonized, the neutrophil is still required in order to ingest and kill the organism. Thus, it is safe to say that all types of acute pyogenic infections, both with the nonencapsulated and encapsulated bacteria, occur more frequently in patients on pharmacologic doses of glucocorticoids.

Superpharmacologic ("Mega-") Doses of Steroids

Here, I refer to doses of steroids in the range from 1 to 2 g of prednisone (30–60 mg/kg, equivalent to doses of 5000–10,000 mg of hydrocortisone) given in some trials every six to eight hours for several days. When dosed in that fashion, secondary infections occur more frequently than in control subjects (24,25). At present, such doses are usually administered as a single daily dose (so called "pulse dose" regimens) over a three- to five- to seven-day period acutely to suppress all immunologically mediated inflammatory processes and/or to provide a variety of dermatological or anticancer effects (26,27). Sustained administration of 2 g of prednisone or its equivalent over a 48-hour period has been shown to suppress all limbs of the immune system and, if continued, will result in an increased rate of infections (24,25). The "pulse dose" approach of single daily doses of up to 2 g of methylprednisolone per day for about a week to patients without underlying systemic diseases is relatively free of infectious side effects (28–30). As the period of therapy extends beyond five days, the frequency of infectious complications will undoubtedly increase. Also, the rate of infection is increased even with pulse dose therapy in patients with an underlying systematic disease such as systemic lupus erythematosus (30).

TYPES OF INFECTIONS EXPECTED IN PATIENTS ON STEROIDS

From the preceding discussion, it should become clear that low, physiologic doses of steroids not only are necessary for patients with inadequate adrenal responses effectively to cope with and survive infections, but that such doses have little if any effect on any limb of the immune system. However, when one initiates physiologic "stress" doses of hydrocortisone (100–200 mg/day, usually given as 50 mg every six to eight hours), one begins to approach the pharmacologic dose range; such doses should be minimized to the period of extreme stress and then promptly and steadily reduced as the patient stabilizes. In fact, it is this author's practice not to use more than 150 mg of hydrocortisone (37.5 mg of prednisone) daily even in patients in highly stressful metabolic/traumatic/infectious situations in order to decrease the likelihood of infections and other metabolic side effects.

When patients are started on pharmacologic doses of steroids (Table 3), immunosuppression occurs fairly rapidly (3,31). In fact, within 12 to 24 hours, circulating leukocytes are affected, and an elevation of the WBC count occurs (2). The elevation of the WBC after steroid administration, especially neutrophils, is accompanied by a rapid decrease of eosinophils (32). The elevation of the neutrophil count is due to a number of factors, including enhanced proliferation and expansion of the neutrophil pool, decreased attachment of neutrophils to endothelial cells (decreased margination, which increases the pool of circulating neutrophils), and inhibition of granulocyte colony stimulating factor, which enhances the proliferation and expansion of the neutrophil pool. Monocytes too are "demarginated" and therefore also have deceased access to peripheral sites of inflammation/infection. High doses of steroids negatively affect both levels and function of the complement system itself (33,34). Pharmacologic doses of steroids must be continued for some weeks before impairment of barrier systems (skin, mucous membrane, etc.) is observed.

Even a single superpharmacologic dose of steroids (1–2 g of prednisone or its equivalent) alters neutrophil, macrophage, and lymphocyte traffic from bone marrow to blood stream to lymphoid tissues as well as to peripheral foci of inflammation and infection. However, such effects are short lived; and as noted earlier, it seems that up to five daily boluses of such superphysiologic amounts of glucocorticoid are well tolerated, not producing a substantial increase in the propensity towards infection.

Pharmacologic doses of steroids for more than four to eight weeks are probably required to substantially impair cellular immunity. Suppression occurs by inhibiting Th-1 lymphocyte-mediated macrophage activation, and disrupting epithelioid cell and giant cell (granuloma) formation, all of which could result in the reactivation of latent facultative infections (tuberculosis and histoplasmosis being the prototypes) (3).

STEROID TREATMENT OF INFECTION

While this chapter has focused primarily on the adverse effects of steroid administration on the host resistance to infections, steroids also have clearly defined indications for use in specific infectious situations. The Infectious Diseases Society of America (IDSA) published guidelines for the systemic use of steroids in the treatment of certain infectious conditions in a well-done article in 1992 (35). A working group of the IDSA classified the strength of data to support recommendations for or against the use of steroid therapy and commented on the quality of evidence available to support a given recommendation. The following infections were felt to have "good evidence" to support a "recommendation for use" of pharmacologic doses of steroids: (i) typhoid fever resulting in critical illness (patient in shock) and (ii) tuberculous pericarditis. Those diseases in which there was "moderate evidence to support a recommendation for use" of pharmacologic doses of steroids included the following: (i) tetanus; (ii) tuberculous meningitis; and (iii) Epstein–Barr virus infection with impending airway obstruction. All the rest of the infectious situations for which steroids have been used in the past either with some data available or which were being used without any supportive evidence were felt to either have "poor evidence to support a recommendation for or against," "moderate evidence to support a recommendation against", or "good evidence to support a recommendation against" steroid use. At the time of publication in 1992, the following illnesses fell into one or the other of those latter categories: septic shock syndrome, tuberculosis with severe constitutional syndromes, *Herpes zoster*, Epstein–Barr viral infection (including hepatitis, pericarditis, and encephalitis), hemorrhagic fever, trichinosis, and Kawasaki disease (35).

Recently, well-done studies have shown the value of dexamethasone administration in both children (36) and adults (37) with meningitis. It is now recommended that such patients receive dexamethasone with or before the first dose of antibiotic (38,39).

Years ago, suprapharmacologic doses of steroids were regularly administered to patients in septic shock; however, controlled trials showed that such treatment did not work (24,25,40). More recently, data has become available in septic shock patients from reasonably well-done studies, which have resulted in a change in the recommendation for steroid use in patients suffering septic shock. A recent meta-analysis (41) and an accompanying editorial (42) put forth the following recommendations: low dose (physiologic/stress doses) steroids should be administered to all patients in septic shock; however, such doses should be continued only in patients with proven adrenal insufficiency. The dose of steroids referred to in the series of meta-analyzed studies is hydrocortisone 50 mg intravenously four times daily (total of 200 mg/day). At the time of steroid administration, a determination of the state of actual or relative adrenal insufficiency should be made; and the aforesaid dose of steroid should be continued beyond an initial two- to three-day period when the results of such testing are available. Only patients with proven adrenal insufficiency should be continued on such doses of hydrocortisone.

Alternate-Day Steroid Therapy

Every patient who requires long-term, pharmacologic doses of a glucocorticoid in order to control a serious inflammatory disorder should have regular attempts made to switch the daily regimen to one where the steroid dose is administered every other day in the morning (3,31). This "alternative-day" dosing schedule reduces the Cushingoid side effects, including reducing the risk of infection (20). For example, a patient requiring 60 mg of prednisone daily to control an autoimmune disease should always be worked, first, toward being dosed once daily in the morning. When stable, such patient should have the every-other day dose slowly (e.g., in 5 mg increments every one to two weeks) but surely reduced. If the patient begins to "flare" with recurrent symptoms of the underlying disease on the "off" day (the day the dose is being reduced), one should pause in terms of further reductions and try adding a nonsteroidal anti-inflammatory agent. In some patients, the symptoms are due to relative adrenal insufficiency rather than the underlying disease, in which case, a pause in further off-day dose reductions will lead to a gradual amelioration of the symptoms (tiredness, muscle aches, low grade fever, etc.). One may even need to increase the "on-day" dose for a brief period before attempting again to reduce the off-day dosage.

Infectious complications in patients able to be transferred to an alternative-day steroid dosing regimen are substantially reduced; for example, delayed hypersensitivity type skin tests are preserved in such patients (20), and therefore underlying Th-1 (cellular immunity) is also probably intact. Such patients also seem quite able to withstand and respond well to the usual types of viral and bacterial infections (20,31).

CONCLUSIONS

Steroids have major inhibitory effects on the nonspecific/innate immune system substantially impairing acute inflammatory cell (mainly neutrophil) access to early sites of infection; thus, not only are the rates of most infections increased in patients on steroids but the accompanying local and systemic signs and symptoms of infections are decreased, making early diagnosis of such episodes difficult. Most infections are caused by the acute pyogenic bacteria, the streptococci and staphylococci. Also adversely affected is the cellular (Th-1) immune system responsible for reacting to and controlling FIP (e.g., the tubercle bacillus); thus, progression and reactivation of such infections, though uncommon, may occur in patients on steroids. Minimal effects are produced by steroids on the humoral (Th-2) immune system. The awareness of the selective actions of steroids on host immunity to infections should assist clinicians in the earlier recognition and treatment of such potentially devastating complications.

REFERENCES

1. Pensabeni-Jasper T, Panush RS. Review: corticosteroid usage: observations at a community hospital. Am J Med Sci 1996; 311(5):234–239.
2. Boumpas DT, Chrousos GP, Wilder RL, Cupps TR, Balow JE. Glucocorticoid therapy for immune-mediated diseases: basic and clinical correlates. Ann Intern Med 1993; 119(12): 1198–1208.
3. Kehrl JH, Fauci AS. The clinical use of glucocorticoids. Ann Allergy 1983; 50(1):2–8.
4. Frey FJ, Speck RF. Glucocorticoids and infection. Schweiz Med Wochenschr 1992; 122(5): 137–146.
5. Sheagren JN. Glucocorticoid action: infectious diseases. In: Schleimer RP, Claman HN, Oronsky AL, eds. Anti-inflammatory Steroid Action: Basic and Clinical Aspects. Orlando, FL: Academic Press, 1989:525–543.
6. Kass EH, Finland M. Adrenocortical hormones in infection and immunity. Annu Rev Microbiol 1953; 7:361–388.
7. Hench PS, Kendall EC, Slocumb CH, Polley HF. Effects of cortisone acetate and pituitary ACTH on rheumatoid arthritis, rheumatic fever and certain other conditions. Arch Med Interna 1950; 85(4):545–666.
8. Kass EH. Hormones and host resistance to infection. Bacteriol Rev 1960; 24:177–185.
9. Franchimont D. Overview of the actions of glucocorticoids on the immune response: a good model to characterize new pathways of immunosuppression for new treatment strategies. Ann N Y Acad Sci 2004; 1024:124–137.
10. Gasque P. Complement: a unique innate immune sensor for danger signals. Mol Immunol 2004; 41(11):1089–1098.
11. Campbell PA. T cell involvement in resistance to facultative intracellular pathogens of the lung. Chest 1993; 103(suppl 2):113S–115S.
12. Ballow M. Primary immunodeficiency disorders: antibody deficiency. J Allergy Clin Immunol 2002; 109(4):581–591.
13. Pruitt BA Jr, McManus AT, Kim SH, Goodwin CW. Burn wound infections: current status. World J Surg 1998; 22(2):135–145.
14. O'Neil KM. Complement deficiency. Clin Rev Allergy Immunol 2000; 19:83–108.
15. Harty JT, Tvinnereim AR, White DW. CD8+ T cell effector mechanisms in resistance to infection. Annu Rev Immunol 2000; 18:275–308; van de Vosse E, Hoeve MA, Ottenhoff TH. Human genetics of intracellular infectious diseases: molecular and cellular immunity against mycobacteria and salmonellae. Lancet Infect Dis 2004; 4(12):739–749.
16. Holland EG, Taylor AT. Glucocorticoids in clinical practice. J Fam Pract 1991; 32(5): 512–519; Stuck AE, Minder CE, Frey FJ. Risk of infectious complications in patients taking glucocorticosteroids. Rev Infect Dis 1989; 11(6):954–963.
17. Ginzler E, Diamond H, Kaplan D, Weiner M, Schlesinger M, Seleznick M. Computer analysis of factors influencing frequency of infection in systemic lupus erythematosus. Arthritis Rheum 1978; 21(1):37–44.
18. Scheinman RI, Cogswell PC, Lofquist AK, Baldwin AS Jr. Role of transcriptional activation of I kappa B alpha in mediation of immunosuppression by glucocorticoids. Science 1995; 270(5234):283–286.

19. Bovornkitti S, Kangsadal P, Sathirapat P, Oonsombatti P. Reversion and reconversion rate of tuberculin skin reactions in connection with the use of prednisone. Dis Chest 1960; 38:51–55.

20. MacGregor RR, Sheagren JN, Lipsett MB, Wolff SM. Alternate-day prednisone therapy. Evaluation of delayed hypersensitivity responses, control of disease and steroid side effects. N Engl J Med 1969; 280(26):1427–1431.

21. Haanaes OC, Bergmann A. Tuberculosis emerging in patients treated with corticosteroids. Eur J Respir Dis 1983; 64(4):294–297.

22. Cupps TR, Gerrard TL, Falkoff RJ, Whalen G, Fauci AS. Effects of in vitro corticosteroids on B cell activation, proliferation, and differentiation. J Clin Invest 1985; 75(2): 754–761.

23. Settipane GA, Pudupakkam RK, McGowan JH. Corticosteroid effect on immunoglobulins. J Allergy Clin Immunol 1978; 62(3):162–166.

24. Hinshaw L, Peduzzi P, Young E, et al. (and the Veterans Administration Systemic Sepsis Cooperative Study Group). Effect of high-dose glucocorticoid therapy on mortality in patients with clinical signs of systemic sepsis. N Engl J Med 1987; 317:659–665.

25. Bone RC, Fisher CJ Jr., Clemmer TP, Slotman GJ, Metz CA, Balk RA. A controlled clinical trial of high-dose methylprednisolone in the treatment of severe sepsis and septic shock. N Engl J Med 1987; 317(11):653–658.

26. Roujeau JC. Pulse glucocorticoid therapy: the "big shot" revisited. Arch Dermatol 1996; 132(12):1499–1502.

27. Sabir S, Werth VP. Pulse glucocorticoids. Dermatol Clin 2000; 18(3):437–446, viii–ix.

28. Mignogna MD, Lo Muzio L, Ruoppo E, Fedele S, Lo Russo L, Bucci E. High-dose intravenous "pulse" methylprednisone in the treatment of severe oropharyngeal pemphigus: a pilot study. J Oral Pathol Med 2002; 31(6):339–344.

29. Friedli A, Labarthe MP, Engelhardt E, Feldmann R, Salomon D, Saurat JH. Pulse methylprednisolone therapy for severe alopecia areata: an open prospective study of 45 patients. J Am Acad Dermatol 1998; 39(4 Pt 1):597–602; Badsha H, Edwards CJ. Intravenous pulses of methylprednisolone for systemic lupus erythematosus. Semin Arthritis Rheum 2003; 32(6):370–377.

30. Chrousos GA, Kattah JC, Beck RW, Cleary PA. Side effects of glucocorticoid treatment: experience of the Optic Neuritis Treatment Trial. JAMA 1993; 269(16):2110–2112.

31. Fauci AS, Dale DC, Balow JE. Glucocorticosteroid therapy: mechanisms of action and clinical considerations. Ann Intern Med 1976; 84(3):304–315.

32. Schleimer RP, Bochner BS. The effects of glucocorticoids on human eosinophils. J Allergy Clin Immunol 1994; 94(6 Pt 2):1202–1213.

33. Packard BD, Weiler JM. Steroids inhibit activation of the alternative-amplification pathway of complement. Infect Immun 1983; 40(3):1011–1014.

34. Engelman RM, Rousou JA, Flack JE III, Deaton DW, Kalfin R, Das DK. Influence of steroids on complement and cytokine generation after cardiopulmonary bypass. Ann Thorac Surg 1995; 60(3):801–804.

35. McGowan JE Jr, Chesney PJ, Crossley KB, LaForce FM. Guidelines for the use of systemic glucocorticosteroids in the management of selected infections. Working Group on Steroid Use, Antimicrobial Agents Committee, Infectious Diseases Society of America. J Infect Dis 1992; 165(1):1–13.

36. Lebel MH, Freij BJ, Syrogiannopoulos GA, et al. Dexamethasone therapy for bacterial meningitis. Results of two double-blind, placebo-controlled trials. N Engl J Med 1988; 319(15):964–971.

37. de Gans J, van de Beek D, European Dexamethasone in Adulthood Bacterial Meningitis Study Investigators. Dexamethasone in adults with bacterial meningitis. N Engl J Med 2002; 347(20):1549–1556.

38. Chaudhuri A. Adjunctive dexamethasone treatment in acute bacterial meningitis. Lancet Neurol 2004; 3(1):54–62.

39. Tunkel AR, Hartman BJ, Kaplan SL, et al. Practice guidelines for the management of bacterial meningitis. Clin Infect Dis 2004; 39(9):1267–1284.
40. Thompson BT. Glucocorticoids and acute lung injury. Crit Care Med 2003; 31(suppl 4): S253–S257.
41. Minneci PC, Deans KJ, Banks SM, Eichacker PQ, Natanson C. Meta-analysis: the effect of steroids on survival and shock during sepsis depends on the dose. Ann Intern Med 2004; 141(1):47–56.
42. Luce JM. Physicians should administer low-dose corticosteroids selectively to septic patients until an ongoing trial is completed. Ann Intern Med 2004; 141(1):70–72.

18

Fever and Rash in the Critical Care Unit

Lee S. Engel, Charles V. Sanders, and Fred A. Lopez
*Department of Medicine, Louisiana State University Health Science Center,
New Orleans, Louisiana, U.S.A.*

INTRODUCTION

There are numerous potential etiologic agents that can cause the syndrome of fever and rash. Skin manifestations may be an early sign of a life-threatening infection. The ability to rapidly identify the cause of fever and rash in critically ill patients is essential for the proper management of the patient and protection of the healthcare worker(s) providing care for that patient.

A rapid method to narrow the potential life-threatening causes of fever and rash has been described by Cunha (1). Patients from the community who are ill enough to be admitted to the critical care unit with fever and rash from outside the hospital will most likely have meningococcemia, Rocky Mountain spotted fever (RMSF), community-acquired toxic shock syndrome (TSS), severe drug reactions, severe bacteremia, *Vibrio vulnificus* septicemia, gas gangrene, arboviral hemorrhagic fevers, dengue infection, or measles (Table 1). Patients who develop fever and rash after admission to the hospital will most commonly have drug reactions, staphylococcal bacteremia from central lines, exacerbations of systemic lupus erythematosis, or postoperative TSS.

The traditional approach to the patient with fever and rash is based on the characteristic appearance of the rash (2,3). The most common types of rash include petechial, maculopapular, vesicular, erythematous, and nodular. Although there can be overlaps in presentation, most causes of fever and rash can be grouped into one specific form of cutaneous eruption (3).

A systematic approach requires a thorough history that includes patient age, seasonality, travel, geography, immunizations, childhood illnesses, sick contacts, medications, and the immune status of the host. A detailed history, physical exam, and characterization of the rash will help the clinician reduce the number of possible etiologies. Appropriate laboratory testing will also assist in delineating the cause of fever and rash in the critically ill patient.

Table 1 Etiology of Rash and Fever Based on Admission Status

Rash and fever on admission to the critical care unit	Rash and fever after admission to the critical care unit
Meningococcemia	Drug reaction
RMSF	Nosocomial acquired toxic shock syndromes
Overwhelming pneumococcal or staphylococcal sepsis	Nosocomial staphylococcal sepsis
TSS	"Surgical" scarlet fever
Epidemic typhus	
Typhoid fever	Cholesterol emboli syndrome
Measles	
Arboviral hemorrhagic fever	
Gas gangrene (*Clostridial myenocrosis*)	
Dengue	
SLE	
Vibrio vulnificus	

Abbreviations: SLE, systemic lupus erythematosis; RMSF, Rocky Mountain spotted fever; TSS, toxic shock syndrome.
Source: Adapted from Ref. 1.

History

A comprehensive history of the events leading up to the development of fever and rash will significantly aid in the determination of the etiology of the illness. Several initial questions should be answered before taking a complete history (4,5).

1. Can the patient or someone who is with the patient provide a history?
2. Does the patient require cardiopulmonary resuscitation?
3. Are special isolation precautions needed?
   For example, patients with meningitis due to *Neisseria meningitidis* will need droplet precautions, whereas patients with *Varicella* infections will need airborne and contact precautions (Table 2). Health care workers should exercise universal precautions with all patients. Gloves should be worn during the examination of the skin whenever an infectious etiology is considered.
4. Are the skin lesions suggestive of a disease process that requires immediate antibiotic therapy?
   Patients with infections suggestive of *N. meningitidis*, RMSF, bacterial septic shock, TSS, or *V. vulnificus* will need urgent medical and possibly surgical treatment to improve their chance of survival.
5. Does the patient have an exotic disease due to travel or bioterrorism?

Agents, such as smallpox and viral hemorrhagic fevers (i.e., Ebola and Marburg) produce a generalized rash, whereas plague and anthrax may produce localized lesions. Again, isolation precautions will need to be addressed (Table 2).

After the preliminary evaluation of the patient, the physician can obtain a more thorough history including history of present illness and previous medical, social, and family histories.

Specific questions about the history of the rash itself are often helpful in determining its etiology (Table 3). Such questions should include time of onset, site of onset,

Table 2 Transmission-Based Precautions for Hospitalized Patients

Standard precautions
Use standard precautions for the care of all patients
Airborne precautions
In addition to standard precautions, use airborne precautions for patients known or
   suspected to have serious illnesses transmitted by airborne droplet nuclei. Examples of such
   illnesses include:
   Measles
   Varicella (including disseminated zoster)[a]
   Tuberculosis[b]
Droplet precautions
In addition to standard precautions, use droplet precautions for patients known or suspected
   to have serious illnesses transmitted by large particle droplets. Examples of such
   illnesses include:
   Invasive *Haemophilus influenzae* type b disease, including meningitis, pneumonia,
      epiglottitis, and sepsis
   Invasive *Neisseria meningitidis* disease, including meningitis, pneumonia, and sepsis
   Other serious bacterial respiratory infections spread by droplet
      transmission, including:
      Diphtheria (pharyngeal)
      Mycoplasma pneumonia
      Pertussis
      Pneumonic plague
   Streptococcal pharyngitis, pneumonia, or scarlet fever in infants and young children
   Serious viral infections spread by droplet transmission, including those caused by:
      Adenovirus
      Influenza
      Mumps
      Parvovirus B19
      Rubella
Contact precautions
In addition to standard precautions, use contact precautions for patients known or suspected
   to have serious illnesses easily transmitted by direct patient contact or by contact with items
   in the patient's environment. Examples of such illnesses include:
   Gastrointestinal, respiratory, skin, or wound infections or colonization with
      multidrug-resistant bacteria judged by the infection control program, based on current
      state, regional, or national recommendations, to be of special clinical and epidemiologic
      significance
   Enteric infections with a low infectious dose or prolonged environmental survival,
      including those caused by:
   Clostridium difficile
   For diapered or incontinent patients: enterohemorrhagic *E. coli* 0157:H7, *Shigella*,
      hepatitis A, or rotavirus
   Respiratory syncytial virus, parainfluenza virus, or enteroviral infections in infants, and
      young children
   Skin infections that are highly contagious or that may occur on dry skin, including:
      Diphtheria (cutaneous)
      Herpes simplex virus (neonatal or mucocutaneous)
      Impetigo
      Major (non-contained) abscesses, cellulitis, or decubiti
      Pediculosis
      Scabies

(Continued)

Table 2 Transmission-Based Precautions for Hospitalized Patients (*Continued*)

Staphylococcal furunculosis in infants and young children
Zoster (disseminated or in the immunocompromised host)
 Viral/hemorrhagic conjunctivitis
 Viral hemorrhagic infections (Ebola, Lassa, or Marburg)

Note: CDC infection control guidelines reprinted from Garner JS and the Hospital Infection Control Practices Advisory Committee.
[a]Certain infections require more than one type of precaution.
[b]See Centers for Disease Control and Prevention.
Source: From Refs. 6 and 7.

change in lesions, symptoms associated with the rash (i.e., itching, burning, numbness, and tingling), provoking factors, previous rashes, and prior treatments.

The physical exam should focus on the patient's vital signs, general appearance, and the assessment of lymphadenopathy, nuchal rigidity, neurological dysfunction, hepatomegaly, splenomegaly, arthritis, and mucosal membrane lesions (Table 4) (3,4). Skin examination to determine type of the rash (Table 5) includes evaluation of distribution pattern, arrangement, and configuration of lesions.

The remainder of this chapter will provide a diagnostic approach to patients with fever and rash based on the characteristics of the rash. Several clinically relevant causes of each type of rash associated with fever are described in brief detail.

Table 3 Fever and Rash: History

Age of patient
Season of the year
Type of prodrome associated with current illness
History of drug or antibiotic allergies
Medications taken with in the past 30 days (prescription or nonprescription)
Drug ingestion
Exposure to febrile or ill persons within the recent past
Prior illness
Occupational exposures
Sun exposures
Recent travel
Exposure to wild or rural habitats
Exposure to insects, arthropods, or wild animals
Exposure to pets
Immunizations
Exposure to sexually transmitted diseases
HIV risk factors (intravenous drug use, unprotected sex, sexual orientation)
Site of rash onset
Factors effecting immunological status (chemotherapy, steroid use,
 hematological malignancy, solid organ or bone marrow transplant,
 asplenia)
Valvular heart disease
Rate of rash development (slow vs. fast)
Direction of rash spread (centrifugal vs. centripetal)
Evolution of rash (Has the rash changed?)
Relationship between rash and fever
Presence or absence of pruritus
Previous treatment of the rash (topical or oral therapies)

Source: Adapted from Refs. 5 and 8.

Table 4 Fever and Rash: Physical Examination

Vital signs
  Temperature
  Pulse
  Respiration
  Blood pressure
General appearance
  Alert
  Acutely ill
  Chronically ill
Signs of toxicity
Adenopathy/location of adenopathy
Presence of mucosal, conjunctival, or genital lesions
hepatosplenomegaly
Arthritis
Nuchal rigidity/Neurological dysfunction
Features of rash
  Type of primary rash lesion (Table 5)
  Presence of secondary lesions
  Presence of desquamation
  Presence of excoriations
  Configuration of individual lesions
  Arrangement of lesions
  Distribution pattern: exposed areas; centripetal vs. centrifugal

Source: Adapted from Refs. 5 and 8.

PETECHIAL AND PURPURIC RASHES

Petechiae are produced by extravasation of red blood cells and are less then 3 mm in diameter. Petechiae appear as small red or brown spots on the skin. Purpura or ecchymoses are lesions that are larger than 3 mm and often form when petechiae coalesce. Neither petechial nor purpuric lesions blanch when pressure is applied.

Infections associated with diffuse petechiae are generally among the most life threatening and require urgent evaluation and management. There are many infectious causes of these lesions (Table 6); several of the most dangerous include meningococcemia, rickettsial infection, and bacteremia (1,3,8).

Table 5 Type of Rash Lesions

Macule	Circumscribed flat lesion that differs from surrounding skin by color. Patches are very large macular lesions
Papule	Circumscribed, solid, elevated skin lesion that is palpable and smaller then 0.5 cm in diameter
Plaque	Large, solid, elevated skin lesion that is palpable and greater the 0.5 cm in diameter, often formed by confluence of papules
Nodule	Circumscribed, solid, palpable skin lesion with depth as well as elevation
Pustule	Circumscribed raised lesion containing pus
Vesicle	Circumscribed elevated, fluid filled lesion less then 0.5 cm in diameter
Bulla	Circumscribed elevated, fluid filled lesion greater then 0.5 cm in diameter

Source: Adapted from Refs. 5 and 9.

Table 6 Etiology of Rash and Fever Based on Type of Rash

Purpura or Petechiae
Meningococcemia
RMSF
Gonococcemia
Staphylococcal/pneumococcal sepsis
Pseudomonal sepsis
Bacterial endocarditis
Typhus
Allergic vasculitis
Echovirus 9
Measles
Centrally Distributed Maculopapular Rash
Viral exanthems (rubeola, rubella, erythema infectiousum, roseola)
Lyme disease
Drug reactions
Peripherally Distributed Maculopapular Rash
Erythema multiforme (Table 7)
Secondary syphilis
Diffuse erythema with desquamation
Scarlet fever
TSS
Scalded skin syndrome
Kawasaki disease
Erlichiosis
TEN
Streptococcus viridans bacteremia
Vesicular, Bullous, or Pustular Rash
Varicella
Herpes zoster
Herpes simplex
Staphylococcus aureus bacteremia
Vibrio vulnificus
Rickettsia akari
Nodular Rash
Erythema Nodosum (Table 8)
Disseminated fungal infections (*Candida, Cryptococcus, Blastomycosis,*
  Histoplasma, Coccidiodes, and *Sporothrix*)
Nocardia
Mycobacteria

Abbreviations: TEN, toxic epidermal necrolysin; RMSF, Rocky Mountain spotted
fever; TSS, toxic shock syndrome.
Source: Adapted from Refs. 1, 3, 5, and 8.

Acute Meningococcemia

N. meningitidis is the leading cause of bacterial meningitis in children and young
adults (10). Bacterial meningitis associated with a petechial or purpuric rash should
always suggest meningococcemia (1). The diagnosis of meningococcemia is more
difficult to make when meningitis is not present.

Meningococcemia can occur sporadically or in epidemics, and is more commonly diagnosed during the winter months. The risk of infection is highest in infants,

asplenic patients, alcoholics, patients with complement deficiency, and persons who live in dormitories (coeds, military personnel, or prisoners). Initial symptoms include cough, headache, sore throat, nausea, and vomiting. Acute meningococcemia progresses rapidly and patients typically appear ill with high spiking fevers, tachypnea, tachycardia, mild hypotension, and a characteristic petechial rash (11,12). Signs and symptoms of meningeal irritation, such as headache, vomiting, and change in conscious state occur in up to 88% of patients with meningococcemia (11,13).

The rash associated with meningococcemia begins within 24 hours of clinical illness. The petechia enlarges rapidly, becoming papular and then purpuric. Lesions most commonly occur on the extremities and trunk but may also be found on the head and mucous membranes (5). The development of lesions on the palms and soles is usually a late finding (1). Purpuric skin lesions have been described in 60% to 100% of meningococcemia cases and are most commonly seen at presentation (Fig. 1) (14,15). Histological studies demonstrate diffuse vascular damage, fibrin thrombi, vascular necrosis, and perivascular hemorrhage in the involved skin and organs. The skin lesions associated with meningococcal septic shock are thought to result from an acquired or transient deficiency of protein C and/or protein S (16). Meningococci are present in endothelial cells and neutrophils, and smears of skin lesions are positive for gram-negative diplococci in many cases (17,18).

The diagnosis of meningococcemia is also aided by culturing the petechial lesions. Blood cultures should be drawn. Admission laboratory data usually demonstrate a leukocytosis and thrombocytopenia. Patients with meningococcemia but without meningitis will have a normal cerebrospinal fluid (CSF) profile. If meningococcal meningitis is present, the CSF culture is usually positive although the gram-stain may be negative. Typically, the CSF-associated glucose is low and the protein elevated.

Chronic Meningococcemia

Chronic meningococcemia is rare, and its lesions differ from those seen in acute meningococcemia. Patients present with intermittent fever, rash, arthritis, and arthralgias occurring over a period of several weeks to months (19,20). The lesions of chronic

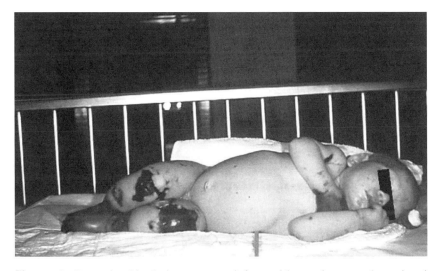

Figure 1 Purpuric skin lesions on an infant with meningococcal septicemia. *Source*: Courtesy of the CDC.

meningococcemia are usually pale to pink colored macules and/or papules typically located around a painful joint or pressure point. Nodules may develop in the lower extremities. The lesions of chronic meningococcemia develop during periods of fever and fade when the fevers dissipate. These lesions (in contrast to those of acute meningococcemia) rarely demonstrate the bacteria on Gram stain or histology (5,8).

Rocky Mountain Spotted Fever

RMSF, the most lethal rickettsial disease in the United States, is caused by *Rickettsia rickettsii* (21–24). Infection occurs after a bite by the tick vector, Dermacentor. RMSF is more common in men, occurs most often between April and September, and is most prevalent in Oklahoma and the southern Atlantic states.

The onset of RMSF can be abrupt with fever, headache, myalgias, shaking chills, photophobia, and nausea. Patients may have periorbital edema, conjunctival suffusion, and localized edema involving the dorsum of the hands and feet (1). A notable clinical finding is a pulse-temperature deficit (i.e., relative bradycardia during fever). Localized abdominal pain secondary to liver involvement, renal failure manifested by acute tubular necrosis, pancreatitis, left ventricular failure, adult respiratory distress syndrome (ARDS), and mental confusion or deafness may also be noted (1).

The rash usually begins about four to five days after the start of the illness. The lesions are initially maculopapular and evolve into petechiae within two to four days. Characteristically, the rash starts on the wrists, forearms, ankles, palms, and soles and then spreads centripetally to involve the arms, thighs, trunk, and face (Fig. 2). Centripetal evolution of the rash occurs 6 to 18 hours after the rash develops. Prompt treatment with tetracycline decreases mortality (25,26).

Routine admission tests may demonstrate a normal or decreased peripheral white blood cell (WBC) count and thrombocytopenia. The total bilirubin and serum transaminases may be elevated. If pancreatitis is present, the serum amylase will be

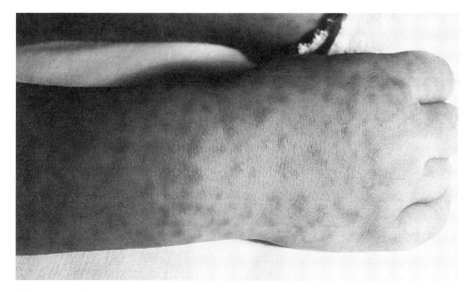

Figure 2 Childs right hand and wrist demonstrating the characteristic spotted rash of Rocky Mountain spotted fever. *Source*: Courtesy of the CDC Public Health Image Library.

elevated. Patients who develop renal failure may demonstrate a rise in blood urea nitrogen (BUN) and creatinine suggestive of prerenal azotemia secondary to intra-vascular volume deficit. When the central nervous system is involved, the CSF profile will demonstrate a mild pleocytosis, normal glucose and protein concentrations, and negative Gram stain and culture. Blood cultures will also be negative in RMSF. Serological studies will demonstrate the presence of antibodies seven to 10 days after symptoms start.

Septic Shock

The yearly incidence of sepsis has been increasing about 9% a year and accounts for 2% of all hospital admissions (27). The peak incidence of septic shock occurs in patients who are in their seventh decade of life (28). Risk factors for sepsis include cancer, immunodeficiency, chronic organ failure, and iatrogenic factors. Sepsis develops from infections of the chest, abdomen, genitourinary system, and primary bloodstream in more than 80% of cases (28,29).

Symmetric peripheral gangrene or purpura fulminans is a cutaneous syndrome associated with septic shock secondary to *N. meningitidis* or *Streptococcus pneumoniae*. This syndrome is usually preceded by petechiae, ecchymosis, purpura, and acrocya-nosis. Acrocyanosis, another cutaneous manifestation of septic shock, is a grayish color of the skin, which occurs on the lips, legs, nose, ear lobes, and genitalia, and does not blanch on pressure. Bacteria are usually absent in smears obtained from these skin lesions.

Sepsis is defined as systemic inflammatory response syndrome with documen-ted infection. Patients with sepsis will therefore have a documented site of infection and display two or more of the following: body temperature $> 38.5°C$ or $< 35°C$; heart rate >90 beats/min; respiratory rate >20 breaths/min; arterial CO_2 tension <32 mmHg; WBC $>12,000/mm^3$ or WBC $<4000/mm^3$; or immature forms $>10\%$. With severe sepsis, patients begin to demonstrate areas of mottled skin, capillary refill time more than three seconds, decreased urine output, changes in mental status, thrombocytopenia, disseminated intravascular coagulation (DIC), cardiac dys-function, and ARDS. When patients can no longer maintain a systemic mean arterial blood pressure of 60 mmHg or require a vasopresser agent, then they are said to be in septic shock. Mortality varies from 35% to 70% depending on patients' age, sex, ethnic origin, co-morbidities, and presence of acute lung injury or ARDS, as well as on whether the infection is nosocomial or polymicrobial, or whether the causative agent is a fungus (28,29). Gram-negative infections are responsible for 25% to 30% of cases of septic shock, whereas gram-positive infections now account for 30% to 50% of the cases of septic shock. Multidrug-resistant bacteria and fungi are increasingly reported as causes of sepsis (28,29).

The diagnosis of septic shock requires a causal link between infection and organ failure (28). Some patients may have clinically obvious infection, such as purpura ful-minans, cellulitis, TSS, pneumonia, or a purulent wound. Without an obvious source of infection, diagnosis will require the recovery of pathogens from blood or tissue cultures. Unfortunately, cultures are negative in 30% of these cases.

Bacterial Endocarditis

Infective endocarditis is classified as acute or subacute based on the tempo and severity of the clinical presentation (30). The characteristic lesion is a vegetation composed of platelets, fibrin, microorganisms, and inflammatory cells on the heart

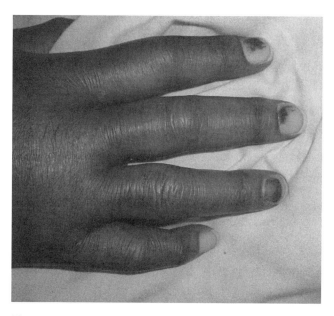

Figure 3 Subungual hemorrhages in an adult patient with Group B streptococcal endocarditis. *Source*: Courtesy of Lee S. Engel.

valve. Conditions associated with endocarditis include injection drug use, poor dental hygiene, long-term hemodialysis, diabetes mellitus, HIV infection, long-term indwelling venous catheters, mitral valve prolapse with regurgitation, rheumatic heart disease, other underlying valvular diseases, and prosthetic valves (31–33). Organisms associated with endocarditis include *Staphylococcus aureus*, viridans streptococci, enterococci, gram-negative bacilli (including the HACEK organisms), and fungi.

Nonspecific symptoms and signs of endocarditis include fever, arthralgias, wasting, unexplained heart failure, new heart murmurs, pericarditis, septic pulmonary emboli, strokes, and renal failure (34). Skin lesions occur less frequently today than they once did but aid in the diagnosis if present (34). Cutaneous manifestations of endocarditis include splinter hemorrhages (Fig. 3), petechiae, Osler's nodes, and Janeway lesions.

Petechiae are the most common skin lesions seen during endocarditis. The petechiae are small, flat, and reddish brown and do not blanch with pressure. They frequently occur in small crops and are usually transient. They are often found on the heels, shoulders, legs, oral mucous membranes, and conjunctiva.

Osler's nodes may be seen in patients with subacute bacterial endocarditis. These nodules are tender, indurated, and erythematous. They occur most commonly on the pads of the fingers and toes, are transient, and resolve without the development of necrosis. The histology of these lesions demonstrates microabscesses and microemboli.

Janeway lesions are small, painless, erythematous macules that are found on the palms and soles. These lesions can be seen with both acute and subacute endocarditis. Histological analysis reveals microabscesses with neutrophil infiltration.

Disseminated Gonococcal Infection

Disseminated gonococcal infections (DGI) result from gonococcal bacteremia and occur in 1% to 3% of patients with untreated *Neisseria gonorrhea*–associated

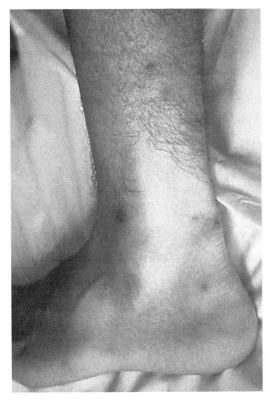

Figure 4 Cutaneous lesions on the left ankle and calf of a patient with disseminated *Neisseria gonorrhea* infection. *Source*: Courtesy of the CDC/Dr. S.E. Thompson, Public Health Image Library.

mucosal infection (35–37). DGI is most often seen in young women during menses or pregnancy (38). Most patients will present with fever, rash, polyarthritis, and teno-synovitis (36).

Skin lesions, which occur in 50% to 70% of patients with DGI, are the most common manifestation (38). The rash usually begins on the first day of symptoms and becomes more prominent with the onset of each new febrile episode (39). The lesions begin as tiny red papules or petechiae (1–5 mm in diameter) that evolve to a vesicular and then pustular form (Fig. 4). The pustular lesions develop a gray, necrotic center with a hemorrhagic base (36,39). The rash of DGI tends to be sparse and widely distributed, and the distal extremities are most commonly involved. Gram stain of the skin lesions rarely demonstrates organisms.

Clinical clues of DGI include the symptoms of fever, rash, and arthritis/teno-synovitis. Early in the infection, blood cultures may be positive; later, synovial joint fluid from associated effusions may yield positive cultures. Smears of the cervix and urethral exudates may also yield positive results.

Capnocytophaga Infection

Capnocytophaga canimorsus is a fastidious gram-negative bacteria that is part of the normal gingival flora of dogs and cats (40,41). Human infections are associated with dog or cat bites, cat scratches, and contact with wild animals (40,41). Predisposing factors include trauma, alcohol abuse, steroid therapy, chronic lung disease, and asplenia (40,41). The clinical syndrome consists of fever, DIC, necrosis of the kidneys and adrenal glands, thrombocytopenia, hypotension, and renal failure. The mortality rate approaches 25%.

Skin lesions occur in 50% of infected patients often progressing from petechiae to purpura to cutaneous gangrene (42). Other dermatologic lesions include macules, papules, painful erythema, or eschars.

Clinical clues include a compatible clinical syndrome and a history of a dog- or cat-inflicted wound. Diagnosis depends on the culture of the bacteria from blood, tissues, or other body fluids. More prompt diagnosis may be made by Gram staining the buffy coat.

Dengue

Dengue is a flavivirus comprised of four serotypes, i.e., DEN-1, DEN-2, DEN-3, and DEN-4. Dengue viruses are transmitted from person to person through infected female *Aedes* mosquitoes. The mosquito acquires the virus by taking a blood meal from an infected human or monkey. The virus incubates in the mosquito for 7 to 10 days before it can transmit the infection. More then 2.5 billion people are at risk for dengue infections worldwide (43).

Dengue fever (also known as breakbone fever or dandy fever) is a short-duration, nonfatal disease characterized by the sudden onset of headache, retro-orbital pain, high fever, joint pain, and rash (43,44). The rash manifests as palpable pinpoint petechiae that begin centrally and spread peripherally (1). Dengue fever lasts about seven days. Recovery from infection provides lifelong immunity to that serotype but does not preclude patients from being infected with the other serotypes of dengue virus, i.e., secondary infections.

Dengue hemorrhagic fever and dengue TSS are two deadly complications of dengue viral infection that occur during secondary infection. Dengue hemorrhagic fever is characterized by hemorrhage, thrombocytopenia, and plasma leakage. Dengue shock syndrome includes the additional complications of circulatory failure and hypotension (43,44).

The incubation period for dengue virus infections is 3 to 14 days. If a patient presents greater than two weeks after visiting an endemic area, dengue is much less likely (45). Laboratory abnormalities include neutropenia followed by lymphocytosis, hemoconcentration, thrombocytopenia, and an elevated aspartate aminotransferase in the serum (46). The diagnosis of dengue virus–associated infection can be accomplished by polymerase chain reaction (PCR), detection of antidengue virus immunoglobulin M (IgM), centrifugation amplification to enhance virus isolation, or flow cytometry for early detection of cultured virus (47).

MACULOPAPULAR RASH

Lyme Disease

Lyme disease is the most common tick vector–associated disease in the United States (48–50). Lyme disease is caused by the spirochete *Borrelia burgdorferi*, which is transmitted by the tick Ixodes. Lyme disease is endemic in the northeastern, mid-Atlantic, north central, and far western regions of the United States. The disease has a bimodal age distribution, with peaks in patients younger than 15 and older than 29 years of age (51). Most infections occur between May and September.

Lyme disease has three stages: early localized, early disseminated, and late disease. Early localized disease is characterized by erythema migrans (EM), which forms 7 to 10 days following the tick bite (52). EM occurs in 60% to 80% of the cases and begins as a small red papule at the site of the bite. The lesion expands centrifugally and can get as large as 70 cm in diameter. The lesion develops central clearing in 30% of cases (Fig. 5). If untreated, the lesions resolve over several weeks. Other symptoms associated with early-localized disease include fatigue, myalgias, arthralgias, headache, fever, and chills.

Early disseminated disease occurs days to weeks after the tick bite. Patients may not recall having had the typical EM rash. Patients at this stage can present with lymphocytic meningitis, cranial nerve palsies, mild pericarditis, atrial-ventricular block, arthritis, generalized or regional adenopathy, conjunctivitis, iritis, hepatitis, and painful radiculoneuritis followed by decreased sensation, weakness, and absent reflexes (48,49,53). Disseminated skin lesions, when present, are similar to EM but smaller and usually multiple in number.

Late disease is characterized by chronic asymmetric oligoarticular arthritis that involves the large joints (most often the knee). The central nervous system may also be affected, manifesting as subacute encephalopathy, axonal polyneuropathy, or leukoencephalopathy.

Diagnosis is based on the history and physical exam. Serology is confirmatory but takes four to six weeks after the onset of symptoms to become positive. CSF should be obtained if neurological signs are present. Synovial fluid can be evaluated if arthritis is present.

Drug Reactions

Drugs cause adverse skin reactions in 2% to 3% of hospitalized patients (54). Classic drug reactions include urticaria, angioedema, exanthems, vasculitis, exfoliative

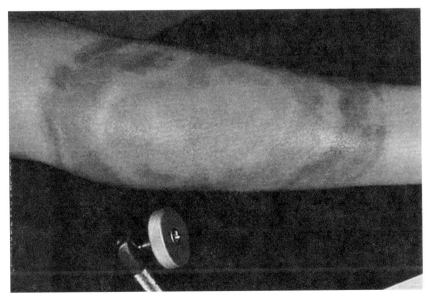

Figure 5 Characteristic rash, erythema migrans, on the arm of a patient with Lyme disease. *Source*: Courtesy of Allen C. Steere, www.forstryimages.org and National Institute of Health, U.S. National Library of Medicine.

dermatitis/erythroderma, erythema multiforme, Stevens–Johnson syndrome, and toxic epidermal necrolysis (TEN) (54,55). There is no predilection for age, gender, or race (8). Diagnosis of a drug reaction is based on a patient's previous reaction to the drug, ruling out alternate etiological causes of the rash, timing of events, drug levels, or evidence of overdose, patient reaction to drug discontinuation, and patient reaction to re-challenge.

Drug Exanthems

Exanthems are the most common skin reaction to drugs. The rash usually appears within the first two weeks after the offending drug is started and resolves within days after the drug is stopped. The rash is often described as morbilliform, macular, and/ or papular eruption. Pruritus is the most common associated symptom of drug-induced rash. Low-grade fever and peripheral blood eosinophilia may also occur in association with drug exanthems.

Erythema Multiforme

Erythema multiforme is an acute, self-limited, peripheral eruptive maculopapular rash that is characterized by a target lesion. Erythema multiforme most often affects persons 20 and 30 years of age and has a predilection for men. The rash begins as a dull-red macular eruption that evolves into papules and the characteristic target lesion. Target lesions are often found on the palms, soles, knees, and elbows. Vesicles and bullae occasionally develop in the center of the papules (8). There are many causes of this disorder (Table 7).

Erythema multiforme is classified as minor or major (8). Bullae and systemic symptoms are absent in erythema multiforme minor. The rash rarely affects the mucous membranes and is usually limited to the extensor surfaces of the extremities. The most common cause of erythema multiforme minor is herpes simplex virus (HSV). Erythema multiforme major is usually caused by drug reactions. Mucous membranes are involved, and the eruptions often become bullous. Fever, cheilosis, stomatitis, balanitis, vulvitis, and conjunctivitis can also occur (54).

Stevens–Johnson Syndrome

Stevens–Johnson syndrome is a blistering disorder that is usually more severe than erythema multiforme (57,58). The causes of Stevens–Johnson syndrome are similar to the etiologies of erythema multiforme (Table 7). Patients with Stevens–Johnson syndrome often present with pharyngitis, malaise, and fever. The syndrome evolves over a few days with the evolution of mucous membrane erosions. Small blisters develop on purpuric or atypical target lesions. The blisters eventually result in skin detachment. Stevens–Johnson syndrome affects less than 10% of the total body surface (54,58).

Toxic Epidermal Necrolysis

TEN is the most serious cutaneous drug reaction and is defined by blistering of over 30% of the total body surface area. More than one mucous membrane is involved. TEN is usually caused by the same drugs that cause erythema multiforme (Table 7), and its onset is acute. A fever greater than 39°C is often present. Intestinal and pulmonary involvement predicts a poor outcome (54,55).

The diagnosis of Stevens–Johnson syndrome and TEN is made by skin biopsy. Sections of frozen skin will demonstrate full-thickness epidermal necrosis. Because extensive skin detachment results in massive transepidermal fluid losses, patients with these maladies are managed similarly to patients who have had extensive burn

Table 7 Causes of Erythema Multiforme

Viral Infections
Herpes simplex 1 and 2
Epstein–Barr virus
Hepatitis A, B, C
Varicella zoster
Parvovirus B19
Bacterial Infections
Hemolytic streptococci
Pneumococcus
Staphylococcus species
Proteus species
Salmonella species
Mycobacterium tuberculosis
Mycobacterium avium complex
Francisella tularensis
Vibrio parahaemolyticus
Yersinia species
Mycoplasma pneumonia
Fungal Infections
Histoplasma capsulatum
Coccidiomycosis
Parasitic Infections
Trichomonas species
Toxoplasma gondii
Antibiotics
Penicillin
Tetracyclines
Erythromycin
Sulfa drugs
Vancomycin
Anticonvulsants
Barbiturates
Carbamazepine
Phenytoin
Antituberculoids
Rafampin
Isoniazid
Pyrizinamide
Other Drugs
Allopurinol
Fluconazole
hydralazine
NSAIDs
Estrogen
Physical factors/contact
Sunlight
Cold
X-ray therapy
Tattooing
Poison ivy
Other factors

(Continued)

Table 7   Causes of Erythema Multiforme (*Continued*)

Pregnancy
Multiple myeloma
Leukemia
Collagen diseases
Idiopathic (50%)

Abbreviations: NSAIDs, nonsteroidal antiinflammatory drugs.
Source: Adapted from Ref. 56.

injuries. Sepsis can occur secondary to microbial colonization of denuded skin. Mortality rates are 5% for Stevens–Johnson syndrome and 50% for TEN (54).

Secondary Syphilis

Syphilis is a systemic disease caused by *Treponema pallidum*. Syphilis is classified into primary, secondary, early latent, late latent, and tertiary stages. The lesion of primary syphilis, the chancre, usually develops about 21 days after infection and resolves in one to two months. Patients with secondary syphilis can present with rash, mucosal lesions, lympadenopathy, and fever. The rash of secondary syphilis may be maculo-papular, papulosquamous, or pustular, and is characteristically found on the palms and the soles (Fig. 6).

The diagnosis of syphilis is based on nontreponemal tests (e.g., Venereal Disease Research Laboratory and Rapid Plasma Reagin) and specific treponemal tests

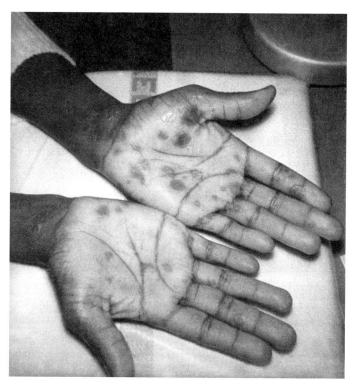

Figure 6   Papulosquamous rash on wrist and hands of patient with secondary syphilis. *Source*: Courtesy of the CDC/Susan Lindsley, Public Health Image Library.

(e.g., fluorescent treponemal antibody absorbed and *T. pallidum* particle agglutination). The nontreponemal tests are used to screen for disease and follow treatment. The specific treponemal tests are used to rule in the diagnosis of syphilis because false-positive nontreponemal tests can occur. Darkfield examination of skin or mucous membrane lesions can be done to diagnose syphilis definitively during the early stages as well.

West Nile Virus

West Nile virus (WNV) is transmitted to humans from the bite of an infected mosquito (59). The virus normally circulates between mosquitoes and birds. The first reported outbreak was in New York in 1999, and since then WNV has spread southward and westward (60–63). WNV has become seasonally endemic, with peak activity for transmission from July to October in temperate zones and from April to December in warmer climates (61,63).

Though most commonly spread by infected mosquitoes, WNV may also be transmitted by organ transplantation, blood transfusion, and breast milk (64–66). Transplacental infection from mother to fetus has also occurred (64).

WNV replicates at the site of inoculation and then spreads to the lymph nodes and bloodstream (67). The majority of human infections, i.e., 80%, are asymptomatic (68). Most patients with symptoms have self-limited West Nile fever. West Nile fever is characterized by acute onset of fever, headache, fatigue, malaise, muscle pain, difficulty concentrating, and neck pain.(69,70). Approximately 57% of patients with West Nile fever will have a transient macular rash on the trunk of the body (69).

Neuroinvasive disease develops in less than 1% of infected patients (68). The clinical severity of WNV encephalitis ranges from disorientation to coma to death (71,72). Advanced age is the most significant risk factor for severe neurologic disease. Risk increases 10 times for persons 50 to 59 years of age and 43 times for persons greater than 80 years of age (61,65). Neuroinvasive disease can present as meningitis, encephalitis, or paralysis (68,70,72,73). Patients with WNV encephalitis or focal neurologic findings will often have persistent deficits for months to years (61,72). Advanced age is the most important risk factor for death. The overall case fatality rate for neuroinvasive WNV disease is 9% (61).

Diagnosis of WNV disease can be made by a high index of clinical suspicion and detection of WNV-specific immunoglobulin M (IgM) in serum or CSF. The serum IgM can persist for up to eight months; therefore, nucleic amplification tests for WNV, such as reverse transcriptase PCR and real-time PCR may be required to prove that the infection is acute (70,74). Neuroinvasive WNV can be diagnosed by the presence of IgM-specific antibody in the CSF. Patients who have been recently vaccinated for yellow fever or Japanese encephalitis or persons recently infected with the St. Louis encephalitis virus or Dengue virus may have false-positive results on IgM antibody tests for WNV (75).

DIFFUSE ERYTHEMATOUS RASHES WITH DESQUAMATION

Toxic Shock Syndrome

TSS is characterized by sudden onset of fever, chills, vomiting, diarrhea, muscle aches, and rash. TSS can rapidly progress to severe hypotension and multiorgan dysfunction. The overall case fatality rate is 5%.

The microbial etiology of TSS is usually *S. aureus*; however, coagulase-negative staphylococci, group A streptococci, and group B streptococci can also produce this syndrome (76–78).

TSS is most commonly seen in menstruating women, women using barrier contraceptive devices, persons who have undergone nasal surgery, and patients with postoperative staphylococcal wound infections (79). Initially, cases associated with menstruation accounted for as many as 91% of the total cases (79). Currently, only half of the reported TSS cases are menstrual (80).

Staphylococcal TSS

Staphylococcal TSS is caused by infection or colonization with toxin-producing bacteria. The most common toxins associated with TSS include toxin 1 and enterotoxin B (81–84). Other toxins that may be involved include enterotoxins A, C, D, E, and H (85).

The clinical presentation of TSS was defined by the Centers for Disease Control and Prevention (CDC) in 1981 (4). All patients with TSS have high fever ($>39°C$), hypotension, and skin manifestations. Patients may also present with headache, vomiting, diarrhea, myalgias, pharyngitis, conjunctivitis, vaginitis, arthralgias, abdominal pain, or encephalopathy (86–89). The syndrome can progress to shock, DIC, ARDS, and renal failure.

The rash of TSS may start as erythroderma that involves both the skin and mucous membranes. The rash is diffuse, red, and macular and may resemble sunburn. The rash can involve the palms and soles. The erythema may be more intense around a surgical wound site. Mucosal involvement can involve the conjunctiva, oropharynx, or vagina (90). One to three weeks after the onset of TSS, the palms and soles may desquamate (Fig. 7) (91).

TSS can be divided into menstrual versus nonmenstrual. The majority of menstrual cases of TSS are associated with tampon use (92). Nonmenstrual cases are caused by abscesses, cellulitis, bursitis, postpartum infections, vaginal infections, sinusitis, burn wounds, insect bites, and surgical procedures (88,93).

The diagnosis of TSS is based on the CDC Diagnostic criteria (4). Although *S. aureus* is isolated from mucosal or wound sites in 80% to 90% of patients with TSS,

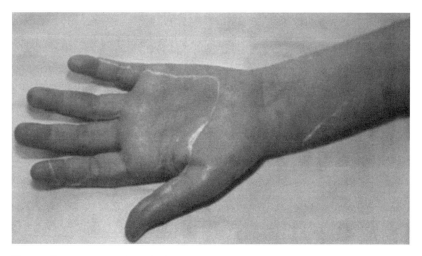

Figure 7   Desquamation of left palm of a patient with toxic shock syndrome. *Source*: Courtesy of the CDC, Public Health Image Library.

this criterion is not required for diagnosis. *S. aureus* is only recovered from blood cultures 5% of the time (92). Other laboratory abnormalities may include hypocalcemia, elevated liver enzymes, elevated creatinine, thrombocytopenia, pyuria, and proteinuria (90).

Streptococcal Toxic Shock Syndrome

The clinical picture of TSS caused by Group A and B streptococcus is similar to that caused by *S. aureus*. Skin and soft-tissue infections are often the source of invasive Group A and B streptococci (76,78). Minor trauma, injuries resulting in hematoma or bruising, surgery, viral infections, and use of nonsteroidal anti-inflammatory drugs are associated with the development of severe streptococcal infections (78). One particular difference from staphylococcal-associated TSS is that streptococci can frequently (60% of the time) be isolated from blood culture (94). The mortality rates for streptococcal TSS are five times higher than those for the staphylococcal TSS (95).

Staphylococcal Scalded Skin Syndrome

Staphylococcal scalded skin syndrome (SSSS) describes a spectrum of superficial blistering skin disorders caused by *S. aureus* strains that produce exfoliative toxins (96). The clinical spectrum of SSSS includes a localized form, bullous impetigo, and a generalized form, pemphigous neonatorum.

The exfoliative toxins are also known as epidermolytic toxins, epidermolysins, and exfoliatins. Production of exfoliative toxin occurs in 5% of all *S. aureus* strains (97,98). The two main exfoliative toxins are ETA and ETB (99–101). More recently, two new toxins, ETC and ETD, have been identified (101).

Bullous impetigo (also known as bullous varicella or measles pemphigoid) presents with a few localized, fragile, superficial blisters that are filled with colorless, purulent fluid (102). The lesions re-epithelialize in five to seven days. This form of SSSS is usually only seen in children. Typically, there are no associated systemic symptoms. The lesions are located in the area of the umbilicus and perineum in infants and over the extremities in older children (103).

The generalized form of SSSS is termed pemphigus neonatorum or Ritter's disease. Risk factors for development in adults include renal dysfunction, lymphoma, and immunosuppression (96,103,104). Patients with pemphigus neonatorum present with fever, erythema, malaise, and irritability. Patients then develop large superficial blisters that rupture easily due to friction (96). A positive Nikolsky sign refers to dislodgement of the superficial epidermis when gently rubbing the skin (105). If untreated, the epidermis will slough off leaving extensive areas of denuded skin that are painful and susceptible to infection. Mucous membranes are not affected in SSSS.

The mortality rate in children remains below 5%. Potentially fatal complications in infants and young children occur because of the loss of protective epidermis. Hypothermia, dehydration, and secondary infections are the leading causes of morbidity and mortality for these age groups affected by generalized SSSS (106). The mortality for adults with generalized SSSS is 60%, probably due to the associated comorbidities, such as renal dysfunction, immunosuppression, or malignancy found in this population (107).

Diagnosis of both generalized and localized SSSS is based on clinical characteristics. A thorough examination looking for foci of infection (pneumonia, abscess, arthritis, endocarditis, sinusitis, etc.) should be undertaken. Unfortunately, in most cases, no focus is ever found (96). Blood cultures are usually negative because toxins are produced at a distant site (103,108).

A number of different tests, including PCR, enzyme-linked immunosorbent assays, radioimmune assays, and reverse latex agglutination assays, can be used to demonstrate toxin production by *S. aureus* (109). The diagnostic challenge is that bacteria must first be isolated. When the diagnosis is uncertain, a skin biopsy may be the optimal test. The biopsy typically reveals mid-epidermal splitting at the level of the zona granulosa without cytolysis, necrosis, or inflammation (110). Staphylococci may be seen in bullous lesions of localized disease but rarely in the bullous lesions of generalized disease (104).

Scarlet Fever

Scarlet fever is the result of infection with a *Streptococcus pyogenes* strain (i.e., Group A streptococcus) that produces a pyrogenic exotoxin (ethrogenic toxin). There are three different toxins, types A, B, and C, which are produced by 90% of these strains. Scarlet fever follows an acute infection of the pharynx/tonsils or skin (8). It is most common in children between the ages of 1 and 10 years (95).

The rash of scarlet fever starts on the head and neck, followed by expansion to the trunk and then extremities (8,111). The rash is erythematous and diffuse, and blanches with pressure. There are numerous papular areas in the rash that produce a sandpaper-type quality. On the antecubital fossa and axillary folds, the rash has a linear petechial character referred to as Pastia's lines (111). The rash varies in intensity but usually fades in four to five days. Diffuse desquamation occurs after the rash fades (111). Diagnosis of scarlet fever can usually be made on a clinical basis. Confirmation of the diagnosis is supported by isolation of Group A streptococci from the pharynx and serologies (95).

Kawasaki Disease

Kawasaki disease (KD) is an acute, self-limited, systemic vasculitis of childhood (112–114). KD was first described by Tomisaku Kawasaki in Japan in 1961 (112) and is the predominant cause of pediatric-acquired heart disease in developed countries (114). The signs and symptoms evolve over the first 10 days of illness and then gradually resolve spontaneously in most children.

The diagnostic criteria for classical KD include the following (112):

1. Fever for five days or more that does not remit with antibiotics and is often resistant to antipyretics.
2. Presence of at least four of the following conditions:
    a. Bilateral (nonpurulent) conjunctivitis.
    b. Polymorphous rash.
    c. Changes in the lips and mouth: reddened, dry, or cracked lips; strawberry tongue; diffuse erythema of oral or pharyngeal mucosa.
    d. Changes in the extremities: erythema of the palms or soles; indurative edema of the hands or feet; desquamation of the skin of the hands, feet, and perineum during convalescence.
    e. Cervical lymphadenopathy: lymph nodes more than 15 mm in diameter.
3. Exclusion of disease with a similar presentation, such as scalded skin syndrome, TSS, viral exanthems, etc.

Other clinical features include intense irritability (possibly due to cerebral vasculitis), sterile pyuria, and upper respiratory symptoms (114). The major morbidity of KD is the development of coronary artery aneurysm(s), which occur in 25% of the cases.

There are no specific or sensitive tests that can be used to diagnose KD. The diagnosis is made by clinical assessment of the above criteria. The cause of KD is unknown; however, an infectious etiology is still being sought. KD has seasonal peaks in the winter and spring months, and focal epidemics occurred in the 1970s and 1980s (115). Treatment with aspirin and intravenous immunoglobulin (IVIG) has reduced the development and severity of coronary artery aneurysms.

Other Causes

Streptococcus viridans bacteremia can cause generalized erythema. Ehrlichiosis can produce a toxic shock-like syndrome with diffuse erythema. Enteroviral infections, graft versus host disease, and erythroderma may all present with diffuse erythema (8).

VESICULAR, BULLOUS, OR PUSTULAR RASHES

Vesicles and bullae refer to small and large blisters. Pustules refer to a vesicle filled with cloudy fluid. The causes of vesiculobullous rashes associated with fever include primary varicella infection, herpes zoster, HSV, smallpox, *S. aureus* bacteremia, gonococcemia, *Vibrio vulnificus*, *Rickettsia akari*, enteroviral infections, parvovirus B19, and HIV infection. Other causes that will not be discussed include folliculitis due to staphylococci, *Pseudomonas aeruginosa*, and *Candida*, but these manifestations would not result in admission to a critical care unit.

Varicella Zoster

Primary infection with varicella (chickenpox) is usually more severe in adults and immunocompromised patients. Although it can be seen year-round, the highest incidence of infection occurs in the winter and spring. The disease presents with a prodrome of fever and malaise one to two days prior to the outbreak of the rash. The rash begins as erythematous macules that quickly develop into vesicles. The characteristic rash is described as "a dewdrop on a rose petal." The vesicles evolve into pustules that umbilicate and crust. A characteristic of primary varicella is that lesions in all stages may be present at one time (8).

Herpes zoster (i.e., shingles) is caused by the reactivation of the varicella-zoster virus (VZV), which lies dormant in the basal root ganglia (116). The incidence of zoster is greatest in older age groups because of a decline in VZV-specific cell-mediated immunity. Herpes zoster also occurs more often in immunosuppressed patients, such as transplant recipients (117–119) and HIV-infected patients (120–122).

Patients often have a prodrome of fever, malaise, headaches, and dysesthesias that precedes the vesicular eruption by several days (123). The characteristic rash usually affects a single dermatome and begins as an erythematous maculopapular eruption that quickly evolves into a vesicular rash (Fig. 8). The lesions then dry and crust over in 7 to 10 days, with resolution in 14 to 21 days (116). Disseminated herpes zoster is seen in patients with solid-organ transplants, hematological malignancies, and HIV infection (120,121,124–128). Thirty-five percent of patients who

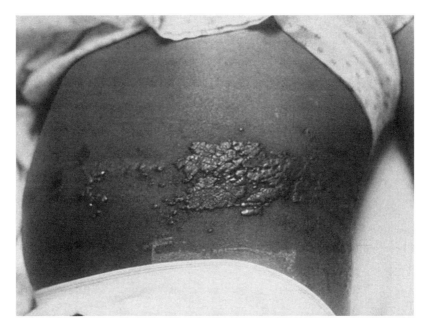

Figure 8 Lower abdomen of a patient with a herpes-zoster outbreak due to varicella-zoster virus. *Source*: Courtesy of the CDC, Public Health Image Library.

have received bone-marrow transplants have reactivation of VZV, and 50% of these patients develop disseminated herpes zoster (126,129,130).

Both immunocompetent and immunocompromised patients can have complications from herpes zoster; however, the risk is greater for immunocompromised patients (131). Complications of herpes zoster include herpes zoster ophthalmalicus (124,132), acute retinal necrosis (133,134), Ramsay Hunt syndrome (135), aseptic meningitis (136), peripheral motor neuropathy (136), myelitis (136,137), encephalitis (136), pneumonitis (131), hepatitis (129), and pancreatitis (126).

The diagnosis of primary varicella infection and herpes zoster is often made clinically. Diagnosis of the neurological complications can be made with CSF PCR assays (138,139). Patients with ocular involvement should be seen promptly by an ophthalmologist.

Smallpox

Smallpox is caused by the variola virus. The last known case of naturally acquired smallpox occurred in Somalia in 1977. The World Health Organization declared that smallpox had been eradicated from the world in 1980 as a result of global vaccination (140,141). The only known repositories for this virus are in Russia and the United States. With the threat of bioterrorism, there is still a remote possibility that this entity would be part of the differential diagnosis of a vesicular rash.

Smallpox usually spreads by respiratory droplets, but infected clothing or bedding can also spread disease (142). The incidence of smallpox is highest during the winter and early spring. The pox virus can survive longer at lower temperatures and low levels of humidity (143,144).

After a 12-day incubation period, smallpox infection presents with a prodromal phase of acute onset of fever (often greater than 40°C), headaches, and backaches

(142). A macular rash develops and progresses to vesicles and then pustules over one to two weeks (145). The rash appears on the face, oral mucosa, and arms first but then gradually involves the whole body. The pustules are 4 to 6 mm in diameter and remain for five to eight days, after which time, they umbilicate and crust. The lesions of smallpox are generally all in the same stage of development (Fig. 9). "Pock" marks are seen in 65% to 80% of survivors. Historically, the case mortality rate was 20% to 50% (142). In the United States, almost nobody under the age of 30 has been vaccinated; therefore this group is largely susceptible to infection.

The diagnosis of smallpox is clinically based on the presence of a characteristic rash that is centrifugal in distribution. After fluid from a vesicle is obtained by someone who has received a smallpox vaccine, laboratory confirmation can quickly be made by electron microscopic examination. Definitive identification in the laboratory is accomplished with viral cell culture, PCR, and restriction fragment–length polymorphism analysis (146).

Herpes Simplex Virus

HSV type 1 (herpes labialis) commonly causes vesicular lesions of the oral mucosa (147). The illness is characterized by the sudden appearance of multiple, often painful, vesicular lesions on an erythematous base. The lesions last for 10 to 14 days. Recurrent infections in the immunocompetent host are usually shorter than the primary infection. In the immunocompromised host, infections can be much more serious. Aside from vesicular eruptions on mucous membranes, the infection can cause keratitis, acute retinal necrosis, hepatitis, esophagitis, pneumonitis, and neurological syndromes (147–156).

HSV-1 can cause sporadic cases of encephalitis characterized by rapid onset of fever, headache, seizures, focal neurological signs, and impaired mental function. HSV-1 encephalitis has a high rate of mortality in the absence of treatment (157).

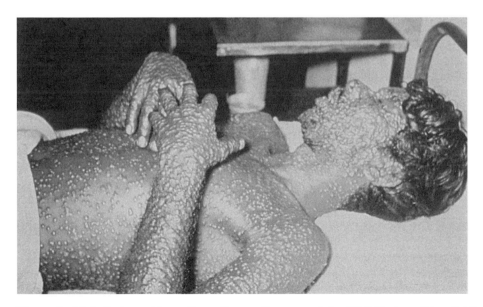

Figure 9 Male Patient with smallpox. *Source*: Courtesy of the CDC/Barbara Rice, Public Health Image Library.

Diagnosis can infrequently be made by culture; PCR analysis of the CSF has become the gold-standard technique for making the diagnosis (158).

S. aureus Bacteremia

S. aureus can cause metastatic skin infections that often manifest as pustules (3). The pustular skin eruption due to this organism is often widespread. Risk factors for bacteremia include older age, diabetes, recent surgery, HIV, hemodialysis, neoplasm, neutropenia, and intravenous drug use (159–164). Bacteremia can lead to metastatic complications, such as endocarditis and arthritis. Risk factors for these metastatic complications include underlying valvular heart disease and prosthetic implants.

V. vulnificus

V. vulnificus is a slightly curved, gram-negative bacillus that is endemic in warm coastal waters around the world. *V. vulnificus* is the leading cause of seafood-related fatalities in the United States (165). There are reports that virtually all oysters and 10% of crabs harvested in the warmer summer months from the Gulf of Mexico are culture positive for *V. vulnificus* (166). Consequently, the illness presents mostly between March and November (167). In the United States, most cases occur in states bordering the Gulf of Mexico or those that import oysters from the Gulf States (168). Risk factors for infection include liver disease (most commonly alcoholic), hemachromatosis, HIV infection, steroid use, malignancy, and achlohydria (165).

    V. vulnificus has been associated with two distinct syndromes: septicemia and wound infection (169,170). A third syndrome of gastrointestinal illness has also been suggested (171). Primary septicemia is a fulminant illness that occurs after the consumption of contaminated raw shellfish. Consumption of raw oysters within 14 days preceding the illness has been reported in 96% of the cases (172). Wound infection occurs after a pre-existing or newly acquired wound is exposed to contaminated seawater.

    The onset of symptoms is abrupt. The most common presenting signs and symptoms are fever, chills, shock, and secondary bullae (170). Skin lesions are seen in 65% of patients and are an early sign of septicemia. The most characteristic skin manifestation is erythema, followed by a rapid development of indurated plaques. These plaques then become violaceous in color, vesiculate, and then form bullae. The necrotic skin eventually sloughs off, leaving large ulcers (Fig. 10) (173). Gangrene of a limb can develop due to blood-vessel occlusion (174).

    Diagnosis is aided by clinical presentation and history. The bacteria can be readily cultured from blood and cutaneous lesions (175). A real-time PCR assay has also been reported (176).

    The mortality rate for septicemia is about 53% and is higher in patients who present with hypotension and leucopenia (177). Median duration from hospitalization to death is about 1.6 days (170). Failure to initiate antibiotics promptly is associated with higher mortality (168). Debridement of involved tissue is usually pursued.

R. akari

Rickettsialpox, which was first described in 1946 in New York City, is caused by *R. akari* (178). *R. akari* infects house mice (*Mus muscaulus*) and is transmitted to humans by the house mouse–associated mite, *Liponyssoides sanguineus* (179).

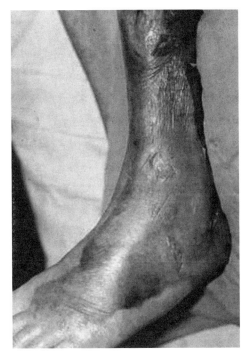

Figure 10 Skin Lesions associated with *Vibrio vulnificus* septicemia in a 75-year-old patient with liver cirrhosis. *Source*: Courtesy of CDC; From Ref. 173.

Most cases have occurred in large metropolitan areas of the northeastern United States (179,180).

Rickettsialpox has an incubation period of 9 to 14 days (181). The initial lesion develops into an eschar at the site of inoculation. Local lymph nodes around the eschar may become enlarged and tender. Approximately one week following the development of the eschar, patients will develop high fever, headaches, malaise, and myalgias. Some patients will have shaking chills and drenching sweats. Thrombocytopenia may also be noted (180). Within three to seven days of the fever, skin eruptions of red macules, papules, and papulovesicles will develop over the body. These lesions number between 20 and 40 and will resolve within a week. The presence of an eschar, the lack of successive crops of vesicles over time, and the presence of thrombocytopenia will help differentiate this entity from VZV infection (180).

Diagnosis has been made by comparing acute and convalescent serum antibody titers. Indirect and direct fluorescent antibody tests using anti–*Rickesttsia rikettsii* antibodies have also been reported (179). The length of the disease course can be reduced with tetracycline, but even untreated patients typically recover without complication (179).

NODULAR RASH

A nodule is a palpable, solid, round, or ellipsoidal lesion that may contain inflammatory cells, organisms (fungi and mycobacterium), or cancer cells (5). Nodules usually result from disease in the dermis.

Erythema Nodosum

Erythema nodosum is an acute inflammatory process involving the fatty-tissue layer and skin. This condition is more common in woman. There are several causes (Table 8), including infections with streptococci, *Chlamydia* species, and hepatitis C (182–186).

The presentation includes fever, malaise, and arthralgias. The characteristic nodules are painful and tender. The nodules commonly develop over the lower legs, knees, and arms (182). Spontaneous resolution usually occurs within six weeks. Diagnosis is often clinical, but biopsy may be needed in atypical cases.

Systemic Fungal Infections

The sudden onset of dermal nodules may indicate disseminated candidiasis. Risk factors for disseminated candidiasis include malignancy, neutropenia, antimicrobial therapy, severe burn injuries, intravenous catheters, and systemic steroid administration (187–189). The lesions are raised erythematous papules or nodules that are discrete, firm, and nontender (189–191).

Other fungi, such as blastomycosis, histoplasmosis, coccidiodomycosis, and sporotrichosis, can also produce skin nodules (5,192). Patients with AIDS may present with umbilicated nodules that resemble *Molluscum contagiousum* but are caused by *Cryptococcus neoformans*.

Table 8 Causes of Erythema Nodosum

Infectious	Non-Infectious
Bacterial infections	Drug reactions
Streptococcus pyogenes	Oral contraceptives
Mycobacterium tuberculosis	Antibiotics
Mycobacterium leprae	Hepatitis B vaccine
Cat scratch disease	Sulfonamides
Chlamydia	Systemic disease
Enteric pathogens (Yersinea,	Systemic lupus erythematosis
Campylobacter, Salmonella)	Ulcerative colitis
Rickettsiae	Crohn's disease
Spirochetes (syphilis)	Leukemia
Systemic fungal infections	Lymphoma
Coccidiodes immitis	Sarcoidosis
Histoplasma capsulatum	Idiopathic (55%)
Blastomycosis	
Parasites	
Amebiasis	
Giardiasis	
Ascaris	
Viral infections	
Hepatitis B	
CMV	
EBV	

Abbreviations: CMV, cytomegalovirus; EBV, Epstein–Barr virus.
Source: Adapted from Ref. 182.

Rheumatic Fever

Rheumatic fever is a late inflammatory complication of acute group A streptococcal pharyngitis (193,194). Rheumatic fever occurs two to four weeks following the pharyngitis. This disease occurs most frequently in children between the ages of four to nine years. The disease is self-limited, but resulting damage to the heart valves may be chronic and progressive, leading to cardiac decompensation and death.

Rheumatic fever is an acute, systemic, febrile illness that can produce a migratory arthritis, carditis, central nervous system deficits, and rash. The diagnosis is based on major and minor criteria (i.e., modified Jones Criteria) (195). The five major criteria are carditis, polyarthritis, chorea, erythema marginatum, and subcutaneous nodules. The three minor criteria are fever, arthralgia, and previous rheumatic fever or rheumatic heart disease.

Arthritis is the most frequent and least specific manifestation (196). Large joints are affected most commonly. The arthritis is migratory, with the joints of the lower extremities affected first, followed by those of the upper extremities.

Carditis associated with rheumatic fever manifests as pericarditis, myocarditis, and endocarditis, most commonly involving the mitral valve, followed by the aortic valve (197,198). Rheumatic heart disease is a late sequela of acute rheumatic fever, occurring 10 to 20 years after the acute attack, and is the most common cause of acquired valvular disease in the world (199). The mitral valve is most commonly affected with resultant mitral stenosis that often requires surgical correction.

Syndenham chorea (chorea minor, St. Vitus' Dance) is a neurological disorder that manifests as abrupt, purposeless, involuntary movements, muscle weakness, and emotional disturbances (200). The abnormal movements disproportionately affect one side of the body and cease during sleep.

Subcutaneous nodules are firm and painless and are seen most often with patients who have carditis (201). The overlying skin is not inflamed. The nodules can be as large as 2 cm and are most commonly located over bony surfaces or near tendons. The nodules may be present for one to four weeks.

Erythema marginatum (202) is a pink or faint-red, nonpruritic rash that affects the trunk and proximal limbs and spares the face. Erythema marginatum occurs early in the disease and may persist or recur. The rash is usually only seen in patients with concomitant carditis.

The diagnosis of rheumatic fever is supported by evidence of preceding Group A streptococcal infection. Evidence of increased antistreptolysin O antibodies, positive throat culture for Group A beta-hemolytic streptococci, positive rapid-direct Group A streptococcus carbohydrate antigen test, or recent scarlet fever along with the presence of one major and two minor or two major criteria is considered adequate to make the diagnosis.

REFERENCES

1. Cunha BA. Rash and fever in the critical care unit. Crit Care Clin 1998; 14(1):35–53.
2. Kingston ME, Mackey D. Skin clues in the diagnosis of life-threatening infections. Rev Infect Dis 1986; 8(1):1–11.
3. Schlossberg D. Fever and rash. Infect Dis Clin North Am 1996; 10(1):101–110.
4. Sanders CV. Approach to the diagnosis of the patient with fever and rash. In: Sanders CV, Nesbitt LTJ, eds. The skin and Infection: A Color Atlas and Text. Baltimore: Williams and Wilkins, 1995:296–304.

5. Weber DJ, Cohen MS, Rutala WA. The acutely ill patient with fever and rash. In: Mandell GL, Bennett JE, Dolin R, eds. Principles and Practice of Infectious Disease. Philadelphia: Elsevier Churchill Livingstone, 2005:729–746.

6. Garner JS. Hospital Infection Control Practices Advisory Committee. Guideline for isolation precautions in hospitals. Infect Control Hosp Epidemiol 1996; 17:53–80.

7. Centers for Disease Control and Prevention. Guidelines for preventing the transmission of *Mycobacterium tuberculosis* in health-care facilities. MMWR Recomm Rep 1994; 43:1–132.

8. McKinnon HD Jr., Howard T. Evaluating the febrile patient with a rash. Am Fam Physician 2000; 62(4):804–816.

9. Nesbitt LTJ. Evaluating the patient with a skin infection-General considerations. In: Sanders CV, Nesbitt LTJ, eds. The Skin and Infection: A Color Atlas and Text. Baltimore: Williams and Wilkins, 1995:1–6.

10. Schuchat A, Robinson K, Wenger JD, et al. Bacterial meningitis in the United States in 1995. Active Surveillance Team. N Engl J Med 1997; 337(14):970–976.

11. Yung AP, McDonald MI. Early clinical clues to meningococcemia. MJA 2003; 178:134–137.

12. van Deuren M, Brandtzaeg P, van der Meer JW. Update on meningococcal disease with emphasis on pathogenesis and clinical management. Clin Microbiol Rev 2000; 13(1):144–166.

13. Pollard AJ, Britto J, Nadel S, et al. Emergency management of meningococcal disease. Arch Dis Child 1999; 80(3):290–296.

14. Mclean S, Caffey J. Endemic purpuric meningococcus bacteremia in early life: the diagnostic value of smears from purpuric lesions. Am J Dis Child 1931; 42:1053–1074.

15. Hill WR, Kinney TD. The cutaneous lesions in acute meningococcemia: a clinical and pathological study. JAMA 1947; 134:513–518.

16. Faust SN, Levin M, Harrison OB, et al. Dysfunction of endothelial protein C activation in severe meningococcal sepsis. N Engl J Med 2001; 345(6):408–416.

17. Bernhard WG, Jordan AC. Purpuric lesions in meningococcal infections: diagnosis from smears and cultures of the purpuric lesions. J Lab Clin Med 1944; 29:273–281.

18. van Deuren M, van Dijke BJ, Koopman RJ, et al. Rapid diagnosis of acute meningococcal infections by needle aspiration or biopsy of skin lesions. BMJ 1993; 306(6887):1229–1232.

19. Gregory B, Tron V, Ho VC. Cyclic fever and rash in a 66-year-old woman. Chronic meningococcemia. Arch Dermatol 1992; 128(12):1645–1648.

20. Ploysangam T, Sheth AP. Chronic meningococcemia in childhood: case report and review of the literature. Pediatr Dermatol 1996; 13(6):483–487.

21. Masters EJ, Olson GS, Weiner SJ, et al. Rocky Mountain spotted fever: a clinician's dilemma. Arch Intern Med 2003; 163(7):769–774.

22. Sexton DJ, Kaye KS. Rocky mountain spotted fever. Med Clin North Am 2002; 86(2):351–360.

23. Thorner AR, Walker DH, Petri WA Jr. Rocky mountain spotted fever. Clin Infect Dis 1998; 27(6):1353–1359.

24. Jacobs RF. Human monocytic ehrlichiosis: similar to Rocky Mountain spotted fever but different. Pediatr Ann 2002; 31(3):180–184.

25. Holman RC, Paddock CD, Curns AT, et al. Analysis of risk factors for fatal Rocky Mountain Spotted Fever: evidence for superiority of tetracyclines for therapy. J Infect Dis 2001; 184(11):1437–1444.

26. Kirkland KB, Marcom PK, Sexton DJ, et al. Rocky Mountain spotted fever complicated by gangrene: report of six cases and review. Clin Infect Dis 1993; 16(5):629–634.

27. Rangel-Frausto MS. The epidemiology of bacterial sepsis. Infect Dis Clin North Am 1999; 13(2):299–312.

28. Annane D, Bellissant E, Cavaillon JM. Septic shock. Lancet 2005; 365(9453):63–78.

29. Alberti C, Brun-Buisson C, Goodman SV, et al. Influence of systemic inflammatory response syndrome and sepsis on outcome of critically ill infected patients. Am J Respir Crit Care Med 2003; 168(1):77–84.

30. Mylonakis E, Calderwood SB. Infective endocarditis in adults. N Engl J Med 2001; 345(18):1318–1330.

31. Strom BL, Abrutyn E, Berlin JA, et al. Risk factors for infective endocarditis: oral hygiene and nondental exposures. Circulation 2000; 102(23):2842–2848.

32. Manoff SB, Vlahov D, Herskowitz A, et al. Human immunodeficiency virus infection and infective endocarditis among injecting drug users. Epidemiology 1996; 7(6):566–570.

33. Brown PD, Levine DP. Infective endocarditis in the injection drug user. Infect Dis Clin North Am 2002; 16(3):645–665.

34. Crawford MH, Durack DT. Clinical presentation of infective endocarditis. Cardiol Clin 2003; 21(2):159–166.

35. Barr J, Danielsson D. Septic gonococcal dermatitis. Br Med J 1971; 1(747):482–485.

36. Holmes KK, Counts GW, Beaty HN. Disseminated gonococcal infection. Ann Intern Med 1971; 74(6):979–993.

37. Kerle KK, Mascola JR, Miller TA. Disseminated gonococcal infection. Am Fam Physician 1992; 45(1):209–214.

38. Handsfield HH. Disseminated gonococcal infection. Clin Obstet Gynecol 1975; 18(1): 131–142.

39. Abu-Nassar H, Hill N, Fred HL, et al. Cutaneous manifestations of gonococcemia. A review of 14 cases. Arch Intern Med 1963; 112:731–737.

40. Krol-van Straaten MJ, Landheer JE, de Maat CE. *Capnocytophaga canimorsus* (formerly DF-2) infections: review of the literature. Neth J Med 1990; 36(5–6):304–309.

41. Lion C, Escande F, Burdin JC. *Capnocytophaga canimorsus* infections in human: review of the literature and case report. Eur J Epidemiol 1996; 12(5):521–533.

42. Kullberg BJ, Westendorp RG, 't Wout JW, et al. Purpura fulminans and symmetrical peripheral gangrene caused by *Capnocytophaga canimorsus* (formerly DF-2) septicemia— a complication of dog bite. Medicine 1991; 70(5):287–292.

43. Guha-Sapir D, Schimmer B. Dengue fever: new paradigms for a changing epidemiology. Emerg Themes Epidemiol 2005; 2(1):1–10.

44. Calisher CH. Persistent emergence of dengue. Emerg Infect Dis 2005; 11(5):738–739.

45. Shirtcliffe P, Cameron E, Nicholson KG, et al. Don't forget dengue! Clinical features of dengue fever in returning travelers. J Roy Coll Physicians Lond 1998; 32(3):235–237.

46. Kalayanarooj S, Vaughn DW, Nimmannitya S, et al. Early clinical and laboratory indicators of acute dengue illness. J Infect Dis 1997; 176(2):313–321.

47. Kao CL, King CC, Chao DY, et al. Laboratory diagnosis of dengue virus infection: current and future perspectives in clinical diagnosis and public health. J Microbiol Immunol Infect 2005; 38(1):5–16.

48. Walker DH. Tick-transmitted infectious diseases in the United States. Annu Rev Public Health 1998; 19:237–269.

49. Taege AJ. Tick trouble: overview of tick-borne diseases. Cleve Clin J Med 2000; 67(4): 241, 245–249.

50. Lyme disease—United States, 1999. Morb Mortal Wkly Rep 2001; 50(10):181–185.

51. Gayle A, Ringdahl E. Tick-borne diseases. Am Fam Physician 2001; 64(3):461–466.

52. Steere AC, Coburn J, Glickstein L. The emergence of Lyme disease. J Clin Invest 2004; 113(8):1093–1101.

53. Edlow JA. Lyme disease and related tick-borne illnesses. Ann Emerg Med 1999; 33(6): 680–693.

54. Roujeau JC, Stern RS. Severe adverse cutaneous reactions to drugs. N Engl J Med 1994; 331(19):1272–1285.

55. Roujeau JC. Clinical heterogeneity of drug hypersensitivity. Toxicology 2005; 209(2): 123–129.

56. Pruksachatkunakorn C, Schachner LA. Erythema Multiforme. www.emedicine.com/derm/topic137.htm, 2005:1–9.

57. Assier H, Bastuji-Garin S, Revuz J, et al. Erythema multiforme with mucous membrane involvement and Stevens-Johnson syndrome are clinically different disorders with distinct causes. Arch Dermatol 1995; 131(5):539–543.

58. Bastuji-Garin S, Rzany B, Stern RS, et al. Clinical classification of cases of toxic epidermal necrolysis, Stevens-Johnson syndrome, and erythema multiforme. Arch Dermatol 1993; 129(1):92–96.

59. Hayes EB, Komar N, Nasci RS, et al. Epidemiology and transmission dynamics of West Nile Virus disease. Emerg Infect Dis 2005; 11(8):1167–1173.

60. Centers for Disease Control and Prevention (CDC). West Nile virus activity—United States, 2005. Morb Mortal Wkly Rep 2005; 54(31):769–770.

61. O'Leary DR, Marfin AA, Montgomery SP, et al. The epidemic of West Nile virus in the United States, 2002. Vector Borne Zoonotic Dis 2004; 4(1):61–70.

62. Petersen LR, Hayes EB. Westward ho?—The spread of West Nile virus. N Engl J Med 2004; 351(22):2257–2259.

63. Zeller HG, Schuffenecker I. West Nile virus: an overview of its spread in Europe and the Mediterranean basin in contrast to its spread in the Americas. Eur J Clin Micro Infect Dis 2004; 23(3):147–156.

64. Hayes EB, O'Leary DR. West Nile virus infection: a pediatric perspective. Pediatrics 2004; 113(5):1375–1381.

65. Kumar D, Prasad GV, Zaltzman J, et al. Community-acquired West Nile virus infection in solid-organ transplant recipients. Transplantation 2004; 77(3):399–402.

66. Stramer SL, Fang CT, Foster GA, et al. West Nile virus among blood donors in the United States, 2003 and 2004. N Engl J Med 2005; 353(5):451–459.

67. Diamond MS, Shrestha B, Mehlhop E, et al. Innate and adaptive immune responses determine protection against disseminated infection by West Nile encephalitis virus. Viral Immunol 2003; 16(3):259–278.

68. Mostashari F, Bunning ML, Kitsutani PT, et al. Epidemic West Nile encephalitis, New York, 1999: results of a household-based seroepidemiological survey. Lancet 2001; 358(9278):261–264.

69. Watson JT, Pertel PE, Jones RC, et al. Clinical characteristics and functional outcomes of West Nile fever. Ann Intern Med 2004; 141(5):360–365.

70. Hayes EB, Sejvar JJ, Zaki, et al. Virology, pathology, and clinical manifestations of West Nile Virus. Emerg Infect Dis 2005; 11(8):1174–1179.

71. Pepperell C, Rau N, Krajden S, et al. West Nile virus infection in 2002: morbidity and mortality among patients admitted to hospital in south-central Ontario. CMAJ 2003; 168(11):1399–1405.

72. Sejvar JJ, Haddad MB, Tierney BC, et al. Neurologic manifestations and outcome of West Nile virus infection. JAMA 2003; 290(4):511–515.

73. Sejvar JJ, Bode AV, Marfin AA, et al. West Nile virus-associated flaccid paralysis. Emerg Infect Dis 2005; 11(7):1021–1027.

74. Tilley PA, Zachary GA, Walle R, et al. West Nile virus detection and commercial assays. Emerg Infect Dis 2005; 11(7):1154–1155.

75. Martin DA, Biggerstaff BJ, Allen B, et al. Use of immunoglobulin M cross-reactions in differential diagnosis of human flaviviral encephalitis infections in the United States. Clin Diagn Lab Immunol 2002; 9(3):544–549.

76. Reich HL, Crawford GH, Pelle MT, et al. Group B streptococcal toxic shock-like syndrome. Arch Dermatol 2004; 140(2):163–166.

77. Todd J, Fishaut M, Kapral F, et al. Toxic-shock syndrome associated with phage-group-I Staphylococci. Lancet 1978; 2(8100):1116–1118.

78. Stevens DL, Tanner MH, Winship J, et al. Severe group A streptococcal infections associated with a toxic shock-like syndrome and scarlet fever toxin A. N Engl J Med 1989; 321(1):1–7.

79. Hajjeh RA, Reingold A, Weil A, et al. Toxic shock syndrome in the United States: surveillance update, 1979–1996. Emerg Infect Dis 1999; 5(6):807–810.

80. Reduced incidence of menstrual toxic-shock syndrome—United States, 1980–1990. MMWR Morb Mortal Wkly Rep 1990; 39(25):421–423.

81. Bergdoll MS, Crass BA, Reiser RF, et al. A new staphylococcal enterotoxin, enterotoxin F, associated with toxic-shock-syndrome *Staphylococcus aureus* isolates. Lancet 1981; 1(8228):1017–1021.

82. Schlievert PM. Staphylococcal enterotoxin B and toxic-shock syndrome toxin-1 are significantly associated with non-menstrual TSS. Lancet 1986; 1(8490):1149–1150.

83. Schlievert PM, Shands KN, Dan BB, et al. Identification and characterization of an exotoxin from *Staphylococcus aureus* associated with toxic-shock syndrome. J Infect Dis 1981; 143(4):509–516.

84. Lee VT, Chang AH, Chow AW. Detection of staphylococcal enterotoxin B among toxic shock syndrome (TSS)- and non-TSS-associated *Staphylococcus aureus* isolates. J Infect Dis 1992; 166(4):911–915.

85. Lehn N, Schaller E, Wagner H, et al. Frequency of toxic shock syndrome toxin- and enterotoxin-producing clinical isolates of *Staphylococcus aureus*. Eur J Clin Micro Infect Dis 1995; 14(1):43–46.

86. Barrett JA, Graham DR. Toxic shock syndrome presenting as encephalopathy. J Infect 1986; 12(3):276–278.

87. Chesney RW, Chesney PJ, Davis JP, et al. Renal manifestations of the staphylococcal toxic-shock syndrome. Am J Med 1981; 71(4):583–588.

88. Herzer CM. Toxic shock syndrome: broadening the differential diagnosis. J Am Board Fam Pract 2001; 14(2):131–136.

89. McKenna UG, Meadows JA III, Brewer NS, et al. Toxic shock syndrome, a newly recognized disease entity. Report of 11 cases. Mayo Clin Proc 1980; 55(11):663–672.

90. Chesney PJ, Davis JP, Purdy WK, et al. Clinical manifestations of toxic shock syndrome. JAMA 1981; 246(7):741–748.

91. Andrews MM, Parent EM, Barry M, et al. Recurrent nonmenstrual toxic shock syndrome: clinical manifestations, diagnosis, and treatment. Clin Infect Dis 2001; 32(10): 1470–1479.

92. Reingold AL, Dan BB, Shands KN, et al. Toxic-shock syndrome not associated with menstruation. A review of 54 cases. Lancet 1982; 1(8262):1–4.

93. Reingold AL, Hargrett NT, Dan BB, et al. Nonmenstrual toxic shock syndrome: a review of 130 cases. Ann Intern Med 1982; 96(6 Pt 2):871–874.

94. Defining the group A streptococcal toxic shock syndrome. Rationale and consensus definition. The Working Group on Severe Streptococcal Infections. JAMA 1993; 269(3): 390–391.

95. Manders SM. Toxin-mediated streptococcal and staphylococcal disease. J Am Acad Dermatol 1998; 39(3):383–398.

96. Ladhani S. Recent developments in staphylococcal scalded skin syndrome. Clin Micro Infect 2001; 7(6):301–307.

97. Adesiyun AA, Lenz W, Schaal KP. Exfoliative toxin production by *Staphylococcus aureus* strains isolated from animals and human beings in Nigeria. Microbiologica 1991; 14(4): 357–362.

98. Dancer SJ, Noble WC. Nasal, axillary, and perineal carriage of *Staphylococcus aureus* among women: identification of strains producing epidermolytic toxin. J Clin Path 1991; 44(8):681–684.

99. Ladhani S, Poston SM, Joannou CL, et al. Staphylococcal scalded skin syndrome: exfoliative toxin A (ETA) induces serine protease activity when combined with A431 cells. Acta Paediatr 1999; 88(7):776–779.

100. Papageorgiou AC, Plano LR, Collins CM, et al. Structural similarities and differences in *Staphylococcus aureus* exfoliative toxins A and B as revealed by their crystal structures. Protein Sci 2000; 9(3):610–618.

101. Prevost G, Couppie P, Monteil H. Staphylococcal epidermolysins. Curr Opin Infect Dis 2003; 16(2):71–76.
102. Lyell A. Toxic epidermal necrolysis (the scalded skin syndrome): a reappraisal. Br J Dermatol 1979; 100(1):69–86.
103. Melish ME. Staphylococci, streptococci and the skin: review of impetigo and staphylococcal scalded skin syndrome. Semin Dermatol 1982; 1:101–109.
104. Beers B, Wilson B. Adult staphylococcal scalded skin syndrome. Int J Dermatol 1990; 29(6):428–429.
105. Moss C, Gupta E. The Nikolsky sign in staphylococcal scalded skin syndrome. Arch Dis Child 1998; 79(3):290.
106. Gemmell CG. Staphylococcal scalded skin syndrome. J Med Micro 1995; 43(5):318–327.
107. Cribier B, Piemont Y, Grosshans E. Staphylococcal scalded skin syndrome in adults. A clinical review illustrated with a new case. J Am Acad Dermatol 1994; 30(2 Pt 2):319–324.
108. Goldberg NS, Ahmed T, Robinson B, et al. Staphylococcal scalded skin syndrome mimicking acute graft-vs.-host disease in a bone marrow transplant recipient. Arch Dermatol 1989; 125(1):85–87.
109. Ladhani S, Robbie S, Garratt RC, et al. Development and evaluation of detection systems for staphylococcal exfoliative toxin A responsible for scalded-skin syndrome. J Clin Microbiol 2001; 39(6):2050–2054.
110. Gentilhomme E, Faure M, Piemont Y, et al. Action of staphylococcal exfoliative toxins on epidermal cell cultures and organotypic skin. J Dermatol 1990; 17(9):526–532.
111. Leyden JJ, Gately LE III. Staphylococcal and streptococcal infections. In: Sanders CV, Nesbitt LTJ, eds. The Skin and Infection: A Color Atlas and Text. Baltimore: Williams and Wilkins, 1995:27–38.
112. Kawasaki T. Acute febrile mucocutaneous syndrome with lymphoid involvement with specific desquamation of the fingers and toes in children. Arerugi 1967; 16(3):178–222.
113. Burns JC, Glode MP. Kawasaki syndrome. Lancet 2004; 364(9433):533–544.
114. Royle J, Burgner D, Curtis N. The diagnosis and management of Kawasaki disease. J Pediatr Child Health 2005; 41(3):87–93.
115. Burns JC, Cayan DR, Tong G, et al. Seasonality and temporal clustering of Kawasaki syndrome. Epidemiology 2005; 16(2):220–225.
116. Morgan R, King D. Shingles: a review of diagnosis and management. Hospital Med (Lond) 1998; 59(10):770–776.
117. Feldman S, Hughes WT, Kim HY. Herpes zoster in children with cancer. Am J Dis Child 1973; 126(2):178–184.
118. Feldhoff CM, Balfour HH Jr., Simmons RL, et al. Varicella in children with renal transplants. J Pediatr 1981; 98(1):25–31.
119. Patti ME, Selvaggi KJ, Kroboth FJ. Varicella hepatitis in the immunocompromised adult: a case report and review of the literature. Am J Med 1990; 88(1):77–80.
120. Veenstra J, van Praag RM, Krol A, et al. Complications of varicella zoster virus reactivation in HIV-infected homosexual men. AIDS 1996; 10(4):393–399.
121. Buchbinder SP, Katz MH, Hessol NA, et al. Herpes zoster and human immunodeficiency virus infection. J Infect Dis 1992; 166(5):1153–1156.
122. Gershon AA, Mervish N, LaRussa P, et al. Varicella-zoster virus infection in children with underlying human immunodeficiency virus infection. J Infect Dis 1997; 176(6):1496–1500.
123. Straus SE, Ostrove JM, Inchauspe G, et al. NIH conference. Varicella-zoster virus infections. Biology, natural history, treatment, and prevention. Ann Intern Med 1988; 108(2):221–237.
124. Galil K, Choo PW, Donahue JG, et al. The sequelae of herpes zoster. Arch Intern Med 1997; 157(11):1209–1213.
125. Levitsky J, Kalil A, Meza JL, et al. Herpes zoster infection after liver transplantation: a case-control study. Liver Transpl 2005; 11(3):320–325.

126. Rogers SY, Irving W, Harris A, et al. Visceral varicella zoster infection after bone marrow transplantation without skin involvement and the use of PCR for diagnosis. Bone Marrow Transplant 1995; 15(5):805–807.

127. Veenstra J, Krol A, van Praag RM, et al. Herpes zoster, immunological deterioration and disease progression in HIV-1 infection. AIDS 1995; 9(10):1153–1158.

128. Rusthoven JJ, Ahlgren P, Elhakim T, et al. Varicella-zoster infection in adult cancer patients. A population study. Arch Intern Med 1988; 148(7):1561–1566.

129. Tojimbara T, So SK, Cox KL, et al. Fulminant hepatic failure following varicella-zoster infection in a child. A case report of successful treatment with liver transplantation and perioperative acyclovir. Transplantation 1995; 60(9):1052–1053.

130. Verdonck LF, Cornelissen JJ, Dekker AW, et al. Acute abdominal pain as a presenting symptom of varicella-zoster virus infection in recipients of bone marrow transplants. Clin Infect Dis 1993; 16(1):190–191.

131. Fleisher G, Henry W, McSorley M, et al. Life-threatening complications of varicella. Am J Dis Child 1981; 135(10):896–899.

132. Pavan-Langston D. Herpes zoster ophthalmicus. Neurology 1995; 45(12 suppl 8): S50–S51.

133. Hellinger WC, Bolling JP, Smith TF, et al. Varicella-zoster virus retinitis in a patient with AIDS-related complex: case report and brief review of the acute retinal necrosis syndrome. Clin Infect Dis 1993; 16(2):208–212.

134. Culbertson WW, Blumenkranz MS, Pepose JS, et al. Varicella zoster virus is a cause of the acute retinal necrosis syndrome. Ophthalmology 1986; 93(5):559–569.

135. Adour KK. Otological complications of herpes zoster. Ann Neurol 1994; 35(suppl): S62–S64.

136. Elliott KJ. Other neurological complications of herpes zoster and their management. Ann Neurol 1994; 35(suppl):S57–S61.

137. Au WY, Hon C, Cheng VC, et al. Concomitant zoster myelitis and cerebral leukemia relapse after stem cell transplantation. Ann Hematol 2005; 84(1):59–60.

138. Burke DG, Kalayjian RC, Vann VR, et al. Polymerase chain reaction detection and clinical significance of varicella-zoster virus in cerebrospinal fluid from human immunodeficiency virus-infected patients. J Infect Dis 1997; 176(4):1080–1084.

139. Cinque P, Bossolasco S, Vago L, et al. Varicella-zoster virus (VZV) DNA in cerebrospinal fluid of patients infected with human immunodeficiency virus: VZV disease of the central nervous system or subclinical reactivation of VZV infection? Clin Infect Dis 1997; 25(3):634–639.

140. Breman JG, Arita I. The confirmation and maintenance of smallpox eradication. N Engl J Med 1980; 303(22):1263–1273.

141. Henderson DA. Smallpox eradication. Public Health Rep 1980; 95(5):422–426.

142. Dixon CW. Smallpox. London: J & A Churchill Ltd., 1962.

143. Huq F. Effect of temperature and relative humidity on variola virus in crusts. Bull World Health Org 1976; 54(6):710–712.

144. Harper GJ. The influence of environment on the survival of airborne virus particles in the laboratory. Arch Gesamte Virusforsch 1963; 13:64–71.

145. Breman JG, Henderson DA. Diagnosis and management of smallpox. N Engl J Med 2002; 346(17):1300–1308.

146. Henderson DA, Inglesby TV, Bartlett JG, et al. Smallpox as a biological weapon: medical and public health management. Working Group on Civilian Biodefense. JAMA 1999; 281(22):2127–2137.

147. Corey L, Spear PG. Infections with herpes simplex viruses (1). N Engl J Med 1986; 314(11):686–691.

148. Frederick DM, Bland D, Gollin Y. Fatal disseminated herpes simplex virus infection in a previously healthy pregnant woman. A case report. J Reprod Med 2002; 47(7): 591–596.

149. Hillard P, Seeds J, Cefalo R. Disseminated herpes simplex in pregnancy: two cases and a review. Obstet Gynecol Surv 1982; 37(7):449–453.

150. Johnson JR, Egaas S, Gleaves CA, et al. Hepatitis due to herpes simplex virus in marrow-transplant recipients. Clin Infect Dis 1992; 14(1):38–45.

151. Kusne S, Schwartz M, Breinig MK, et al. Herpes simplex virus hepatitis after solid organ transplantation in adults. J Infect Dis 1991; 163(5):1001–1007.

152. Liesegang TJ. Herpes simplex virus epidemiology and ocular importance. Cornea 2001; 20(1):1–13.

153. Muller SA, Herrmann EC Jr., Winkelmann RK. Herpes simplex infections in hematologic malignancies. Am J Med 1972; 52(1):102–114.

154. Priya K, Mahalakshmi B, Malathi J, et al. Prevalence of herpes simplex virus, varicella zoster virus and cytomegalovirus in HIV-positive and HIV-negative patients with viral retinitis in India. Eur J Clin Micro Infect Dis 2004; 23(11):857–858.

155. Remeijer L, Osterhaus A, Verjans G. Human herpes simplex virus keratitis: the pathogenesis revisited. Ocular Immunol Inflamm 2004; 12(4):255–285.

156. Siegal FP, Lopez C, Hammer GS, et al. Severe acquired immunodeficiency in male homosexuals, manifested by chronic perianal ulcerative herpes simplex lesions. N Engl J Med 1981; 305(24):1439–1444.

157. Tyler KL. Herpes simplex virus infections of the central nervous system: encephalitis and meningitis, including Mollaret's. Herpes 2004; 11(suppl 2):57A–64A.

158. DeBiasi RL, Kleinschmidt-DeMasters BK, Weinberg A, et al. Use of PCR for the diagnosis of herpes virus infections of the central nervous system. J Clin Virol 2002; 25(suppl 1):S5–S11.

159. Gopal AK, Fowler VG Jr., Shah M, et al. Prospective analysis of *Staphylococcus aureus* bacteremia in non-neutropenic adults with malignancy. J Clin Oncol 2000; 18(5): 1110–1115.

160. Gottlieb GS, Fowler VG Jr., Kong LK, et al. *Staphylococcus aureus* bacteremia in the surgical patient: a prospective analysis of 73 postoperative patients who developed *Staphylococcus aureus* bacteremia at a tertiary care facility. J Am Coll Surg 2000; 190(1):50–57.

161. Marr KA, Kong L, Fowler VG, et al. Incidence and outcome of *Staphylococcus aureus* bacteremia in hemodialysis patients. Kidney Int 1998; 54(5):1684–1689.

162. Petti CA, Fowler VG Jr. *Staphylococcus aureus* bacteremia and endocarditis. Cardiol Clin 2003; 21(2):219–233.

163. Shah MA, Sanders L, Lanclos K, et al. *Staphylococcus aureus* bacteremia in patients with neutropenia. South Med J 2002; 95(7):782–784.

164. Tumbarello M, de Gaetano DK, Tacconelli E, et al. Risk factors and predictors of mortality of methicillin-resistant *Staphylococcus aureus* (MRSA) bacteremia in HIV-infected patients. J Antimicrob Chemo 2002; 50(3):375–382.

165. Mitra AK. *Vibrio vulnificus* infection: epidemiology, clinical presentations, and prevention. South Med J 2004; 97(2):118–119.

166. Ruple AD, Cook DW. *Vibrio vulnificus* indicator bacteria in shellstock and commercially processed oysters. J Food Prot 1992; 55:667–671.

167. Hill MK, Sanders CV. Localized and systemic infection due to *Vibrio* species. Infect Dis Clin North Am 1987; 1(3):687–707.

168. Klontz KC, Lieb S, Schreiber M, et al. Syndromes of *Vibrio vulnificus* infections. Clinical and epidemiologic features in Florida cases, 1981–1987. Ann Intern Med 1988; 109(4): 318–323.

169. Chiang SR, Chuang YC. *Vibrio vulnificus* infection: clinical manifestations, pathogenesis, and antimicrobial therapy. J Microb Immun Infect 2003; 36(2):81–88.

170. Haq SM, Dayal HH. Chronic liver disease and consumption of raw oysters: a potentially lethal combination—a review of *Vibrio vulnificus* septicemia. Am J Gastro 2005; 100(5): 1195–1199.

171. Levine WC, Griffin PM, Gulf Coast Vibrio Working Group. Vibrio infections on the Gulf Coast: results of first year of regional surveillance. J Infect Dis 1993; 167(2):479–483.

172. Howard RJ, Bennett NT. Infections caused by halophilic marine *Vibrio* bacteria. Ann Surg 1993; 217(5):525–530.

173. Hsueh PR, Lin CY, Tang HJ, et al. *Vibrio vulnificus* in Taiwan. Emerg Infect Dis 2004; 10(8):1363–1368.

174. Wickboldt LG, Sanders CV. *Vibrio vulnificus* infection. Case report and update since 1970. J Am Acad Dermatol 1983; 9(2):243–251.

175. Koenig KL, Mueller J, Rose T. *Vibrio vulnificus*. Hazard on the half shell. West J Med 1991; 155(4):400–403.

176. Chen CY, Wu KM, Chang YC, et al. Comparative genome analysis of *Vibrio vulnificus*, a marine pathogen. Genome Res 2003; 13(12):2577–2587.

177. Morris JG Jr. *Vibrio vulnificus*—a new monster of the deep? Ann Intern Med 1988; 109(4):261–263.

178. Greenberg M, Pellitteri OJ, Jellison WL. Rickettsialpox-a newly recognized rickettsial disease. Am J Public Health 1947; 37:860–868.

179. Kass EM, Szaniawski WK, Levy H, et al. Rickettsialpox in a New York City hospital, 1980 to 1989. N Engl J Med 1994; 331(24):1612–1617.

180. Krusell A, Comer JA, Sexton DJ. Rickettsialpox in North Carolina: a case report. Emerg Infect Dis 2002; 8(7):727–728.

181. Brettman LR, Lewin S, Holzman RS, et al. Rickettsialpox: report of an outbreak and a contemporary review. Medicine 1981; 60(5):363–372.

182. Cribier B, Caille A, Heid E, et al. Erythema nodosum and associated diseases. A study of 129 cases. Int J Dermatol 1998; 37(9):667–672.

183. Blomgren SE. Conditions associated with erythema nodosum. NY State J Med 1972; 72(18):2302–2304.

184. James DG. Erythema nodosum. Br Med J 1961; 5229:853–857.

185. Puavilai S, Sakuntabhai A, Sriprachaya-Anunt S, et al. Etiology of erythema nodosum. J Med Assoc Thai 1995; 78(2):72–75.

186. Vesey CM, Wilkinson DS. Erythema nodosum: a study of seventy cases. Br J Dermatol 1959; 71(4):139–155.

187. Maksymiuk AW, Thongprasert S, Hopfer R, et al. Systemic candidiasis in cancer patients. Am J Med 1984; 77(4D):20–27.

188. Bodey GP. Fungal infection and fever of unknown origin in neutropenic patients. Am J Med 1986; 80(5C):112–119.

189. Bodey GP. Candidiasis in cancer patients. Am J Med 1984; 77(4D):13–19.

190. Balandran L, Rothschild H, Pugh N, et al. A cutaneous manifestation of systemic candidiasis. Ann Intern Med 1973; 78(3):400–403.

191. Jacobs MI, Magid MS, Jarowski CI. Disseminated candidiasis. Newer approaches to early recognition and treatment. Arch Dermatol 1980; 116(11):1277–1279.

192. Radentz WH. Opportunistic fungal infections in immunocompromised hosts. J Am Acad Dermatol1920(6):989–1003.

193. Hahn RG, Knox LM, Forman TA. Evaluation of poststreptococcal illness. Am Fam Physician 2005; 71(10):1949–1954.

194. Stollerman GH. Rheumatic fever in the 21st century. Clin Infect Dis 2001; 33(6): 806–814.

195. Guidelines for the diagnosis of rheumatic fever. Jones Criteria, 1992 update. Special Writing Group of the Committee on Rheumatic Fever, Endocarditis, and Kawasaki Disease of the Council on Cardiovascular Disease in the Young of the American Heart Association. JAMA 1992; 268(15):2069–2073.

196. Feinstein AR, Spagnuolo M. The clinical patterns of acute rheumatic fever: a reappraisal. Medicine 1962; 41:279–305.

197. Stollerman GH. Rheumatic fever. Lancet 1997; 349(9056):935–942.

198. Hilario MO, Andrade JL, Gasparian AB, et al. The value of echocardiography in the diagnosis and follow up of rheumatic carditis in children and adolescents: a 2 year prospective study. J Rheumatol 2000; 27(4):1082–1086.
199. McCallum AH. Natural history of rheumatic fever and rheumatic heart disease. Ten-year report of a co-operative clinical trial of A.C.T.H., Cortisone, and aspirin. Br Med J 1965; 5462:607–613.
200. Swedo SE. Sydenham's chorea. A model for childhood autoimmune neuropsychiatric disorders. JAMA 1994; 272(22):1788–1791.
201. Baldwin JS, Kerr JM, Kuttner AG, et al. Observations on rheumatic nodules over a 30-year period. J Pediatr 1960; 56:465–470.
202. Burke JB. Erythema marginatum. Arch Dis Child 1955; 30(152):359–365.

19

Tropical Infections in the Critical Care Unit[a]

David R. Tribble
Department of Enteric Diseases, Infectious Diseases Directorate, Naval Medical Research Institute, Silver Spring, Maryland, U.S.A.

Kenneth F. Wagner
Independent Consultant, Infectious Diseases and Tropical Medicine, Islamorada, Florida, U.S.A.

EPIDEMIOLOGY OF INFECTIONS IN INTERNATIONAL TRAVELERS

International travel brings a world of experiences and opportunities but also carries a degree of health risks that can often be prevented or better managed if appropriate pre-travel preparation is undertaken. Retrospective case series of traveler health risks have documented the wide range of health problems that may be associated with international travel (1). Both noninfectious and infectious diseases are well represented with the predominant causes of death being accidents (motor vehicle and drowning) and cardiovascular related in younger and older travelers, respectively (2). Infections account for significant morbidity and mortality both during and after international travel, particularly into developing tropical regions (1,3). There is a predominance of enteric transmission as the most common route of infection with the usual clinical syndrome being traveler's diarrhea (1,3). Food- and water-borne infections such as typhoid fever, cholera, hepatitis A, and uncommonly agents of traveler's diarrhea occasionally result in critical illness in travelers. The most common life-threatening infection in returning travelers is malaria, and this will be emphasized in this chapter.

The determinants of infectious risk and potential etiologies in a returning traveler are based on relative incidence of the infection, regional distribution, traveler predisposition, and specific aspects of the traveler's itinerary or activities. Steffen et al. calculated incidences (per 100,000 travelers) of various infectious diseases in returning European travelers from developing regions (1). Severe diarrhea was the most common illness (12,998) followed by diarrhea with fever (1940), acute respiratory tract infection with fever (1261), giardiasis (660), hepatitis (446), amebiasis (427), gonorrhea (330), and malaria (97). Notably absent in this study were

---

[a]The opinions and assertions contained herein are those of the authors and do not reflect the official policy of the Department of Navy, Department of Defense, or the U.S. Government.

typhoid and cholera, which have been reported in other retrospective surveys at rates of approximately 5/100,000 and <0.5/100,000, respectively (4–7). The regional distribution of infections must take into account "globally" distributed infections seen in most developing regions [i.e., tuberculosis (TB) and typhoid] versus focally distributed infections (i.e., schistosomiasis, Ebola virus, etc.). Variable distribution for vectors (i.e., lack of Anopheline mosquitoes in highland areas or certain urban centers and focal distribution of snail intermediate host in schistosomiasis) should also be considered. The individual traveler's predisposition can be divided into traveler-specific risks (i.e., increased risk of enteric infections with achlorhydria, failure to use proper malarial prophylaxis, no personal protective measures used to avoid arthropod exposures, immunocompromised, and lack of immunoprophylaxis) and itinerary-specific risks [i.e., purpose of travel (leisure, business, or humanitarian), prolonged duration in rural area, adventurous travel using local food and water, outdoor camping, swimming in fresh water, and unprotected sexual contact]. Applying exposure risk assessment allows appropriate inclusion of specific infections for diagnostic consideration while also focusing the differential diagnosis.

Several excellent reviews and retrospective series discuss returning travelers and immigrants with fever (8–17). A more recent series from Australia investigated the etiology of returning febrile travelers requiring hospitalization (18). Malaria was the most common cause accounting for 27% of the patients followed by lower respiratory tract infections (24%) and febrile gastroenteritis (14%). No description of illness severity was provided. Hospitalization typically occurred soon upon return from a trip with a median of six-and-a-half days (53% and 81% within one week and one month, respectively). This chapter will focus on returning travelers with potentially life-threatening infections. Table 1 details the general diagnostic considerations applicable to any potential infected critically ill returning traveler. A management algorithm for returning travelers with severe infections is detailed in Figure 1.

Table 1 General Considerations in Potentially Infected Critically Ill Returning Travelers

Diagnostic consideration	Comments
Accurate traveler- and itinerary-specific risk assessment	Obtain detailed history of sites visited, activities, and potential infectious exposures
Calculate approximate incubation period	Incubation periods: short (<10 day); intermediate (10–14 day); prolonged (>21 day). A minimum period of 5–7 day before considering malaria. Incubation period exceeding three weeks rules out arboviral etiologies
Avoid narrow focus on "tropical infections"	Avoid becoming so focused on the international travel history that common community-acquired infections such as pneumococcal pneumonia, staphylococcal infections, etc. are not considered
Use concomitant signs and/or symptoms	Narrow the differential diagnosis using clinical progression and specific findings (i.e., diarrhea, rash, or respiratory complaints)
Rule out malaria	Always consider and perform diagnostic testing to evaluate for malaria if a traveler has been in a malarious region with an appropriate incubation period

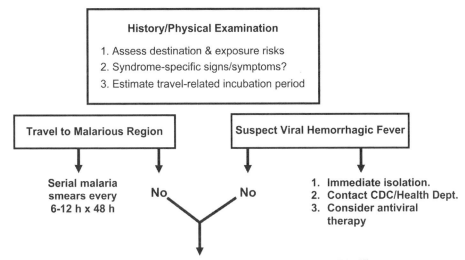

Figure 1 Initial evaluation of returning travelers with severe infections.

Given the wide diversity of infectious etiologies, space does not permit a comprehensive discussion of all diagnostic and therapeutic modalities.

MALARIA

Malaria is caused by four different species of *Plasmodium*; however, *P. falciparum* is the predominant cause of mortality due to malaria (19). Data from 1997 to 2002 collected through the GeoSentinel global sentinel surveillance identified malaria in 3.7% of all returning travelers seeking medical care (20). The majority of the cases were caused by *P. falciparum* at 60% followed by *P. vivax* at 24% (20). Falciparum malaria cases had more commonly traveled to sub-Saharan Africa (89%) with the majority (80%) presenting within four weeks of trip return. Among the falciparum malaria cases, 60% were hospitalized with 2.4% diagnosed with cerebral malaria and 2.3% with severe complicated noncerebral malaria. There was a 9% case fatality rate among the severe malaria cases. Case fatality rate for U.S. travelers with falciparum malaria from 1966 to 1987 was 3.8% (21). Recent U.S. traveler case fatality rate estimate for 1985 to 2001 was 1.3% for *P. falciparum* infections (22). Mortality from *P. falciparum* in returning travelers to the United States from 1959 to 1987 demonstrated several important features including the failure to use any or use incorrect malaria chemoprophylaxis (90%) and diagnostic/therapeutic delay (40%) even after physician evaluation highlighting the preventable aspect to these deaths (21). In a more recent series, cerebral malaria was the most common complication in 48% followed by renal failure (44%), acute respiratory distress (32%), anemia (21%), disseminated intravascular coagulation (DIC) (11%), and splenic rupture (5%) (22). Deaths were considered preventable in 85% and were commonly related to both patient-related decisions/actions and contributing medical errors (22).

The current recommendations for malaria prophylaxis entail a consideration of regional antimalarial drug resistance to include whether or not the traveler visits a chloroquine sensitive or resistant region or an area with documented mefloquine resistance (23). There is no universally effective regimen as evidenced by *P. falciparum* mefloquine resistance in Thai-Burmese and Thai-Cambodian borders, breakthrough falciparum malaria in U.S. troops in Somalia on either doxycycline or mefloquine, and reports of chloroquine resistance in *P. vivax* in Indonesia (24–28). There is a lack of sensitive predictive historical or physical findings (fever pattern, symptom duration, temperature, splenomegaly, or thrombocytopenia); therefore, malaria cannot be ruled out on historical or physical findings alone (22,29,30). Falciparum malaria will often present without the classical features of cyclical fever and the malarial paroxysm (initial chill lasting approximately 15 minutes to a few hours followed by high fever for two to six hours, then diaphoresis and extreme fatigue) (31). Commonly seen is a febrile nondescript illness without apparent cyclical nature. Other presenting features may include severe anemia, thrombocytopenia, central nervous system (CNS) dysfunction such as coma or seizures, pulmonary edema, or dysentery (14,23).

The diagnosis of malaria rests primarily on prompt consideration and serial examination of peripheral blood smears. Rapid diagnostic tests offer the promise of bringing the diagnosis nearer to the bedside as well as providing simple procedures less reliant upon technician expertise (32). Nonmicroscopic immunochromatographic rapid tests are rapid and simple to perform; however, challenges remain with variable sensitivity (>100 parasites/μL), negative results requiring microscopic confirmation, and cost concerns (32). Rapid diagnosis of malaria is critical due to the semiquantitative relationship between level of parasitemia and mortality: <25,000 parasites/μL = 0.2% mortality, 25 to 100,000 parasites/μL = 1.1% mortality, 100 to 500,000 parasites/μL = 14.8% mortality, and >500,000 parasites/μL = 72% mortality (33). A qualified laboratory is a necessity based on the lack of clinical predictors. Standard methods are thick and thin peripheral blood Giemsa or Wright stained smears obtained serially (every six to eight hours over 24 hours usually a minimum of three smears). Appropriate expertise and timely referral to a reference laboratory if necessary is critical.

The management of malaria is reliant on prompt recognition and initiation of effective therapy with a blood schizonticide to rapidly reduce parasitemia (34). After recognizing that the patient has malaria, the next steps are to differentiate species between *P. falciparum* and nonfalciparum malaria. If the traveler with falciparum malaria reports travel limited to chloroquine-susceptible regions (Central America, Haiti, and possibly limited areas in the Middle East), then chloroquine therapy can be used (intravenous and oral available). Given the widespread chloroquine resistance, monotherapy should only be used in areas where treatment efficacy has been recently demonstrated and not for severe malaria (25,35). Severe malaria should be managed with parenteral antimalarial therapy given the potential for erratic absorption through the gastrointestinal tract (36). Recommended treatment modalities currently available are from the cinchona alkaloid class [quinine dihydrochloride (intravenous or intramuscular) or quinidine gluconate (intravenous)] or artemisinin derivatives [artesunate (intravenous) or artemether (intramuscular)] (34,36). The artemisinins more rapidly clear parasitemia with equivalent efficacy to intravenous quinine even with rectal delivery (37–40). In the U.S., the only licensed drug for intravenous therapy is quinidine gluconate often combined with a second blood schizonticide for radical cure (such as tetracycline) (Table 2) (41). Loading doses are used to rapidly attain effective drug levels with the exception of quinine or quinidine loading in patients who have been receiving quinine, mefloquine, or quinidine (34). Monitoring of the QRS and QTc intervals is needed during quinidine therapy due to the potential for systemic hypotension or QT prolongation (42).

Exchange transfusion is occasionally used for severe malaria when parasitemia levels exceed 10% or if the patient has altered mental status, nonvolume overload pulmonary edema, or renal complications (43). It is usually continued until the parasite load is <1% (usually 8–10 units). IV quinidine should not be delayed for an exchange transfusion and can be given concurrently. There is no randomized controlled trial to assess efficacy of exchange transfusions, and no survival benefit was demonstrated in a meta-analysis when compared with antimalarial chemotherapy alone (44). Corticosteroids have been shown in controlled trials of severe malaria to not only lack efficacy as adjunctive therapy but also to be deleterious (45). Renal failure and/or lactic acidosis can contribute to life-threatening metabolic acidosis. Hemofiltration has been demonstrated to have lower mortality as compared to peritoneal dialysis in the management of acute renal failure secondary to severe malaria (46).

Early recognition and directed therapy of complicated malaria cases are critical to successful management. All severe or complicated malaria should be managed in an intensive care setting. Severe or complicated malaria includes the following: (i) hyperparasitemia (>5%), (ii) altered level of consciousness (cerebral malaria; r/o hypoglycemia), (iii) circulatory shock (typically due to gram-negative sepsis),

Table 2 Severe Malaria Treatment Regimens Available in the United States[a]

Drug	Adult dosage	Pediatric dosage
Parenteral administration All severe malaria Quinidine gluconate plus one of the below	10 mg salt/kg load (max 600 mg) in normal saline over 1–2 hr then 0.02 mg salt/kg/min continuous infusion for at least 48–72 hr or 24 mg salt/kg load over 4 hr, followed by 12 mg salt/kg infused over 4 hr every 8 hr starting 8 hr after loading dose for at least 48–72 hr. Switch to PO quinine sulfate 650 mg q8h when parasite density <1% and patient can take PO meds to complete 7 day Rx	Same as for adults, do not exceed adult dose
Doxycycline[b]or	100 mg IV q12h and switch when pt can take PO meds to complete 7 day Rx	Same as for adults if ≥45 kg <45 kg give 4 mg/kg q12h
Clindamycin	10 mg base/kg load followed by 5 mg base/kg q8h. Switch when pt can take PO meds to complete 7 day Rx	Same as adult

[a]Comments: see pages 6 and 7, 401–402.
[b]Benefits of tetracycline therapy versus the possibility of dental staining in children less than 9-yrs old must be considered. Health care providers needing assistance with the diagnosis or management of suspected cases of malaria may call the Centers for Disease Control and Prevention CDC Malaria Hotline: 770-488-7788 (M-F, 8 AM–4:30 PM, Eastern Time). Emergency consultation after hours, call: 770-488-7100 and request to speak with a CDC Malaria Branch clinician.

(iv) prolonged hyperthermia, (v) high output gastrointestinal losses, (vi) pulmonary involvement [adult respiratory distress syndrome (ARDS)], (vii) cardiac involvement (ischemia or congestive failure), (viii) hepatitis, (ix) renal failure, and (x) hypoglycemia (34). Proposed criteria for intensive care unit (ICU) admission for patients with severe malaria include base excess <0.8, high level parasitemia (nonendemic area >10% and endemic area >20%), Glasgow Coma Score ≤8, blood glucose <2.2 mmol/L, urine output <0.5 mL/kg/hr, or pulmonary edema (36). Clinical monitoring is directed at symptom and sign resolution and microbiologic clearance. The following are important endpoints when caring for a patient with malaria:

1. Clinical symptoms should be improving within 48 to 72 hours.
2. Parasitemia should be monitored approximately every 12 hours and should be reduced by 75% within 48 hours on therapy.
3. Failure to show clinical or microbiologic resolution suggests one or more of the following problems:
   a. Secondary complication such as bacterial superinfection [not limited to developing areas; observed in 14% of returning travelers with severe malaria (47)];
   b. Problems with medication administration;
   c. Antimalarial resistance.

CRITICAL CARE INFECTIOUS DISEASE SYNDROMES

Severe Pneumonia or ARDS

Severe pneumonia or ARDS in the United States is most commonly caused by community-acquired respiratory pathogens such as *Streptococcus pneumoniae* and *Legionella pneumophila* or as a complication of bacterial sepsis (48,49). If the patient has recently traveled into developing regions of the world, then it becomes important to broaden the differential diagnoses. TB is highly prevalent throughout much of the world and may present with an extensive pulmonary infiltrate with hypoxia and hemoptysis or with miliary or disseminated disease (50–52). A fulminant presentation of miliary TB may occur in children with meningeal involvement in up to two-thirds, and also may be seen in older adults (50,51). The clinical presentation of severe tuberculous pneumonia may be indistinguishable from other causes of bacterial pneumonia. Miliary TB commonly has nonspecific presenting symptoms with the most common signs being fever, tachypnea, rales, and altered mental status, less commonly presenting with ARDS and DIC. Because mortality rates reach as high as 21% in miliary TB, it is important to consider TB in the differential diagnosis, initiate respiratory isolation, obtain diagnostic clinical specimens (i.e., sputum, bronchial washings, etc.), consider associated diseases such as HIV infection, realize the potential for multidrug resistance, and provide early initiation of 4-drug anti-tuberculous regimen (i.e., isoniazid, rifampin, pyrazinamide, and ethambutol/streptomycin) (53,54).

S. pneumoniae is the most common cause of life-threatening bacterial pneumonia in the United States and is very common throughout the world (49). Specific associated risks (i.e., chronic lung disease and HIV) should increase the suspicion of pneumococcal disease, but their absence does not assist in exclusion because pneumococcal pneumonia is very common in previously healthy people. The global problem of penicillin-resistant pneumococci, which is now seen in the United States, requires the initial antibiotic selection to include a respiratory fluoroquinolone or an advanced macrolide plus a beta-lactam antibiotic (such as cefotaxime, ceftriaxone, ampicillin-sulbactam, or ertapenem) in severe hospitalized cases with no prior anti-biotic use as well as vancomycin if CNS involvement or a more severe clinical pre-sentation is suspected (55). *L. pneumophila* has been documented as a cause of severe pneumonia in travelers often in association with exposure to whirlpool spas on cruise ships (56). In one of the outbreaks involving 50 cruise ship passengers, the risk of acquiring Legionnaire's disease increased by 64% for every hour spent in the spa water (56). The diagnosis of *L. pneumophila* can be difficult and requires prior consideration so that the microbiology lab can process clinical respiratory specimens on selective media (57). Urine antigen testing can provide a more rapid diagnosis of *L. pneumophila* serogroup one (most common isolate—approximately 80%) with sensitivity of 80% and specificity >99% (57). Preferred treatment of severe Legionnaire's disease is with azithromycin or a respiratory fluoroquinolone for at least 10 days ± rifampin 300 mg IV. Influenza has also been well documented to cause focal outbreaks among travelers often associated with air travel (58). Epidemic influenza varies in seasonality based on the geographic region—Northern hemi-sphere (December–April), Southern hemisphere (May–September), and tropical regions (year long). The diagnosis of influenza is based on clinical features (abrupt onset, high fevers, myalgias, and respiratory symptoms), virus isolation, antigen detection, and/or serology. Antiviral therapies have documented efficacy in influ-enza A (amantadine, rimantadine, and neuraminidase inhibitors) and influenza A and B (neuraminidase inhibitors) therapy. Consideration should be given to poten-tial secondary bacterial pneumonia with *Staphylococcus aureus or S. pneumoniae* that may require antibiotic therapy.

Other less common causes of respiratory infections or syndromes in travelers include hantaviral pulmonary syndrome (HPS), *Burkholderia pseudomallei* (melioi-dosis), plague, histoplasmosis and atypical manifestations of malaria, typhoid fever, leptospirosis, rickettsial diseases, and some protozoal (amebiasis)/helminthic (schisto-somiasis and fascioliasis) infections (52). HPS was first described in an outbreak in the Southwestern United States (59). Hantaviruses have a global distribution and typically manifest clinically with hemorrhagic and/or renal disease. Less common clinical features with HPS providing helpful differentiation from more common causes of severe respiratory infections include sore throat and cough (dif-fering from influenza) and radiographic evidence of lobar infiltrates (differing from bacteremic pneumococcal pneumonia) (60). The presence of dizziness, nausea or vomit-ing, a lack of cough, thrombocytopenia, decreased serum bicarbonate, and hemoconcentration identified all HPS patients in a series of patients presenting with ARDS (60). More recent studies have confirmed these findings as clinical pre-dictors of HPS (61). Ribavirin [loading dose of 33 mg/kg (max 2 g), followed by 16 mg/kg (max 1 g) given every six hours for four days and by 8 mg/kg (max 0.5 g) given every eight hours for three days] has been demonstrated in a controlled clinical trial to significantly reduce mortality (sevenfold) in hantaviral hemorrhagic fever with renal syndrome, although efficacy was not demonstrated in a rando-mized controlled trial for HPS (62,63). *B. pseudomallei* (melioidosis) has rarely been reported as a cause of fulminant disease in travelers from Southeast Asia and Australia and more commonly presents as a chronic granulomatous illness resembling TB (64). The spectrum of disease in melioidosis ranges from an asymp-tomatic illness to chronic debilitating illness (such as with lung abscess) to fulmi-nant septicemia. Currently recommended antibiotic therapy for melioidosis is ceftazidime with the additional requirement of prolonged oral therapy with chlor-amphenicol, doxycycline, and cotrimoxazole to prevent relapse (64,65). Plague may present in either a bubonic (tender, fluctuant adenopathy with systemic illness), septicemic, or pneumonic form. No recent occurrence of plague in international travelers has been reported. However, as there are recent concerns over plague importation from India, awareness of areas with endemic/potentially epidemic plague (India, Viet Nam, Myanmar, Zaire, and Madagascar) is important (66,67). Symptoms in patients with plague can range from a mild febrile illness with a bubo to fulminant sepsis. Rapid institution of appropriate therapy (gentamicin 2 mg/kg loading dose then 1.7 mg/kg every eight hours) is critical given the potential for rapid deterioration and the extreme contagiousness via respiratory spread. Acute pulmonary histoplasmosis has recently been observed as an etiology of acute febrile respiratory illness among travelers returning from Mexico (68). In this large outbreak among college students, the apparent exposure to *Histoplasma capsulatum* was temporary residence at a hotel where maintenance projects were underway. Other endemic mycoses, such as coccidioidomycosis and penicilliosis, are also considerations in the differential diagnosis in returning travelers (69).

The newly identified coronavirus, which emerged as the etiology of the severe acute respiratory syndrome (SARS) in the spring of 2003, must be considered in returning travelers from Far East destinations or areas with known SARS activity (70,71). SARS frequently presents similar to other etiologies of severe atypical pneumonia; however, a proposed clinical prediction rule yielded a sensitivity of 90% with specificity of 62% during an epidemic setting prior to more definitive reverse transcriptase polymerase chain reaction (RT-PCR) testing (72). A first step in prediction was a history of potential contact with a SARS patient and an illness accompanied by fever, myalgias, and malaise. The second step supporting SARS was the finding of an abnormal chest radiograph (diffuse haziness or consolidation), lymphopenia, and thrombocytopenia with an inverse likelihood with age >65 years or <18 years, sputum production, abdominal pain, sore throat, rhinorrhea, or leukocytosis. This rule was applied in one epidemic setting and requires further validation in other clinical settings; however, SARS should be considered in appropriate settings with application of rapid diagnostic tests, infection control practices, and therapeutic considerations (72–74).

Coma and Meningoencephalitis

Infections may result in CNS dysfunction either indirectly as a systemic infection as in typhoid fever or directly through CNS invasion. A returning traveler presenting with one or more of the following signs/symptoms with or without fever must be evaluated for CNS infection: meningismus, altered mental status (delirium, lethargy, obtundation, or coma), seizures, severe headache, photophobia, or focal neurologic findings (75). Common tropical infections such as malaria (cerebral malaria), typhoid, and TB should remain high on the differential diagnosis. The diagnostic approach including CNS imaging studies [computed tomography (CT) or magnetic resonance imaging scans (MRI)] with cerebrospinal fluid (CSF) analysis will be similar to the approach used in nontravelers. The incubation period is particularly important when trying to decide if certain etiologic agents need to be considered. Travelers presenting within two to three weeks post-travel from developing regions may have acquired regional arboviruses causing meningoencephalitis or meningococcal disease whereas incubation periods exceeding two to three weeks require inclusion of TB, African trypanosomiasis, and rabies.

Endemic or sporadic meningococcal disease varies between one to three and 10 to 25 cases per 100,000 persons in developed and developing regions, respectively (76).

In addition to this increased endemic risk for travelers, there is also the potential of epidemic meningococcal disease (primarily serogroup A) with attack rates as high as 1000/100,000 as seen in the meningococcal belt of sub-Saharan Africa (76). Rapid diagnosis using CSF analysis (neutrophilic pleocytosis, elevated protein, low glucose, and gram-negative diplococci) with prompt institution of antibiotic therapy is critical because treated meningococcal meningitis carries mortality rates in the range of 5% to 15% (77).

Herpes simplex–1 encephalitis is the most common cause of sporadic viral encephalitis seen by clinicians in the United States; however, endemic arboviruses such as California group bunyaviral encephalitis are also not uncommon (78). Additionally, international travel into developing regions with potential mosquito exposure further broadens the differential diagnosis. Knowledge of the regional arboviral threats, such as Japanese encephalitis in rural areas of eastern Asia and the Indian subcontinent and Rift Valley Fever in Egypt and central/southern Africa, will allow appropriate inclusion/exclusion of arboviral threats (79–81). Flavivirus encephalitis occurs in both developed and developing countries with regional threats such as Japanese Encephalitis in South and Southeast Asia, Murray Valley Encephalitis in Australia and New Guinea, West Nile Encephalitis across many areas including Africa, Southwest Asia, Europe, and North America, and St. Louis Encephalitis throughout the Americas (82). These viral encephalitides have much higher rates of asymptomatic infection as compared to CNS illness and may present with a meningitis syndrome rather than encephalitis. Human rabies is often transmitted in developing urban areas through contact with rabid dogs and cats unlike the wild animal reservoir in the United States (83). Patients presenting with a compatible clinical syndrome for rabies (respiratory and/or gastrointestinal prodromal symptoms followed by acute neurologic symptoms, furious or paralytic, leading to coma) should have a thorough travel history focusing on any animal contact. Diagnostic testing, virus-specific fluorescent material in skin biopsy, serum or CSF antirabies antibodies, and/or virus isolation in saliva, should be used in appropriate settings with prompt initiation of isolation precautions and postexposure immunoprophylaxis (83). Emergent threats such as the Nipah virus in Malaysia in 1998 to 1999 further add to the differential diagnosis for returning travelers with encephalitis (84). An open-label trial reported a 36% reduction in mortality for acute Nipah virus encephalitis when treated with intravenous ribavirin (85). Eosinophilic meningoencephalitis (CSF leukocytosis with ≥10% eosinophils) is a clinical syndrome with relatively limited etiologies including parasites (*Angiostrongylus cantonensis*, *Gnathostoma spinigerum*, migrating ascarids, and schistosomiasis), coccidiomycosis, and hypersensitivity reaction (drug related) (86). The travel and exposure history will greatly assist in the inclusion/exclusion of parasitic etiologies.

Acute Abdomen

Returning travelers presenting with an acute abdomen are most likely to have common conditions seen in nontravelers such as appendicitis, cholecystitis, diverticulitis, or peptic ulcer with perforated viscus (87). Two common diseases in indigenous populations, enteric fever and amebic liver abscess, occur occasionally in immigrants and less commonly in native travelers (87–89). Both of these diseases may present with an acute abdomen secondary to severe abdominal pain from uncomplicated disease or as a result of complicated disease such as cyst rupture in amebiasis or bowel perforation in enteric fever. Risk factors for intestinal perforation in typhoid fever were a short duration of symptoms (within two weeks of illness onset), inadequate antibiotic therapy, male gender, and leukopenia in a case–control study in Turkey (90). Enteric fever is most commonly due to *Salmonella typhi* but also can be caused by *S. paratyphi* or *Brucella* species (91,92). In the United States, the total number of typhoid fever cases has decreased. A larger proportion (69%) has been imported during foreign travel especially from Mexico and India (93). Typhoid fever may also present with other clinical syndromes requiring ICU admission including ARDS, lower gastrointestinal bleeding, splenic rupture, and coma (90,92,94,95). Confirmatory diagnosis of typhoid fever requires blood culture isolation, which is positive in approximately 80% of cases or approximately 90% with bone marrow culture (92,96). Stool and urine cultures are occasionally positive, 37% and 7%, respectively, but do not constitute definitive evidence of systemic infection. Widespread multidrug-resistant *S. typhi* (resistant to ampicillin, chloramphenicol, and trimethoprim-sulfamethoxazole (TMP-SMX) has been documented in many areas of Asia, Africa, and the Middle East requiring the use of fluoroquinolones as first line therapy, or alternatives such as 3rd-generation cephalosporins or azithromycin (89,92,97,98). Adjunctive therapy with high-dose corticosteroids has been shown to decrease mortality in severely ill typhoid fever patients with delirium, obtundation, coma, or shock (99). The majority (95%) of amebic liver abscesses will present within the first two to five years after leaving the endemic region (88,100,101). Diarrhea is present in less than half with amebic trophozoites or cysts in <30%. The differential diagnosis must also include bacterial liver abscess, echinococcal cyst, and hepatoma. Ultrasound and CT imaging will assist in defining the hepatic lesions, and highly sensitive and specific serology will often confirm extraintestinal amebiasis (often negative in the first seven days) (88). Therapy with parenteral metronidazole results in mortality rates of <1% in uncomplicated liver abscesses (88). However, complicated amebic liver abscesses with extension into the thoracic cavity, peritoneum, or pericardium have case fatality rates of 6.2%, 18.4%, and 29.6%, respectively (100).

Dysentery and Severe Gastrointestinal Fluid Losses

Dysentery is characterized by a toxic appearance, fever, lower abdominal pain, tenesmus, and frequent small volume loose stools containing blood and/or mucus with large numbers of fecal leukocytes on microscopic exam. Etiologies of dysentery can be divided into amebic (*Entamoeba histolytica*) versus bacillary [*Shigella* spp. especially *S. dysenteriae* and *S. flexneri*, *Campylobacter jejuni*, nontyphoidal *Salmonella* spp., *Yersinia enterocolitica*, enteroinvasive *Escherichia coli*, and enterohemorrhagic *E. coli* (EHEC)] (102). Shigellosis is the most common etiology and is associated with fatality rates as high as 9% in indigenous populations in endemic regions and 20% during *S. dysenteriae* epidemics (103). Complications can include bacteremia, intestinal perforation, dehydration, toxic megacolon, ileus, rectal prolapse, hemolytic uremic syndrome (also well documented with EHEC strains such as O157:H7), and altered consciousness and seizures. Predictive factors associated with increased risk of death in shigellosis (age <1 year, diminished serum total protein, thrombocytopenia, and altered consciousness) reflect the importance of sepsis in shigellosis-related deaths (104). Diarrhea-related mortality in noninflammatory diarrhea has been significantly reduced globally with the institution of oral rehydration therapy. Dysenteric-related deaths have not been significantly reduced and require antimicrobial therapy and supportive intensive care in addition to appropriate rehydration (102,103,105,106). The majority of noninflammatory diarrhea cases in returning travelers present as mild or moderate illness due to bacterial agents such as Enterotoxigenic *E. coli*, *C. jejuni*, and, less commonly, protozoal agents such as *Giardia lamblia*. Noninflammatory diarrhea due to cholera may present in a returning traveler with life-threatening dehydrating illness with profound fluid and electrolyte deficits (107). Imported *Vibrio cholerae* is rare in the United States; however, an appreciation of regional risks of epidemic strains (El Tor in South/Central America and Africa, non-O1 *V. cholerae* O139 in Southeast Asia and the Indian subcontinent) is important (107).

Fulminant Hepatitis

Fulminant hepatitis manifests as severe acute liver failure with jaundice and hepatic encephalopathy (108). Viral hepatitis accounts for the majority ($\sim$75%) of fulminant hepatitis and may be either early onset (within first eight weeks) or late onset (8–12 weeks) after jaundice develops (108–111). Hepatitis B accounts for 30% to 60% with coinfection with delta virus in 30% to 40% that has been demonstrated to increase disease severity (112). Hepatitis A only accounts for <0.1% of causes of fulminant hepatitis, although overall hepatitis A represents the most commonly acquired agent of viral hepatitis (50–60% in most series) (109). Hepatitis C association with fulminant non-A, non-B hepatitis has been reported in Japan but is very uncommon in Western countries (113,114). Hepatitis E, a virus transmitted via an enteric route, has an increased fatality rate in pregnant women (115). Early indicators of a poor prognosis and the potential need for liver transplantation in viral hepatitis include age <11 or >40 years, duration of jaundice before onset of encephalopathy >7 days, serum bilirubin >300 µmol/L, and prothrombin time >50 seconds (116). Early diagnosis of acute hepatitis is important given evidence of specific benefit from antiviral therapies including lamivudine in acute hepatitis B and interferon therapy for hepatitis C (117–121). Other less common causes of fulminant hepatitis include Yellow fever virus and leptospirosis. Yellow fever virus endemic zones are updated on a regular basis and available (as are cholera and plague endemic zones) through the weekly centers for disease control and prevention (CDC) publication (the Blue Sheet). A resurgence in yellow fever in Africa and South America emphasizes the continued threat from this agent for unvaccinated travelers (122). Severe Yellow fever is fatal in greater than 50% of cases and continues to be a cause of deaths in returning travelers (123–126). Leptospirosis has widespread distribution and is usually transmitted to humans through contact with surface water contaminated with urine from infected animals (127). Travelers returning with leptospirosis typically present with a mild or moderate illness. The spectrum of disease includes fulminant hepatitis, meningoencephalitis, hemorrhagic manifestations, pulmonary manifestations including ARDS, and renal failure (127–132). Leptospirosis should be considered in most severely ill returning travelers. A recent randomized controlled trial demonstrated equal efficacy of seven-day intravenous therapy with ceftriaxone (1 g daily) and penicillin G (1.5 million U every six hours) in severe leptospirosis (133). However, case fatality was 5.8% with 10% requiring dialysis and 22% experiencing respiratory failure.

Fever with Eosinophilia

Eosinophilia in the returning traveler is not uncommon and requires an initial assessment of the absolute eosinophil count (eosinophilia >450/mm^3), consideration if travel related (i.e., check pretravel differential white blood cell counts) and the most likely parasite based on travel destination, duration of stay, and exposure history (134). Critically important is a determination of whether the eosinophilia is related to the patient's current symptoms because most causes of eosinophilia in travelers result in either asymptomatic or mild disease, although the predictive value of peripheral eosinophilia has limitations (135). A tenet of tropical infectious diseases is that patients may present with multiple infections; an acutely ill traveler with moderate eosinophilia may have malaria as the cause of the symptoms and asymptomatic hookworm infection as the etiology of the eosinophilia. Infectious etiologies of fever and eosinophilia that may present with potentially life-threatening illnesses include acute schistosomiasis (acute serum sickness-like disease termed Katayama fever or acute neurologic sequelae of myelitis or encephalitis), visceral larva migrans, tropical pulmonary eosinophilia, acute fascioliasis, and acute trichinosis (134). Schistosomiasis is the most common of these infections with reported high infection rates (mean 77%) in groups of travelers exposed to fresh water in endemic regions occasionally resulting in severe acute infection approximately four to eight weeks postexposure (136–138). Definitive diagnosis of schistosomiasis requires identification of the ova in stool, urine, or tissue specimens. The acute hypersensitivity syndromes of schistosomiasis occurring prior to ova deposition or ectopic distribution of the schistosome ova (such as in the CNS) necessitate the use of sensitive serologic methods for diagnosis (139). Specific therapy with praziquantel is highly efficacious in the low worm density infections seen in travelers (139). The acute hypersensitivity syndromes often require adjunctive corticosteroid therapy.

Toxic Appearance and Fever

Patients with a toxic appearance with fever often present difficult diagnostic dilemmas. As has already been discussed, malaria must be ruled out. Other potential diagnoses already discussed such as typhoid fever, early shigellosis, leptospirosis, and anicteric hepatitis remain in the differential diagnosis. This group of conditions can be further subdivided into the presence or absence of a rash. The presence of a hemorrhagic rash is somewhat helpful in narrowing the differential to arboviral, rickettsial, and meningococcal etiologies, but even this is not completely reliable. Maculopapular rashes can be either the common exanthem of that illness (i.e., measles) or an earlier stage in an evolving exanthem (i.e., rickettsial or meningococcal disease). Rickettsial diseases are usually in the differential for critically ill patients with fever and rash. There has been increasing recognition of rickettsial infections as etiologies of serious travel-associated infections (140,141). The majority of imported rickettsial disease in travelers is due to *Rickettsia africae*, the spotted fever group agent of African tick bite fever, and less commonly, *R. conorii*, the spotted fever group agent of boutonneuse fever, both which typically present as mild and self-limited illnesses (140,142–145). Scrub typhus has reported case fatality rates in indigenous populations of 15% and rarely has caused life-threatening disease in returning travelers (146). These reports highlight the importance of including rickettsial agents in the differential diagnosis and consideration of empiric therapy with doxycycline. Rapid responses to doxycycline therapy within 24 hours support the diagnosis, and the lack of response should prompt alternative diagnoses. Sexually transmitted diseases such as secondary syphilis, disseminated gonococcal infection, or acute retroviral syndrome may rarely present in this manner and need consideration. Measles has significant morbidity with the most common complication, pneumonitis, resulting in mortality rates of 2% to 15% in children and <1% in adults

(147,148). A study of hospitalized adults with complications of typical measles revealed pneumonitis rates of approximately 50% with respiratory failure and mechanical ventilation in 18% (149).

Dengue fever is, by far, the most common arboviral etiology of nonspecific febrile illness in returning travelers (122,150,151). Global estimates of 150 million cases of classic dengue fever and 250,000 cases of dengue hemorrhagic fever/dengue shock syndrome (DHF/DSS), continued regional spread in the Western hemisphere, and the urban peridomestic transmission from infected *Aedes aegypti* (also *A. albopictus*) mosquito vectors make dengue fever a prominent consideration in returning travelers with fever (152). As with other arboviral etiologic agents of viral hemorrhagic fever (VHF), illness onset with an elapsed time exceeding three weeks (two weeks with dengue) from the potential exposure effectively rules out these agents (153). Dengue fever may be caused by any one of the four serotypes with the relative risk of severe disease (DHF/DSS) 100-fold higher during the second dengue infection then with the first (152). Dengue fever rarely presents with life-threatening infection in U.S. travelers probably due to the lack of prior dengue infections. In West Africa, Lassa fever is endemic, causing 100,000 to 300,000 human infections and approximately 5000 deaths each year (154). Other than in regions where it is endemic, Lassa fever is encountered rarely. To date, approximately 20 cases of imported Lassa fever have been reported worldwide with one death in the United States in 2004 after travel to West Africa (154). Etiologies of VHF that have been known to cause person-to-person transmission (Lassa virus, Ebola virus, Marburg virus, and Crimean-Congo hemorrhagic fever virus) are particularly important because specific recommendations are available for patient management and proper containment of these potentially deadly viruses (153,155,156). VHF is characterized by fever, nonspecific symptoms (i.e., pharyngitis, myalgias, respiratory symptoms, headache, and malaise), and in severe cases, shock and hemorrhagic manifestations (153,155–158). These viruses have distinct geographic distributions, variable case fatality rates, and potential therapeutic options as detailed in Table 3. Nosocomial transmission has been documented for each of these agents and is primarily transmitted through direct contact or aerosolization of blood or body fluids

Table 3 Viral Hemorrhagic Fever Etiologies Associated with Nosocomial Spread

Virus	Geographic region	Case fatality rate (%)	Therapeutic options
Lassa	West Africa	1–2	Ribavirin (efficacy in clinical trial)[a]
Ebola	Zaire, Sudan	65–88	Supportive care
Marburg	East and Central Africa	23	Supportive care
CCHF	Eastern Europe, Eastern Mediterranean, Asia, and Africa	15–70	Ribavirin (in vitro evidence/no controlled trial)

[a]Ribavirin dosing regimen—30 mg/kg loading dose IV (max 2 g) then 16 mg/kg (max 1 g/dose) q6h × 4 day, then 8 mg/kg (max 500 mg) q8h × 6 day; ribavirin prophylaxis in close contacts—(unproven regimen) 5 mg/kg TID × 2–3 wks.
Abbreviation: CCHF, Congo Crimean hemorrhagic fever.

Table 4 General Considerations in the Management of Suspected Viral Hemorrhagic Fever

Steps	Action
1	Rapid assessment to determine if VHF suspect (fever within 3 wk of exposure plus travel to endemic region or direct contact with potentially infected blood or body fluids)
2	Isolate immediately (main focus is avoidance of blood/body fluid exposure—refer to CDC guidelines for specific details)
3	Rule out more common illness such as malaria and typhoid fever (refer to guidelines for proper specimen handling)
4	Contact local/state health dept. and the CDC [tel: (404) 639-1510 during normal working hours; after hours (404) 639-2888]
5	If clinical syndrome/exposure history supportive of Lassa fever or CCHF, consider ribavirin therapy (also consider prophylaxis for high risk contacts)

Note: All suspected cases of VHF should be reported immediately to local and state health departments and to CDC [Special Pathogens Branch, (404) 639–2888]. Consult the Special Pathogens Branch before obtaining or sending specimens to CDC for confirmatory testing. State health departments should also be notified before sending specimens to CDC. For links to state health departments visit the "Information Networks and Other Information Sources."
Abbreviation: VHF, viral hemorrhagic fever.
Source: From Ref. 160.

from often terminally ill infected patients (153,159). Table 4 summarizes the general concepts from the CDC in properly managing a suspected VHF patient. Recent interim CDC guidance provides updates on VHF transmission and infection control precautions with specific focus on patient care practices, environmental procedures, reporting, specimen handling, human remains handling, and postexposure management (http://www.cdc.gov/ncidod/hip/Blood/VHFinterimGuidance05_19_05.pdf). Consideration should also be given to postexposure prophylaxis based on the infectious agent such as ribavirin in imported Lassa fever cases (157). In the event this situation were to arise, the medical personnel must obtain the CDC references in the Morbidity and Mortality Weekly Report in order to have all specific guidelines.

REFERENCES

1. Steffen R, Rickenbach M, Wilhelm U, Helminger A, Schar M. Health problems after travel to developing countries. J Infect Dis 1987; 156:84–91.
2. Hargarten SW, Baker TD, Guptill K. Overseas fatalities of United States citizen travelers: an analysis of deaths related to international travel. Ann Emerg Med 1991; 20:622–626.
3. Steffen R. Travel medicine—prevention based on epidemiological data. Trans R Soc Trop Med Hyg 1991; 85:156–162.
4. Taylor DN, Pollard RA, Blake PA. Typhoid in the United States and the risk to the international traveler. J Infect Dis 1983; 148:599–602.
5. Steffen R, Schar G, Mosimann J. Salmonella and Shigella infections in Switzerland, with special reference to typhoid vaccination for travellers. Scand J Infect Dis 1981; 13: 121–127.
6. Synder JD, Blake PA. Is cholera a problem for US travelers? JAMA 1982; 247: 2268–2269.
7. Morger H, Steffen R, Schar M. Epidemiology of cholera in travellers, and conclusions for vaccination recommendations. Br Med J (Clin Res Ed) 1983; 286(6360):184–186.

8. Saxe SE, Gardner P. The returning traveler with fever. Infect Dis Clin North Am 1992; 6:427–439.

9. Maguire JH. Epidemiologic considerations in the evaluation of undifferentiated fever in a traveler returning from Latin America or the Caribbean. Curr Clin Top Infect Dis 1993; 13:26–56.

10. Doherty JF, Grant AD, Bryceson AD. Fever as the presenting complaint of travellers returning from the tropics. Qjm 1995; 88:277–281.

11. Felton JM, Bryceson AD. Fever in the returning traveller. Br J Hosp Med 1996; 55:705–711.

12. Humar A, Keystone J. Evaluating fever in travellers returning from tropical countries. Bmj 1996; 312:953–956.

13. Schwartz MD. Fever in the returning traveler. Part II: A methodological approach to initial management. Wilderness Environ Med 2003; 14:120–130.

14. D'Acremont V, Ambersin AE, Burnand B, Genton B. Practice guidelines for evaluation of fever in returning travelers and migrants. J Travel Med 2003; 10(suppl 2):S25–S52.

15. Schwartz MD. Fever in the returning traveler, part one: A methodological approach to initial evaluation. Wilderness Environ Med 2003; 14:24–32.

16. Antinori S, Galimberti L, Gianelli E. Prospective observational study of fever in hospitalized returning travelers and migrants from tropical areas, 1997–2001. J Travel Med 2004; 11:135–142.

17. Blair JE. Evaluation of fever in the international traveler. Unwanted "souvenir" can have many causes. Postgrad Med 2004; 116:13–20, 29.

18. O'Brien D, Tobin S, Brown GV, Torresi J. Fever in returned travelers: review of hospital admissions for a 3-year period. Clin Infect Dis 2001; 33:603–609.

19. Warrell DA. Management of severe malaria. Parassitologia 1999; 41:287–294.

20. Leder K, Black J, O'Brien D. Malaria in travelers: a review of the GeoSentinel surveillance network. Clin Infect Dis 2004; 39:1104–1112.

21. Greenberg AE, Lobel HO. Mortality from *Plasmodium falciparum* malaria in travelers from the United States, 1959 to 1987. Ann Intern Med 1990; 113:326–327.

22. Newman RD, Parise ME, Barber AM, Steketee RW. Malaria-related deaths among U.S. travelers, 1963–2001. Ann Intern Med 2004; 141:547–555.

23. Centers for Disease Control and Prevention, *Health Information for International Travel* 2005–2006. Atlanta: U.S. Department of Health and Human Services, Public Health Service, 2005.

24. Baird JK. Chloroquine resistance in *Plasmodium vivax*. Antimicrob Agents Chemother 2004; 48:4075–4083.

25. Baird JK. Effectiveness of antimalarial drugs. N Engl J Med 2005; 352:1565–1577.

26. Breman JG, Alilio MS, Mills A. Conquering the intolerable burden of malaria: what's new, what's needed: a summary. Am J Trop Med Hyg 2004; 71:1–15.

27. Farooq U, Mahajan RC. Drug resistance in malaria. J Vector Borne Dis 2004; 41: 45–53.

28. White NJ. Antimalarial drug resistance. J Clin Invest 2004; 113:1084–1092.

29. Svenson JE, Gyorkos TW, MacLean JD. Diagnosis of malaria in the febrile traveler. Am J Trop Med Hyg 1995; 53:518–521.

30. Svenson JE, Mac Lean JD, Gyorkos TN, Keystone J. Imported malaria. Clinical presentation and examination of symptomatic travelers. Arch Intern Med 1995; 155: 861–868.

31. Kean BH, Reilly PC Jr. Malaria - the mime. Recent lessons from a group of civilian travellers. Am J Med 1976; 61:159–164.

32. Moody A. Rapid diagnostic tests for malaria parasites. Clin Microbiol Rev 2002; 15: 66–78.

33. Field JW. Blood examination and prognosis in acute falciparum malaria. Trans R Soc Trop Med Hyg 1949; 43:33–48.

34. Severe falciparum malaria. World Health Organization, Communicable Diseases Cluster. Trans R Soc Trop Med Hyg 2000; 94(suppl 1):S1–S90.
35. D'Alessandro U. Treating severe and complicated malaria. BMJ 2004; 328:155.
36. Njuguna P, Newton C. Management of severe falciparum malaria. J Postgrad Med 2004; 50:45–50.
37. Awad MI, Alkadeu AM, Behrens RH, Baraka OZ, Eltayeb IB. Descriptive study on the efficacy and safety of artesunate suppository in combination with other antimalarials in the treatment of severe malaria in Sudan. Am J Trop Med Hyg 2003; 68(2):153–158.
38. Barnes KI, Mwenechanya J, Tembo M. Efficacy of rectal artesunate compared with parenteral quinine in initial treatment of moderately severe malaria in African children and adults: a randomised study. Lancet 2004; 363:1598–1605.
39. Newton PN, Angus BJ, Chierakul W. Randomized comparison of artesunate and quinine in the treatment of severe falciparum malaria. Clin Infect Dis 2003; 37:7–16.
40. Aceng JR, Byarugaba JS, Tumwine JK. Rectal artemether versus intravenous quinine for the treatment of cerebral malaria in children in Uganda: randomised clinical trial. BMJ 2005; 330:334.
41. Miller KD, Greenberg AE, Campbell CC. Treatment of severe malaria in the United States with a continuous infusion of quinidine gluconate and exchange transfusion. N Engl J Med 1989; 321:65–70.
42. Phillips RE, Warrel DA, White NJ, Looareesuwan S, Karbwang J. Intravenous quinidine for the treatment of severe falciparum malaria. Clinical and pharmacokinetic studies. N Engl J Med 1985; 312:1273–1278.
43. Phillips P, Nantel S, Benny WB. Exchange transfusion as an adjunct to the treatment of severe falciparum malaria: case report and review. Rev Infect Dis 1990; 12:1100–1108.
44. Riddle MS, Jackson JL, Sanders JW, Blozes DL. Exchange transfusion as an adjunct therapy in severe Plasmodium falciparum malaria: a meta-analysis. Clin Infect Dis 2002; 34:1192–1198.
45. Warrell DA, Looareesuwan S, Warrell MJ. Dexamethasone proves deleterious in cerebral malaria. A double-blind trial in 100 comatose patients. N Engl J Med 1982; 306:313–319.
46. Phu NH, Hien TT, Mai NT. Hemofiltration and peritoneal dialysis in infection-associated acute renal failure in Vietnam. N Engl J Med 2002; 347:895–902.
47. Bruneel F, Hocqueloux L, Alberti C. The clinical spectrum of severe imported falciparum malaria in the intensive care unit: report of 188 cases in adults. Am J Respir Crit Care Med 2003; 167:684–689.
48. Cohen J, Brun-Buisson C, Torres A, Jorgensen J. Diagnosis of infection in sepsis: an evidence-based review. Crit Care Med 2004; 32:S466–S494.
49. Mandell LA. Epidemiology and etiology of community-acquired pneumonia. Infect Dis Clin North Am 2004; 18:761–776, vii.
50. Kim JH, Langston AA, Gallis HA. Miliary tuberculosis: epidemiology, clinical manifestations, diagnosis, and outcome. Rev Infect Dis 1990; 12:583–590.
51. Maartens G, Willcox PA, Benatar SR. Miliary tuberculosis: rapid diagnosis, hematologic abnormalities, and outcome in 109 treated adults. Am J Med 1990; 89:291–296.
52. Jindal SK, Aggarwal AN, Gupta D. Adult respiratory distress syndrome in the tropics. Clin Chest Med 2002; 23:445–455.
53. Treatment of tuberculosis. MMWR Recomm Rep 2003; 52:1–77.
54. Guidelines for preventing the transmission of Mycobacterium tuberculosis in health-care facilities, 1994. Centers for Disease Control and Prevention. MMWR Recomm Rep 1994; 43:1–132.
55. File TM Jr., Garan J, Blasi F. Guidelines for empiric antimicrobial prescribing in community-acquired pneumonia. Chest 2004; 125:1888–1901.
56. Jernigan DB, Hofmann J, Cetron MS. Outbreak of Legionnaires' disease among cruise ship passengers exposed to a contaminated whirlpool spa. Lancet 1996; 347:494–499.

57. Ruf B, Schurmann D, Horbach I, Fehrenbach FJ, Pohle HD. Prevalence and diagnosis of Legionella pneumonia: a 3-year prospective study with emphasis on application of urinary antigen detection. J Infect Dis 1990; 162:1341–1348.
58. Moser MR, Bender TR, Margolis HS, Noble GR, Kendel A, Ritter DG. An outbreak of influenza aboard a commercial airliner. Am J Epidemiol 1979; 110:1–6.
59. Haemorrhagic fever with renal syndrome: memorandum from a WHO meeting. Bull World Health Organ 1983; 61:269–275.
60. Moolenaar RL, Dalton C, Lipman HB. Clinical features that differentiate hantavirus pulmonary syndrome from three other acute respiratory illnesses. Clin Infect Dis 1995; 21:643–649.
61. Chapman LE, Ellis BA, Koster FT. Discriminators between hantavirus-infected and -uninfected persons enrolled in a trial of intravenous ribavirin for presumptive hantavirus pulmonary syndrome. Clin Infect Dis 2002; 34:293–304.
62. Huggins JW, Hsiang CM, Cosgrift TM. Prospective, double-blind, concurrent, placebo-controlled clinical trial of intravenous ribavirin therapy of hemorrhagic fever with renal syndrome. J Infect Dis 1991; 164:1119–1127.
63. Mertz GJ, Miedzinski L, Goade D. Placebo-controlled, double-blind trial of intravenous ribavirin for the treatment of hantavirus cardiopulmonary syndrome in North America. Clin Infect Dis 2004; 39:1307–1313.
64. White NJ. Melioidosis. Lancet 2003; 361:1715–1722.
65. Sookpranee M, Boonma P, Susaengrat W, Bhuripanyo K, Punyagupta S. Multicenter prospective randomized trial comparing ceftazidime plus co-trimoxazole with chloramphenicol plus doxycycline and co-trimoxazole for treatment of severe melioidosis. Antimicrob Agents Chemother 1992; 36:158–162.
66. Dennis DT, Chow CC. Plague. Pediatr Infect Dis J 2004; 23:69–71.
67. Krishna G, Chitkara RK. Pneumonic plague. Semin Respir Infect 2003; 18:159–167.
68. Morgan J, Cano MV, Feikin DR. A large outbreak of histoplasmosis among American travelers associated with a hotel in Acapulco, Mexico, spring 2001. Am J Trop Med Hyg 2003; 69:663–669.
69. Panackal AA, Hajjeh RA, Cetron MS, Warnock DW. Fungal infections among returning travelers. Clin Infect Dis 2002; 35:1088–1095.
70. Lee N, Hui D, Wu A. A major outbreak of severe acute respiratory syndrome in Hong Kong. N Engl J Med 2003; 348:1986–1994.
71. Tsang KW, Ho PL, Ooi GC. A cluster of cases of severe acute respiratory syndrome in Hong Kong. N Engl J Med 2003; 348:1977–1985.
72. Leung GM, Rainer TH, Lau FL. A clinical prediction rule for diagnosing severe acute respiratory syndrome in the emergency department. Ann Intern Med 2004; 141:333–342.
73. Poon LL, Wong OK, Chan KH, Chu CM, Yuen KY. Rapid diagnosis of a coronavirus associated with severe acute respiratory syndrome (SARS). Clin Chem 2003; 49:953–955.
74. Cheng VC, Tang BS, Wu AK. Medical treatment of viral pneumonia including SARS in immunocompetent adult. J Infect 2004; 49:262–273.
75. Day JN, Lalloo DG. Neurological syndromes and the traveller: an approach to differential diagnosis. J Neurol Neurosurg Psychiatr 2004; 75(suppl 1):i2–9.
76. Riedo FX, Plikaytis BD, Broome CV. Epidemiology and prevention of meningococcal disease. Pediatr Infect Dis J 1995; 14:643–657.
77. van de Beek D, de Gans J, Spanjaard L, Weisfelt M, Reitsma JB, Vermeulen M. Clinical features and prognostic factors in adults with bacterial meningitis. N Engl J Med 2004; 351:1849–1859.
78. Toltzis P. Viral encephalitis. Adv Pediatr Infect Dis 1991; 6:111–136.
79. Rift Valley fever—Egypt, 1993. MMWR 1994; 43:693, 699–700.
80. Macdonald WB, Tink AR, Ouvrier RA. Japanese encephalitis after a two-week holiday in Bali. Med J Aust 1989; 150:334–336, 339.
81. Thisyakorn U, Thisyakorn C, Wilde H. Japanese encephalitis and international travel. J Travel Med 1995; 2:37–40.

82. Solomon T. Flavivirus encephalitis. N Engl J Med 2004; 351:370–388.

83. Hankins DG, Rosekrans JA. Overview, prevention, and treatment of rabies. Mayo Clin Proc 2004; 79:671–676.

84. Goh KJ, Tan CT, Chew NK. Clinical features of Nipah virus encephalitis among pig farmers in Malaysia. N Engl J Med 2000; 342:1229–1235.

85. Chong HT, Kamarulzaman A, Tan CT. Treatment of acute Nipah encephalitis with riba- virin. Ann Neurol 2001; 49:810–813.

86. Lim JM, Lee CC, Wilder-Smith A. Eosinophilic meningitis caused by *Angiostrongylus cantonensis*: a case report and literature review. J Travel Med 2004; 11:388–390.

87. Silen W. The acute abdomen in the tropics. In: Silen W, ed. Cope's Early Diagnosis of the Acute Abdomen. 18 ed. New York: Oxford University Press, 1991:268–277.

88. Ravdin JI. Amebiasis. Clin Infect Dis 1995; 20:1453–1464; quiz 1465–1466.

89. Crump JA, Luby SP, Mintz ED. The global burden of typhoid fever. Bull World Health Organ 2004; 82:346–353.

90. Hosoglu S, Aldemir M, Akalin S, Geyik MF, Tacyildiz IH, Loeb M. Risk factors for enteric perforation in patients with typhoid fever. Am J Epidemiol 2004; 160:46–50.

91. Young EJ. An overview of human brucellosis. Clin Infect Dis 1995; 21:283–289; quiz 290.

92. Parry CM, Hien TT, Dougan G, White NJ, Farrar JJ. Typhoid fever. N Engl J Med 2002; 347:1770–1782.

93. Ryan CA, Hargrett-Bean NT, Blake PA. Salmonella typhi infections in the United States, 1975–1984: increasing role of foreign travel. Rev Infect Dis 1989; 11:1–8.

94. Buczko GB, McLean J. Typhoid fever associated with adult respiratory distress syn- drome. Chest 1994; 105:1873–1874.

95. Gilman RH. General considerations in the management of typhoid fever and dysentery. Scand J Gastroenterol Suppl 1989; 169:11–18.

96. Gilman RH, Terminel M, Levine MM, Hernandez-Mendoza P, Hornick RB. Relative efficacy of blood, urine, rectal swab, bone-marrow, and rose-spot cultures for recovery of Salmonella typhi in typhoid fever. Lancet 1975; 1:1211–1213.

97. Gupta A. Multidrug-resistant typhoid fever in children: epidemiology and therapeutic approach. Pediatr Infect Dis J 1994; 13:134–140.

98. Steinberg EB, Bishop R, Haber P. Typhoid fever in travelers: who should be targeted for prevention? Clin Infect Dis 2004; 39:186–191.

99. Hoffman SL, Punjabi NH, Kumala S. Reduction of mortality in chloramphenicol-trea- ted severe typhoid fever by high-dose dexamethasone. N Engl J Med 1984; 310: 82–88.

100. Adams EB, MacLeod IN. Invasive amebiasis. II. Amebic liver abscess and its complica- tions. Medicine (Baltimore) 1977; 56:325–334.

101. Adams EB, MacLeod IN. Invasive amebiasis. I. Amebic dysentery and its complications. Medicine (Baltimore) 1977; 56:315–323.

102. Thielman NM, Guerrant RL. Clinical practice. Acute infectious diarrhea. N Engl J Med 2004; 350:38–47.

103. Kotloff KL, Winickoff JP, Ivanoff B. Global burden of Shigella infections: implications for vaccine development and implementation of control strategies. Bull World Health Organ 1999; 77:651–666.

104. Bennish ML, Harris JR, Wojtyniak BJ, Struelens M. Death in shigellosis: incidence and risk factors in hospitalized patients. J Infect Dis 1990; 161:500–506.

105. Guerrant RL, Van Gilder T, Steiner TS. Practice guidelines for the management of infec- tious diarrhea. Clin Infect Dis 2001; 32:331–351.

106. DuPont HL. Guidelines on acute infectious diarrhea in adults. The Practice Parameters Committee of the American College of Gastroenterology. Am J Gastroenterol 1997; 92:1962–1975.

107. Kaper JB, Morris JG Jr., Levine MM. Cholera. Clin Microbiol Rev 1995; 8:48–86.

108. Pappas SC. Fulminant viral hepatitis. Gastroenterol Clin North Am 1995; 24: 161–173.

109. O'Grady J. Management of acute and fulminant hepatitis A. Vaccine 1992; 10(suppl 1): S21–S23.
110. Tibbs CJ, Williams R. Liver transplantation for acute and chronic viral hepatitis. J Viral Hepat 1995; 2:65–72.
111. Williams R, Riordan SM. Acute liver failure: established and putative hepatitis viruses and therapeutic implications. J Gastroenterol Hepatol 2000; 15:G17–G25.
112. Smedile A, Farci P, Verme G. Influence of delta infection on severity of hepatitis B. Lancet 1982; 2:945–947.
113. Wright TL, Hsu H, Donegan E. Hepatitis C virus not found in fulminant non-A, non-B hepatitis. Ann Intern Med 1991; 115:111–112.
114. Yanagi M, Kaneko S, Unoura M. Hepatitis C virus in fulminant hepatic failure. N Engl J Med 1991; 324:1895–1896.
115. Schwartz E, Jenks NP, Van Damme P, Galun E. Hepatitis E virus infection in travelers. Clin Infect Dis 1999; 29:1312–1314.
116. O'Grady JG, Alexander GJ, Hayllar KM, Williams R. Early indicators of prognosis in fulminant hepatic failure. Gastroenterology 1989; 97:439–445.
117. Nakhoul F, Gelman R, Green J, Khankin E, Baruch Y. Lamivudine therapy for severe acute hepatitis B virus infection after renal transplantation: case report and literature review. Transplant Proc 2001; 33:2948–2949.
118. Alberti A, Boccato S, Vario A, Benvegnu L. Therapy of acute hepatitis C. Hepatology 2002; 36:S195–S200.
119. Poynard T, Regimbeau C, Myers RP. Interferon for acute hepatitis C. Cochrane Database Syst Rev 2002; (1):CD000369.
120. Kondili LA, Osman H, Mutimer D. The use of lamivudine for patients with acute hepatitis B (a series of cases). J Viral Hepat 2004; 11:427–431.
121. Santantonio T. Treatment of acute hepatitis C. Curr Pharm Des 2004; 10:2077–2080.
122. Gubler DJ. The changing epidemiology of yellow fever and dengue, 1900 to 2003: full circle? Comp Immunol Microbiol Infect Dis 2004; 27:319–330.
123. Fatal yellow fever in a traveler returning from Venezuela, 1999. MMWR 2000; 49: 303–305.
124. Monath TP. Yellow fever: an update. Lancet Infect Dis 2001; 1:11–20.
125. Fatal yellow fever in a traveler returning from Amazons, Brazil, 2002. JAMA 2002; 287:2499–2500.
126. Tomori O. Yellow fever: the recurring plague. Crit Rev Clin Lab Sci 2004; 41:391–427.
127. Antony SJ. Leptospirosis—an emerging pathogen in travel medicine: a review of its clinical manifestations and management. J Travel Med 1996; 3:113–118.
128. van Crevel R, Speelman P, Gravekamp C, Terpstra WJ. Leptospirosis in travelers. Clin Infect Dis 1994; 19:132–134.
129. Farr RW. Leptospirosis. Clin Infect Dis 1995; 21:1–6.
130. Marotto PC, Nascimento CM, Eluf-Neto J. Acute lung injury in leptospirosis: clinical and laboratory features, outcome, and factors associated with mortality. Clin Infect Dis 1999; 29(6):1561–1563.
131. Yang CW, Wu MS, Pan MJ. Leptospirosis renal disease. Nephrol Dial Transplant 2001; 16 (suppl 5):73–77.
132. Vieira SR, Brauner JS. Leptospirosis as a cause of acute respiratory failure: clinical features and outcome in 35 critical care patients. Braz J Infect Dis 2002; 6:135–139.
133. Panaphut T, Domrongkitchaiporn S, Vibhagool A, Thinkamrop B, Susaengrat W. Ceftriaxone compared with sodium penicillin g for treatment of severe leptospirosis. Clin Infect Dis 2003; 36:1507–1513.
134. Weller PF. Eosinophilia in travelers. Med Clin North Am 1992; 76:1413–1432.
135. Schulte C, Krebs B, Jelinek T, Nothdurft HD, von Sonnenburg F, Loscher T. Diagnostic significance of blood eosinophilia in returning travelers. Clin Infect Dis 2002; 34: 407–411.

136. Visser LG, Polderman AM, Stuiver PC. Outbreak of schistosomiasis among travelers returning from Mali, West Africa. Clin Infect Dis 1995; 20:280–285.

137. Cooke GS, Lalvani A, Gleeson FV, Conlon CP. Acute pulmonary schistosomiasis in travelers returning from Lake Malawi, sub-Saharan Africa. Clin Infect Dis 1999; 29:836–839.

138. Acute schistosomiasis in U.S. travelers returning from Africa. MMWR 1990; 39: 141–142, 147–148.

139. Ross AG, Bartley PB, Sleigh AC. Schistosomiasis. N Engl J Med 2002; 346:1212–1220.

140. Jensenius M, Fournier PE, Raoult D. Rickettsioses and the international traveler. Clin Infect Dis 2004; 39:1493–1499.

141. Palau LA, Pankey GA. Mediterranean spotted fever in travelers from the United States. J Travel Med 1997; 4:179–182.

142. Font-Creus B, Bella-Cueto F, Espejo-Arenas E. Mediterranean spotted fever: a cooperative study of 227 cases. Rev Infect Dis 1985; 7:635–642.

143. African tick-bite fever among international travelers—Oregon, 1998. MMWR 1998; 47:950–952.

144. Jensenius M, Fournier PE, Vene S. African tick bite fever in travelers to rural sub-Equatorial Africa. Clin Infect Dis 2003; 36:1411–1417.

145. Jackson Y, Chappuis F, Loutan L. African tick-bite fever: four cases among Swiss travelers returning from South Africa. J Travel Med 2004; 11:225–228.

146. Watt G, Strickman D. Life-threatening scrub typhus in a traveler returning from Thailand. Clin Infect Dis 1994; 18:624–626.

147. Duke T, Mgone CS. Measles: not just another viral exanthem. Lancet 2003; 361: 763–773.

148. Perry RT, Halsey NA. The clinical significance of measles: a review. J Infect Dis 2004; 189(suppl 1):S4–S16.

149. Wong RD, Goetz MB. Clinical and laboratory features of measles in hospitalized adults. Am J Med 1993; 95:377–383.

150. Jelinek T. Dengue fever in international travelers. Clin Infect Dis 2000; 31:144–147.

151. Lindback H, Lindback J, Tegnell A, Janzon R, Vene S, Ekdahl K. Dengue fever in travelers to the tropics, 1998 and 1999. Emerg Infect Dis 2003; 9:438–442.

152. Wilson ME. Breakbone basics: dengue fever in the 1990s. Infect Dis Clin Pract 1996; 5:376–379.

153. Centers for Disease Control and Prevention. Update: management of patients with suspected viral hemorrhagic fever—United States. JAMA 1995; 274:374–375.

154. Imported Lassa fever—New Jersey, 2004. MMWR Morb Mortal Wkly Rep 2004; 53:894–897.

155. Management of patients with suspected viral hemorrhagic fever. MMWR 1988; 37(suppl 3): 1–16.

156. Isaacson M. Viral hemorrhagic fever hazards for travelers in Africa. Clin Infect Dis 2001; 33:1707–1712.

157. Haas WH, Breuer T, Pfaff G. Imported Lassa fever in Germany: surveillance and management of contact persons. Clin Infect Dis 2003; 36:1254–1258.

158. Smego RA Jr., Sarwari AR, Siddiqui AR. Crimean-Congo hemorrhagic fever: prevention and control limitations in a resource-poor country. Clin Infect Dis 2004; 38: 1731–1735.

159. Weber DJ, Rutala WA. Risks and prevention of nosocomial transmission of rare zoonotic diseases. Clin Infect Dis 2001; 32:446–456.

160. CDC. www.cdc.gov/doc.do/id/0900f3ec80226c7a.

20

HIV/AIDS in the Critical Care Unit

Larry I. Lutwick

Department of Infectious Diseases, VA New York Harbor Health Care System, and State University of New York Downstate Medical School, Brooklyn, New York, U.S.A.

INTRODUCTION

In a previous chapter written on this topic (1), the authors spent the great majority of the text discussing the variety of infectious diseases as causes for the HIV-infected individual to require intensive care. Written at the beginning of the highly active anti-retroviral therapy (HAART) combination drug era, it could not yet reflect the changes in HIV/AIDS care that would soon result. The commonly used anti-retroviral agents are listed in Table 1 (2). This therapy by "slowing and then stopping the virus train" (Table 2) resulted in suppression of viral replication and at least partial immune reconstitution in many individuals. The sum and substance of this therapy was to dramatically decrease the mortality of individuals with HIV/AIDS primarily by the prevention of the great host of opportunistic infections from profound defects in cellular immune function.

Recent reviews of the utilization of intensive care units (3,4) have not clearly shown a diminution in ICU admissions, but rather a switch from admissions related to opportunistic infections to illnesses either totally unrelated to HIV disease and/or ones linked to antiretroviral therapy.

Because of these dramatic changes, the issue of this chapter has rotated 180° from that time period where opportunistic infections such as pneumocystosis, cryptococcal meningitis, cerebral toxoplasmosis, and a variety of disseminated bacterial, viral, fungal, and protozoal infections took central stage. Instead, much of the potentially life-threatening issues related to the HIV now revolve around complications of this life-saving antiretroviral treatment, although not anywhere close to the same degree. Although a great majority of the treatment-limiting toxicities associated with the nucleoside analog reverse transcriptase inhibitors (NRTIs) is not in itself life threatening (5), serious potentially fatal drug reactions such as lactic acidosis, hepatic necrosis, neuromuscular weakness, and hypersensitivity reactions do occur. This chapter reflects these changes and concentrates on these intensive care–requiring adverse events. It is vital to understand that despite these uncommon adverse effects

Table 1 Commonly Used Antiretroviral Agents[a]

Drug	Also referred to as	Usual dosing
Nucleoside RTIs[b]		
Zidovudine	AZT, Retrovir	300 mg twice daily
Lamivudine	3TC, Epivir	150 mg twice daily
Stavudine	D4T, Zerit	40 mg twice daily
Didanosine	DDI, Videx	200 mg twice daily
Abacavir	Ziagen	300 mg twice daily
Tenofovir	Viread	300 mg once daily
Emtricitabine	FTC, Emtriva	200 mg once daily
Non-nucleoside RTIs		
Efavirenz	Sustiva	600 mg at bedtime
Nevirapine	Viramune	200 mg twice daily After
Protease Inhibitors[c]		once daily × 2 weeks
Amprenavir	Agenerase	1200 mg twice daily
Atazanavir	Reyataz	400 mg once daily
Ritonavir	Norvir	100 mg once or twice daily
Indinavir	Crixivan	800 mg three times daily
Lopinavir	Kaletra	Two tablets twice daily
Nelfinavir	Viracept	1250 mg twice daily
Tipranavir	Aptivus	500 mg twice daily

[a]Dose adjustment of some drugs, particularly the nucleoside analog reverse transcriptase inhibitors (NRTIS), are required in renal insufficiency situations.
[b]Several fixed combinations of NRTIs are available to decrease pill burden including Combivir (Zidovudine/ Lamivudine), Truvada (Tenofovir/ Emtricitabine), and Trizivir (Zidovudine/Lamivudine/Abacavir).
[c]Lengthening the half-life of many of the protease inhibitors can be accomplished by the use of ritonavir. Lopinavir comes as a fixed combination with ritonavir, the others require the second drug separately.
Abbreviations: RTIs, reverse transcriptase inhibitors. AZT, azidothynidine; 3TC, 2′-deoxy-3′-thiacytidine; D4T, 2′,3′-didehydro-3′-deoxy thynidine; DDI, 2′,3′-dideoxyinosine; FTC, 5′-fluoro-1-(DP.55)-2-(hydroxyethyl)-1,3-oxathiolan-5-cytosine

of therapy, antiretroviral treatment has metamorphosized a rapidly fatal disease into a chronic condition with long-term survivals.

HAART ATTACKS

Mitochondrial Toxicity

Mechanisms of Injury

Mitochondrial dysfunction caused by a nucleoside analog NRTI was first described in 1988 in individuals being treated with high-dose zidovudine (6). Initial investigations led to the postulate that NRTIs inhibited the activity of mitochondrial DNA

Table 2 The Allegory of the Train: HIV Therapy

HIV infection can be considered to be a train heading uphill towards a deep ravine
When it crashes into the ravine, intensive care with major morbidity and mortality results
The speed of the train is the HIV RNA level
The distance between the train and the ravine is the CD4 cell count
Antiretroviral therapy can stop the train (virological response)
When it stops, as it is heading uphill, the train starts to roll backwards (immunological response)

(mtDNA) polymerase–gamma, which produced a depletion in levels of mtDNA and subsequent drop in mitochondrial RNA and protein levels (7). Indeed the enzyme appears to be much more preferentially inhibited by NRTIs as compared to the other cellular DNA polymerase accounting for this more specific effect on cellular DNA synthesis. The evaluation of different NRTIs has revealed varying degrees of effect on DNA polymerase–gamma with zalcitabine, didanosine, and stavudine being the most potent and much more effective than lamuvidine, which is more inhibitory than tenofovir and zidovudine, and abacavir being the least inhibitory (8).

The mitochondrion, a cellular organelle, has the function of producing ATP, the major source of cellular energy. There are 100 to 1000 mitochondria per cell, and mtDNA is a 16.5 kilobase circular DNA encoding for 13 proteins involved in oxidative phosphorylation to produce ATP as well as ribosomal and transfer RNAs (9). As noted by Dagan et al. (10), the various manifestations of NRTI mitochondrial toxicity appear to be remarkably similar to a number of recognized mitochondrial diseases of genetic origin (Table 3).

The inhibition of DNA polymerase–gamma appears not the only effect on mitochondrial function. Other effects, as reviewed by Gerschenson and Brinkman (8), include increased oxidative stress, effects on the mitochondrial uncoupling protein, increased cytokine production, and promotion of programmed mitochondrial death (apoptosis). Notably, as well, is the effect that HIV itself has on mitochondrial apoptosis (11). The HIV-specific proteins that have been reported to be involved in mitochondrial apoptosis include the HIV gp120 envelope protein, the soluble HIV viral protein R (Vpr), the regulatory Tat protein, and HIV-transactivating region RNA.

Cell culture models have been developed to study NRTI-related mitochondrial dysfunction. As reviewed by Hoschele (12), the use of cell lines such as those of T-lymphoblastoid, neuronal, hepatic, and myocyte derivation may be quite useful in screening newer antiretroviral agents.

Lactic Acidosis

The spectrum of increased serum lactic acid is one of the most prominent adverse events related to antiretroviral therapy, having its basis in mitochondrial toxicity. In 1991, Lai et al. described a case of severe lactic acidosis associated with fatty liver and fulminant liver failure that occurred in an individual treated with didanosine (13). Subsequently, in association with a number of the NRTI drugs, elevated lactic acid

Table 3 Some Genetic Diseases of Mitochondrial Function

Disease	Alper's Syndrome
Genetic mutation	DNA polymerase–gamma deficiency
Symptoms	Liver failure, lactic acidosis, ataxia, hypotonia, myopathy
Disease	Leigh disease
Genetic mutation	Point mutations primarily in ATPase6 gene in mtDNA
Symptoms	Lactic acidosis, hypotonia, cardiomyopathy, early death
Disease	MELAS
Genetic mutation	Point mutations in mtDNA coding for transfer RNA
Symptoms	Myopathy, lactic acidosis, cardiomyopathy, diabetes

Abbreviation: MELAS, mitochondrial encephalopathy, lactic acidosis, stroke-like symptoms.
Source: From Ref. 10.

levels and hepatotoxicity have been described with additional features that might include lipoatrophy, pancreatitis, peripheral neuropathy, and myopathy (skeletal or cardiac) (14,15).

The hyperlactatemia syndrome is now recognized to occur in several forms from a subclinical frequent entity to symptomatic disease ranging from a mild-to-moderate form with a good prognosis to one with substantial mortality.

The subclinical form is less specifically linked to NRTI use. It is found, in one study, to occur in 8.7% of people taking antiretroviral therapy and 2% of therapy-naive HIV-infected individuals (16). The range in reviews is generally from 8% to 18% of treated individuals (14). This entity, which is associated with serum lactate levels between 2.1 and 5.0 mmol/L, normal arterial pH, normal liver function abnormalities, and no extrahepatic manifestations, is often transient and poorly predictive of more serious consequences. Only 5% of these asymptomatic patients were found to subsequently require treatment for either symptoms or a more elevated lactate level (>5 mmol/L) (16).

In some patients, mildly elevated lactic acid levels can be associated with symptoms including nausea, vomiting, abdominal pain, and fatigue. Antecedent weight loss may also be seen. Usually associated with NRTI use, especially stavudine or didanosine, this entity has lactate levels usually less than 5 mmol/L without acidosis Incidence rates of this disorder are 8 to 14 cases/1000 treated patient years (14). Most of these individuals respond promptly to discontinuance of the particular NRTI(s), substituting an NRTI with less potential towards mitochondrial injury such as lamivudine, tenofovir, or abacavir or using other non-NRTI drugs. John and Mallal (17) have reviewed whether this entity is distinct by itself, or whether it will progress to overt lactic acidosis if no interventions are done.

The overt lactic acidosis syndrome (LAS) is also strongly linked to NRTI therapy especially stavudine and/or didanosine and presents with the same constellation of symptoms with, in addition, hepatic aminotransferase elevations and in some cases liver failure. The incidence of this ICU care–requiring disorder is between 1 and 4 cases per 1000 patient treatment years.

In addition to the liver, involvement of other organs in LAS such as the lung, pancreas, and/or kidney is also common. Here the lactate levels are higher, as high as 70 mmol/L, median about 15 (15), and acidosis is present with low arterial pH and decreased serum bicarbonate. Female gender, pregnancy, and a higher body mass appear to be cofactors (18). In this disorder, it has been observed that there is a poor correlation between the degree of liver injury and the height of aminotransferase elevations (17). Importantly, promptly stopping the NRTI medication(s) here does not assure resolution. Case fatality rates of overt NRTI-associated lactic acidosis are over 50% with multiorgan (including the liver) and cardiovascular collapse intervening. A straight-line association has been reported between serum lactate levels and mortality rate (18).

In LAS, after the culprit NRTI has been discontinued, close monitoring of the acid–base status and cardiovascular status is needed. It is generally recommended (2) that intravenous fluids are administered to serve to assist in liver and kidney clearance of lactate and for cardiovascular support. In severe cases, hemodialysis or hemofiltration, or mechanical ventilation, may be necessary. Intravenous sodium bicarbonate infusions have been utilized as well, although LAS cases associated with encephalopathy or coma may trigger or compound a respiratory acidosis (14,17).

The administration of "specific" treatment for NRTI-associated lactic acidosis has been suggested and utilized in an effort to bolster cellular oxidative phosphorylation to produce more ATP. A variety of cellular cofactors in the biochemical energy pathways has been used as treatment modalities in LAS. These include riboflavin, thiamine, l-carnitine, and coenzyme Q, and the treatments have been associated with anecdotal success. No controlled trial, however, has established the efficacy of any of these treatments nor has the dosage schedule been well defined.

In survivors, after interruption of the lactic acidosis, it may take a number of weeks for the lactate levels to totally normalize (14). It is probably best to reinstitute a HAART regimen not containing potentially offending RTIs, although recurrences appear to be low when low-risk RTIs, such as tenofovir, lamivudine, or abacavir, are utilized. Caution should be used upon reinstitution of RTI therapy with frequent monitoring.

It remains unclear if serum lactate screening is a useful tool in preventing LAS as the positive predictive value is quite low (16).

HIV-Associated Ascending Neuromuscular Weakness

Related to the more classically recognized LAS associated with NRTI therapy is a rapidly progressive neuromuscular weakness syndrome. First reported in 1999 (19), the affected individuals manifest impressive, ascending muscle weakness, which can develop over a period of days to weeks. Presenting similarly to the Guillan–Barre syndrome, this antiretroviral therapy–related complication can progress to overt respiratory muscle paralysis and death.

As defined by the HIV Neuromuscular Syndrome Study Group (20), the criteria used in the diagnosis are fourfold:

1. The onset of new extremity weakness with a neuromuscular cause in a patient infected with HIV;
2. The disease may or may not involve sensory nerves;
3. The disease may be acute (less than two weeks) or subacute (greater than two weeks); and
4. The process involves both the lower and the upper extremities or just the lower extremities.

The classifications as possible, probable, and definite are shown in Table 4.

In Simpson et al.'s review of this entity (20), 69 individuals were identified with an approximately equal gender mix and classification as definite, probable, or possible in 27, 19, and 23 individuals, respectively. The similar number of men and women

Table 4 Classification of HIV-Associated Neuromuscular Weakness Syndrome

Possible:
Progessive weakness suggestive of muscle or nerve disease and
  other causes of weakness present or
  no documentation of medical evaluation to exclude these confounding conditions
Probable:
Appropriate clinical features of neuromuscular weakness and
  documented medical and/or neurological examinations to exclude other causes of weakness
Definite:
Features of probable HANWS and Electrophysiological and/or pathological confirmation
  of the typical pathology

Abbreviation: HANWS, HIV-associated ascending neuromuscular weakness.
Source: From Ref. 20.

reflect an increased risk of these mitochondrial diseases among women. The groups did not have any significant differences in considering age, HIV infection parameters (HIV RNA levels, CD4 cell count), or measurement of severity of acidosis (pH, lactate, and bicarbonate concentrations in the blood).

Not unexpectedly, in addition to the neuromuscular symptomatology, systemic manifestations of hyperlactatemia were found in many but not in all of the group. Specifically, nausea, vomiting, and abdominal pain were reported in 56% of the 69 patient cohort. Of these, two-thirds had documented elevated levels of venous lactate. The antiretroviral agent used most often at the time of presentation of HANWS was stavudine, which was on board in 89% of the definite cases and 88% of all cases.

Based on the definition of this syndrome, all individuals had some degree of extremity weakness. In the available data, it was shown that the weakness was acute in 14 of 22 definite assessable cases for this variable and subacute in 8 cases. The subacute cases had a range from 17 to 60 days. In the overall cohort, however, the progression of disease was from 1 to 200 days. Other findings associated with HANWS in this series included the bulbar manifestations of eye muscle plegias, facial nerve palsy, dysarthria, and dysphagia. Additionally, a total of 32% of the cohort reported some degree of sensory nerve involvement, which was numbness, paresthesias, and/or dysesthesias. Neuromuscular studies in definite cases revealed primarily a sensorimotor polyneuropathy usually axonal in most, but pure myopathy and mixed neuropathy/myopathy were also found.

Histological analysis, done in some cases, included nerve and muscle biopsies. Six of the nine nerves biopsies revealed axonal degeneration or demyelination, whereas the other three manifested some degree of inflammation. Muscle biopsy found muscle fiber atrophy with or without inflammation in some cases. Importantly, evidence of dysfunction of the muscle mitochondria was found. These pathological and/or biochemical manifestations of the mitochondrial toxicity include ragged red fibers, poorly defined mitochondria with dense irregular granules and disorganized cristae, and drops of 60% or more in the amount of mtDNA isolated, and the activities of the mitochondrial respiratory chain enzymes decreased (20).

The relationship of the disease to antiretroviral therapy is quite variable. It is important to note that the symptoms can occur after therapy was discontinued as occurred in 25 patients in this cohort, whereas only four of those with evidence of lactic acidosis had the therapeutic regimen discontinued prior to the onset of compatible symptoms. In those with information regarding follow-up, 36% had evidence of improvement (from mild improvement to total resolution) in the neurological status over a median time of almost four months. The National Institutes of Health guide (2) states that any recovery that occurs may take months. Residuae, however, was more the rule, usually manifest as severe extremity paresis. Of the group as a whole (20), 16% developed enough muscle weakness to necessitate respiratory support and 16% died. Of those with a fatal outcome, six had elevated lactate levels and two were in the definite HIV-associated ascending neuromuscular weakness (HANWS) group. It is not clear if any medicinal therapeutic intervention such as those described for the treatment of the lactic acid syndrome had any positive effect but, of note, the use of corticosteroids seemed to correlate with increased mortality. Rechallenge of the patient with the offending agent, as with the LAS, is not recommended.

Simpson et al. (20) have discussed the observation that there was often a delay from the discontinuation of antiretroviral therapy to the development of neurological disease. This discontinuation was often because of the recognition of lactic acidemia, so that it is important to watch for neurological disease even after the systemic symptoms of lactic acidemia lessen or even resolve.

To be complete, it should be noted that a number of other and comparatively less severe neuromuscular syndromes associated with mitochondrial toxicity are described in HIV/AIDS (21). These include antiretroviral-associated distal symmetric polyneuropathy and a proximal muscle myopathy. Although both entities can be associated with HIV infection itself, several of the antiretroviral nucleoside RTIs have been linked, including stavudine and didanosine in the neuropathy and zidovudine and stavudine in the myopathy.

Hepatic Necrosis

In a 2006 report on suspected drug-induced liver fatalities reported to a World Health Organization database (22), four antiretroviral agents were listed among the top 10 drugs associated with acute hepatic deaths. Stavudine and didanosine were listed as a likely part of their association with the LAS discussed previously, and lamivudine was listed in its role as a therapeutic agent for HIV and/or hepatitis B and the role it may play in exacerbation of hepatitis B virus infections when the drug is stopped in HIV or hepatitis B therapy. Nevirapine, however, a non-nucleoside analog RTI has also been associated with a risk of acute hepatic necrosis independent of the effects associated with the above nucleoside RTIs.

It has been observed that severe, life threatening, and fatal incidence of hepatotoxicity have been described in HIV-infected individuals treated with nevirapine as part of a therapeutic regimen (23–25). Overall, the risk of any hepatic event, regardless of the severity, is highest in the first six weeks of nevirapine therapy but remains higher as compared to controls through the first 18 weeks of treatment. Close monitoring of patients for clinical symptoms and abnormal aminotransferases should occur during this time period. As with the cutaneous reactions seen with nevirapine, to minimize the risk nevirapine dosing is begun as a 200 mg/day lead-in for 14 days prior to full 200 mg twice daily. As compared to non-nevirapine–containing regimens, nevirapine is associated with an 8% rate of elevated serum aminotransferase alanine aminotransferase (ALT) and aspartate aminotransferase (AST) levels of greater than fivefold above normals (6.2% in controls), with symptomatic liver events observed in about 4.0% (1.2% of controls).

Symptomatic liver inflammation occurs particularly in certain cohorts. Symptoms include nausea, vomiting, muscle aches, fatigue, and abdominal pain. About half of the episodes are associated with rash (2). These include individuals with elevated pretreatment levels of aminotransferases, with co-existing hepatitis B and/or C virus infection, and women and those in whom pretreatment CD4 cell count is higher. In addition to a cofactor for the production of liver cell damage, hepatitis C appears to predispose to higher nevirapine plasma levels (over 6 μg/mL). The combination of chronic hepatitis C and these higher nevirapine levels was associated with much higher risks of hepatic toxicity (26).

Females have an almost threefold higher incidence of symptomatic liver disease than men in the first six weeks of therapy. In combining gender and CD4 cell count variables (27), 11% of women with a CD4 cell counts above 250/cmm at time of initiation of therapy had symptomatic hepatic events as compared to 0.9% in those with CD4 cell counts below this amount. In men, 6.3% developed symptomatic liver disease when pretreatment CD4 count was over 400 as compared to 2.3% when the count was below that number. Because of these observations, nevirapine should be avoided in female patients whose CD4 cell count is above 250. When nevirapine is used together with a protease inhibitor (PI) as part of antiretroviral therapy, an increased risk of hepatotoxicity may also occur (28). Although pregnancy has also been considered to be a risk factor for hepatic disease from nevirapine, a Brazilian retrospective study of the use of nevirapine during pregnancy (29) in 197 women found no serious liver toxicity.

Most of the life-threatening, intensive care–requiring toxicities of antiretroviral therapy occur only in those receiving the medication for a therapeutic reason and not for postexposure prophylaxis (PEP). Serious hepatic as well as other toxic effects of nevirapine, however, have been also reported in individuals taking the drug as part of PEP. In 2001, the CDC (30) reported two cases of severe hepatic disease in health care workers taking nevirapine as part of PEP with one leading to liver transplantation. The report also reviewed 20 other reports of severe PEP-related nevirapine toxicity, of which 14 involved the liver.

In the presence of hepatotoxicity, antiretroviral therapy including nevirapine should be discontinued as well as stopping all other hepatotoxic agents if possible. Care must be taken regarding stopping lamivudine and tenofovir in those who are chronically infected with hepatitis B virus. Patients should not be rechallenged with nevirapine (2). It should be noted that hepatic injury can progress even after the nevirapine has been discontinued.

Despite the potential for serious liver disease (as well as serious cutaneous disease discussed below), a number of reasons remain why this agent remains an important part of HAART in many HIV-infected individuals world wide. These reasons include (31):

1. The drug is chemically stable in environmental conditions, whereas other antiretrovirals are not;
2. Symptomatic liver disease has not been reported in HIV-infected children, and nevirapine is available in a liquid formulation, whereas many other antiretrovirals are not; and
3. With lower rates of nevirapine liver toxicities in patients with lower CD4 cell counts, resource-poor countries starting patients at lower CD4 cell levels are likely to see less hepatotoxicity.

Abacavir Hypersensitivity Reaction

The antiretroviral NRTI abacavir has been relatively free of mitochondrial dysfunction and liver necrosis. Even before release, during Phase II dose-ranging clinical trials, the medication was found to be associated with an idiosyncratic reaction characterized by a relatively insidious onset of a mélange of potential symptoms including fever, gastrointestinal manifestations (nausea, vomiting, and abdominal pain), respiratory symptoms (cough and shortness of breath), and exanthem. These nonspecific symptoms resolved on discontinuation of the abacavir but returned in hours if the drug was reintroduced. The incidence of the reaction, based on 1302 cases in 30,595 individuals who were enrolled in prerelease clinical trials and expanded access programs was found to be 4.3% (32). A frequency of up to 9% has been reported in clinical trials (2).

Two reviews have summarized the manifestations of this drug complication (32,33). The onset of abacavir hypersensitivity reaction (ASHR) generally occurs with six weeks of initiation of abacavir, with a median time of 11 days; 5.2%, however, began more than three months after abacavir initiation. The symptoms, being nondiagnostic by themselves, can be highly suggestive when occurring together, especially without another etiology being found and the characteristic observation that the symptoms became worse with each consecutive dose of abacavir being administered (33). A list of potential symptom complex reactions in descending order of frequency is shown in Table 5. The risk of ASHR does not appear to relate to age, gender, history of allergy or atopy, or the type of concomitant antiretroviral therapy. It has been suggested that a higher incidence of more severe ASHR may occur when the drug is administered as 600 mg once daily as compared to 300 mg twice daily (2).

Fever is clearly the most common manifestation of ASHR, although chills are uncommon (11%). The second most common symptom is rash, usually nonpruritic and generally described as maculopapular or urticarial and usually thought to be mild or moderate in severity. Vesicles or bullae (see below) are usually not seen. It is important to note (33) that rash is not usually the first symptom to occur and is most often an incidental observation on exam and not the reason for coming to a health care deliverer. It also should be noted, in this regard, that a nonspecific rash may occur in as many as 10% of patients treated with this NRTI and as an isolated finding, if mild, does not necessitate discontinuance of the drug.

Gastrointestinal complaints are more common than respiratory ones, but the combination of fever, respiratory symptoms, and muscle aches produces a syndrome reminiscent of influenza. Most chest radiograms are unremarkable. Despite being referred to as a hypersensitivity reaction and one that may be associated with an urticarial rash, evidence of bronchospasm is quite unusual (less than 1%) (33). Occasional biochemical abnormalities are seen, each in 10% of cases, which resolve with discontinuation of the drug. These abnormalities include elevated ALT, AST, creatinine, and creatine phosphokinase, as well as leucopenia and/or thrombocytopenia.

In addition to the observation that symptoms worsen with each successive dose of the drug, it is the constellation of symptoms occurring that most strongly lends the diagnosis its credence. For example (33), 50% of cases involved symptoms in three or four organ systems (fever, cutaneous, gastrointestinal, and respiratory)

Table 5 Frequency of Symptoms Reported in Cases of Abacavir Hypersensitivity Reaction

Symptom	Percentage of cases
Fever	78
Rash	66
Malaise or fatigue	46
Nausea and/or vomiting	46
Muscle or joint pain	27
Headache	23
Diarrhea	22
Itching	19
Abdominal pain	13
Shortness of breath	12
Cough	10
Edema	8
Low blood pressure	7
Sore throat	6
Influenza-like illness	6

Source: From Ref. 32.

and the diagnosis should be highly considered when fever, malaise, nausea, and vomiting is combined with an exanthem.

If ASHR is believed to be manifest, the appropriate response should be stopping the medication. The use of symptomatic therapy should be avoided and could make the resolution of symptoms upon stopping the abacavir harder to assess. Furthermore, the health care deliverer should emphasize to the affected patient that any unused abacavir prescription should be returned to the clinician or pharmacy for disposal to avoid accidental restarting. A warning card or medical alert bracelet should be given to the patient. It is this rechallenge, although confirming the diagnosis of ASHR, that can lead to substantial morbidity and mortality.

Overall, the signs and symptomatology of a rechallenge with abacavir after discontinuance for ASHR are not unlike the initial episode but with more severity. Rechallenge manifestations, however, more likely result in hypotension, tachycardia, azotemia, and lethargy, and in the absence of aggressive intensive care unit interventions, may result in death. The reaction, although not IgE mediated, can mimic anaphylaxis (2). In the Hetherington et al.'s report (32), 19 deaths related to abacavir use were reported with an overall death rate of 3 per 10,000 treatment courses. Despite issues with rechallenge, only 6 of the 19 deaths occurred following this event and in the five cases where the information was available, symptoms recurred within 24 hours and as quickly as 10 minutes or less. The other 13 deaths occurred during the initial reaction but some, perhaps much, of the mortality was contributed by fatal co-morbidities. Hetherington et al. (32) also noted that 11 of the 19 deaths occurred in a situation where respiratory symptoms were part of the initial ASHR. The risk of symptoms occurring after rechallenge when the abacavir was discontinued for reasons other than ASHR is quite low (34).

In investigations of the histocompatibility loci, Mallal et al. (35) and Hetherington et al. (36) both found a strong association between abacavir hypersensitivity in Caucasians (not dark-skinned patients) and the HLA-B-5701 allele. The combination of human leukocyte antigen (HLA)-B-5701 and polymorphism in heat shock protein-Hom (HSP1AL) has greater predictive accuracy than HLA B-5701 by itself (37). This association has been confirmed by other groups. The mechanism involved in ASHR has not been well characterized. In one study, King et al. (38) found a significant association between interleukin-4 production and the idiosyncratic reaction. Evidence of functional activation of T cells was also observed in ASHR patients as compared to control cells as manifested by expression of CD28 and the chemokine macrophage inflammatory protein 1-beta.

Stevens–Johnson Syndrome/Toxic Epidermal Necrosis

Stevens–Johnson syndrome (SJS) and toxic epidermal necrosis (TEN) are variants of the same process, presenting as severe mucosal erosions with widespread erythematous, cutaneous macules, or atypical targets. Disease is usually accompanied by fever, erosive oral lesions, conjunctivitis, facial edema, and muscle/joint pains. The skin lesions often become confluent and show a positive Nikolsky sign (superficial layers of skin slipping free from the lower layers with slight pressure). In SJS, the area of epidermal detachment involves less than 10% of the total body skin area; transitional SJS-TEN is defined by an epidermal detachment between 10% and 30%; TEN is defined by a detachment greater than 30%. Full-thickness epidermal necrosis is observed on pathological examination. The incidence of TEN is estimated to be 1 to 1.4 cases per million inhabitants per year. The incidence of SJS is probably of the same order (one to three cases per million inhabitants per year).

SJS–TEN is essentially drug-induced. A few cases are related to infective agents (such as *Mycoplasma pneumoniae*), and a few other cases remain unexplained. The most common medications associated with SJS–TEN are the antibacterial sulfonamides (related to HIV care as trimethoprim/sulfamethoxazole (SXT) used for pneumocystosis treatment or with primary or secondary prevention), anticonvulsant agents, some nonsteroidal anti-inflammatory drugs, and allopurinol. Prior to the introduction of nevirapine, SXT was the medication most associated with SJS–TEN in the Western world (39), whereas thiacetazone (an antituberculosis medication) was most associated with this disease in Africa (40). HIV infection dramatically increases the risk especially when the antiretroviral drug, nevirapine, is used. These ICU-requiring illnesses have been reported to occur in about 3 per 1000 HIV-infected patients treated with nevirapine (42), and the risk of severe reactions may be higher in women.

In one European multicenter study where SJS–TEN was actively detected (41), 246 cases of the disease were reported. Of these, 18 (7.3%) were infected with HIV and exposure to nevirapine was present in 15 (83%) of the HIV-infected cohort and all but one of these had received other components of HAART. In this group of 15, the cutaneous reaction began from 10 to 240 days after nevirapine was begun (median 12 days). Importantly, 10 of the 15 were still taking the once daily lead-in dose when the reaction began, which is said to decrease the risk of this serious reaction (42). Conflicting data exist on the use of corticosteroids to prevent the rash during the lead-in period, but it does not appear to do so and may increase the risk. Likewise, antihistamines do not appear to be effective in preventing the nevaripine rash. A longer lead-in period may decrease the risk of STS–TEN, as suggested by Anton et al. (43) where 100 mg daily doses were increased 100 mg weekly to reach the 400 mg/day dose.

That SJS–TEN is a life-threatening illness is reflected by a mortality rate of 23% in this study overall, with 2 of 18 deaths in the HIV cohort. Management revolves around permanent discontinuation of the nevirapine if a rash is severe, if it is combined with constitutional symptoms, and if it is associated with elevated serum aminotransferases. Mild rashes are common with nevirapine, as an isolated finding, and do not by themselves require discontinuation of the medication. Liver disease may be a confounding variable, as decreased clearance of nevirapine is linked to longer serum half-life of the drug. Corticosteroid use is controversial (2) but generally not employed due to high mortality rates and poor wound healing. Likewise, other immunological modulations such as intravenous immunoglobulin (44) remain debated. Whether another non-nucleoside analog RTI can be substituted for nevirapine after SJS–TEN is uncertain but the class might be avoided unless no other therapeutic options remain (2). Aggressive symptomatic management of SJS–TEN in the ICU setting may include aggressive local wound care (as in a burn unit), intravenous hydration, parenteral nutrition, and pain management.

HEART ATTACKS

HIV-associated cardiac disease can present in a variety of ways including dilated cardiomyopathy and pericardial effusion (45). The cardiomyopathy can be infectious (related to HIV itself or other opportunistic pathogens) or drug related (cocaine, doxorubicin, and interferon), and the pericardial involvement can be related to a variety of pathogens or malignancies. The dilated cardiomyopathy has been estimated to occur in 15.9 patients per 1000 HIV infected otherwise asymptomatic individuals (46). Pericardial effusions have been reported to occur at a frequency of 11% per year (47), often spontaneously resolving.

With effective HAART, direct HIV effects and the impact of opportunistic infections have decreased in treated individuals. Cardiac disease, however, can be impacted by part of the HIV-treatment regimen, most notably the third group of drugs besides nucleoside and non-nucleoside RTIs, the PIs.

These effective HIV drugs, at least a great majority of them, have significant metabolic effects related to disturbances in glucose metabolism primarily related to insulin resistance (48) as well as elevated lipids (49).

In one five-year study involving 221 HIV-infected individuals (50), those treated with a PI were 5 times more likely to have hyperglycemia, 6.1 more times more likely to have elevated triglycerides, and 2.8 more times to have elevated cholesterol levels. These effects were independent of the degree of HIV suppression. Indeed, even a short interruption from PI therapy (mean seven weeks) produced a lower cholesterol, low density lipoprotein cholesterol, and triglyceride (51).

As reviewed by Fisher and colleagues (52), independent of the type of HAART used, an increased risk of ischemic heart disease is found in HIV-infected individuals. In analyzing the contribution of PIs in the development of myocardial infarction in HIV-infected persons, an increased, yet nonsignificant, risk was found (risk factor 1.69, 2.56, and 6.5 in three studies (53–55) but larger retrospective studies did not clearly demonstrate an increased risk of ischemic cardiac disease in those taking PIs as compared to non-PI–containing regimens (56, 57). In support of a somewhat increased risk of atherosclerotic vascular disease in those taking PIs (58), one study found that atherosclerosis measured by ultrasonography could correlate with PI use. The clinical impact of the findings requires consideration of the use of cardiovascular disease prevention as a primary preventive measure but not necessarily abandoning PI therapy.

REFERENCES

1. Lutwick LI, Lavkan A, Greenbaum D. Infections in AIDS patients. In: Cunha BA, ed. Infectious Disease in Critical Care. New York: Marcel Dekker, 1998:599–643.
2. Department of Health and Human Services: Guidelines for the Use of Antiretroviral Agents in HIV-1–Infected Adults and Adolescents.
   < aidsinfo.nih.gov/ContentFiles/AdultandAdolescentGL.pdf > Updated Oct 6, 2005.
3. Narasimhan M, Posner AJ, DePaol VA, et al. Intensive care in patients with HIV infection in the era of highly active antiretroviral therapy. Chest 2004; 125:1800–1804.
4. Morris A, Masur H, Huang L. Current issues in critical care of the human immunodeficiency virus-infected patient. Crit Care Med 2006; 34:42–49.
5. Palacios R, Santos J, Camino X, et al. Treatment-limiting toxicities associated with nucleoside analogue reverse transcriptase inhibitor therapy: a prospective, observational study. Curr Ther Res Clin Exp 2005; 66:117–129.
6. Gertner E, Thurn JR, Williams DN, et al. Zidovudine-associated myopathy. Am J Med 1989; 86:814–818.
7. Kakuda T. Pharmacology of nucleoside and nucleoside reverse transcriptase inhibitor-induced mitochondrial toxicity. Clin Ther 2000; 22:685–708.
8. Gerschenson M, Brinkman K. Mitochondrial dysfunction in AIDS and its treatment. Mitochondrion 2004; 4:763–777.
9. Stryer K, ed. Biochemistry. New York: WH Freeman and Co., 1988:397–426.

10. Dagan T, Sable C, Bray J, Gerschenson M. Mitochondrial dysfunction and antiretroviral nucleoside analog toxicities: what is the evidence? Mitochondrion 2002; 1:397–412.
11. Arnoult D, Violett L, Petit F, et al. HIV-1 triggers mitochondrial death. Mitochondrion 2004; 4:255–260.
12. Hoschele D. Cell culture models for the investigation of NRTI-induced mitochondrial toxicity. Relevance for the prediction of clinical toxicity. Toxicology In Vitro. 2006; 20: 535–54.
13. Lai KK, Gang DL, Zawacki JK, Cooley TP. Fulminant hepatic failure associated with 2′, 3′dideoxyinosine. Ann Intern Med 1991; 115:283–284.
14. Ogedegbe A-E, Thomas DL, Diehl AM. Hyperlactataemia syndromes associated with HIV therapy. Lancet Infect Dis 2003; 3:329–337.
15. Calza L, Manfredi R, Chiodo F. Hyperlactateaemia and lactic acidosis in HIV-infected patients receiving antiretroviral therapy. Clin Nutrition 2005; 24:5–15.
16. Moyle GJ, Datta D, Mandalia S, et al. Hyperlactataemia and lactic acidosis during antiretroviral therapy: relevance, reproducibility and possible risk factors. AIDS 2002; 16: 1341–1349.
17. John M, Mallal S. Hyperlactataemia syndrome in people with HIV infection. Curr Opin Infect Dis 2002; 15:23–29.
18. Falco V, Rodriquez D, Ribera E, et al. Severe nucleoside-associated lactic acidosis in human immunodeficiency virus-infected patients: report of 12 cases and review of the literature. Clin Infect Dis 2002; 34:838–846.
19. Verma A, Roland M, Jayaweere D, Kett D. Fulminat neuropathy and lactic acidosis associated with nucleoside analog therapy. Neurology 1999; 53:1365–1369.
20. Simpson D, Estanislao L, Evans S, et al. HIV-associated neuromuscular weakness syndrome. AIDS 2004; 18:1403–1412.
21. Estanislao L, Thomas D, Simpson D. HIV neuromuscular disease and mitochondrial function. Mitochondrion 2004; 4:131–139.
22. Bjornsson E, Olsson R. Suspected drug-induced liver fatalities reported to the WHO database. Dig Liver Dis 2006; 38:33–38.
23. Cattelan AM, Erne E, Stalino A, et al. Severe hepatic failure related to nevirapine treatment. Clin Infect Dis 1999; 29:455–456.
24. Prakash M, Poreddy V, Tiyyagura L, Bonacini M. Jaundice and hepatocellular damage associated with nevirapine therapy. Am J Gastroenterol 2001; 96:1571–1574.
25. Pollard RB, Robinson P, Dransfield K. Safety profile of nevirapine, a nonnucleoside reverse transcriptase inhibitor for the treatment of human immunodeficiency virus infection. Clin Therap 1998; 20:1071–1092.
26. Gonzales de Requena D, Nunez M, Jimenez-Nacher I, Soriano V. Liver toxicity caused by nevirapine. AIDS 2005; 19:621–623.
27. Reisler K. High hepatotoxicity rate seen among HAART patients. AIDS Alert 2001; 16:118–119.
28. De Maat MMR, Mathot RAA, Veldkam AI, et al. Hepatotoxicity following nevirapine-containing regimens in HIV-1-infected individuals. Pharmacological Res 2002; 46:295–300.
29. Joao EC, Calvet GA, Menezes JA, et al. Nevirapine toxicity in a cohort of HIV-1-infected pregnant women. Am J Obstet Gynecol 2006; 194:199–202.
30. Centers for Disease Control and Prevention: Serious adverse events attributed to nevirapine regimens for postexposure prophylaxis after HIV exposures – Worldwide, 1997–2000. MMWR 2001; 49:1153–1156.
31. Food and Drug Administration Center for Drug Evaluation and Research: FDA public health advisory for nevirapine (Viramune). http://www.fda.gov/cder/drug/advisory/Nevirapine.htm.
32. Hetherington S, McGuirk S, Powell G, et al. Hypersensitivity reactions during therapy with the nucleoside reverse transcriptase inhibitor abacavir. Clin Ther 2001; 23:1603–1614.
33. Clay PG. The abacavir hypersensitivity reaction: a review. Clin Therap 2001; 24:1502–1514.

34. Loeliger AE, Steel H, McGuirk S, et al. The abacavir hypersensitivity reaction and interruptions in therapy. AIDS 2001; 15:1325–1326.

35. Mallal S, Nolan D, Witt C, et al. Association between presence of HLA-B*5701, HLA-DR7, and HLA-DQ3 and hypersensitivity to HIV-1 reverse-transcriptase inhibitor abacavir. Lancet 2002; 359:727–732.

36. Hetherington S, Hughes AR, Mosteller M, et al. Genetic variations in HLA-B region and hypersensitivity reactions in abacavir. Lancet 2002; 359:1121–1122.

37. Martin AM, Nolan D, Gaudieri S, et al. Predisposition to abacavir hypersensitivity conferred by HLA-B*5701 and a haplotypic Hsp70-Hom variant. Proc Natl Acad Sci USA 2004; 101:4180–4185.

38. King D, Tomkins S, Waters A, et al. Intracellular cytokines may model immunoregulation of abacavir hypersensitivity in HIV-infected subjects. J Allergy Clin Immunol 2005; 115: 1081–1087.

39. Carr A, Tindall B, Penny R, Cooper DA. Patterns of multiple-drug hypersensitivities in HIV-infected patients. AIDS 1993; 7:1532–1533.

40. Nunn P, Kibuga D, Gathua S, et al. Cutaneous hypersensitivity reactions due to thiacetazone in HIV-1 seropositive patients treated for tuberculosis. Lancet 1991; 337:627–630.

41. Fagot J-P, Mockenhaupt M, Bouwes-Bavinck J-N, et al. Nevirapine and the risk of Steven-Johnson syndrome or toxic epidermal necrolysis. AIDS 2001; 15:1843–1848.

42. Barner A, Myers M. Nevirapine and rashes. Lancet 1998; 351:1133.

43. Anton P, Soriano V, Jimenez-Nacher I, et al. Incidence of rash and discontinuation of nevirapine using two different escalating initial doses. AIDS 1999; 13:524–525.

44. Claes P, Wintzen M, Allard S, et al. Nevirapine-induced toxic epidermal necrolysis and toxin hepatitis treated successfully with a combination of intravenous immunoglobulins and N-acetylcysteine. Eur J Intern Med 2004; 15:255–258.

45. Barbaro G, Fisher SD, Luipshultz SE. Pathogenesis of HIV-associated cardiovascular complications. Lancet Infect Dis 2001; 1:115–124.

46. Lipshultz SE. Dilated cardiomyopathy in HIV-infected patients. N Engl J Med 1998; 339:1153–1155.

47. Silva-Cardoso J, Moura B, Martins L, et al. Pericardial involvement in human immunodeficiency virus infection. Chest 1999; 115:418–422.

48. Walli R, Herfort O, Michl GM, et al. Treatment with protease inhibitors associated with peripheral insulin resistance and impaired glucose tolerance in HIV-1-infected patients. AIDS 1998; 12:F167–F173.

49. Behrens G, Dejam A, Schmidt H, et al. Impaired glucose tolerance, beta cell function, and lipid metabolism in HIV patients under treatment with protease inhibitors. AIDS 1999; 13:F63–F70.

50. Tsiodras S, Mantzonos C, Hammer S, Samore M. Effects of protease inhibitors on hyperglycemics, hyperlipidemia, and lipodystrophy: a 5-year cohort study. Arch Intern Med 2000; 160:2050–2056.

51. Hatano H, Miller KD, Yoder CP, et al. Metabolic and anthropometric consequences of interruption of highly active antiretroviral therapy. AIDS 2000; 14:1935–1942.

52. Fisher SD, Miller TL, Lipshultz SE. Impact of HIV and highly active antiretroviral therapy on leukocyte adhesions molecules, arterial inflammation, dyslipidemia, and atherosclerosis. Atherosclerosis 2006; 185:1–11.

53. Holmberg SD, Moorman AC, Williamson JM, et al. Protease inhibitors and cardiovascular outcomes in patients with HIV-1. Lancet 2002; 360:1747–1748.

54. Mary-Kraus M, Cotte L, Simon A, et al. The Clinical Epidemiology Group from the French Hospital Database. Increased risk of myocardial infarction with duration of protease inhibitor therapy in HIV-infected men. AIDS 2003; 17:2479–2486.

55. Coplan PM, Nikas A, Japour A, et al. Incidence of myocardial infarction in randomized clinical trials of protease inhibitor-based antiretroviral therapy: an analysis of four different protease inhibitors. AIDS Res Hum Retroviruses 2003; 19:449–455.

56. Klein D, Hurley LB, Quesenberry CP, Sidney S. Do protease inhibitors increase the risk for coronary heart disease in patients with HIV-1 infection? J Acquir Immune Defic Syndr 2002; 30:471–477.
57. Bozzette SA, Ake CF, Tam HK, et al. Cardiovascular and cerebrovascular events in patients treated for human immunodeficiency virus infection. N Engl J Med 2003; 348:702–710.
58. de Saint Marftin, Vandhuick O, Guillo P, et al. Premature atherosclerosis in HIV-positive patient and cumulated time of exposure to antiretroviral therapy (SHIVA study). Atherosclerosis. 2006; 185:361–367.

21
Infections in Cirrhosis in the Critical Care Unit

Laurel C. Preheim

*Departments of Medicine, Medical Microbiology and Immunology,
Creighton University School of Medicine, University of Nebraska
College of Medicine, and VA Medical Center, Omaha, Nebraska, U.S.A.*

INTRODUCTION

Cirrhosis is characterized by fibrosis of the hepatic parenchyma with regenerative nodules surrounded by scar tissue. It can result from a variety of chronic, progressive liver diseases. The clinical manifestations vary widely from asymptomatic disease (up to 40% of patients) to fulminant liver failure. Cirrhosis is a major cause of morbidity worldwide. In the United States, cirrhosis has an estimated prevalence of 360 per 100,000 population and accounts for approximately 30,000 deaths annually. The majority of cases in the United States are due to alcoholic liver disease or chronic infection with hepatitis B or C viruses.

Infection is a common complication of cirrhosis (reviewed in Refs. 1–4). A Danish death registry study (5) examined long-term survival and cause-specific mortality in 10,154 patients with cirrhosis between 1982 and 1993. The results revealed an increased risk of dying from respiratory infection (fivefold), from tuberculosis (15-fold), and other infectious diseases (22-fold) when compared to the general population. In a recent prospective study (6), 20% of cirrhotic patients admitted to the hospital developed an infection while hospitalized. The mortality among patients with infection was 20% compared to 4% mortality in those who remained uninfected. Of patients admitted to the critical care unit, 41% became infected. The most common bacterial infections seen in cirrhotic patients are urinary tract infections (12–29%), spontaneous bacterial peritonitis (SBP) (7–23%), respiratory tract infections (6–10%), and primary bacteremia (4–11%) (7). The increased susceptibility to bacterial infections among cirrhotic patients is related to impaired hepatocyte and phagocytic cell function as well as the consequences of parenchymal destruction (portal hypertension, ascites, and gastroesophageal varices).

It should be noted that the usual signs and symptoms of infection may be subtle or absent in individuals who have advanced liver disease. Thus a high index of suspicion is required to ensure that infections are not overlooked in this patient population, especially in those who are hospitalized. Occasionally fever may be due to cirrhosis itself (8), but this must be a diagnosis of exclusion made only when appropriate diagnostic tests, including cultures, have been unrevealing.

ROLE OF THE LIVER IN HOST DEFENSE AGAINST INFECTION

The liver plays an important role in host defense against infection. Cirrhosis can adversely affect a number of these host defenses. The mechanisms identified in human and experimental animal studies include depression of reticuloendothelial system clearance of organisms from the bloodstream (9); impairment of chemotaxis, phagocytosis, and intracellular killing by polymorphonuclear leukocytes (PMNL) and monocytes (10–12); reduction in serum bactericidal activity and opsonic activity (13,14); depression of serum complement (15–17); dysregulation of cytokine synthesis and metabolism (18); and reduced protective efficacy of type-specific antibody (19) and granulocyte colony-stimulating factor (20).

CLASSIFICATION OF LIVER DISEASE SEVERITY

Patients who have cirrhosis are at increased risk for both community-acquired and nosocomial infections, the majority of which are bacterial. The incidence of infection is highest for patients with the most severe liver disease (6,21–23). Accurate assessment for risk of infection is dependent upon proper classification of the extent of liver disease. The Child–Pugh scoring system of liver disease severity (24) is based upon five parameters: serum bilirubin, serum albumin, prothrombin time, ascites, and encephalopathy. A total score is derived from the sum of the points for each of these five parameters. Patients with chronic liver disease are placed in one of three classes (A, B, or C). Despite having some limitations, the modified Child–Pugh scoring system continues to be used by many clinicians to assess the risk of mortality in patients with cirrhosis (Table 1).

SPONTANEOUS BACTERIAL PERITONITIS

Pathogenesis

SBP is the infection of ascitic fluid with no identifiable abdominal source for the infection. SBP is perhaps the most characteristic bacterial infection in cirrhosis,

Table 1 Modified Child–Pugh Classification of Liver Disease Severity

Parameter	Points assigned		
	1	2	3
Ascites	None	Slight	Moderate/severe
Encephalopathy	None	Grade 1–2	Grade 3–4
Bilirubin (mg/dL)	<2.0	2.0–3.0	>3.0
Albumin (mg/L)	>3.5	2.8–3.5	<2.8
Prothrombin time (seconds increased)	1–3	4–6	>6.0
	Total score		*Child–Pugh class*
	5–6		A
	7–9		B
	10–15		C

occurring in as many as 20% to 30% of cirrhotic patients who are admitted to the hospital with ascites (6,21,23). SBP occurs when normally sterile ascitic fluid is colonized following an episode of transient bacteremia. Aerobic gram-negative bacilli, especially *Escherichia coli*, cause approximately 75% of SBP infections. Aerobic gram-positive cocci, including *Streptococcus pneumoniae*, *Enterococcus faecalis*, other streptococci, and *Staphylococcus aureus*, are responsible for most other SBP cases (25,26). Because enteric bacteria predominate in SBP it is thought that the gut is the major source of organisms for this infection. Several mechanisms have been proposed to explain the movement of organisms from the intestinal lumen to the systemic circulation (reviewed in Ref. 1). Cirrhosis-induced depression of the hepatic reticuloendothelial system (RES) impairs the liver's filtering function, allowing bacteria to pass from the bowel lumen to the bloodstream via the portal vein. Cirrhosis also is associated with a relative increase in aerobic gram-negative bacilli in the jejunum. A decrease in mucosal blood flow due to acute hypovolemia or drug-induced splanchnic vasoconstriction may compromise the intestinal barrier to enteric flora, thereby increasing the risk of bacteremia. Finally, bacterial translocation may occur with movement of enteric organisms from the gut lumen through the mucosa to the intestinal lymphatics. From there bacteria can travel through the lymphatic system and enter the bloodstream via the thoracic duct. It is assumed that SBP caused by nonenteric organisms also is due to bacteremia secondary to another site of infection with subsequent seeding of the peritoneum and ascitic fluid (Fig. 1).

Decreased opsonic activity of ascitic fluid also increases the risk of SBP in patients with cirrhosis. Immunoglobulin, complement, and fibronectin are important opsonins in ascitic fluid, and patients with low protein concentrations in their ascitic fluid are especially predisposed to SBP (27,28). Patients with ascitic fluid protein concentrations below 1 g/dL have a sevenfold increase in the incidence of SBP when compared to patients with higher protein concentrations in ascites (27).

Other risk factors have been associated with SBP, including gastrointestinal bleeding, fulminant hepatic failure, and invasive procedures such as the placement of peritoneovenous shunts for the treatment of ascites. An elevated bilirubin level also is correlated with a high risk of peritonitis in patient with cirrhosis (28).

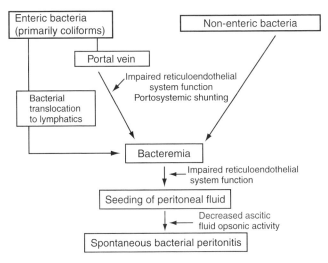

Figure 1 Pathogenic mechanisms underlying spontaneous bacterial peritonitis. *Source*: Adapted from Ref. 1.

Diagnosis

Classic signs and symptoms of peritonitis, including fever, chills, abdominal pain, and increasing ascites may or may not be present in cirrhotic patients who have SBP. Abdominal symptoms may be absent in up to one-third of cases. Patients with SBP may present with encephalopathy, gastrointestinal bleeding, or increasing renal insufficiency. Therefore a high index of suspicion must be maintained in all cases of cirrhotic patients who have ascites and are acutely ill.

A diagnostic paracentesis must be performed on all patients suspected to have SBP. A cell count of greater than $250 \, PMNL/mm^3$ of ascitic fluid is highly suggestive of infection. Gram stain of centrifuged ascitic fluid will reveal organisms in approximately 30% of cases. The fluid should be cultured both aerobically and anaerobically. Inoculating some fluid directly into blood culture bottles increases the yield of positive cultures. But this nonquantitative culture technique also increases the risk of false positives if any skin flora contaminant is introduced into the blood culture bottle at the bedside.

As indicated previously, aerobic gram-negative enteric bacilli are the most frequent isolates from ascitic fluid cultures in SBP. Anaerobes are uncommon causes of SBP, and their presence in ascitic fluid should raise suspicions for bowel perforation. If ascitic fluid cultures yield polymicrobial flora, *Candida albicans* (or other yeast), or *Bacteroides fragilis* one should suspect a secondary peritonitis caused by an acute abdominal infection.

Treatment

Historically SBP has been a severe, frequently fatal infection. In the past few decades mortality rates have dropped from over 90% in the 1970s to the current 20%–40% mortality for patients who have their first diagnosis of SBP. Earlier detection and treatment and the use of non-nephrotoxic antibiotics has contributed to the increased short-term survival. The most common causes of death in patients with SBP are liver failure, gastrointestinal bleeding, and renal failure. One of the greatest threats to long-term survival is recurrence of SBP, which can occur in 70% of patients (29).

Previously aminoglycosides, alone or in combination with beta-lactam antibiotics, were widely used to treat SBP. However, the risk of aminoglycoside nephrotoxicity in cirrhotic patients has limited the usefulness of this class of agents (30). Expanded-spectrum cephalosporins are active against most of the strains of enteric gram-negative pathogens that cause SBP. Cefotaxime has been shown effective in a number of trials with regimens of 2 g administered every eight hours for five days (26) or 2 g every 12 hours for a mean of nine days (31). In a more recent study (32) 24 of 33 cirrhotic patients (73%) with SBP had clinical and bacteriologic cures after receiving 1 g of ceftriaxone every 12 hours for five days. With prolonged treatment using ceftriaxone or with a change to another antibiotic according to susceptibility, SBP resolved in seven of the nine patients who had not responded by day 5 of therapy. Study patients had an overall hospital mortality of only 12%. The authors concluded that antibiotic therapy for SBP can be discontinued if the polymorphonuclear differential count in ascitic fluid is less than $250 \, cells/mm^3$ on day 5 of treatment (32).

Other parenteral antibiotics that have been reported effective for the treatment of SBP include aztreonam (500 mg every eight hours) (33), cefonicid (2 g every 12 hours) (34), and amoxicillin-clavulanic acid (35). Several small trials have involved the use of oral antibiotics. These included intravenous followed by oral therapy with amoxicillin-clavulanic acid (36) or ciprofloxacin (37) and oral ofloxacin (38). While some experts recommend that patients with moderate symptoms and a positive response to a short course of intravenous antibiotics could benefit from therapy with oral fluoroquinolones (29), others have found the supporting evidence to be inconclusive (39).

Deterioration of renal function is the most sensitive predictor of in-hospital mortality in patients with SBP (40). In a randomized, multicenter comparative study, patients with SBP who received intravenous albumin for plasma volume expansion plus cefotaxime had less renal impairment and significantly lower mortality (22%) than those receiving cefotaxime alone (41%) (41). The dose of albumin used in this study was 1.5 g/kg of body weight at the time of diagnosis followed by 1 g/kg on day 3.

Prophylaxis

The use of prophylactic antibiotics decreases the incidence and mortality of bacterial infections, including SBP, in patients who are hospitalized with cirrhosis and ascites (7). Cirrhotic patients who recover from SBP also are at increased risk of subsequent episodes. The one-year probability of recurrence of SBP in this population has been estimated to approach 70% (42). Antibiotics reported effective in preventing SBP have included trimethoprim/sulfamethoxazole (43) and, more commonly, fluoroquinolones such as norfloxacin, ofloxacin, and ciprofloxacin (7,44–46). A major concern regarding repeated or prolonged courses of antibiotic prophylaxis is selection for resistant bacterial pathogens. There are a growing number of recent reports of the development of SBP or other infections caused by fluoroquinolone-resistant organisms, including *E. coli*, *Pseudomonas* spp., and methicillin-resistant *S. aureus* (MRSA), in cirrhotic patients on fluoroquinolone prophylaxis (7,47,48). Thus the use of prophylactic antibiotics should be restricted to patients at greatest risk of SBP, weighing the increased risk of inducing resistant bacteria against the benefits of preventing infection.

URINARY TRACT INFECTIONS

Urinary tract infections account for 25%–40% of infections in hospitalized cirrhotic patients (21,23,49). The majority of these patients have asymptomatic bacteriuria, but approximately one-third have symptomatic infections (23). The incidence of significant bacteriuria ($>10^5$ colony forming units/mL) is higher in women than in men and does not correlate with the severity of the underlying liver disease or with the age of the patient (49). The presence of an indwelling urinary catheter increases the risk of infection. The most common pathogens are *E. coli* and other aerobic gram-negative coliforms. Asymptomatic bacteriuria does not require treatment, particularly in patients with an indwelling urinary catheter. A urine culture should be obtained on any cirrhotic patient suspected to have a urinary tract infection. Antibiotic therapy, when indicated, should be guided by microbiologic susceptibility testing of the urinary isolate. Antibiotic options for empiric therapy of symptomatic infections include fluoroquinolones or expanded-spectrum penicillins or cephalosporins. Indwelling urinary catheters should be removed as soon as possible to reduce the risk of infection.

BACTEREMIA

Cirrhosis predisposes patients to systemic bloodstream infections due to intrahepatic blood shunting and impaired bacterial clearance from the portal blood. Bacteremia has been reported to occur in approximately 9% of hospitalized cirrhotic patients (50) and accounts for 20% of the infections diagnosed during their hospital stay (23). The incidence of bacteremia increases with the severity of liver disease. The most commonly identified sources of bacteremia have been SBP, urinary tract infections, pneumonia, soft tissue infections, and biliary tract infections (50,51). The pathogens identified in blood cultures from bacteremic patients mirror those responsible for the primary source infections. *E. coli*, *Klebsiella pneumoniae*, *Aeromonas hydrophila*, and other enteric gram-negative aerobes are common causes of bacteremic infections. Most gram-positive bacteremias are due to *S. aureus*, *S. pneumoniae*, or other aerobic streptococcal species. Bloodstream infection is associated with a poor prognosis despite appropriate antibiotic therapy. Mortality rates commonly exceed 50% (50,52). Poor outcome is independent of the type of bacteremia (52), but in-hospital mortality has been correlated with the absence of fever, an elevated serum creatinine, and marked leukocytosis (51). Cirrhotic patients with suspected bacteremia should receive empiric therapy directed against the most common gram-negative and gram-positive pathogens in this setting. Antibiotic selection should take into consideration local microbial susceptibility patterns. Usual therapeutic options would include expanded-spectrum cephalosporins, piperacillin/tazobactam, or a fluoroquinolone such as levofloxacin or moxifloxacin.

Cirrhotic patients who undergo endoscopic procedures for gastrointestinal hemorrhage or transhepatic procedures are at increased risk of bacteremia. Endoscopic variceal sclerotherapy or band ligation for bleeding esophageal varices is associated with a reported risk of bacteremia ranging from 5% to 30% (53–55). Although the bacteremia associated with these procedures may be brief, cirrhotic patients are susceptible to infections from transient bacteremia. Gastrointestinal hemorrhage itself is an independent risk factor for bacteremia and other infections in cirrhotic patients. Antibiotic administration has been shown to reduce infectious complications and mortality in cirrhotic patients who are hospitalized for gastrointestinal hemorrhage (56–59). Antibiotic prophylaxis is recommended for all cirrhotic inpatients with gastrointestinal bleeding (60,61). Fluoroquinolone antibiotics were used in most trials with a median treatment duration of seven days.

PNEUMONIA

Respiratory tract infections account for approximately 20% of the infectious diseases that are diagnosed in hospitalized cirrhotic patients (21,23,62). *S. pneumoniae* continues to rank first among bacterial pathogens causing community-acquired pneumonia in adults (63). Chronic liver disease has long been recognized as a risk factor for bacteremic pneumococcal pneumonia (64). The mortality rate for pneumococcal bacteremia in cirrhotic patients may exceed 50% despite appropriate antibiotic therapy (65). Other organisms commonly responsible for community-acquired pneumonia include *Mycoplasma pneumoniae*, *Chlamydia pneumoniae*, *Legionella pneumophila*, and *Haemophilus influenzae*. Cirrhosis has been associated with an increased risk of severe *Acinetobacter baumannii* community-acquired pneumonia (66). Sputum and blood samples should be obtained for appropriate diagnostic studies, including Gram stain (sputum) and cultures (sputum and blood). Appropriate empiric therapy while awaiting the results of cultures and other tests would include an expanded-spectrum cephalosporin plus a macrolide or a beta-lactam/betalactamase-inhibitor plus a macrolide or a fluoroquinolone (67).

Table 2 Risk Factors for Nosocomial Pneumonia Due to
Resistant Bacteria

Antimicrobial therapy in preceding 90 days
Current hospital stay ≥5 days
High frequency of antibiotic resistance in the community
  or hospital unit
Hospitalization ≥2 days in preceding 90 days
Residence in nursing home or extended care facility
Home infusion therapy (including antibiotics)
Chronic dialysis within 30 days
Home wound care
Family member with multidrug-resistant pathogen
Immunosuppressive disease and/or therapy

Source: Adapted from Ref. 67.

Hospital-acquired pneumonia may be caused by a wide variety of bacteria. Common pathogens include aerobic gram-negative bacilli, such as *Pseudomonas aeruginosa*, *E. coli*, *K. pneumoniae*, *Serratia marcescens*, *Enterobacter* species, *Proteus* species, and *Acinetobacter* species. *S. aureus* and *S. pneumoniae* predominate among gram-positive pathogens, and the incidence of MRSA nosocomial pneumonia is increasing. A number of risk factors have been identified for nosocomial pneumonia caused by multidrug-resistant bacteria (Table 2) (68).

Recommended initial empiric antibiotic therapy for nosocomial pneumonia in patients with no risk factors for multidrug-resistant pathogens or *P. aeruginosa* would be ceftriaxone or a fluoroquinolone or ampicillin/sulbactam or ertapenem. Patients with any risk factors listed in Table 2 or with onset of nosocomial pneumonia after four days of hospitalization are more likely to have infection due to multidrug-resistant pathogens. Initial empiric therapy in such cases should include an antipseudomonal cephalosporin (e.g., cefepime) or antipseudomonal carbapenem (e.g., imipenem) or piperacillin/tazobactam plus an antipseudomonal fluoroquinolone (ciprofloxacin or levofloxacin) plus vancomycin or linezolid if MRSA risk factors are present or there is a high incidence locally (68). Due to increased risks of aminoglycoside-induced nephrotoxicity and ototoxicity, the use of these agents should be avoided in cirrhotic patients if possible (30).

OTHER INFECTIONS

Vibrio Infections

Vibrio bacteria are gram-negative halophilic inhabitants of marine and estuarine environments. Typical infections caused by these organisms include gastroenteritis, wound infections, and septicemia. Infection usually occurs following consumption of contaminated food or water or by cutaneous inoculation through wounds. The most common pathogens include *Vibrio cholerae*, *V. parahaemolyticus*, and *V. vulnificus*. Preexisting liver disease is a major risk factor for *Vibrio* infections and has been associated with a fatal outcome in both wound infections and primary septicemia (69). *V. vulnificus*, the most virulent of the noncholera vibrios, can rapidly invade the bloodstream from the gastrointestinal tract. Classic clinical features of *V. vulnificus* sepsis include the abrupt onset of chills and fever followed by hypotension with subsequent development of disseminated skin lesions within 36 hours of onset. The skin lesions progress to hemorrhagic vesicles or bullae and then to necrotic ulcers (70). This syndrome is highly associated with a history of consuming raw oysters. The mortality rate exceeds 50%. Recommended antibiotic therapy includes using an expanded-spectrum cephalosporin plus a tetracycline (e.g., cefotaxime or ceftazidime plus doxycycline) or a fluoroquinolone (e.g., ciprofloxacin) (70).

Endocarditis

Infective endocarditis is a relatively unusual complication of cirrhosis. In the past *E. coli* and *S. pneumoniae* were commonly implicated in these infections. More recent studies have identified *S. aureus* as the most common pathogen along with other gram-positive bacteria such as the viridans streptococci and *Enterococcus* species (71,72). *Streptococcus bovis* biotypes [recently reclassified as *Streptococcus gallolyticus* (*S. bovis* I), *Streptococcus lutetiensis* (*S. bovis* II/1), and *Streptococcus pasteurianus* (*S. bovis* II/2)] are emerging as another important cause of bacteremia and endocarditis in patients with chronic liver disease (73,74). Endocarditis caused by *S. bovis* is commonly associated with bivalvular involvement and a high rate of embolic events.

Spontaneous Bacterial Empyema

Spontaneous bacterial empyema is an infection of a preexisting hydrothorax in cirrhotic patients. Although the majority of these patients have ascites, the presence of ascites is not a prerequisite for spontaneous bacterial empyema. SBP is present in approximately half of patients who develop empyema. The most common causes of spontaneous bacterial empyema include *E. coli*, *K. pneumoniae*, streptococci, including *Enterococcus* species, and *S. bovis*. A diagnostic thoracentesis is recommended in patients with cirrhosis who develop pleural effusions and signs and symptoms of infection (75).

REFERENCES

1. Navasa M, Rimola A, Rodés J. Bacterial infections in liver disease. Semin Liver Dis 1997; 17:323–333.
2. Navasa M, Rodés J. Bacterial infections in cirrhosis. Liver Int 2004; 24:277–280.
3. Johnson DH, Cunha BA. Infections in cirrhosis. Infect Dis Clin N Am 2001; 15:363–371.
4. Vilstrup H. Cirrhosis and bacterial infections. Romanian J Gastroenterol 2003; 12:297–302.
5. Sørensen HT, Thulstrup AM, Mellemkjar L, et al. Long-term survival and cause-specific mortality in patients with cirrhosis of the liver: a nationwide cohort study in Denmark. J Clin Epidemiol 2003; 56:88–93.
6. Deschênes M, Villeneuve J. Risk factors for the development of bacterial infections in hospitalized patients with cirrhosis. Am J Gastroenterol 1999; 94:2193–2197.
7. Soares-Weiser K, Brezis M, Tur-Kaspa R, et al. Antibiotic prophylaxis of bacterial infections in cirrhotic inpatients: a meta-analysis of randomized controlled clinical trials. Scand J Gastroenterol 2003; 38:193–200.
8. Singh N, Yu VL, Wagener MM, et al. Cirrhotic fever in the 1990s: a prospective study with clinical implications. Clin Infect Dis 1997; 24:1135–1138.
9. Rimola A, Soto R, Bory F, et al. Reticuloendothelial system phagocytic activity in cirrhosis and its relation to bacterial infections and prognosis. Hepatology 1984; 4:53–58.
10. Rajkovic IA, Williams R. Abnormalities of neutrophil phagocytosis, intracellular killing, and metabolic activity in alcoholic cirrhosis and hepatitis. Hepatology 1986; 6:252–262.

11. Gentry MJ, Snitily MU, Preheim LC. Phagocytosis of *Streptococcus pneumoniae* measured in vitro and in vivo in a rat model of carbon tetrachloride-induced liver cirrhosis. J Infect Dis 1995; 171:350–355.
12. Gentry MJ, Snitily MU, Preheim LC. Decreased uptake and killing of *Streptococcus pneumoniae* within the lungs of cirrhotic rats. Immunol Infect Dis 1996; 6:43–47.
13. Fierer J, Finley F. Serum bactericidal activity against *Escherichia coli* in patients with cirrhosis of the liver. J Clin Invest 1979; 63:912–921.
14. Lister PD, Mellencamp MA, Preheim LC. Serum-sensitive *Escherichia coli* multiply in cirrhotic serum. J Lab Clin Med 1992; 120:633–638.
15. Mellencamp MA, Preheim LC. Pneumococcal pneumonia in a rat model of cirrhosis: effects of cirrhosis on pulmonary defense mechanisms against *Streptococcus pneumoniae*. J Infect Dis 1991; 163:102–108.
16. Homann C, Varming K, Hogasen K, et al. Acquired C3 deficiency in patients with alcoholic cirrhosis predisposes to infection and increased mortality. Gut 1997; 40:544–549.
17. Alcantara RB, Preheim LC, Gentry MJ. The role of pneumolysin's complement-activating activity during pneumococcal bacteremia in cirrhotic rats. Infect Immun 1999; 67:2862–2866.
18. Baudouin B, Roucloux I, Crusiaux A, et al. Tumor necrosis factor α and interleukin 6 plasma levels in infected cirrhotic patients. Gastroenterology 1993; 104:1492–1497.
19. Preheim LC, Mellencamp MA, Snitily MU, Gentry MJ. Effect of cirrhosis on the production and efficacy of pneumococcal capsular antibody in a rat model. Am Rev Respir Dis 1992; 146:1054–1058.
20. Preheim LC, Snitily MU, Gentry MJ. Effects of granulocyte colony-stimulating factor in cirrhotic rats with pneumococcal pneumonia. J Infect Dis 1996; 174:225–228.
21. Caly WR, Strauss E. A prospective study of bacterial infections in patients with cirrhosis. J Hepatol 1993; 18:353–358.
22. Yoshida H, Hamada T, Inuzuka S, et al. Bacterial infections in cirrhosis, with and without hepatocellular carcinoma. Am J Gastroenterol 1993; 88:2067–2071.
23. Borzio M, Salerno F, Piantoni L, et al. Bacterial infection in patients with advanced cirrhosis: a multicentre prospective study. Digest Liver Dis 2001; 33:41–48.
24. Pugh RN, Murray-Lyon IM, Dawson JL, et al. Transection of the oesophagus for bleeding oesophageal varices. Br J Surg 1973; 60:646–649.
25. Rimola A, Navasa M, Arroyo V. Experience with cefotaxime in the treatment of spontaneous bacterial peritonitis in cirrhosis. Diagn Microbiol Infect Dis 1995; 22:141–145.
26. Runyon BA, McHutchison JG, Antillon MR, et al. Short-course versus long-course antibiotic treatment of spontaneous bacterial peritonitis. Gastroenterology 1991; 100: 1737–1742.
27. Runyon BA. Low-protein-concentration ascitic fluid is predisposed to spontaneous bacterial peritonitis. Gastroenterology 1986; 91:1343–1346.
28. Andreu M, Sola R, Sitges-Serra A, et al. Risk factors for spontaneous bacterial peritonitis in cirrhotic patients with ascites. Gastroenterology 1993; 104:1133–1138.
29. Rimola A, Garcia-Tsao G, Navasa M, et al. Diagnosis, treatment and prophylaxis of spontaneous bacterial peritonitis: a consensus document. J Hepatol 2000; 32:142–153.
30. Westphal J, Jehl F, Vetter D. Pharmacological, toxicologic, and microbiological considerations in the choice of initial antibiotic therapy for serious infections in patients with cirrhosis of the liver. Clin Infect Dis 1994; 18:324–335.
31. Rimola A, Salmerón JM, Clemente G, et al. Two different dosages of cefotaxime in the treatment of spontaneous bacterial peritonitis in cirrhosis: results of a prospective, randomized, multicenter study. Hepatology 1995; 21:674–679.
32. Franca AVC, Giordano HM, Seva-Pereira T, et al. Five days of ceftriaxone to treat spontaneous bacterial peritonitis in cirrhotic patients. J Gastroenterol 2002; 37:119–122.
33. Ariza J, Xiol X, Esteve M, et al. Aztreonam vs. cefotaxime in the treatment of gram-negative spontaneous peritonitis in cirrhotic patients. Hepatology 1991; 14:91–98.
34. Gómez-Jimenez J, Ribera E, Gasser I, et al. Randomized trial comparing ceftriaxone with cefonicid for treatment of spontaneous bacterial peritonitis in cirrhotic patients. Antimicrob Agents Chemother 1993; 37:1587–1592.

35. Grange JD, Amiot X, Grange V, et al. Amoxicillin-clavulanic acid therapy of spontaneous bacterial peritonitis: a prospective study of twenty-seven cases in cirrhotic patients. Hepatology 1990; 11:360–364.

36. Ricart E, Soriano G, Novella MT, et al. Amoxicillin-clavulanic acid versus cefotaxime in the therapy of bacterial infections in cirrhotic patients. J Hepatol 2000; 32:596–602.

37. Terg R, Cobas S, Fassio E, et al. Oral ciprofloxacin after a short course of intravenous ciprofloxacin in the treatment of spontaneous bacterial peritonitis: results of a multicenter randomized study. J Hepatol 2000; 33:564–569.

38. Navasa M, Follo A, Llovet JM, et al. Randomized, comparative study of oral ofloxacin versus intravenous cefotaxime in spontaneous bacterial peritonitis. Gastroenterology 1996; 111:1011–1107.

39. Soares-Weiser K, Brezis M, Leibovici L. Antibiotics for spontaneous bacterial peritonitis in cirrhotics. Cochrane Database Syst Rev 2001; (3): 1–16. Art. No.: CD002232.

40. Follo A, Llovet JM, Navasa M, et al. Renal impairment after spontaneous bacterial peritonitis in cirrhosis: incidence, clinical course, predictive factors, and prognosis. Hepatology 1994; 20:1495–1501.

41. Sort P, Navasa M, Arroyo V, et al. Effect of intravenous albumin on renal impairment and mortality in patients with cirrhosis and spontaneous bacterial peritonitis. N Engl J Med 1999; 341:403–409.

42. Titó L, Rimola A, Ginés P, et al. Recurrence of spontaneous bacterial peritonitis in cirrhosis: frequency and predictive factors. Hepatology 1988; 8:27–31.

43. Singh N, Gayowski T, Yu VL, et al. Trimethoprim-sulfamethoxazole for the prevention of spontaneous bacterial peritonitis in cirrhosis. Ann Intern Med 1995; 122:595–598.

44. Ginés P, Rimola A, Planas R, et al. Norfloxacin prevents spontaneous bacterial peritonitis recurrence in cirrhosis: results of a double-blind, placebo-controlled trial. Hepatology 1990; 12:716–724.

45. Grange J, Roulot D, Pelletier G, et al. Norfloxacin primary prophylaxis of bacterial infections in cirrhotic patients with ascites: a double-blind randomized trial. J Hepatol 1998; 29:430–436.

46. Fernández J, Navasa M, Gómez J, et al. Bacterial infections in cirrhosis: epidemiological changes with invasive procedures and norfloxacin prophylaxis. Hepatology 2002; 35:140–148.

47. Campillo B, Dupeyron C, Richardet J, et al. Epidemiology of severe hospital-acquired infections in patients with liver cirrhosis: effect of long-term administration of norfloxacin. Clin Infect Dis 1998; 26:1066–1070.

48. Ortiz J, Vila MC, Soriano G, et al. Infections caused by *Escherichia coli* resistant to norfloxacin in hospitalized cirrhotic patients. Hepatology 1999; 29:1064–1069.

49. Rabinovitz M, Prieto M, Gavaler JS, et al. Bacteriuria in patients with cirrhosis. J Hepatol 1992; 16:73–76.

50. Kuo CH, Changchien CS, Yang CY, et al. Bacteremia in patients with cirrhosis of the liver. Liver 1991; 11:334–339.

51. Barnes PF, Arevalo C, Chan LS, et al. A prospective evaluation of bacteremic patients with chronic liver disease. Hepatology 1988; 8:1099–1103.

52. Thulstrup AM, Sørensen HT, Schønheyder HC, et al. Population-based study of the risk and short-term prognosis for bacteremia in patients with liver cirrhosis. Clin Infect Dis 2000; 31:1357–1361.

53. Selby WS, Norton ID, Pokorny CS, et al. Bacteremia and bacterascites after endoscopic sclerotherapy for bleeding esophageal varices and prevention by intravenous cefotaxime: a randomized trial. Gastrointest Endosc 1994; 40:680–684.

54. Rolando N, Gimson A, Philpott-Howard J, et al. Infectious sequelae after endoscopic sclerotherapy of oesophageal varices: role of antibiotic prophylaxis. J Hepatol 1993; 18: 290–294.

55. Kulkarni SG, Parikh SS, Dhawan PS, et al. High frequency of bacteremia with endoscopic treatment of esophageal varices in advanced cirrhosis. Indian J Gastroenterol 1999; 18:143–145.

56. Rimola A, Bory F, Teres J, et al. Oral, nonabsorbable antibiotics prevent infection in cirrhotics with gastrointestinal hemorrhage. Hepatology 1985; 5:463–467.

57. Soriano G, Guarner C, Thomás A, et al. Norfloxacin prevents bacterial infection in cirrhotics with gastrointestinal hemorrhage. Gastroenterology 1992; 103:1267–1272.

58. Pauwels A, Mostefa-Kara N, Debenes B, et al. Systemic antibiotic prophylaxis after gastrointestinal hemorrhage in cirrhotic patients with a high risk of infection. Hepatology 1996; 24:802–806.

59. Hsieh W, Lin H, Hwang S, et al. The effect of ciprofloxacin in the prevention of bacterial infection in patients with cirrhosis after upper gastrointestinal bleeding. Am J Gastroenterol 1998; 93:962–966.

60. Soares-Weiser K, Brezis M, Tur-Kaspa R, et al. Antibiotic prophylaxis for cirrhotic patients with gastrointestinal bleeding. Cochrane Database Syst Rev 2002; (2):1–34, Art. No. CD002907.

61. Hirota WK, Petersen K, Baron TH, et al. American Society for Gastrointestinal Endoscopy. Guidelines for antibiotic prophylaxis for GI endoscopy. Gastrointest Endosc 2003; 58:475–482.

62. Silverio RH, Perini RF, Arruda CB. Bacterial infection in cirrhotic patients and its relationship with alcohol. Am J Gastroenterol 2000; 95:1290–1293.

63. Mandell LA. Epidemiology and etiology of community-acquired pneumonia. Infect Dis Clin N Am 2004; 18:761–776.

64. Austrian R, Gold J. Pneumococcal bacteremia with especial reference to bacteremic pneumococcal pneumonia. Ann Intern Med 1964; 60:759–776.

65. Gransden WR, Eykyn SJ, Phillips I. Pneumococcal bacteremia: 325 episodes diagnosed at St. Thomas's Hospital. Br Med J 1985; 290:505–508.

66. Chen M, Hsueh P, Lee L, et al. Severe community-acquired pneumonia due to *Acinetobacter baumannii*. Chest 2001; 120:1072–1077.

67. File TM, Garau J, Blasi F, et al. Guidelines for empiric antimicrobial prescribing in community-acquired pneumonia. Chest 2004; 125:1888–1901.

68. Niederman MS, Craven DE, Bonten MJ, et al. Guidelines for the management of adults with hospital-acquired, ventilator-associated, and healthcare-associated pneumonia. Am J Respir Crit Care Med 2005; 171:388–416.

69. Hlady WG, Klontz KC. The epidemiology of *Vibrio* infections in Florida, 1981–1993. J Infect Dis 1996; 173:1176–1183.

70. Chiang S, Chuang Y. *Vibrio vulnificus* infection: clinical manifestations, pathogenesis, and antimicrobial therapy. J Microbiol Immunol Infect 2003; 36:81–88.

71. McCashland TM, Sorrell MF, Zetterman RK. Bacterial endocarditis in patients with chronic liver disease. Am J Gastroenterol 1994; 89:924–927.

72. Hsu, Chen RJ, Chu SH. Infective endocarditis in patients with liver cirrhosis. J Formos Med Assoc 2004; 103:355–358.

73. Gonzalez-Quintela A, Martinez-Rey C, Castroagudin JF, et al. Prevalence of liver disease in patients with *Streptococcus bovis* bacteremia. J Infect 2001; 42:116–119.

74. Tripodi MF, Adinolfi LE, Ragone E, et al. *Streptococcus bovis* endocarditis and its association with chronic liver disease: an underestimated risk factor. Clin Infect Dis 2004; 38:1394–1400.

75. Xiol X, Castellví JM, Guardiola J, et al. Spontaneous bacterial empyema in cirrhotic patients: a prospective study. Hepatology 1996; 23:719–723.

22

Infections Associated with Diabetes in the Critical Care Unit

Larry I. Lutwick
Department of Infectious Diseases, VA New York Harbor Health Care System, and State University of New York Downstate Medical School, Brooklyn, New York, U.S.A.

INFECTION AND DIABETES

As reviewed succinctly by Rajbhandari and Wilson (1), it appears to be the case that there is a measurable increased incidence of infection in those who are diagnosed with diabetes. Indeed, they cite one study of U.S. factory workers that reported that 28% of workers with diabetes took 10 or more sick-days annually related to infection as compared to 10% of controls without diabetes (2). Additionally, certain specific pathogens appear to be more prevalent in the diabetic cohort, notably *Staphylococcus aureus* and *Candida* species.

The mechanism of increased infection rate in diabetics is multifactorial including direct effects of diabetes on the immune system. Among the defects found (1) have been a variety of polymorpholeukocyte function including those involving adherence, chemotaxis, and intracellular oxidative killing as well as impairment in aspects of cell-mediated immunity and monocyte function. Infection itself also produces increasing degrees of glucose intolerance. Indeed, it has been pointed out by many clinicians that a rising blood glucose is one of the earliest signs of an underlying infection.

This review concentrates specifically on a number of infections that often require intensive care and in which diabetes is most commonly associated with severe disease. The topic will be divided into those recognized and reported throughout the world and reported primarily in the developed world and those reported almost exclusively in parts of the developing world. The former category will consist of emphysematous pyelonephritis (EPN), gangrenous cholecystitis, rhinocerebral mucormycosis, and Fournier's gangrene. Malignant otitis externa, a locally invasive *Pseudomonas aeruginosa* of the external ear canal causing temporal bone osteomyelitis and cranial nerve involvement, is clearly a serious condition also linked to diabetes, but is not classically in need of intensive care unit care. Gangrenous cholecystitis, a more serious form of acute cholecystitis usually needing emergency cholecystectomy, is another entity that is at increased risk in the diabetic patient (3). The tropical group disorders discussed are melioidosis and tropical diabetic hand syndrome (TDHS).

LIFE-THREATENING INFECTION CHARACTERISTIC OF DIABETICS

Emphysematous Pyelonephritis

Urinary tract infections in the diabetic appear to be more common than in the nondiabetic host, though few prospective cohort observations assess this. Stapleton (4), in reviewing this topic, cited a number of observations that suggest that asymptomatic bacteriuria and symptomatic urinary tract infections are more common in the diabetic (especially the female diabetic). As an example, one study found that the incidence of urinary tract infections in postmenopausal women was twice as high in those who were diabetic (5). The same group (6) subsequently reported that during 1773 person-years of follow-up of postmenopausal women, 138 symptomatic urinary tract infections occurred (incidence, 0.07 per person-year) with diabetes being an independent predictor of infection (hazard ratio $= 3.4$; 95% confidence interval: 1.7–7.0). Another study found that asymptomatic bacteriuria occurred four times more frequently in the diabetic (7). Complications of these lower tract infections are more common in the diabetic including Candida infections as well as emphysematous cystitis and pyelonephritis (3).

EPN, a kidney infection associated with gas in and around the renal parenchyma, was first described by Kelly and MacCallum at the end of the 19th century (8) in a patient with pneumaturia. The infection is an acute necrotizing infection of the kidney itself. It is a relatively uncommon infection that continues to be associated with a high degree of morbidity and mortality. Although quite uncommon when one considers the overall number of urinary tract infections found in the diabetic host, 70% to 90% of cases of this entity occur in the diabetic (9). Most diabetic patient with EPN, but not all, have issues with adequate glucose control but not necessarily manifesting ketoacidosis (10). In those individuals without diabetes, the most common comorbidity is obstructive uropathy, but polycystic kidney disease, end stage nephropathies, and immunosuppression have been linked to it (11). Obstructive uropathy is generally found in a great majority of nondiabetics who develop EPN, and 50% of diabetics (11).

EPN, being more common in women, reflects the increased number of urinary tract infections in women as compared to men, diabetic or not. The left kidney appears to be the more common side affected (60%), and bilateral involvement occurs in the remaining 5% of cases (10). Its clinical presentation is similar to that of the more common acute pyelonephritis (nonemphysematous) with fever and chills associated with flank, costovertebral angle, and/or abdominal pain. More prominent symptoms can suggest EPN such as lethargy, confusion, low platelet count, increasing azotemia, and overt shock, all symptoms suggesting an ongoing sepsis syndrome. One uncommon but helpful physical finding is the presence of crepitation over the patient's flank with or without a clearly palpable mass (12).

The EPN is diagnosed radiographically (13) by visualizing gas in the renal parenchyma and the perinephric space. The gas is thought to be produced by the fermentation of the high tissue concentrations of glucose by the etiologic microorganisms. The gas can dissect further the subcapsular and perinephric spaces and can be found in the contralateral retroperitoneal space whether the other kidney is affected or not (11). It may even dissect along the psoas margin into the scrotal sac and the spermatic cord. The standard abdominal radiogram can reveal mottled collections of gas in and around the renal parenchyma. Radiographic staging has been proposed by Michaeli et al. (14):

> Stage 1: Gas in either the renal tissue or the pericapsular areas
> Stage 2: Gas in both the parenchyma and the pericapsular areas
> Stage 3: Extension through Gerota's fascia (the renal capsule) and/or bilateral disease

Nephrolithiasis may also be visualized, which may have been a significant comorbidity in the development of the EPN. Ultrasound and/or computed tomography (CT) may also reveal the gas patterns. Ultrasound is not as good as CT for elucidating the gas patterns and is a more operator-dependent procedure. CT is generally considered to be the diagnostic test of choice because it can well define the extent and amount of gas, can assess destruction of the renal tissue by the process, and can be useful in assisting the placement of one or more catheters for drainage. The destruction of the renal parenchyma may in part be due to infection per se but swelling of the kidney in its capsule, which may impair blood supply and/or renal vessel thrombosis, may play a role. Additionally, CT is an excellent technique for following the response to therapy as carbon dioxide is usually rapidly absorbed and prolonged persistence implies poor response (13).

Gas may be found entirely in the collecting system of a kidney, a condition referred to as emphysematous pyelitis. It can present similarly, albeit often less severely, is usually associated with diabetes as well, and generally has a lower degree of morbidity and mortality, but is not inconsequential, however. Gas may also be found entirely in the urinary bladder, so called emphysematous cystitis. This entity, which also can be linked with the diabetic host, is much more often associated with pneumaturia and can also be linked to fistulae from the colon or vagina communicating with the urinary bladder. This can be associated with either a malignant or nonmalignant process (i.e., diverticulitis).

The microbiology of EPN is quickly obvious on culture, but antimicrobial therapy should not be delayed awaiting culture results. The process is overwhelming due to the facultative enteric gram-negative bacilli, the most common of which in most studies is *Escherichia coli*, the most common cause of urinary tract infections overall. Other gram-negative bacilli to be commonly linked to EPN are *Proteus mirabilis* and *Enterobacter aerogenes*. In Shokeir's report (10), of the 15 patients who had blood cultures done, all of them grew the same bacterium (or bacteria as mixed infections may occur) that was also isolated from urine culture. Occasionally other gram-negative bacilli such as *P. aeruginosa* (a bacterium inherently more resistant to antimicrobials than some of the others) may be isolated, more often in cases associated with recurrent urinary tract infections in the past and with multiple courses of antimicrobial agents. Rarely, diverse organisms such as the yeasts, *Candida albicans* or *Cryptococcus neoformans*, anaerobic streptococci, and the phylogenetically confused *Pneumocystis carinii* have been reported to be associated with EPN (14).

The therapy needed for EPN has generally been considered to be active antimicrobial therapy, glucose control, and nephrectomy (10). Even with these modalities, an overall mortality rate of 30% to 40% may be found. In some less severe cases, however, medical therapy alone or combined with percutaneous drainage has been successful (15–17).

The initial choice of empirical antimicrobial agents, prior to culture results, can be quite vital in assisting in a favorable outcome. Rational choice requires the following:

1. Considering the common resistance pattern of gram-negative bacilli to antimicrobials in the geographic area of the patient. As an example, the

sensitivity to a fluoroquinolone may be much lower in New York City than in Kalamazoo.

2. Knowing the patient's history of antimicrobial sensitivity. If it is reported that a patient is allergic to an antimicrobial that might be considered for use then it is important to assess what the manifestation of allergy is. For example, nausea and vomiting after receiving an oral antimicrobial does not preclude its use especially parenterally. Likewise, a nonspecific drug–associated rash (maculopapular nonurticarial eruption) does not predict serious IgE-associated anaphylaxis if used again. Indeed, the incidence of anaphylaxis following no previous reaction to penicillin use is not different from after a nonspecific rash from penicillin.

3. Being cognizant of the so-called banana peel syndrome. This euphemism suggests broader initial antimicrobial therapy for individuals who are seriously ill, "one foot in the grave and the other on a banana peel." This does not at all preclude the narrowing of the spectrum of the therapy once the antimicrobial resistance pattern of the pathogen is known.

Rhinocerebral Zygomycosis

Rhinocerebral zygomycosis (RCZ, also referred to as rhinocerebral mucormycosis) is an acute and often fatal fungal infection of the nasal mucosa and adjacent cerebral parenchymal and vascular tissues. Although this infection can occur in seemingly healthy individuals, RCZ is, in general, linked to diabetics. The diabetic state is classically one with ketoacidosis. As an example, in a Mexican series of 22 cases of RCZ (of 36 cases of zygomycosis overall), 20 were in diabetics (18). In the diabetic cases, 10 had ketoacidosis, one had hyperosmolar coma, and nine were "stable." Other reviews report that between 60% and 80% of cases of RCZ had diabetes, with half of these with ketoacidosis. These organisms are associated with a ketone reductase system that facilitates the growth of the molds in high glucose, acidotic, and ketotic milieu (19).

The other two cases in the Mexican series had myelodysplasia and chronic renal failure as cofactors. Indeed, acute leukemia is associated with RCZ as well, and additional cases have been linked to severe malnutrition, steroid therapy, desferrioxamine toxicity, and severe burns. The demographics of other forms of zygomycosis (pulmonary, cutaneous, and disseminated) are much less likely to be associated with the diabetic state. *Rhizopus* species are the most commonly isolated agents of this severe infection, followed by *Absidia*, *Rhizomucor* and *Cunninghamella*. Laboratory confirmation of the identity of the organism is the only way to differentiate among the fungi. They are ubiquitous fungi that are common inhabitants of decaying matter. As an example, *Rhizopus* spp. can be recovered frequently from moldy bread.

The spores of these fungi causing RCZ gain entry to the body through the respiratory tract and presumably are deposited on the nasal turbinates. Normal human serum can inhibit the growth of *Rhizopus*. In contrast, serum obtained from patients with diabetic ketoacidosis is not inhibitory and may actually enhance fungal growth (20). Once the ubiquitous fungus begins to grow, the wide, nonseptate, right angle branching hyphae invade tissue and have a special affinity for blood vessels. Direct penetration and growth through the arterial blood vessel wall explain the propensity for thrombosis and tissue necrosis, major hallmarks of the pathology of this infection. Lymphatic vessels and nerves can also be directly invaded. Progressive infection dissects the internal elastic lamina from media of the artery, leading to extensive endothelial damage and thrombosis, causing infarction in the tissues supplied.

It appears clear that early recognition of the initial signs and symptoms of RCZ are quite important in management. The infection begins at the nasal mucosa and spreads quickly (within days) to the adjacent paranasal sinuses, the orbit, and via direct extension to the brain through the ethmoid bone or along penetrating vessels. The method of penetration into the brain may also be via the cribriform plate, which is thin and also has preformed pathways in the form of olfactory nerves passing through it, the roof of orbit, which is also very thin, or through the retro-orbital region. Cavernous sinus thrombosis and/or carotid artery involvement may occur.

Initial symptoms of RCZ include some degree of fever, altered vision, and facial swelling. In a patient with diabetic ketoacidosis, an alert diagnostician should suspect RCZ when the altered mental status of diabetic ketoacidosis does not improve within a day or so of correction of the metabolic abnormalities. Other symptoms include facial pain, headache, and nasal stuffiness. In a large review of 114 cases (21), no symptom was reported in more than 44% of affected individuals. On physical examination, invasion of the nasal mucosa with associated tissue infarction can produce a necrotic, black eschar, which may be visible. Early on, these lesions are visible in about 20% of patients, but close to 40% will develop them at some time (22). More lesions will be seen with the use of endoscopic examination as compared to routine rhinoscopy. Dark necrotic epistaxis may be the only visual finding (22). It is important to note that biopsy of this area may not demonstrate the organism, only infarction, because the fungi are generally found deeper in the tissue. Other physical signs of RCZ are facial edema and multiple cranial nerve palsies, as the infection spreads into the orbital apex. The orbital apex syndrome is associated with unilateral ptosis, proptosis, visual loss, complete ophthalmoplegia, maxillary and ophthalmic nerve anesthesia, and anhidrosis (23).

Plain roentgenograms of the sinuses and orbits can reveal sinusoidal mucosal thickening, with or without air-fluid levels. Erosion of bone through the walls of the sinuses or into the orbit can be found as the disease progresses. Destruction of bone in this region is often dramatically revealed by CT. Abnormalities in soft tissues involved in the disease process can also be visualized by CT scans and can be used to guide surgical intervention. If disease is seen, nasal endoscopy with biopsy from tissue is mandatory. The specimen should be sent for fungal staining (a 10% KOH mount may reveal the hyphal elements), fungal culture, and histopathology. Fixed tissue can be stained with hematoxylin and eosin, and fungal hyphae can be seen with this routine histologic stain. Grocott methenamine-silver or periodic acid-Schiff staining also adequately demarcates fungal elements in tissue in most cases.

Despite the availability of a variety of new azole antifungal medications (such as itraconazole and voriconazole) and echinocandins (caspofungin and micafungin), the standard drug for RCZ has remained to be amphotericin B (24). Because the agents of zygomycosis are relatively refractory to medical treatment, the maximum tolerated dose of the drug is used, typically 1.0 to 1.5 mg/kg/day. This dosage range is usually associated with renal function abnormalities, which can limit the use of the drug. There are some successful outcomes in patients with RCZ when treated with lipid preparations of amphotericin B (25). In RCZ, the recommended dose of lipid formulations of amphotericin B is 5 mg/kg daily. A new, broad-spectrum triazole, posaconazole (not yet commercially available in the United States), has been shown to be active in a murine model of zygomycosis (26).

Although patients recover from RCZ using antifungal therapy alone, these are clearly the exception, and aggressive surgical débridement of necrotic tissue is advisable. As reviewed by Sugar (24), some patients may recover with minimally disfiguring surgery. A medical-surgical approach, however, improves the chances of success. Repeated operations may be required for satisfactory removal of continuously appearing necrotic tissue. Major reconstructive surgery may also be necessary during convalescence if the patient survives. Although hyperbaric oxygen therapy has been utilized, this therapy is not routinely recommended at present (24).

Two factors determine the outcome in all patients: early diagnosis and resolution of predisposing problems (24). The overall mortality rate has been about 50% (24), although higher survival rates, up to 80% (2), have been reported more recently. This compares with survival rates of about 12% in 1961 (27). Yohai et al. (21) reported that treatment within six days of symptom onset produced a survival rate of about 80%, whereas delay for more than 12 days after onset of symptoms resulted in a ~40% survival rate. Diabetics (where the underlying hyperglycemia and ketosis can be reversed) had a 77% survival as compared with a rate of 34% in nondiabetics (21). Similar numbers have been reported in other studies (28).

Fournier's Gangrene

Necrotizing fasciitis was characterized by the Confederate Army surgeon Joseph Jones in the postwar period of 1871. When the process, a necrotizing, gas-producing infection spreading quickly along the fascial planes, involves the perineum (and scrotum in the male patient), it is referred to as Fournier's gangrene. It was first described by Alfred Jean Fournier, a Parisian venereologist, in 1843 (29).

Although single organisms (such as the Group A beta-hemolytic streptococcus) can be associated with necrotizing fasciitis, Fournier's gangrene is clearly a polymicrobial process including gram-positive cocci such as streptococci and facultative gram negative bacilli such as *E. coli* and *Proteus* as well as a variety of strict anaerobic bacteria including *Bacteroides*, *Peptostreptococcus*, and *Fusobacterium*. The process has been historically associated with diabetes among other risk factors. Other factors that may predispose to this progressive, destructive process include alcoholism, local pathology (such as rectal abscesses, hidradenitis, and urinary tract infections with strictures), blunt local trauma, postsurgical complications, and the injection of illicit drugs into the superficial penile veins (30). In one relatively recent report, diabetes was second only to perianal pathology as a predisposing cause of Fournier's gangrene (31).

An uncommon problem leading to intensive care for antimicrobial and surgical interventions has been estimated to occur in 1 in 7500 hospital admissions (32) or 1% of urological admissions in another (33). Usually initially beginning as pain and/or pruritus in or around the scrotum with fever and chills, the process quickly manifests as a cellulitic area in the scrotum or peritoneum with very prominent pain and marked systemic toxicity. This progresses quickly to prominent soft tissue swelling of the genitalia usually with subcutaneous crepitus. These changes can spread superiorly to the anterior abdominal wall, inferiorly to the anterior thighs and posteriorly to the perianal areas (33). Dark purple patches develop in the area and progress to extensive scrotal necrosis. At this point, local pain dramatically decreases, probably related to destruction of the sensory nerves. If it is not treated immediately, gangrenous sloughing of the tissue will ensue.

Radiographically, the detection of gas in the scrotal and perineal tissues increases from the yield by palpation of crepitus on examination (64%) (34) to 90%

on the standard X ray (30). The pattern of gas is sometimes referred to as a "honey-comb" scrotum. An ultrasonic examination of the scrotum (30) demonstrates prominent thickening of the scrotal skin with subcutaneous gas. Scrotal hernias can demonstrate gas on the scrotal ultrasound, but it is the gas in the hernial sac, not in the scrotal skin. Additional findings can be peritesticular fluid collections.

Treatment must include aggressive broad-spectrum antimicrobial therapy aimed at gram-positive cocci, facultative enteric gram negative, and strict anaerobes. The foul odor of the process supports a prominent role of anaerobes in the necrotic infection. Usual regimens include those aimed at usual bowel flora (antipseudomonal penicillins, carbapenems, or a combination such as ampicillin/sulbactam plus an aminoglycoside, aztreonam, or fluoroquinolone). Surgical intervention usually necessitates debridement of the scrotal sac and, often, bilateral orchiectomy. As in many necrotic deep tissue infections, after debridement extensive restorative and reconstructive surgery may be needed.

LIFE-THREATENING INFECTION CHARACTERISTIC OF DIABETICS IN THE TROPICS

Most reviews regarding critical care for infections in diabetics do not focus or even mention infections that are exclusively (or almost so) described in the tropics. Two of these will be discussed here, melioidosis and TDHS. Neither of these infections is well known in the developed world. Melioidosis is particularly relevant because it is considered to be a class B bioterrorism infection.

Melioidosis

The causal organism, *Burkholderia pseudomallei*, has, as many before it, gone through many name changes from *Loefflerella* or *Pfeifferella whitmori* and *Bacillus* or *Pseudomonas pseudomallei* to, in 1992, its current designation. The genus is named after Walter Burkholder who first characterized *Burkholderia cepacia* as a phyto-pathogen responsible for a root rot of onions. *B. pseudomallei* is a motile, aerobic, and nonspore-forming gram-negative bacillus.

Although primarily an intracellular organism, it readily grows on most solid media resulting in prominently wrinkled (rugose) colonies that may manifest an earthy-like aroma. Selective media are available for isolation as well. Gram stain of the bacillus can reveal the safety pin bipolar appearance often seen with *Yersinia pestis*. There are some *B. pseudomallei*–like organisms that are much less virulent. Formerly considered to be a separate biotype, these L-arabinoside assimilators are now classified as *Burkholderia thailandensis* and account for about a quarter of soil isolates in Thailand (35). *B. pseudomallei* is a hard-core survivalist organism nutritionally versatile to persist in triple-distilled water for long periods of time (36).

The organism exists in nature as an environmental saprophyte that lives in the soil and surface water in endemic areas (Southeast Asia and northern, tropical Australia), particularly in rice paddies (37–39). In endemic countries, the organism exists primarily in focal areas and is not equally distributed throughout the landscape. Sporadic cases have been reported to be acquired in parts of Africa and the Americas. Two recent outbreaks in Australia have also implicated potable water supplies rather than surface water as a potential source of the infection (40,41).

Melioidosis is a disease of rainy season in these endemic areas (37,42). It mainly affects people who have direct contact with soil and water. Many have an underlying predisposing condition such as diabetes (which overall is the most common risk factor), renal disease, cirrhosis, thalassemia, alcohol dependence, immunosuppressive therapy, chronic obstructive lung disease, and cystic fibrosis (42). Melioidosis may present at any age, but peaks in the fourth and fifth decades of life, affecting men more than women. In addition, although severe fulminating infection can and does occur in healthy individuals, severe disease and fatalities are much less common in those without risk factors.

Infection in humans is usually acquired by inoculation in an open wound or inhalation of aerosolized soil or water and not generally by ingestion. Although inhalation of aerosolized organisms causing pneumonia clearly occurs, pneumonia has also occurred following well-documented skin injuries (43), suggesting that the lung involvement can be related to bacteremic spread as well.

The incubation period after significant exposure to *B. pseudomallei* can be as short as one day but averages about nine days; however, because of "latency" (the mechanism of which is unclear) it can be up to 29 years. Recrudescent infections in veterans of the Vietnam War have given rise to the nickname "Vietnamese Time Bomb" (44). Despite the risk of reactivation, documented American cases were fairly uncommon as compared to the individuals exposed in Vietnam. An Australian study, in fact, suggested that only 3% of melioidosis infections were related to reactivation, and 97% to acute disease (45).

Melioidosis presents mostly as a febrile illness, ranging from an acute fulminant septicemia to a chronic debilitating localized infection to an unknown subclinical infection. As virtually every organ can be affected, melioidosis has been termed a "great imitator" of many other infectious diseases (46). The majority of infected patients are asymptomatic. The most commonly recognized presentation of melioidosis is pneumonia with high fever, myalgias, and chest pain. Although the cough can be nonproductive, respiratory secretions may be purulent, significant in quantity, and associated with intermittent hemoptysis. The process can be rapidly fatal with bacteremia and hypotension.

In addition to an acute pneumonia which may result in intensive care unit admission, chronic pulmonary infection may also be caused by *B. pseudomallei*, either as a continuum for acute disease or as reactivation years later. The presentation is quite similar to reactivation tuberculosis with upper lobe involvement associated with productive cough, weight loss, and hemoptysis.

Acute melioidosis septicemia is the most severe complication of the infection. It presents as a typical sepsis syndrome with hypotension, high cardiac output, and low systemic vascular resistance. In many cases, a primary focus in the soft tissues or lung can be found. The syndrome, usually in patients with risk factor comorbidities, is characteristically associated with multiple abscesses involving the cutaneous tissues, the lung, the liver and spleen, and a very high mortality rate of 80% to 95%. With prompt optimal therapy, the case fatality rate can be decreased to 40% to 50%.

In acute severe melioidosis, there is the rapid progression of respiratory failure that is due to acute respiratory distress syndrome and/or pneumonia. It has been suggested that the acute respiratory distress syndrome (ARDS) to melioidosis sepsis is more rapid in progression than with other bacteria and may be related to the intracellular interactions of the bacillus and the leukocyte (47). Bacteremia without shock/hypotension has a substantially better prognosis.

Abscesses can be found in many organs. Two organs that are particularly relevant in disease are the prostate and the parotid gland. Acute prostatic abscess may cause urinary retention. Residual prostatic abscess appears to be a potential focus for reactivation infection or relapse and unlike other visceral collection of melioidosis, unless the abscesses are large and accessible, ought to be definitively drained as needed. The purulent material obtained is yellow to tan in color and odorless. In focal melioidosis without bacteremia, the mortality rate is 4% to 5%.

The melioidosis bacillus is intrinsically insensitive to many antimicrobials. *B. pseudomallei* is usually inhibited by tetracyclines, chloramphenicol, trimethoprim-sulfamethoxazole (SXT), antipseudomonal penicillins, carbapenems, ceftazidime, and amoxicillin/clavulanate or ampicillin/sulbactam. Ceftriaxone and cefotaxime have good in vitro activity but poor efficacy (M35), and cefepime does not appear to be equivalent to ceftazidime in a mouse model (48).

Samuel and Ti (49) have reviewed the randomized and quasirandomized trials comparing melioidosis treatment and found that the formerly standard therapy of chloramphenicol, doxycycline, and SXT combination had a higher mortality rate than therapy with ceftazidime, imipenem/cilastatin, or amoxicillin/clavulanate (or ampicillin/sulbactam). The betalactam-betalactamase inhibitor therapy, however, seemed to have a higher failure rate. A more prolonged oral phase of treatment is used to decrease the risk of late relapse with a total period of therapy of 20 weeks. During the oral therapy phase, the conventional standard regimen appears to be equivalent to any newer therapies. Table 1 lists current treatment recommendations (50).

Tropical Diabetic Hand Syndrome (TDHS)

In the developed world, diabetic infections of the lower extremity remain a significant cause of morbidity leading to disability, prolonged hospital stays, and amputations of

Table 1 Treatment of *Burkholderia pseudomallei* Infection[a]

Initial parenteral therapy for severe infection (usual 14 day minimum)
Ceftazidime[b]: 40 mg/kg IV every 8 hrs (typical adult dose 2 g)
or
Imipenem/cilastatin[c]: 20 mg/kg IV every 6–8 hrs (typical adult dose 1 g) (note: IV amoxicillin/clavulanate or ampicillin/sulbactam can be used in every 4 hrs dosing but is associated with a higher failure rate)
Follow-up oral therapy (to complete 20 wks of treatment) (note: in mild, localized disease, oral therapy can be used for the entire 20 wks)
Doxycycline: 2 mg/kg orally (PO) every 12 hrs (typical adult dose 100–200 mg)
and
Trimethoprim-sulfamethoxazole (fixed 1:5 combination): typical adult dose two double strength (trimethoprim 320/sulfamethoxazole 1600) PO every 12 hrs
and
Chloramphenicol: 10 mg/kg PO every 6 hrs for the first 8 wks (typical adult dose 500–1000 mg) or (especially in children or pregnant women)
Amoxicillin/clavulanate (fixed combination 2:1): 10 mg/kg amoxicillin/5 mg/kg clavulanate PO every 8 hrs (typical adult dose 1000 mg/500 mg)
and
Amoxicillin: 10 mg/kg PO every 8 hrs (typical adult dose 1000 mg)

[a]Dosing may require adjustments in renal or hepatic dysfunction.
[b]Ceftriaxone and cefotaxime have good in vitro activity but a higher mortality rate and should not be used. No human data is found for cefepime.
[c]Meropenem, 1 g or 25 mg/kg IV every eight hours, may be used in lieu of imipenem/cilastatin.

toes, feet, and sometimes lower legs. It is not common, however, that such infections result in intensive care unit stays. Both in the developed and developing world, the most relevant risk factor in the diabetic appears to be an underlying peripheral neuropathy. This denervation of the sensory nerves of the foot impairs the perception of traumatic events (including ill-fitting shoes), resulting in the development of calluses, cracking soles, fissures, and other direct breakdown of the protective skin to produce ulcerations and infection. When combined with large and small vessel peripheral vascular disease and changes in polymorphonuclear leukocyte function associated with hyperglycemia, a range of infection may develop from cellulitis to deeper soft tissue infections to osteomyelitis related to deeper contiguous spread of infection (51).

In parts of the tropical world, however, a similar but even more aggressive infection, requiring intensive care unit, has been recognized. This severe and limb- and even life-threatening upper extremity sepsis is TDHS. This condition is far less recognized in the developed world but is a significant cause of both morbidity as well as mortality in parts of the African continent (52,53) and has been described in India as well (54).

Although a report of a similar syndrome was initially described in the United States (55), the African experience was first published in 1984 from Nigeria (56). In this study, 3% of 152 consecutive hospitalized diabetics were found to develop ulcerations of the hand and frank gangrene of the extremity. All of the five patients had progressive disease associated with initial trivial hand trauma. Importantly, none of the individuals had clinical evidence of either peripheral neuropathy or peripheral vascular disease. As reviewed by Abbas et al. who have published extensively regarding this entity, cases have been reported from a number of areas of the African continent including Tanzania, Kenya, and Libya (53). Many of the earlier studies were primarily descriptive so that risk factors were difficult to clearly elucidate, but proposed risk factors included insect bites or other minimal hand trauma, adult-onset diabetes, female gender, delayed seeking of medical care, poor glucose control, low socioeconomic status, and living near a coastal area.

In 2001, a case–control study of TDHS was reported from Das-es-Salaam, Tanzania (a coastal city) involving 31 patients and 96 control diabetics (52). Despite the previously postulated risk factors, this study found that on logistic regression analysis independent risk factors were low body mass index, type 1 diabetes, and peripheral neuropathy. The initial wounds reflected the spectrum of hand injuries including insect bites, burns, other traumatic injuries, and nonspecific papules. At the time of presentation of TDHS, more than 80% had had purulent hand ulcerations and almost 30% rapidly progressed to frank gangrene. Thirteen percent of the total needed arm amputation for progressive gangrene despite glucose control and antimicrobial therapy, and another 13% died from unbridled sepsis despite aggressive therapy.

In a subsequent report expanding the numerator of involved cases published in 2002 (57), 72 individuals fitting the case definition were included. The case definition was unchanged from previous reports and was any adult diabetic (greater than 18 years old) who had sought medical attention with cellulitis or other deeper infection of the hand with or without gangrene. Here 61% had type 2 diabetes, with an average age of 52 years (range 20–89), median interval of five years since the diagnosis of diabetes (two weeks to 19 years), low median body mass index, and generally high glucose levels. Of note, only 10 (14%) had evidence of peripheral neuropathy. In this study (57), at the time of presentation, each of the affected individuals had ulcerations with 85 of them purulent in nature, 32% had deep ulcerations involving bone, and a quarter already had localized or progressive gangrenous changes. The median time to presentation from perceived onset of symptoms was two weeks but was as short as two days and as long as 252 days.

In most of the reports regarding TDHS, little, if any, microbiological information is given, which could reflect the lack of adequate microbiological support. The Centers for Disease Control and Prevention report, from the same Tanzanian authors, however, notes that superficial swab cultures all revealed polymicrobial growth reflective of the pathogens often found in Meleney's synergistic gangrene. These organisms included gram-positive cocci such as staphylococci and streptococci and gram-negative bacilli such as *Klebsiella pneumoniae*, *E. coli*, and *P. aeruginosa*. No anaerobic flora were noted but were likely to be present.

It was felt that these superficial swabs were inadequate to guide the choice of antimicrobial agents and advised tissue biopsy cultures in this regard. In this study, half of the individuals required surgery, and of this, 44% had gangrene, and about half of these needed amputation of digits, hand or arm. More than half of the group able to be followed up had enough impaired hand function to affect their activities of daily living, and many reported severe, ongoing neuropathic pain.

REFERENCES

1. Rajbhandari SM, Wilson RM. Unusual infections in diabetes. Diabetes Res Clin Pract 1998; 39:123–128.
2. Wilson RM. Pickup J, Williams G, eds. Textbook of Diabetes. 2. Oxford: Blackwell, 1991: 813–831.
3. Fagan SP, Awad SS, Rahwan K, et al. Prognostic factors for the development of gangrenous cholecystitis. Am J Surg 2003; 186:481–485.
4. Stapleton A. Urinary tract infections in patients with diabetes. Am J Med 2002; 113(1A): 80S–84S.
5. Boyko E, Fihn S, Scholes D, et al. Diabetes mellitus and the risk of acute urinary tract infection among post-menopausal women. Diabetes Care 2002; 25:1778–1783.
6. Jackson SL, Boyko EJ, Scholes D, et al. Predictors of urinary tract infection after menopause: a prospective study. Am J Med 2004; 117:903–911.
7. Geerlings SE, Stolk RP, Camps MJ, et al. Asymptomatic bacteriuria may be considered a complication in women with diabetes. Diabetes Care 2000; 23:744–749.
8. Kelly HA, MacCallum WG. Pneumaturia. JAMA 1898; 31:375.
9. McDermid, Watterson J, van Eeden SF. Emphysematous pyelonephritis: case report and review of the literature. Diabetes Res Clin Pract 1999; 44:71–75.
10. Skokeir AA, El-Azav M, Mohsen T, El-Diasty T. Emphysematous pyelonephritis: a 15-year experience with 20 cases. Urology 1997; 49:343–346.
11. Stone SC, Mallon WK, Childs JM, Docherty SD. Emphysematous pyelonephritis: clues to rapid diagnosis in the emergency department. J Emerg Med 2005; 28:315–319.
12. Bonoan JT, Mehra S, Cunha BA. Emphysematous pyelonephritis. Heart Lung 1997; 26: 501–503.
13. Narlawar RS, Raut AA, Nagar A, et al. Imaging features and guided drainage in emphysematous pyelonephritis: a study of 11 cases. Clin Radiol 2004; 59:192–197.
14. Michaeli J, Mogle MJ, Heiman PS, Cains HS. Emphysematous pyelonephritis. J Urol 1984; 131:203–207.
15. Najjar M, Gouda HE, Rodriguez P, Ahmed S. Successful medical management of emphysematous pyelonephritis. Am J Med 2002; 113:262–263.
16. Chen MT, Huang CN, Chou YH. Percutaneous drainage in the treatment of emphysematous pyelonephritis: a 10 year experience. J Urol 1997; 157:1569–1573.
17. Cardinael AS, De Blay V, Gilbeau JP. Emphysematous pyelonephritis: successful treatment with percutaneous drainage. Am J Roentgenol 1995; 164:1554–1555.

18. Rangel-Guerra RA, Martinez HR, Saenz C, et al. Rhinocerebral and systemic mucormycosis. Clinical experience with 36 cases. J Neurol Sci 1996; 143:19–30.

19. Anand VK, Alemar G, Griswold JA. Intracranial complications of Mucormycosis: an experimental model and clinical review. Laryngoscope 1992; 102:656–662.

20. Gale GR, Welch A. Studies of opportunistic fungi: I. Inhibition of *R. oryzae* by human sera. Am J Med Sci 1961; 45:604–612.

21. Yohai RA, Bullock JD, Aziz AA, Mardert RJ. Survival factors in rhino-orbital-cerebral mucormycosis. Surv Ophthalmol 1994; 39:3–22.

22. Hendrickson RG, Olshaker J, Duckett O. Rhinocerebral mucormycosis: a case of a rare, but deadly disease. J Emerg Med 1999; 17:641–645.

23. Schwartz JC. Rhinocerebral mucormycosis. Three case reports and subject review. J Emerg Med 1985; 3:11–19.

24. Sugar AM. Agents of mucormycosis and related species. In: Mandell GL, Bennett JE, Dolin R, eds. Mandell, Douglas and Bennett's: Principles and Practice of Infectious Diseases. Philadelphia, PA: Elsevier, Churchill, Livingstone, 2005:2973–2984.

25. Strasser MD, Kennedy RJ, Adam RD. Rhinocerebral mucormycosis: therapy with amphotericin B lipid complex. Arch Intern Med 1996; 156:337–339.

26. Sun QN, Najvar LK, Bocanegra R, et al. In vivo activity of posaconazole against Mucor spp. in an immunosuppressed mouse model. Antimicrob Agents Chemother 2003; 46: 2310–2312.

27. Ferry AP. Cerebral mucormycosis (phycomycosis). Ocular findings and review of the literature. Surv Ophthalmol 1961; 6:1–24.

28. Blitzer A, Lawson W, Meyers BR, Biller HF. Patient survival factors in paranasal sinus mucormycosis. Laryngoscope 1980; 90:635–648.

29. Efem SE. The features and aetiology of Fournier's gangrene. Postgrad Med J 1994; 70: 568–571.

30. Morrison D, Blaivas M, Lyon M. Emergency diagnosis of Fournier's gangrene with bedside ultrasound. Am J Emerg Med 2005; 23:544–547.

31. Capitan Manion C, Tejido Sanchez A, Suarez Charneco A, et al. Fournier's gangrene. A serious infectious disease. Eur Urol Suppl 2003; 2:18.

32. Bejanga BI. Fournier's gangrene. Br J Urol 1979; 51:312–316.

33. Hejase MJ, Simonin JE, Bihrle R, Coogan CL. Genital fournier's gangrene: experience with 38 patients. Urology 1996; 47:734–739.

34. Smith MD, Angus BJ, Wuthiekanun V, White NJ. Arabinose assimilation defines a nonvirulent biotype of *Burkholderia pseudomallei*. Infect Immun 1997; 65:4319–4321.

35. White NJ. Melioidosis. Lancet 2003; 361:1715–1722.

36. Chaowagul W, White NJ, Dance DA, et al. Melioidosis: a major cause of community-acquired septicemia in northeastern Thailand. J Infect Dis 1989; 159:890–899.

37. Wuthiekanun V, Smith MD, Dance DAB, White NJ. The isolation of *Pseudomonas pseudomallei* from soil in northeastern Thailand. Trans R Soc Trop Med Hyg 1995; 89:41–43.

38. Strauss JM, Groves MG, Mariappan M, et al. Melioidosis in Malaysia. II. Distribution of *Pseudomonas pseudomallei* in soil and surface water. Am J Trop Med Hyg 1969; 18: 698–702.

39. Currie BJ, Fisher DA, Howard DM, et al. Endemic melioidosis in tropical northern Australia: a 10-year prospective study and review of the literature. Clin Infect Dis 2000; 31:981–986.

40. Currie BJ, Mayo M, Anstey NM, et al. A cluster of melioidosis cases from an endemic region is clonal and is linked to the water supply using molecular typing of *Burkholderia pseudomallei* isolates. Am J Trop Med Hyg 2001; 65:177–179.

41. Leelarasamee A, Bovornkitti S. Melioidosis: review and update. Rev Infect Dis 1989; 11: 413–425.

42. Suputtamongkol Y, Chaowagul W, Chetchotisakd P, et al. Risk factors for melioidosis and bacteremic melioidosis. Clin Infect Dis 1999; 29:408–413.

43. Currie BJ, Fisher DA, Howard DM, et al. The epidemiology of melioidosis in Australia and Papua New Guinea. Acta Trop 2000; 74:121–127.

44. Goshorn RK. Recrudescent pulmonary melioidosis. A case report involving the so-called "Vietnamese Time Bomb." Indiana Med 1987; 80:247–249.

45. Currie BJ, Fisher DA, Anstey NM, Jacups SP. Melioidosis: acute and chronic disease relapse and reactivation. Trans R Soc Trop Med Hyg 2000; 94:301–304.

46. Poe RH, Vassalo CL, Domm BM. Melioidosis: the remarkable imitator. Am Rev Respir Dis 1971; 104:427–431.

47. Puthucheary SD, Vadivelu J, Wong KT, Ong GSY. Acute respiratory failure in melioidosis. Singapore Med J 2001; 42:117–121.

48. Ulett GC, Hirst R, Bowden B, et al. A comparison of antibiotic regimens in the treatment of acute melioidosis in a mouse model. J Antimicrob Chemother 2003; 51:77–81.

49. Samuel M, Ti TY. Interventions for treating melioidosis (Cochrane Review). In: The Cochrane Library, Issue 4. Chichester, U.K.: John Wiley & Sons, Ltd., 2003.

50. Tolaney P, Lutwick LI. Melioidosis. In: Lutwick LI, Lutwick SM, eds. Bioterror: The Weaponization of Infectious Diseases. Towana, NJ: Humana Press. In press.

51. Lipsky BA. A current approach to diabetic foot infections. Curr Infect Dis Rep 1999; 1:253–260.

52. Abba ZG, Lutale J, Gill VG, Archibald LK. Tropical diabetic hand syndrome: risk factors in an adult diabetes population. Int J Infect Dis 2001; 5:19–23.

53. Abbas ZG, Gill GV, Archibald LK. The epidemiology of diabetic limb sepsis: an African perspective. Diabetic Med 2002; 19:895–899.

54. Bajaj S, Bajaj AK. Tropical diabetic hand syndrome—Indian experience. J Assoc Physicians India 1999; 47:1118–1119.

55. Mann RJ, Peacock M. Hand infections in patients with diabetes mellitus. J Trauma 1977; 17:376–380.

56. Akintewe TA. The diabetic hand—5 illustrative case reports. Br J Clin Pract 1984; 38: 368–371.

57. Centers for Disease Control and Prevention. Tropical diabetic hand syndrome-Dar es Salaam, Tanzania, 1998-2002. Morbid Mortal Wkly Rep 2002; 51:969–970.

23

Infection in Organ Transplant Patients in the Critical Care Unit

Patricia Muñoz
Clinical Microbiology and Infectious Diseases Department, Hospital General Universitario "Gregorio Marañón," Universidad Complutense, Madrid, Spain

Almudena Burillo
Department of Clinical Microbiology, Hospital Madrid-Montepríncipe, Madrid, Spain

Emilio Bouza
Clinical Microbiology and Infectious Diseases Department, Hospital General Universitario "Gregorio Marañón," Universidad Complutense, Madrid, Spain

INTRODUCTION

Solid organ transplant (SOT) recipients may require intensive care unit (ICU) admissions for different reasons in different moments of their evolution, and infection is the most important one. Between 5% and 50% of transplantation candidates must await transplantation in an ICU and, after the procedure, most of them spend a mean of four to seven days there for life support (1–6). If the ICU stay is prolonged due to postsurgical complications, the probability of acquiring a nosocomial infection increases significantly.

Most ICU days will take place during the period of deepest immunosuppression (7), but transplant recipients may require readmission to the ICU at any time due to infectious and noninfectious complications such as severe rejection, bleeding, organ dysfunction, etc. In fact, infections are the most common indication for admission of transplant recipients in emergency departments (35%), and severe sepsis (11.7%) is the most common reason for ICU utilization (8). Figures regarding infection and ICU admission show that one-half of all febrile days in liver recipients occur in the ICU, and 87% of these are caused by infection (9).

In a multicentric study in Italy, it was shown that most centers are not supported by an ICU exclusively dedicated to transplantation (10). Accordingly, many of these patients will be cared by physicians not always familiar with the specific problems posed by the transplant population. Our aim is to provide information and guidelines regarding most frequently encountered clinical scenarios relevant to critically ill infected SOT recipients. This chapter deals with the etiology, approach, and outcome of most common infectious complications intensive care specialists may

459

find when taking care of SOT recipients. Where no solid data were available, perspectives based on our own experience and opinion are presented.

INFLUENCE OF THE TYPE OF TRANSPLANTATION AND OF THE TIME AFTER TRANSPLANTATION

The incidence of infection after a heart transplantation (HT) ranges from 30% to 60% (with a related mortality of 4–15%), and the rate of infectious episodes per patient is 1.73 in a recent series (11). Infections are more frequent and severe than those occurring in renal transplant recipients, but less frequent than those occurring after liver or lung transplantation. The type of SOT and the time after transplantation may be useful clues to the clinician because, unless unexpected exposure has occurred, there is a timetable according to which different infections occur postorgan transplantation (12,13). According to it, although, for example, pneumonia can occur at any point in the posttransplant course, the etiology will be very different at very different points in time.

Importance of the Underlying Disease and Type of Transplantation

The type of organ transplanted, the degree of immunosuppression, the need for additional antirejection therapy, and the occurrence of technical or surgical complications all impact on the incidence of infection posttransplant.

Within each type of transplantation there are patients in which the risk of infection is greater. In HT, patients with prior ischemic cardiomyopathy experience more surgical complications, longer postoperative mechanical assistance, and are more susceptible to *Pneumocystis jiroveci* pneumonia (14,15) (Table 1). Incidence of infection is higher in pediatric thoracic transplantation than in adult patients (16).

After orthotopic liver transplantation (OLT), patients with prior fulminant liver disease fared the worst ICU course and cirrhotics the best (17). Thrombocytopenia

Table 1 Risk Factors for Infections in Heart Transplant Patients

Preoperative period	Intraoperative period	Postoperative period
Pulmonary hypertension not responsive to vasodilators	Prolonged operative time	Prolonged stay in intensive care unit
Critically ill status and mechanically ventilated patients at time of transplanation	Complicated surgical procedure	Mediastinal complications and need for reintervention
Renal insufficiency	Need for large number of blood transfusions	Prolonged hospitalization
Cardiac cachexia	Need for ventricular assist devices	Prolonged antibiotic use
Prior sternotomy	Presence of pathogens in the transplant allograft	Renal insufficiency
Donor's CMV positive serology		Induction therapy with with OKT3[R]
Older age		Immunosuppressive drugs and treatment of allograft rejection
Repeated hospital admissions		Immunosuppression due to concomitant viral infections
Lack of pathogen-specific immunity		Retransplanation
Latent infections in the donor or the recipient		

Abbreviations: CMV, cytomegalovirus.

of $< 50 \times 10^9$/L for three days is frequent after liver transplantation and as such was not found to be an important contributor to bleeding. The unique associated event identified for significant bleeding was sepsis (HR, hazard rate 34.80; 95% CI, confidence interval 1.47–153.40) (18). If severely ill patients with end-stage liver disease are selected appropriately, liver transplant outcomes are similar to those observed among subjects who are less ill and are transplanted electively from home (19).

Following lung transplantation, patients with obstructive lung disease, double lung transplant, or cystic fibrosis have a longer stay in the ICU and a higher risk of infection (2,20,21).

The type of SOT also determines the complexity of the surgery, the intensity of immunosuppression, and the most likely sites of infection. Lung and HT recipients are especially susceptible to thoracic infections, whereas intra-abdominal complications predominate in OLT or pancreas recipients. Patients receiving alentuzumab are more prone to suffer fungal infections (22).

Certain infections are characteristic of a particular type of transplantation, e.g., infections related to circulatory support devices (intra-aortic balloon pumps, ventricular assistance devices, and total artificial hearts) in heart transplant recipients (23–25) or endotipsitis in cirrhotic patients (26). Infections such as insertion site sepsis, endocarditis, pneumonia, candidiasis, or sternal infection may complicate 38% of support courses. Lung transplant recipients are admitted to the ICU most commonly due to respiratory deterioration requiring mechanical ventilation (59%) or due to suspicion of sepsis (35%) (27).

The use of extended donors does not seem to increase the risk of poor outcome (28). Some characteristics have been found to have a negative impact on liver graft survival (elderly donor with hypertension combined with the presence of metabolic acidosis, or a prolonged ICU donor stay) (29).

Time of Appearance of Infection after Transplantation

All SOT recipients share a number of conditions (end-stage organ failure, surgery, immunosuppressive regimens, etc.) that bring along a predictable time line of posttransplant infectious complications. The time of appearance of infection after transplantation is an essential component of the evaluation of the etiology of infection. Early infections occurring within the first month after transplantation are generally similar to nontransplant patients who have undergone major surgery in the same body area. Intermediate infections (two to six months) are usually caused by opportunistic microorganisms, such as cytomegalovirus (CMV), fungi, and multiresistant bacteria. Finally, late infections (after six months) may be caused either by common community pathogens in healthy patients or by opportunistic microorganisms in patients with chronic rejection (Table 2).

Early Infections

In the first month after SOT, patients are very susceptible to ventilator-associated pneumonia, IV catheter-related infections, surgical wound infection, or urinary tract infection (UTI) usually due to bacterial or candidal infections. Some of these may not be evident during the initial examination, which should be frequently repeated. If the patient is still intubated and the chest X ray does not reveal infiltrates, the possibility of tracheobronchitis or bacterial sinusitis should be considered. Staphylococci or enterobacteriaceae will cause most early infections. Gram positives predominate if quinolone prophylaxis is given. Herpetic stomatitis and infections transmitted with the allograft or present in the recipient may also appear at this time.

Table 2 Chronology of Most Common Infections or Causative Microorganisms in Severely Ill Solid Organ Transplant Recipients

Chronology of infection	Most common syndromes

Early infection (first month)	Bacterial infections
	  Pneumonia
	  Surgical wound infection
	  Deep infections near the surgical area
	  Intra-abdominal abscesses
	  Urinary tract infection
	  Catheter-related infection
	  Bloodstream infection
	  Antibiotic associated diarrhea
	Viral infections
	  Herpes simplex stomatitis
	  HHV-6 infections
	  Primary CMV disease
	Infections transmitted with the allograft
	Invasive aspergillosis or candidiasis

Intermediate infections (2–6 month)	Opportunistic infections: bacterial, tuberculosis, nocardiosis, invasive aspergillosis, other fungal infections, viral diseases, toxoplasmosis
Late infections (after sixth month)	Common community-acquired infections Respiratory tract infections Urinary tract infections Varicella-zoster infections CMV, adenovirus Other opportunistic microorganisms: listeriosis, Cryptococcus, *Pneumocystis jiroveci*

Abbreviations: HHV-6, human herpesvirus–6; CMV, cytomegalovirus.

Bleeding or anastomosis dehiscences may require a new surgical intervention. Prolonged ICU stay due to central nervous system (CNS) lesions or organ failure usually implies involvement of more resistant species such as vancomycin resistant enterococci (VRE), *Acinetobacter*, *Pseudomonas*, methicillin resistant *Staphylococcus aureus* (MRSA) or *Candida* (30). *Aspergillus* may also cause early infection in patients requiring prolonged admission to the ICU and who are especially difficult to diagnose (31).

Intermediate Period

From the second to the sixth month, patients are susceptible to opportunistic pathogens that take advantage of the immunosuppressive therapy. In this period we may expect infection with immunomodulatory viruses and with opportunistic pathogens (*Pneumocystis jiroveci*, *Listeria monocytogenes*, and *Aspergillus* species). Most life-threatening infections occur within the first three months. CMV is the most common pathogen after SOT. When no prophylaxis is given, 30% to 90% of patients will show laboratory data of "CMV infection" and 10% to 50% may develop associated clinical manifestations (CMV disease). However, CMV disease is readily diagnosed at present and seldom requires ICU admission. In our experience, only gastrointestinal and respiratory CMV has required ICU admission. Cultures for human herpesvirus (HHV)–6 should be ordered in patients with leukopenia. Some bacterial infections such as listeriosis may appear at this time as primary sepsis or meningitis.

Tuberculosis and nocardiosis are also characteristic of this second period (32). Aspergillosis (IA) may be encountered in patients with risk factors or massive exposure (33) and toxoplasmosis in seronegative recipients of a seropositive allograft (34).

Late Period

From the sixth month onwards SOT patients are susceptible to community-acquired infections if chronic rejection is not present. Herpes zoster virus, bacterial pneumonia, and UTI predominate. At this time, fever of unknown origin should be managed almost as in immunocompetent hosts. However, the aforementioned opportunistic infections may complicate this late period in patients with chronic viral infection, such as hepatitis B or C, which may progress to end-stage organ dysfunction and/or cancer. Patients requiring chronic hemodialysis, malignancy, or with late rejection are also susceptible to opportunistic infections (*Cryptococcus neoformans*, *P. jiroveci*, *L. monocytogenes*, etc.) in this timeframe (35).

Anamnesis and Physical Examination

Risk factors for infection should be carefully sought in all SOT patients admitted to the ICU because they may suggest an etiology and a clinical syndrome. The pretransplantation history, e.g., serological status against microorganisms such as CMV, hepatitis virus, *Toxoplasma*, etc., may yield valuable information. Previous infections or colonization, exposure to tuberculosis, contact with animals, raw food ingestion, gardening, prior antimicrobial therapy or prophylaxis, vaccines or immunosuppressors, and contact with contaminated environment or persons should be recorded (36,37). History of residence or travel to endemic areas of regional mycosis (38) or *Strongyloides stercoralis* may be essential to recognize these diseases (39). Exposure to ticks may be essential to diagnose entities such as human monocytic ehrlichiosis, which may be potentially lethal in immunosuppressed patients (40). Diagnosis may be confirmed by polymerase chain reaction (PCR) for *Ehrlichia chaffeensis*, serology, and by in vitro cultivation of *E. chaffeensis* from peripheral blood.

Certain complications may increase the risk of bacterial and fungal infection in the early posttransplant period. They include long operation (over eight hours), blood transfusion in excess of 3 L, allograft dysfunction, pulmonary or neurological problems, diaphragmatic dysfunction, renal failure, hyperglycemia, poor nutritional state, and thrombocytopenia (17,41–44). Intraoperative hypothermia increased the incidence of early CMV infection in liver transplant recipients (45). Blood cell transfusions have been associated with an increased risk of ventilator-associated pneumonia (46), and leukocyte reduction of all administered blood products during OLT was associated with an improved outcome demonstrated by both a decreased incidence of acute cellular rejection and length of hospital stay (47). Critically ill orthotopic liver transplant patients with kidney failure managed with a conservative anticoagulation policy and continuous venovenous hemofiltration (CVVH) have a much better outcome than acute renal failure (ARF) without orthotopic liver transplantation (OLTX) (48).

Fever in critically ill transplant recipients should be considered an emergency. In our opinion, a basic tenet of the management of a SOT with fever is that physical examination data should be directly obtained by the ID consultant, not relying on second hand information. This may be more useful than many expensive and time-consuming tests.

The oral cavity is frequently forgotten and may disclose previously unnoticed herpetic gingivo-stomatitis or ulcers. Within the exploration of the thoracic area, the consultant should visualize the entry sites of all intravascular devices, even if they "have just been cleansed." It should be remembered that the presence of inflammatory signs is suggestive of infection, although their absence does not exclude infection. Sepsis, without local signs, may be the initial sign of postsurgical mediastinitis. When the sternal wound remains closed, a positive epicardial pacer wire culture may be a clue to sternal osteomyelitis (49). Although unusual after SOT, cardiac auscultation and echography may help to detect endocarditis (50), and physical examination may occasionally disclose the existence of pneumonia, or empyema before abnormal radiological signs become evident.

The abdominal examination is always essential, especially in OLT recipients. The surgical wound is also a common site of infection and a cause of fever. Its presence requires rapid debridement and effective antimicrobial therapy and should prompt the exclusion of adjacent cavities or organ infection. The presence of ascites should be immediately analyzed and properly cultured to exclude peritonitis. We recommend bedside inoculation in blood-culture bottles due to its higher yield of positive results. Examination of the iliac fossa is particularly important after kidney transplantation. Tenderness, erythema, fluctuance, or increase in the allograft size may indicate the presence of a deep infection or rejection. Ultrasound or computed tomography (CT)–guided aspiration may facilitate the diagnosis. The possibility of colonic perforation in steroid-treated patients or gastrointestinal CMV disease should always be considered in intra-abdominal infections. It is important to remember that even very severe intestinal CMV disease may occur in patients with negative antigenemia, especially in patients on mycophenolate mofetil (MMF) (51).

Finally, skin and retinal examination are "windows" at which the physician may look in and obtain quite useful information on the possible etiology of a previously unexplained febrile episode. We have analyzed the value of ocular lesions in the diagnosis and prognosis of patients with tuberculosis, bacteremia, and sepsis (52,53). Cutaneous or subcutaneous lesions are a valuable source of information and frequently allow a rapid diagnosis. Viral and fungal infections are the leading causes of skin lesions in this setting. The entire skin surface should be inspected and palpated in SOT recipients with unexplained fever. The biopsy of nodules, subcutaneous lesions, or collections may lead to the immediate diagnosis of invasive mycoses and infections caused by *Nocardia* or Mycobacteria, among others.

An aggressive diagnostic approach is necessary when dealing with febrile compromised ICU hosts because it has been shown or documented that many infectious complications remain undiagnosed. In a recent study, complete agreement between pre- and postmortem diagnoses took place in only 58% of a total 149 patients. Two-thirds of all missed diagnoses were infectious, and disagreement was particularly prominent in the transplant population (complete agreement 17% and major error in 61%) in comparison with trauma patients (complete agreement 86%) or cardiac surgery group (69%). The majority of the missed diagnoses were fungal infections. Longer ICU stays increased the rate of error (31).

Approximately 25% of febrile episodes do not present with an evident focal origin and do not permit a straight syndromic approach (54). Therefore, it is essential to know the patient's antecedents, type of transplantation, and time after surgery. We systematically recommend to our residents to go over the viral, bacterial, fungal, and parasitic etiologies that should be excluded.

MOST COMMON CLINICAL SYNDROMES

Pneumonia

Pneumonia accounts for 30% to 80% of infections suffered by SOT recipients and for a great majority of episodes of fever in the ICU (41% of all febrile infections during the first seven days of ICU stay and 14% of those after seven days) (9). Pneumonia is among the leading causes of infectious mortality in this population. The incidence of pneumonia is higher in the early postoperative period, especially in the patients who require prolonged ventilation. The clinical presentation and the differential diagnosis are similar to those in other critical patients.

The incidence of bacterial pneumonia is highest in recipients of heart–lung (22%) and liver transplants (17%), intermediate in recipients of heart transplants (5%), and lowest in renal transplant patients (1–2%). The crude mortality of bacterial pneumonia in solid organ transplantation has exceeded 40% in most series (55).

Pneumonias occur in 13% to 34% of liver transplant recipients. Singh et al. have recently analyzed 40 OLT who developed lung infiltrates in the ICU (35). The etiology was pulmonary edema 40%, pneumonia 38%, atelectasis 10%, acute respiratory distress syndrome (ARDS) 8%, contusion 3%, and unknown 3%. The signs that suggest an infectious origin were clinical pulmonary infection score (CPIS) score >6 (73% vs. 6%), abnormal temperature (73% vs. 28%), and creatinine level >1.5 mg/dL (80% vs. 50%) (35). Methicillin resistant *Staphylococcus aureus*, *Pseudomonas aeruginosa*, and Aspergillus caused 70% of all pneumonias in the ICU (9). All *Aspergillus* and 75% of MRSA pneumonias, but only 14% of the gram-negative pneumonias, occurred within 30 days of transplantation. *Legionella*, *Toxoplasma gondii*, and *CMV* may also cause pneumonia in this setting (7,56).

Pneumonia is the most common infection following HT. Gram-negative pneumonia in the early posttransplant period is associated with significant mortality. In a recent multicentric prospective study performed in Spain, the incidence of pneumonia after HT was 15.6 episodes/100 HT (57). Most cases occurred in the first month after transplantation. Etiology could be established in 61% of the cases. Bacteria caused 91% of the cases, fungi 9%, and virus 6%. In another study, opportunistic microorganisms caused 60% of the pneumonias, nosocomial pathogens 25%, and community-acquired bacteria and mycobacteria 15% (58). Gram-negative rods caused early pneumonias (median nine days), gram-positive cocci (11 days), fungi (80 days), *Mycobacterium tuberculosis* and *Nocardia* spp. (145 days), and virus (230 days). *Legionella* should always be included in the differential diagnosis (59–62). Pneumonia increases the risk of mortality after HT (odds ratio (OR) 3.7, IC 95% 1.5–8.1, $P < 0.01$).

Lung infections are very common in lung and heart–lung transplant recipients. These patients have particular predisposing factors because the allograft is in contact with the outside environment, and have an impaired mucociliary clearance, ischemic lymphatic interruption, and abolition of the cough reflex distal to the tracheal or bronchial anastomoses. In fact, the anastomosis is especially vulnerable to invasion with opportunistic pathogens including gram-negative bacilli (Pseudomonas), staphylococci, or fungus. Lung transplant recipients with underlying cystic fibrosis may be prone to suffer infections caused by multiresistant microorganisms such as *Burkholderia cepacia*. In this group of patients perioperative antimicrobials are chosen on the basis of surveillance cultures. Pathogens transmitted from the donor may also cause pneumonia in this setting.

Pneumonia is less common after renal transplantation (8–16%), although it remains a significant cause of morbidity (63–65).

Most Common Pathogens in Transplant Patients with Pneumonia

We have already mentioned some data on the etiology of pneumonia in SOT recipients, but we will now review in more detail some of the most common groups of pathogens.

Bacteria. Although bacterial pneumonia may occur any time after transplantation, the period of greater risk is the first month after the procedure. Need for

Table 3 Probable Etiology of Pneumonia in Relation to the Type and Progression of the Infiltrates

Radiologic pattern	Acute[a]	Subacute
Consolidation	Bacteria (*Streptococcus pneumoniae* gram-negative rods, Legionella, staphylococci) Embolisms Hemorrhage CMV	Aspergillus, Nocardia, tuberculosis, drugs, *Pneumocystis jiroveci*, Legionella, HSV, VVZ, Toxoplasma
Interstitial	Edema, Transfusions (Bacteria)	Virus, *P. jiroveci*, drugs (Fungi, Nocardic, tuberculosis)
Nodular	(Bacteria, edema)	Fungi, Nacardia, tuberculosis (*P. jiroveci, CMV*)

[a]Acute: require attention in < 24 hr. Less common possibilities are among brackets.
Abbreviations: CMV, cytomegalovirus; HSV, herpes simplex virus; VVZ, virus waucella zoster.

mechanical ventilation and intensive care in this period are among the causes. The etiology will depend on the moment after transplantation, length of previous hospital stay, the days on ventilation, previous use of antimicrobial agents, and clinical and radiological manifestations (Table 3). Gram-negative rods predominate (*P. aeruginosa*, *Acinetobacter* spp., and *Enterobacteriaceae*) but gram-positive cocci (*S. aureus, S. pneumoniae*) account for a significant proportion of cases, as we mentioned before.

Legionella has been reported in 2% to 27% of SOT recipients with pneumonia (66–68). Most common species implicated are *Legionella pneumophila* and *L. micdadei* (69,70). A prodrome of influenza-like symptoms is followed by a sometimes "explosive" pneumonia with patchy lobular or interstitial infiltrates on chest radiograph. High fever, hypothermia, abdominal pain, and mental status changes are sometimes seen. Pneumonia is the most common presentation, but some patients have just fever (62). Other manifestations have also been described such as liver abscesses, pericarditis, cellulitis, peritonitis, or hemodialysis fistula infections (71). Infiltrate is usually lobar, but *Legionella* has to be included in the differential diagnosis of lung nodules, cavitating pneumonia, and lung abscess (59). Legionella infections can be overlooked unless specialized laboratory methodology (cultures on selective media, urinary antigen) is applied routinely on all cases of pneumonia (60). Routine culture of the water supply for *Legionella* is recommended in all transplant centers and ICUs with cases of Legionellosis (72). The use of impregnated filter systems may help prevent nosocomial Legionellosis in high-risk patient care areas (73).

The frequency of *M. tuberculosis* disease in receptors of solid organ transplantation in most developed countries ranges from 1.2% to 6.4%, but in transplant patients living in areas of high-level endemicity it might reach up to 15% (32,74–76). Although there is a huge regional variability, in general SOT incidence is 20 to 74 times higher than in the general population, with a mortality rate of up to 30%. The most frequent form of acquisition of tuberculosis after transplantation is the reactivation of latent tuberculosis in patients with previous exposure. Tuberculosis develops a mean of nine months after transplantation (0.5–13 months). Risk factors for early onset are nonrenal transplant, allograft rejection, immunosuppressive therapy with

(OKT3$^{®}$) anti-CD$_3$ monoclonal antibodies or anti-T cell antibodies, and previous exposure to *M. tuberculosis*. Clinical presentation is frequently atypical and diverse, with unsuspected and elusive sites of involvement. A large series of tuberculosis (TBC) in transplant recipients described pulmonary involvement in 51% of patients, extrapulmonary tuberculosis in 16%, and disseminated infection in 33% (32). In lungs, radiographic appearance may vary between focal or diffuse interstitial infiltrates, nodules, pleural effusion, or cavitary lesions. Manifestations include fever of unknown origin, allograft dysfunction, gastrointestinal bleeding, peritonitis, or ulcers. In transplant patients, *M. tuberculosis* infection was also described in skin, muscle, osteoarticular system, CNS, genitourinary tract, lymph nodes, larynx, adrenal glands, and thyroid (32,77). Ocular lesions may be an early way to detect dissemination (52). Coinfection with other pathogens is not uncommon. Treatment requires control of interactions between antituberculous drugs and immunosuppressive therapy. A high index of suspicion is recommended.

Rhodococcus equi (78) and *Nocardia* (79–83) are well-known causes of respiratory tract infection in transplant recipients. However, they usually present in a subacute form and rarely require ICU admission. These infections usually occur more than three months posttransplantation. Radiologically, they may appear as multiple and bilateral nodules, possibly due to their long-term silent evolution. The incidence of nocardiosis has been significantly reduced since the widespread use of cotrimoxazole prophylaxis. *Nocardia farcinica* may be resistant to cotrimoxazole prophylaxis and cause particularly aggressive disease (79).

R. equi is an opportunistic pathogen, which usually causes cavitated pneumonia in HIV-positive patients, but SOT recipients may be affected as well. Infection occurs usually late (median of 49 months after transplantation), and the lungs are primarily involved in most cases. Infection presents as a lung nodule in half of the patients. Clinicians should consider *R. equi* when evaluating a solid organ recipient with an asymptomatic lung nodule, particularly when cultures fail to identify Mycobacteria, *Nocardia*, or fungal organisms. Clinical microbiology laboratories should be alerted when a *R. equi* infection is suspected, because it could be mistaken for a contaminant diphtheroid and will not respond to the standard empirical therapy.

Fungal infections have been reported to occur in 5% to 20% of SOT recipients, and although they are decreasing proportionally, they increase in absolute figures as more transplantation procedures are performed each year. Rates vary according to the type of transplant recipient and are greatly influenced by the degree of immunosuppression, the use of prophylaxis, the rate of surgical complications, and rate of renal failure among the transplant population. Fungal pathogens more likely to cause pneumonia in this population are *Aspergillus*, *P. jiroveci*, *Candida* spp., and *Cryptococcus* spp.

Different types of transplantations imply differences in fungal infections (84). A recent series prospectively collected in Spain reported the incidence of invasive IA in SOT recipients, which ranged from 0.3% in kidney transplant to 3.9% in pancreas recipients (85). In lung and heart–lung transplantation, the incidence of fungal infections, most notably IA, ranged from 14% to 35% if no prophylaxis was provided, but has significantly decreased because aerosolized amphotericin B is given to these patients (86,87). In single lung transplant patients, invasive IA more commonly affects the native lung than the transplanted lung and may arise immediately postoperatively due to preexistent disease in pretransplant immunosuppressed patients. In lung and heart–lung transplant recipients the types of disease presentation include bronchial anastomosis dehiscence, vascular anastomosis erosion, bronchitis, tracheobronchitis, invasive lung disease, aspergilloma, empyema, disseminated disease, endobronchial stent obstruction, and mucoid bronchial impaction. Kramer et al. have described a distinct form of IA after lung transplantation: ulcerative tracheobronchitis, a semi-invasive disease involving the anastomosis site, and the large airways (88). Risk factors include CMV infection, obliterative bronchitis, rejection, and increased immunosuppression.

In HT, *Aspergillus* is the predominant fungal isolate and accounts for 38% of all lung nodular lesions (89). It appears a median of 50 ± 63 days after HT (90). We found that postoperative hemodialysis, CMV disease, reoperation, and other episodes of IA in the ward close to the transplantation date are the major risk factors for IA in this population. The use of oral itraconazole is an effective way of preventing this infection.

In liver transplantation, *Aspergillus* infection is less common when compared to lung or heart–lung transplant recipients, but is more commonly found than in kidney transplant recipients. In liver transplant recipients, IA usually is an early event, and most patients were still in the ICU with evidence of organ dysfunction when the disease was diagnosed (76,91). Retransplantation is also an independent risk factor (91,92), although IA may happen in low-risk patients if an overload exposure has occurred (33). Accordingly, ICUs caring for transplant patients should maintain a good quality of air control (93). Aspergillus may appear late after transplantation, mainly in patients with a neoplastic disease (94).

Pulmonary involvement is described in 90% of the cases, but CNS or disseminated manifestations may predominate (95). The isolation of *Aspergillus* from any SOT recipient sample is always a warning clue. Although the lung is the primary site of infection, other presentations have also been described (surgical wound, primary cutaneous infection, infection of a biloma, endocarditis, endophthalmitis, etc.).

Scedosporium species are increasingly recognized as significant pathogens, particularly in immunocompromised hosts. These fungi now account for ~25% of all non-Aspergillus mold infections in organ transplant recipients (96). *Scedosporium* species are generally resistant to amphotericin B. *Scedosporium prolificans*, in particular, is also resistant to most currently available antifungal agents. We found that 46% of *Scedosporium* infections in organ transplant recipients were disseminated and that patients may occasionally present with shock and sepsis-like syndrome (97). Fungemia is especially frequent when *S. prolificans* is involved. Overall, mortality rate for *Scedosporium* infections in transplant recipients in our study was 58%. When adjusted for disseminated infection, voriconazole as compared to amphotericin B was associated with a lower mortality rate that approached statistical significance ($p = 0.06$).

P. jiroveci (former *P. carinii*) is now rarely seen in SOT receiving prophylaxis. Before prophylaxis, incidence was around 5%, although it has been described to reach up to 80% in lung transplant recipients. *P. jiroveci* pneumonia was diagnosed a median of 75 days after transplant (range, 37–781 days). Clinical presentation was acute (less than 48 hours) with fever (89%), shortness of breath (84%), dry cough (74%), and hypoxia (63%). CMV was isolated from lung or blood in 74% of patients. Chest X ray usually showed interstitial pneumonia (84%). Some patients required ventilatory support. Mortality was 26%. Older age was the only significant poor prognostic factor (61 years vs. 49 years; $p < 0.03$) (15). Weekend prophylaxis (one double-strength tablet, 160/800 mg, every 12 hours on Saturdays and Sundays) has shown practically universal efficacy, also eliminating cases of Listeria or Nocardia infections.

C. neoformans affects the lung in 55% of SOTs with cryptococcosis (98). However, the disease is uncommon and appears a median of 24 months after transplantation (1 month to 17 years). An immune reconstitution syndrome–like entity may occur in organ transplant recipients with *C. neoformans* infection. This entity may be interpreted as failure of therapy. Immunomodulatory agents may have a role as adjunctive therapy in such cases (99).

Although Candida is frequently recovered from the lower respiratory tract of ventilated patients, *Candida pneumonia* is exceedingly rare (100). It has been reported in lung transplant recipients, and the diagnosis requires histological confirmation, because the recovery of Candida may represent colonization. In these patients, infection with Candida may be associated with very severe complications such as the necrosis of bronchial anastomoses (101–104).

CMV was the most common organism infecting the lungs in solid transplant recipients, but the incidence has significantly decreased with the widespread use of prophylaxis. CMV may be the sole causative agent of pneumonia after SOT or appear as a copathogen when other microorganisms are isolated (61). CMV pneumonitis commonly adopts a diffuse interstitial radiological appearance, but focal and even nodular infiltrates are described in up to one-third of patients. CMV may cause severe pneumonia with ARDS requiring ICU admission. In a recent study, in kidney transplant recipients, including 21 patients in this situation, it was found that among 13 surviving patients, the numbers of CD4+ and CD8+ T cells and their ratio increased as the patients recovered. In eight nonsurviving patients, the numbers of CD4+ and CD8+ T cells and their ratio was similar to day 0. It was concluded that the variations of CD4+ and CD8+ T lymphocytes and their ratio are useful indicators of the severity of disease and the outcome of patients with CMV infections accompanying ARDS after renal transplantation. Nevertheless, it may be helpful to evaluate the efficiency of ongoing treatment methods in these patients.(105) Herpes simplex (106,107) and virus vamcella zoster (VVZ) may also cause pneumonia in the transplant population. human herpes virus 6 (HHV)-6 has been reported to cause diverse clinical symptoms including fever, skin rash, pneumonia, bone marrow suppression, encephalitis, and rejection.

The respiratory viruses, particularly respiratory syncytial virus, influenza, para-influenza, adenovirus, and picornaviruses, are increasingly recognized as significant pathogens in these populations. Adenovirus may also cause pneumonia, occasionally with dysfunction of the allograft (108). Respiratory syncytial virus and influenza have been found to be the most common of the respiratory viruses causing severe infections in transplant recipients (109–115). New antiviral medications may bring improved outcomes of picornavirus infections in this population. Finally, a new virus, the human metapneumovirus, has recently been described and may be a significant respiratory pathogen in immunocompromised transplant recipients (116). Respiratory viruses may be associated with high morbidity, particularly in lung transplant recipients, and may appear as "culture-negative" pneumonia. Molecular methods such as reverse transcription-PCR assays allow the identification of respiratory viruses in bronchoalveolar lavage (BAL) specimens (117). Advances in prevention, particularly with regard to infection control practices, and to a lesser extent treatment, have had a substantial impact on the frequency and outcomes of this infection.

Considering the high mortality that some of these pathogens engender, the prompt detection of the etiology is of the utmost importance. As with other critical patients, differentiating pneumonia from other etiologies of pulmonary infiltrates can be extremely difficult. In liver transplant patients, a CPIS score >6, abnormal temperature, and renal failure (serum creatinine >1.5 mg/dL) were significant predictors of pneumonia (35). It is important to bear in mind that some drugs, such as sirolimus, may cause pulmonary infiltrates (118). Patients may develop dyspnea, cough, fatigue, and sometimes fever. Characteristic radiological changes are bilateral lower zone haziness. The presentation ranges from insidious to fulminant, and usually there is a rapid response to sirolimus withdrawal.

Chest X rays of transplant recipients with pneumonia predominantly show alveolar or interstitial infiltrates of variable extension. However, nodular lesions are not uncommon. The differential diagnosis of a lung nodule in a normal host includes many malignant and benign processes. However, in immunosuppressed patients the most common causes are potentially life-threatening opportunistic infections that may be treated and prevented. We have detected single or multiple lung nodules on the chest radiograph in 10% of our HT patients (89). *Aspergillus* infection was detected early after transplantation (median 38 days, range 23–158), whereas *Nocardia asteroides* and *Rhodococcus* infections developed only later (median 100 days, range 89–100). Nodules due to CMV occurred 16 to 89 days after HT (median 27 days). Patients with *Aspergillus* were, overall, more symptomatic and were the only ones in our series to present neurological manifestations and hemoptysis. CT is more sensitive than standard chest X ray in identifying the number of lesions and may assist guided biopsy.

Etiologic diagnosis is mandatory considering that only 50% of the empirical treatments of pneumonia in HT patients are appropriate (58). For this reason, fast diagnostic procedures that guide antimicrobial treatment are necessary. Etiologic diagnosis may be performed by using different techniques, so this requires careful tailoring to each single patient. Once pneumonia is identified, blood cultures, respiratory samples for culture of bacteria, mycobacteria, fungi and viruses, and urine for *Legionella* and *S. pneumoniae* antigen detection must be sent to the laboratory (if possible, before starting antimicrobials). The rate of expected bacteremia in patients with pneumonia is 16% to 29% (119). Demonstration of pathogenic microorganisms (*M. tuberculosis*, *Legionella*, *Cryptococcus* spp., *R. equi*, or *P. jiroveci*) in a sputum sample is diagnostic. PCR techniques may help improve diagnostic sensitivity (74). A bronchoscopic sample with bronchial biopsy is preferable for CMV, *Aspergillus*, or *P. jiroveci* pneumonia. If pleural fluid is present it should also be analyzed. In our series of nodular lesions in HT patients, etiological diagnosis was established within a median of eight days (1–24). A median of 1.8 invasive techniques per patient was necessary to achieve the diagnosis. Overall diagnostic yield was 60% for transtracheal aspiration, 70% for BAL, and 75% for transthoracic aspiration. BAL was the first positive technique in 58% of the patients. The only complications were a minor pneumothorax after a transbronchial biopsy and minor hemoptysis after a transthoracic needle aspiration. Direct microscopic examination of the respiratory samples (Gram stain, potassium hydroxide, or cotton blue preparations) was positive in three out of five cases of IA and in three out of four cases of Nocardiosis (89). A serum sample should also be submitted. Pneumonia is the infection with the highest related mortality rate, and this is also true for SOT recipients, so prompt empirical therapy is highly recommended for patients in critical condition after obtaining adequate samples. The selection of the empirical therapy will be guided by the characteristics of the patient and the clinical situation.

Postsurgical Infections

Complications in the proximity of the surgical area must always be investigated. Surgical problems leading to devitalized tissue, anastomotic disruption, or fluid collections markedly predispose the patient to potentially lethal infection. In the early posttransplantation period, renal and pancreas transplant recipients may develop peri-graft hematomas, lymphoceles, and urinary fistula. Liver transplant recipients are at risk for portal vein thrombosis, hepatic vein occlusion, hepatic artery thrombosis, and biliary stricture formation and leaks. Heart transplant recipients are at risk for medias-tinitis and infection at the aortic suture line, with resultant mycotic aneurysm, and lung transplantation recipients are at risk for disruption of the bronchial anastomosis.

Intra-abdominal Infection

In OLT recipients intra-abdominal infections may be responsible for 50% of bacter-ial complications and cause significant morbidity (120); they include intra-abdominal abscesses, biliary tree infections, and peritonitis. In nonabdominal transplantations, intra-abdominal infections may be caused by preexisting problems such as biliary tract lithiasis, diverticulitis, CMV disease, etc.

Risk factors for intra-abdominal complications after OLT include prolonged duration of surgery, transfusion of large volumes of blood products, use of a choledo-chojejunostomy (rous-en-Y) instead of a choledochostomy (duct-to-duct) for biliary anastomosis, repeat abdominal surgery of the biliary tract, dehiscence or obstruction, intra-abdominal hematomas, vascular problems of the allograft (for example the throm-bosis of the hepatic artery or the ischemia of the biliary tract may create the apparition of cholangitis and liver abscesses), and CMV infection. Occasionally, the complications will appear after the performance of some procedure such as a liver biopsy or a cholan-giography. These infections may be bacteremic, and in fact, OLT recipients show the highest rate of secondary bloodstream infections. Most common microorganisms include Enterobacteriaceae, enterococci, anaerobes, and Candida.

In a series published by Singh et al. biliary tree was the origin of 9% of infec-tions associated with fever in the ICU (9). Biliary anastomosis leaks may result in peritonitis or perihepatic collections, cholangitis, or liver abscesses (121–123). OLT recipients are especially predisposed to suffer cholangitis. Recent data suggest that duct-to-duct biliary anastomosis stented with a T-tube tends to be associated with more postoperative complications (124). A percutaneous aspirate with culture of the fluid is required to confirm infection. Culture of T-tube is unreliable because it may only reflect colonization.

Hepatic abscess is frequently associated with hepatic artery thrombosis (125). In one series, median time from transplant to hepatic abscess was 386 days (range 25–4198). Clinical presentation of hepatic abscess was similar to that described in nonimmunosuppressed patients. Occasionally the only manifestations are unex-plained fever and relapsing subacute bacteremia. In fact 40% to 45% of the liver abscesses are associated with bacteremia. Prolonged antibiotic therapy, drainage, and even retransplantation may be required to improve the outcome in these patients. Catheter drainage was successful in 70% of cases. Mortality rate was 42% (126). Ultrasonography and CT of the abdomen are the normal techniques to identify intra-abdominal or biliary infections. However, sterile fluid collections are exceedingly common after liver transplantation, so an aspirate is necessary to estab-lish infection.

Mediastinitis

In heart and lung transplant recipients the possibility of mediastinitis (2–9%) should be considered. HT patients have a higher risk of postsurgical mediastinitis and sternal osteomyelitis than other heart surgical patients (127). It may initially appear merely as fever or bacteremia of unknown origin. Inflammatory signs in the sternal wound, sternal dehiscence, and purulent drainage may appear later. The most commonly involved microorganisms are staphylococci, but gram-negative rods represent at least a third of the cases. Mycoplasma, mycobacteria, and other less common pathogens should be suspected in "culture-negative" wound infections (Thaler, 1992 #7537; Levin, 2004 #5135). A bacteremia of unknown origin during the first month after HT should always suggest the possibility of mediastinitis. Risk factors are prolonged hospitalization before surgery, early chest reexploration, low output syndrome in adults, and the immature state of immune response in infants. Therapy consists of surgical debridement and repair, and antimicrobial therapy given for three to six weeks.

Urinary Tract Infections

Urinary tract infections are the most common form of bacterial complication affecting renal transplant recipients (128,129). The incidence in patients not receiving prophylaxis has been reported to vary from 5% to 36% in recent series (130,131). However, it is not a common cause of ICU admission. The most common pathogens include Enterobacteriaceae, enterococci, staphylococci, and Pseudomonas. However, other less frequent microorganisms, like *Salmonella*, *Candida*, or *Corynebacterium urealyticum* pose specific management problems in this population. It is also important to remember the possibility of infection caused by unusual pathogens such as *Mycoplasma hominis*, *M. tuberculosis*, or BK and JC viruses. Unless another source of fever is readily apparent, any febrile kidney transplant patient with an abrupt deterioration of renal function should be treated with empiric antibacterial therapy aimed at gram-negative bacteria, including *P. aeruginosa*, after first obtaining blood and urine cultures (132). Prolonged administration of antimicrobial therapy has been classically recommended for the treatment of early infections, although no double-blind, comparative study is available (128).

Gastrointestinal Infections

Gastrointestinal symptoms are present in up to 51% of HT patients in recent series, although only 15% are significant enough to warrant endoscopic, radiologic, or surgical procedures. Possible manifestations include gastrointestinal bleeding, diarrhea, abdominal pain, jaundice, nausea or vomiting, odynophagia, or dysphagia. Hepatobiliary, peptic ulcer, and pancreatic complications are the most prevalent. Peritonitis, intra-abdominal infections, and *Clostridium difficile* colitis accounted for 5% of all febrile episodes in OLT in the ICU (9). Abdominal pain and/or diarrhea are detected in up to 20% of organ transplant recipients (119). CMV and *C. difficile* are the most common causes of infectious diarrhea in SOT patients.

CMV may involve the whole gastrointestinal tract, although duodenum and stomach are the most frequent sites involved (133). Infection of the upper gastrointestinal tract with CMV used to be a major cause of morbidity in transplant patients (134). In one series 53 out of 201 heart transplant patients had persistent upper gastrointestinal symptoms (abdominal pain, nausea, and vomiting). Of these 53 patients, 16 (30.2%) had diffuse erythema or ulceration of the gastric mucosa (14), esophagus (1), and duodenum (1) with biopsy results that were positive for CMV on viral cultures (incidence, 8%). All patients with positive biopsy results were treated with intravenous ganciclovir. Recurrence developed in six patients (37.5%) and required repeated therapy with ganciclovir. None of the 16 patients died as a result of gastrointestinal CMV infection. Other possible presentation symptoms are fever and gastrointestinal bleeding. Differential diagnosis should include diverticulitis, intestinal ischemia, cancer, and Epstein-Barr Virus (EBV)-associated lymphoproliferative disorders. A particular gastric lymphoma called mucosa-associated lymphoid tissue lymphoma may develop in renal transplant patients. It usually responds to the eradication of *Helicobacter pylori* (135). PCR is an accurate method for the detection of CMV in the mucosa of the gastrointestinal (GI) tract (136).

The natural history of CMV disease associated with solid organ transplantation has been modified as a result of the widespread use of potent immunosuppressants and antiviral prophylaxis, and late severe forms are now detected (137). Hypogammaglobulinemia may also justify severe or relapsing forms of CMV after solid organ transplantation (138).

C. difficile should be suspected in patients who present with nosocomial diarrhea. It is more common in transplant populations who frequently receive antimicrobial agents, and up to 20% to 25% of patients may experience a relapse (139–141). Incidence of *C. difficile* infection is increasing, even taking into account improved diagnosis and increased awareness. Most infections occur early after transplantation (140). The most important factor in the pathogenesis of disease is exposure to antibiotics that disturb the homeostasis of the colonic flora. Nosocomial transmission has also been described. SOT recipients have many risk factors for developing *C. difficile*-associated diarrhea (CDAD): surgery, frequent hospital admissions, antimicrobials exposure, and immunosuppression.

Most common clinical presentation is diarrhea, but clinical presentation may be unusually severe (142,143). In a recent series 5.7% of the kidney or pancreas transplant recipients developed fulminant CDAD that presented with toxic megacolon, and underwent colectomy. One of them died; the other patient survived after colectomy (144). Absence of diarrhea is a poor prognostic factor. In these cases significant leukocytosis may be a very useful clue. The infection may be demonstrated with a rectal swab. Occasionally patients present with an acute abdomen (145) or inflammatory pseudotumor (146).

The reference method for diagnosis is the cell culture cytotoxin test, which detects the presence of toxin B in a cellular culture of human fibroblasts (147), but recovering *C. difficile* in culture allows the performance of a "second-look" cell culture assay that enhances the potential for diagnosis (148). CDAD may pose important diagnostic problems in the transplant setting. Clinical presentation may be atypical and sometimes quite severe, differential diagnosis with other entities causing diarrhea in this population is required (CMV, adenovirus), and relapses may be difficult to manage. *C. difficile* colitis may occur in coincidence with CMV gastrointestinal infection, which may complicate the diagnosis (139).

The first step in managing diarrhea and colitis caused by *C. difficile* is discontinuation of the antibiotic therapy that precipitated the disease, whenever possible. About 15% to 25% of patients respond within a few days. Patients with severe disease should be treated with oral metronidazole or vancomycin. Oral metronidazole (500 mg tid or 250 mg every six hours) and oral vancomycin (125 mg every six hours) administered for 10 to 14 days have similar therapeutic efficacy, with response rates near 90% to 97%. When oral administration is not feasible, IV metronidazole should be used, because IV vancomycin is not effective. Nearly all patients respond to treatment in about five days. Comparison of metronidazole's activity with that of vancomycin in patients with moderately severe disease shows similar response rates. The former is preferred because of its reduced risk of vancomycin-resistance induction and lower cost. However, recent reports of very severe clinical forms suggest that vancomycin may be preferable for these especially virulent strains.

C. difficile strains resistant to metronidazole and with intermediate resistance to vancomycin have been described. The administration of probiotics such as *Saccharomyces boulardii*, or *Lactobacillus* sp. for prophylaxis of CDAD remains controversial, and we do not recommend it in critical patients because the occurrence of severe invasive disease by *S. boulardii* has been described (149).

As mentioned, a substantial proportion of patients (10–25%) have a relapse usually 3 to 10 days after treatment has been discontinued, even with no further antibiotic therapy. Relapse usually results from either a failure to eradicate *C. difficile* spores from the colon or due to reinfection from the environment. Nearly all patients respond to another course of antibiotics if given early. The frequency of relapses does not seem to be affected by the antibiotic selected for treatment, the dose of these drugs, or the duration of treatment.

Multiple relapses may be difficult to manage. Several measures have been suggested: gradual tapering of the dosage of vancomycin over one to three months, administration of "pulse-dose" vancomycin, use of anion-exchange resins to absorb *C. difficile* toxin A, administration of vancomycin plus rifampin, or administration of immunoglobulins.

Infectious enteritis is especially frequent in intestinal transplant recipients (39%). Viral agents are the cause in two-thirds of the cases. In a recent series there were 14 viral enteritis (one CMV, eight rotavirus, four adenovirus, and one Epstein–Barr virus), three bacterial (*C. difficile*), and three protozoal infections (one *Giardia lamblia* and two Cryptosporidium). The bacterial infections tended to present earlier than the viral infections, and the most frequent presenting symptom was diarrhea (150).

Immunosuppressive drugs, such as MMF, cyclosporine A, tacrolimus, and sirolimus, are all known to be associated with diarrhea. Rarely, graft-versus-host disease, lymphoproliferative disorder, de novo inflammatory bowel disease (IBD), or colon cancer may present as diarrhea. Flare-up of preexisting IBD is also not uncommon after LT. However, the cause of acute diarrhea remains unidentified in one of three patients (151).

Neurological Focality

The detection of CNS symptoms in a SOT recipient should immediately arouse the suspicion of an infection (152). Fever, headache, altered mental status, seizures, focal neurological deficit, or a combination of them should prompt a neuroimaging study (119). Noninfectious causes include immunosuppressive-associated leukoencephalopathy (153), toxic and metabolic etiologies, and stroke and malignancies (154). Therapy with OKT3 monoclonal antibody has been related to the production of acute aseptic meningitis [cerebrospinal fluid (CSF) pleocytosis with negative cultures, fever, and transient cognitive dysfunction]. Infectious progressive dementia has been related to JC virus, Herpes simplex, CMV, and EBV.

The most common cause of meningoencephalitis in organ transplant recipients is herpes viruses, followed by *L. monocytogenes*, *C. neoformans*, and *T. gondii*. HHV-6 is a neurotropic ubiquitous virus known to cause febrile syndromes and exanthema subitum in children. Less commonly, and particularly in organ transplant recipients, it may cause hepatitis, bone marrow suppression, interstitial pneumonitis, and meningoencephalitis (155). In a recent review, HHV-6 encephalitis occurs a median of 45 days (range 10 days to 15 months) after transplantation. Mental status changes, ranging from confusion to coma (92%), seizures (25%), and headache (25%) were the predominant clinical presentations. Focal neurologic findings were present in only 17% of the patients. Twenty-five percent of the patients had fever, occasionally reaching 40° C. CSF pleocytosis was generally lacking. Magnetic resonance images of the brain may reveal multiple bilateral foci of signal abnormality (nonenhancing involving both gray and white matter). HHV-6 can be detected in CSF by PCR or by viral isolation. HHV-6 viremia was documented in 78% of the patients. Overall mortality in patients with HHV-6 encephalitis was 58% (7 of 12); 42% (5 of 12) of the deaths were caused by HHV-6. Cure was documented in seven of eight patients who received ganciclovir or foscarnet for seven days, compared with 0% (zero of four) in those who did not receive these drugs or received them for < seven days ($P = 0.01$) (156). A growing body of evidence suggests that the more important effect of HHV-6 and HHV-7 reactivation on the outcomes of liver transplantation may be mediated indirectly by their interactions with CMV (157). HHV-6 viremia is an independent predictor of invasive fungal infection (158).

Cytomegalovirus infection of the CNS is quite uncommon in SOT recipients. It may affect the brain (diffuse encephalitis, ventriculoencephalitis, and cerebral mass lesions) or the spinal cord (transverse myelitis and polyradiculomyelitis). Diagnosis is very difficult and should be based on clinical presentation, results of imaging, and virological markers. The most specific diagnostic tool is the detection of CMV DNA by PCR in the CSF. Treatment should be initiated promptly if CMV infection is suspected. Antiviral therapy consists of intravenous ganciclovir, intravenous foscarnet, or a combination of both. Cidofovir is the treatment of second choice. Patients who experience clinical improvement or stabilization during induction therapy should be given maintenance therapy (159). Encephalitis caused by herpes simplex virus (HSV) has also been described (160,161).

Among causes of encephalitis, West Nile virus has emerged as an important cause of several outbreaks of febrile illness and encephalitis in North America over the past few years. In a recent report 11 transplant recipients with naturally acquired West Nile Encephalitis (WNE) were identified (four kidney, two stem cell, two liver, one lung, and two kidney/pancreas). Ten patients developed meningoencephalitis, which in three cases was associated with acute flaccid paralysis. All patients had CSF pleocytosis and WNV-specific immunoglobulin M in the CSF and/or serum. Magnetic resonance images of the brain were abnormal in seven of eight tested patients, and electroencephalograms were abnormal in seven of seven, with two showing periodic lateralized epileptiform discharges. Nine of 11 patients survived infection, but three had significant residual deficits. This viral infection should be considered in all transplant recipients who present with a febrile illness associated with neurological symptoms (162–164).

L. monocytogenes infections can occur at almost any time, although the most common occurrence is two to six months posttransplant (165). The incidence has significantly been reduced because prophylaxis with cotrimoxazole is used (15). Listeria infections may present as isolated bacteremia or with associated meningitis (166,167). OLT recipients may present with acute hepatitis (168). Brainstem encephalitis or rhomboencephalitis have been characteristically described in patients with Listeriosis, in which cranial nerve palsies or pontomedullary signs may be observed. Cerebritis/abscess due to *L. monocytogenes*, without meningeal involvement, is less common (169).

Incidence of cryptococcosis after organ transplantation is 0.3% to 6% (170–172). Cryptococcus is mostly a cause of meningitis, pneumonia, and skin lesions (173–176). However, more uncommon sites of infection have been also described in immunocompromised patients such as hepatic cryptococcosis in a heart transplant recipient (177). The patient developed fever, dyspnea, and signs of liver damage. Diagnosis was made with liver biopsy and with cryptococcal antigen in serum (177). Cryptococcosis is usually a late disease after transplantation, although rare fulminant early cases have been reported (178). CSF analysis usually reveals moderate pleocytosis. CSF cryptococcal antigen is positive in most patients. In a recent series 83 transplant recipients with cryptococcosis were analyzed. Patients with central nervous system infection (69% vs. 16%, $P = 0.00001$), disseminated infection (82.7% vs. 20%, $P = 0.00001$), and fungemia (29% vs. 8%, $P = 0.046$) were more likely to receive regimens containing amphotericin B than fluconazole as primary therapy. Survival at six months tended to be lower in patients whose CSF cultures at two weeks were positive compared to those whose CSF cultures were negative (50% vs. 91%, $P = 0.06$) (98).

Focal brain infection (seizures or focal neurologic abnormalities) may be caused by *Listeria*, *T. gondii*, fungi (*Aspergillus*, *Mucorales*, phaeohyphomycetes, or dematiaceous fungi), posttransplantation lymphoproliferative disease or *Nocardia*. Brain abscesses are relatively uncommon (0.6%) in SOT patients, and most of them (78%) are caused by Aspergillus (179), followed by *T. gondii* and *N. asteroides*.

Aspergillus brain abscesses usually occur in the early posttransplantation period. Most of the patients present with simultaneous lung lesions that allow an easier diagnostic way. Overall, disseminated *Aspergillus* disease has been described in 9% to 36% of kidney recipients, 15% to 20% of lung recipients, 20% to 35% of heart recipients, and 50% to 60% of liver recipients with IA (95,180). Disseminated infection with CNS involvement occurred in 17% of the cases studied in Spain. Clinical manifestations of CNS IA include alteration of mental status, diffuse CNS depression, seizures, evolving cerebrovascular accidents, and headache (95,181). The CSF is almost always sterile.

Toxoplasmosis was more prevalent when prophylaxis with cotrimoxazole was not provided (34,182). The incidence is higher in heart transplant recipients. The disease usually occurred within three months posttransplantation, with fever, neurological disturbances, and pneumonia as the main clinical features. Chorioretinitis may also be found (183,184). Diagnosis was established by serology and by direct examination, culture, or PCR of biological samples. In heart transplant recipients the diagnosis may be provided by the endomyocardial biopsy (185). The lesions of *T. gondii* are usually multiple, have preferential periventricular localization, and demonstrate ring enhancement. The donor was the likely source of transmission to most recipients (186). The mortality rate was high (around 60%). Obstructive urinary tract lithiasis involving sulfadiazine crystals has been described (187). Disseminated toxoplasmosis should be considered in the differential diagnosis of immunocompromised patients with culture-negative sepsis syndrome, particularly if combined with neurologic, respiratory, or unexplained skin lesion (188).

Other parasitic infections such as Chagas disease, neurocysticercosis, schistosomiasis, and strongyloidiasis are exceedingly less common (189).

Nocardiosis is usually observed between one and six months posttransplantation. The clinical presentation of nocardiosis includes pneumonia, CNS focal lesions, and cutaneous involvement (190–193). Brain abscesses due to Nocardia are multiple in up to 40% of the cases and may demonstrate ring enhancement. Diagnosis may be reached by direct observation of biological samples using modified Ziehl-Neelsen staining or Gram stain.

BSI, Catheter-Related Infections, and Infective Endocarditis

As other patients requiring intensive care, catheter-related bloodstream infections (CRBSI) are a potential threat for severe infection after SOT. In a recent study performed by our group in heart transplant recipients, CRBSI accounted for 16% of BSI in this population (194). In heart transplant recipients the incidence of bloodstream infection is 15.8%. Bloodstream infection (BSI) episodes were detected a median of 51 days after transplantation. The main BSI origins were lower respiratory tract (23%), urinary tract (20%), and catheter-related-BSI (16%). Gram-negative organisms predominated (55.3%), followed by gram-positive (44.6%). We found a clear relationship between time of onset and some characteristics of the BSI. During the first month after transplantation, 95% of the BSI were nosocomially acquired, and the main origins were intravenous (IV) catheter (32%), surgical site, and lower respiratory tract (LRT) (18% each). From month 2 to month 6, 70% of the BSI were nosocomially acquired, and the main origins were urinary tract infection (UTI) and LRT (25% each). After the sixth month, only 22% of the BSI episodes were nosocomial, and the most common portals of entry were LRT (33%), primary bacteremia (22%), and urinary tract infection UTI (17%) ($p = 0.1$). Mortality was 59.2%, with 12.2% directly attributable to BSI. Independent risk factors for BSI after HT were hemodialysis (OR 6.5; 95% CI 3.2–13), prolonged ICU stay (OR 3.6; 95% CI 1.6–8.1), and viral infection (OR 2.1; 95% CI 1.1–4). BSI was a risk factor for mortality (OR 1.8; 95% CI 1.2–2.8) (194).

CRBSI caused 15% of the febrile episodes of liver transplant recipients in the ICU (9). Although only 37% of the bacterial infections after liver transplantation occur more than 100 days after transplant, 60% of the cases of primary bacteremia after liver transplantation occur late (195). The incidence of BSI after OLT is 0.28 episodes/patient. BSI accounted for 36% of all major infections. Intravascular catheters were the most frequent source, and methicillin-resistant *S. aureus* was the most frequent pathogen causing bloodstream infections. In recent years a shift toward a higher importance of gram-negative microorganisms causing bacteremia has been observed (194,196). Gram-negative CRBSI, mainly if more than one case is detected, should always prompt exclusion of a nosocomial hazard, such as contamination of the infusate or transmission by the health-care workers (197,198).

Seventy percent of the catheter-related and all bacteremias due to intra-abdominal infections occurred ≤90 days, whereas 75% of the bacteremias due to biliary source occurred >90 days after transplantation. Length of initial posttransplant ICU stay ($p = 0.014$) and readmission to the ICU ($p = 0.003$) were independently significant predictors of bloodstream infections. Forty percent of the candidemias occurred within 30 days of transplantation and were of unknown portal, whereas the portal in all candidemias occurring >30 days posttransplant was known (catheter, hepatic abscess, and urinary tract). Mortality in patients with bloodstream infections was 52% (15/29) versus 9% (9/101) in patients without bloodstream infections ($p = 0.0001$). In conclusion, intravascular catheters (and not intra-abdominal infections) have emerged as the most common source of BSI after OLT (199).

In another study, primary (catheter-related) bacteremia (31%; 9 of 29 patients), pneumonia (24%; 7 of 29 patients), abdominal and/or biliary infections (14%; 4 of 29 patients), and wound infections (10%; 3 of 29 patients) were the predominant sources of bacteremia (200).

Most important risk factors for CRBSI is the length of catheterization. Most catheters used in critically ill SOT patients are short-termed. They include central venous catheters, temporary hemodialysis catheters, peripheral venous catheters, and arterial cannulas. The site of central venous catheterization (internal jugular vein vs. the subclavian vein) does not seem to have an impact on the incidence of related infections as long as catheterization is performed by experienced personnel (201). *S. aureus* nasal carriage is associated with a higher risk of bacteremia (54); active surveillance cultures to detect colonization and implementation of targeted infection control interventions have proved to be effective in curtailing new acquisition of *S. aureus* colonization and in decreasing the rate of *S. aureus* infection in this population (202). Strict adherence to prophylactic guidelines may help reduce the incidence of these infections.

Infective endocarditis is a rare event in SOT population (1.7–6%), but it may be an underappreciated sequela of hospital-acquired infection in transplant patients (50). The spectrum of organisms causing infective endocarditis was clearly different in transplant recipients than in the general population; 50% of the infections were due to *Aspergillus fumigatus* or *S. aureus*, but only 4% were due to viridans streptococci. Fungal infections predominated early (accounting for 6 of 10 cases of endocarditis within 30 days of transplantation), while bacterial infections caused most cases (80%) after this time. In 80% (37) of the 46 cases in transplant recipients, there was no underlying valvular disease. Seventy-four percent (34) of the 46 cases were associated with previous hospital-acquired infection, notably venous access device and wound infections. Three patients with *S. aureus* endocarditis had had an episode of *S. aureus* bacteremia more than three weeks prior to the diagnosis of endocarditis and had received treatment for the initial bacteremia of less than the duration of 14 days. The overall mortality rate was 57% (26 of 46 patients died), with 58% (15) of the 26 fatal cases not being suspected during life (50). CMV, toxoplasma, and parvovirus B19 may cause myocarditis in this population. Therapy of established infections is similar to that of other immunosuppressed patients.

Fever of Unknown Origin

Undoubtedly, the most common alarm sign suggesting infection is fever. In transplant recipients, fever has been defined as an oral temperature of 37.8°C on at least two occasions during a 24-hour period (9). Antimetabolite immunosuppressive drugs, MMF and azathioprine, are associated with significantly lower maximum temperatures and leukocyte counts (203). However, it is important to remember that fever and infections do not always come together. The absence of fever does not exclude infection. In fact, 40% of the liver recipients with documented infection (mainly fungal) were afebrile in a recent series (35). Absence of febrile response has been found to be a predictor of poor outcome in liver transplant recipients with bacteremia (200). In that series, the independent factors predictive of greater mortality were ICU stay at the time of bacteremia (100% vs. 47%; $P = 0.005$), absence of chills (0% vs. 53%; $P = 0.005$), lower temperature at the onset of bacteremia (99.2 F vs. 101.5 F; $P = 0.009$), lower maximum temperature during the course of bacteremia (99.3 F vs. 102 F, $P = 0.008$), greater serum bilirubin level (7.6 vs. 1.5 mg/dL; $P = 0.024$), presence of abnormal blood pressure (80% vs. 16%; $P = 0.0013$), and greater prothrombin time (15.6 seconds vs. 13.3 seconds; $P = 0.013$).

A major difference with immunocompetent critical patients is that the list of potential etiological agents is much longer and is influenced by time elapsed from transplantation. CMV (as main offender or as copathogen) should be considered in practically all-infectious complications in this population. Accordingly, a sample for CMV antigenemia (or PCR if available) should always be obtained. Other viruses such as adenovirus, influenza A, or HHV-6 may also cause severe infections after SOT and can be recovered from respiratory samples or blood. If indicated, invasive diagnostic procedures should be performed rapidly and a serum sample stored.

Bacterial infections must always be considered and urine and blood cultures obtained before starting therapy. Diagnosis of catheter-related infections without removing the devices may be attempted in stable patients. Lysis centrifugation blood cultures and hub and skin cultures have a high negative predictive value (204). The first steps for diagnosis of pneumonia should include a chest X ray and culture of expectorated sputum or bronchoaspirate (submitted for virus, bacteria, mycobacteria, and fungus). A CT scan or ultrasonography may also be ordered to exclude the presence of collections in the proximity of the surgical area. Lumbar puncture and cranial CT (including the paranasal sinus) must be performed if neurological symptoms or signs are detected. In case of diarrhea, *C. difficile* should be investigated. Cultures and PCR for detection of *M. tuberculosis* should be ordered for all transplant recipients with suspicion of infection.

Fungal infections should be aggressively pursued in colonized patients and in patients with risk factors. Early stages of fungal infection may be very difficult to detect (95,205). Isolation of *Candida* or *Aspergillus* from superficial sites may indicate infection. Fundi examination, blood and respiratory cultures and *Aspergillus* and *Cryptococcus* antigen detection tests must be performed.

Parasitic infections are uncommon, but toxoplasmosis and leishmaniasis should be considered if diagnosis remains elusive. Serology or bone marrow cultures usually provide the diagnosis. The possibility of a *Toxoplasma* primary infection should be considered when a seronegative recipient receives an allograft from a seropositive donor. HT recipients are more susceptible to toxoplasmosis, which may be transmitted with the allograft and occasionally requires ICU admission. The risk of primary toxoplasmosis (R-D+) is over 50% in HT, 20% after liver transplantation, and < 1% after kidney transplantation. Patients with toxoplasmosis have fever, altered mental status, focal neurological signs, myalgias, myocarditis, and lung infiltrates. Allograft-transmitted toxoplasmosis is more often associated with acute disease (61%) than with reactivation of latent infection (7%). Lethal cases associated to hemophagocytic syndrome have been described (206). Leishmaniasis is another parasitic infection that should be excluded, though it is exceedingly uncommon after SOT. It may present as fever, pancytopenia, and splenomegaly.

Multimodality imaging such the use of combined indium-labeled WBC scintigraphy and CT allowed the detection of infection within retained left ventricular assist device tubing in a heart transplant recipient with a diagnosis of fever of unknown origin (207).

Noninfectious Causes of Fever

Both infectious and noninfectious causes of fever should be considered when approaching a febrile SOT patient. In a recent series, 87% of the febrile episodes detected in OLT in the ICU were due to infections, and 13% were noninfectious (9). Rejection, malignancy, adrenal insufficiency, and drug fever were the most common noninfectious causes.

Fever is common in the first 48 hours after surgery and after certain procedures. If it is not persistent or accompanied by other signs or symptoms it should not trigger any diagnostic action. Acute rejection accounts for 4% to 17% of the noninfectious febrile episodes (208). It is usually related to an impairment of the allograft function and requires histological confirmation. It is more common in the first six months, especially in the first 16 days after transplantation in one study (209). It is important to remember that severe graft rejection and increased immuno-suppression could stimulate cooperatively active CMV (210,211).

Malignancy, mainly lymphoproliferative disease, is relatively common after SOT and may initially present as a febrile episode (80%) (212). It usually occurs longer after transplantation (208). Acute adrenal insufficiency should be excluded in SOT patients admitted to an ICU because of sepsis or surgery, mainly when corticos-teroids have been withdrawn and drugs that accelerate the degradation of cortisol (phenytoin and rifampin) are administered (213). However, although analytical adrenal insufficiency is frequent in SOT patients, prospective studies suggest that supplemental steroids are not needed in most cases even under stress (214–216). Another setting of potential adrenal insufficiency is renal transplants that return to dialysis (217,218). Occasionally, lymphoproliferative disease may present with adre-nal insufficiency after liver transplantation (219).

Drugs such as OKT3, antithymocyte globulin (ATG), everolimus, antimicro-bials, interferon, anticonvulsants, etc. may also cause fever in this population (220). The temporal relationship with the drug is usually a diagnostic clue. New induction therapies such as basiliximab are related to fewer side effects and fewer CMV infections (221).

Other causes of noninfectious fever include thromboembolic disease, hema-toma reabsorption, pericardial effusions, tissue infarction, hemolytic uremic syndrome, and transfusion reaction. Noncardiogenic pulmonary edema (pulmonary reimplantation response) is a common finding after lung transplantation (50–60%) and may occasionally lead to a differential diagnosis with pneumonia. It gives rise to prolonged mechanical ventilation and ICU stay but does not affect survival (222).

MANAGEMENT

Diagnostic Approach

As we mentioned before, the diagnostic approach to a critically ill SOT with sus-pected infection should take into account the time onwards from transplantation (Table 1) and previous complications such as episodes of rejection, surgical or tech-nical problems, reactivation of a latent infection, etc

The findings provided by the anamnesis and physical examination (see previous parts of this chapter) may suggest a focus causative of the fever (pneumonia, wound infection, etc.). In this situation, a list of possible pathogens as well as necessary samples and tests for diagnosis should be elaborated. In most cases, analytical and imaging studies will also be ordered. Samples for culture should be obtained before starting empirical antimicrobial therapy.

In a recent study, 79% of the infections associated with fever in the liver recipi-ents in the ICU were bacterial, 9% viral, and 9% fungal. Accordingly, blood cultures are practically always needed. Bacteremia is present in 45% of the febrile critical SOT patients, and its origin must always be investigated. In liver recipients the most com-mon sources are IV devices, lung, biliary tree, and wound infections. Accordingly, the entry site of the catheters must be examined. MRSA and *P. aeruginosa* caused 65% of the bacteremias in ICU patients (7). Lack of febrile response in bacteremic OLT reci-pients portended a poorer outcome (195).

In heart transplant recipients, the main BSI origins were lower respiratory tract, urinary tract, and CRBSI, which should always be investigated (194). If focal signs of infections are present, appropriate samples must be sent to the laboratory (catheter tips, wound exudate, CSF, etc.) as in any other critical patient. When a collection of fluid or pus is to be sampled, aspirated material provides more valuable information.

Length of stay in the ICU is also a determinant factor, which may help find the origin of the infection. Pneumonia is more common in the first seven days of ICU stay, while CRI incidence tripled after the first week.

Information on some of the most severe infections may be obtained rapidly when the clinician and the microbiology laboratory communicate effectively and the best specimen type and test are selected. Antigen detection tests for adenovirus, HSV, Influenza A, respiratory syncytical virus (RSV), rotavirus etc., are available. Most common herpesviruses can be easily cultured and detected. Gram stain requires expertise but may provide valuable rapid information (five minutes) on the quality of the specimen and whether gram-negative or positive rods or cocci are present. It may reveal yeasts and occasionally molds, parasites, *Nocardia*, and even mycobacteria. The amount of material and the number of organisms limit detection sensitivity. Continuous agitation blood cultures have significantly reduced the detection time to less than 24 hours for bacterial isolates.

Direct testing of specimens with antigen assays are mainly used for CSF samples (*Neisseria meningitidis*, *S. pneumoniae*, and *C. neoformans*). Group A streptococci, *C. difficile*, and *C. trachomatis* antigen detection tests are also available. Specific stains for *Legionella* direct fluorescence assay (DFA) and *Bordetella pertussis* are offered by most laboratories. *Legionella* urinary antigen test will be very useful in pneumonias caused by *L. pneumophila* serotype 1, and *S. pneumoniae* antigenuria can also be rapidly investigated. HIV infection, *Brucella*, and syphilis are some of the infections that can be rapidly diagnosed serologically.

Acid-fast stain and fluorochrome stains for mycobacteria or *Nocardia* require a more prolonged laboratory procedure (30–60 minutes). New techniques, such as PCR and quantification of interferon-gamma, have been developed to achieve more rapid and accurate diagnoses. *M. tuberculosis* complex PCR is very effective in smear-positive specimens. In smear-negative samples sensitivity is ~70% (74).

Fungal elements may be rapidly detected in wet mounts with potassium hydroxide or immunofluorescent Calcofluor white stain. An India ink preparation allows the identification of encapsulated *C. neoformans*, particularly in CSF in approximately 50% of patients. The latex agglutination test or enzyme immunoassay (EIA) cryptococcal antigen have greater sensitivity. Fluorescent antibody stains or toluidine blue O permits the detection of *P. jiroveci*. Antigen detection for *Histoplasma capsulatum* is quite sensitive, and the detection of *Aspergillus* antigen is useful, although its efficiency is lower than in hematological patients (223–225).

Management

Fever is not harmful by itself, and accordingly it should not be systematically eliminated. In fact, it has been demonstrated that fever enhances several host defense mechanisms (chemotaxis, phagocytosis, and opsonization) (119). Besides, antibiotics may be more active at higher body temperatures. If provided, antipyretic drugs should be administered at regular intervals to avoid recurrent shivering and an associated increase in metabolic demand.

After obtaining the previously mentioned samples, empiric antibiotics should be promptly started in all transplant patients with suspicion of infection and toxic or unstable situation. They are also recommended if a focus of infection is apparent, in the early posttransplant setting in which nosocomial infection is very common, or when there has been a recent increase of immunosuppression. In a stable patient without a clear source of infection further diagnostic testing should carried out and noninfectious causes considered.

We have recently demonstrated that only 58.5% of patients with BSI received appropriate empirical antimicrobial therapy. Inadequate treatment was related to a longer hospital stay, a higher mean risk of CDAD, a higher mean overall mortality rate, and a higher risk of infection-related mortality (226). So once blood cultures are obtained, empirical broad-spectrum antimicrobials guided by the clinical condition of the patient and the presumed origin should be promptly started. When results of blood cultures are available, antibiotics should be adjusted according to susceptibility patterns of the isolates. This antibacterial de-escalation strategy attempts to balance the need to provide appropriate, initial antibacterial treatment while limiting the emergence of antibacterial resistance.

The selection of the antimicrobial should be based on the likely origin of the infection, prevalent bacterial flora, rate of antimicrobial resistance, and previous use of antimicrobials by the patient. In our series of bacteremia in HT recipients gram-negative microorganisms predominated (55.3%), followed by gram-positive microorganisms (44.6%). Gram-negatives accounted for 54% of infections in the first month, 50% during months 2 to 6, and 72% of infections occurring afterwards ($p = 0.3$) (194).

The possibility of drug interactions mainly with cyclosporine and tacrolimus is very real and impacts significantly on the choice of antimicrobial. There are three categories of antimicrobial interaction with cyclosporine and tacrolimus. First, the antimicrobial agent (e.g., rifampin, isoniazid, and nafcillin) upregulates the metabolism of the immunosuppressive drugs, resulting in decreased blood levels and an increased possibility of allograft rejection. Second, the antimicrobial agent (e.g., the macrolides erythromycin, clarithromycin, and to a lesser extent azithromycin, or the azoles ketoconazole, itraconazole, and to a lesser extent fluconazole) down-regulates the metabolism of the immunosuppressive drugs, resulting in increased blood levels and an increased possibility of nephrotoxicity and overimmunosuppression. And last, there may be synergistic nephrotoxicity, when therapeutic levels of the immunosuppressive agents are combined with therapeutic levels of aminoglycosides, amphotericin, and vancomycin, and high therapeutic doses of trimethoprim-sulfamethoxazole and fluoroquinolones.

Outcome of Febrile Processes of SOT Recipients in the ICU

SOT patients have higher risk of dying after an ICU admission than the general population, and in most series it is a poor prognostic factor (227,228). However, the overall prognosis is better than that of bone marrow recipients (229–231). The overall ICU mortality of SOT patients was 18% in a recent series, and infection was the major cause of death (disseminated mycoses, hepatitis C virus (HCV), multi-organic failure, hepatic artery thrombosis with sepsis, and primary nonfunction of the graft).

Mortality of febrile liver recipients at 14 days (24% vs. 0%, $p = 0.001$) and at 30 days (34% vs. 5%, $p = 0.001$) was significantly higher in the ICU, as compared to non-ICU patients (9). Mortality of OLT with lung infiltrates in the ICU was 28%. Pneumonia, creatinine level $> 1.5\,mg/dL$, higher blood urea nitrogen, and worse acute physiology and chronic health evaluation (APACHE) neurological score were predictors of poor outcome (35). The need for mechanical ventilation was an independently significant predictor of mortality (7). Infection was a risk factor for early renal dysfunction (232). Need for preoperative ICU care was predictive of an increased risk of death in OLT patients waiting for retransplantation (228).

Infection is also a leading cause of death in heart recipients (30% of early deaths, 45% of deaths from one to three months, and 9.7% thereafter) (233). Overall, 31% of the patients with pneumonia died (*Aspergillus* 62%; CMV 13%; nosocomial bacteria 26%). Mortality was 100% in patients requiring mechanical ventilation (7 out of 13 *Aspergillus*, 5 out of 11 *P. carinii*, 1 out of 8 CMV) (58). From 51 lung transplant recipients who required admission to the ICU at the Duke University Medical Center, 53% required mechanical ventilation, and 37% died (59% of those requiring mechanical ventilation) (234). In other series, mortality of lung transplant recipients requiring admission to a medical intensive care unit (MICU) was 37%. A preadmission diagnosis of bronchiolitis obliterans syndrome, APACHE III scores, nonpulmonary organ system dysfunction, initial serum albumin level, and duration of mechanical ventilation are important prognostic factors (27). Mortality of renal transplant recipients in the ICU was 11% in a recent series, and infection caused six out of seven deaths (235).

PREVENTION

Organ transplant patients admitted to the ICU should receive all measures available to prevent nosocomial infection. The first one could be "avoid the admission to the unit itself," which has been demonstrated to be a very stress-inducing situation for transplant recipients (236). In one recent study it was determined the proportion of liver transplant patients who could be extubated immediately after surgery and transferred to the surgical ward without intervening ICU care. Of 147 patients, 36 patients did not meet postsurgical criteria for early extubation, and 111 patients were successfully extubated. Eighty-three extubated patients were transferred to the surgical ward after a routine admission to the postoperative care unit. Only three patients who were transferred to the surgical ward experienced complications that required a greater intensity of nursing care. A learning curve detected during the three-year study period showed that attempts to extubate increased from 73% to 96%, and triage to the surgical ward increased from 52% to 82% without compromising patient safety. The protocol resulted in a one-day reduction in ICU use in 75.5% of study subjects (237). The same approach can be extended to the use of IV catheters or indwelling bladder catheters, which should be withdrawn as soon as possible.

Other measures such as selective gastrointestinal decontamination (238), use of gowns, or high efficiency particulate air filters (HEPA) filters have not demonstrated so clearly an impact on the reduction of mortality or even nosocomial infections.

REFERENCES

1. Miller LW, Naftel DC, Bourge RC, et al. Infection after heart transplantation: a multi-institutional study. Cardiac Transplant Research Database Group. J Heart Lung Transplant 1994; 13(3):381–392.

2. Plöchl W, Pezawas L, Artemiou O, Grimm M, Klepetko W, Hiesmayr M. Nutritional status, ICU duration and ICU mortality in lung transplant recipients. Intens Care Med 1996; 22(11):1179–1185.

3. Hsu J, Griffith BP, Dowling RD, et al. Infections in mortally ill cardiac transplant recipients. J Thorac Cardiovasc Surg 1989, 98:506–509.

4. Cisneros Alonso C, Montero Castillo A, Moreno González E, García García I, Guillén Ramírez F, García Fuentes C. Complications of liver transplant in intensive care. Experience in 130 cases. Rev Clin Esp 1991; 189(6):264–267.

5. Plevak DJ, Southorn PA, Narr BJ. Intensive-care unit experience in the Mayo liver transplantation program: the first 100 cases. Mayo Clin Proc 1989; 64:433–445.

6. Bindi ML, Biancofiore G, Pasquini C, et al. Pancreas transplantation: problems and prospects in intensive care units. Minerva Anestesiol 2005; 71(5):207–221.

7. Singh N, Gayowski T, Wagener MM. Intensive care unit management in liver transplant recipients: beneficial effect on survival and preservation of quality of life. Clin Transpl 1997; 11(2):113–120.

8. Trzeciak S, Sharer R, Piper D, et al. Infections and severe sepsis in solid-organ transplant patients admitted from a university-based ED. Am J Emerg Med 2004; 22(7): 530–533.

9. Singh N, Chang FY, Gayowski T, Wagener M, Marino IR. Fever in liver transplant recipients in the intensive care unit. Clin Transpl 1999; 13(6):504–511.

10. Viscoli C, Dimitri P, Di Domenico S, Mannelli S, Dodi F, Veroni L. Infectious complications in liver transplant in Italy: current status and prospectives. Recenti Prog Med 2001; 92(1):16–31.

11. Montoya JG, Giraldo LF, Efron B, et al. Infectious complications among 620 consecutive heart transplant patients at Stanford University Medical Center. Clin Infect Dis 2001; 33(5):629–640.

12. Rubin RH. The prevention and treatment of infectious disease in the transplant patient: where are we now and where do we need to go? Transpl Infect Dis 2004; 6(1):1–2.

13. Rubin RH, Marty FM. Principles of antimicrobial therapy in the transplant patient. Transpl Infect Dis 2004; 6(3):97–100.

14. Martinelli L, Rinaldi M, Pederzolli C, et al. Different results of cardiac transplantation in patients with ischemic and dilated cardiomyopathy. Eur J Cardiothorac Surg 1995; 9(11):644–650.

15. Muñoz P, Muñoz RM, Palomo J, Rodríguez Creixéms M, Muñoz R, Bouza E. *Pneumocystis carinii* infections in heart transplant patients. Twice a week prophylaxis. Medicine (Baltimore) 1997; 76:415–422.

16. Edwards LB, Keck BM. Thoracic organ transplantation in the US. Clin Transpl 2002:29–40.

17. Detre KM, Belle SH, Carr MA, et al. A report from the NIDDK Liver Transplantation Database. Clin Transpl 1989:129–141.

18. Ben Hamida C, Lauzet JY, Rezaiguia-Delclaux S, et al. Effect of severe thrombocytopenia on patient outcome after liver transplantation. Intens Care Med 2003; 29(5): 756–762.

19. Aggarwal A, Ong JP, Goormastic M, et al. Survival and resource utilization in liver transplant recipients: the impact of admission to the intensive care unit. Transplant Proc 2003; 35(8):2998–3002.

20. Wiebe K, Wahlers T, Harringer W, vd Hardt H, Fabel H, Haverich A. Lung transplantation for cystic fibrosis—a single center experience over 8 years. Eur J Cardiothorac Surg 1998; 14(2):191–196.

21. Madden BP, Kamalvand K, Chan CM, Khaghani A, Hodson ME, Yacoub M. The medical management of patients with cystic fibrosis following heart–lung transplantation. Eur Respir J 1993; 6(7):965–970.

22. Nath DS, Kandaswamy R, Gruessner R, Sutherland DE, Dunn DL, Humar A. Fungal infections in transplant recipients receiving alemtuzumab. Transplant Proc 2005; 37(2): 934–936.

23. Argenziano M, Catanese KA, Moazami N, et al. The influence of infection on survival and successful transplantation in patients with left ventricular assist devices. J Heart Lung Transplant 1997; 16(8):822–831.

24. Fischer SA, Trenholme GM, Costanzo MR, Piccione W. Infectious complications in left ventricular assist device recipients. Clin Infect Dis 1997; 24(1):18–23.

25. Masters RC, Hendry PJ, Davies RA, et al. Cardiac transplantation after mechanical circulatory support: a canadian perspective. Ann Thorac Surg 1996; 61:1734–1739.

26. Bouza E, Muñoz P, Rodriguez C, et al. Endotipsitis: an emerging prosthetic-related infection in patients with portal hypertension. Diagn Microbiol Infect Dis 2004; 49(2):77–82.

27. Pietrantoni C, Minai OA, Yu NC, et al. Respiratory failure and sepsis are the major causes of ICU admissions and mortality in survivors of lung transplants. Chest 2003; 123(2):504–509.

28. Lardinois D, Banysch M, Korom S, et al. Extended donor lungs: eleven years experience in a consecutive series. Eur J Cardiothorac Surg 2005; 27(5):762–767.

29. Cuende N, Miranda B, Canon JF, Garrido G, Matesanz R. Donor characteristics associated with liver graft survival. Transplantation 2005; 79(10):1445–1452.

30. Ostrowsky BE, Venkataraman L, EM DA, Gold HS, DeGirolami PC, Samore MH. Vancomycin-resistant enterococci in intensive care units: high frequency of stool carriage during a non-outbreak period. Arch Intern Med 1999; 159(13):1467–1472.

31. Mort TC, Yeston NS. The relationship of pre mortem diagnoses and post mortem findings in a surgical intensive care unit [see comments]. Crit Care Med 1999; 27(2):299–303.

32. Singh N, Paterson DL. *Mycobacterium tuberculosis* infection in solid-organ transplant recipients: impact and implications for management. Clin Infect Dis 1998; 27(5):1266–1277.

33. Muñoz P, Guinea J, Pelaez T, Duran C, Blanco JL, Bouza E. Nosocomial invasive aspergillosis in a heart transplant patient acquired during a break in the HEPA air filtration system. Transpl Infect Dis 2004; 6(1):50–54.

34. Muñoz P, Arencibia J, Rodriguez C, et al. Trimethoprim-sulfamethoxazole as toxoplasmosis prophylaxis for heart transplant recipients. Clin Infect Dis 2003; 36(7):932–933 (author reply 3).

35. Singh N, Gayowski T, Wagener MM, Marino IR. Pulmonary infiltrates in liver transplant recipients in the intensive care unit. Transplantation 1999; 67(8):1138–1144.

36. Papanicolaou GA, Meyers BR, Meyers J, et al. Nosocomial infections with vancomycin-resistant *Enterococcus faecium* in liver transplant recipients: risk factors for acquisition and mortality. Clin Infect Dis 1996; 23(4):760–766.

37. Duchini A, Goss JA, Karpen S, Pockros PJ. Vaccinations for adult solid-organ transplant recipients: current recommendations and protocols. Clin Microbiol Rev 2003; 16(3):357–364.

38. Braddy CM, Heilman RL, Blair JE. Coccidioidomycosis after renal transplantation in an endemic area. Am J Transplant 2006; 6(2):340–345.

39. Martín-Rabadán P, Muñoz P, Palomo J, Bouza E. Strongyloidiasis: the Harada-Mori test revisited. Clin Microbiol Infection 1999; 5:374–376.

40. Tan HP, Stephen Dumler J, Maley WR, et al. Human monocytic ehrlichiosis: an emerging pathogen in transplantation. Transplantation 2001; 71(11):1678–1680.

41. Lafayette RA, Paré G, Schmid CH, King AJ, Rohrer RJ, Nasraway SA. Pretransplant renal dysfunction predicts poorer outcome in liver transplantation. Clin Nephrol 1997; 48(3):159–164.

42. Deschênes M, Belle SH, Krom RA, Zetterman RK, Lake JR. Early allograft dysfunction after liver transplantation: a definition and predictors of outcome. National Institute of Diabetes and Digestive and Kidney Diseases Liver Transplantation Database. Transplantation 1998; 66(3):302–310.

43. Reilly J, Mehta R, Teperman L, et al. Nutritional support after liver transplantation: a randomized prospective study [see comments]. JPEN 1990; 14(4):386–391.

44. Gurakar A, Hassanein T, Van Thiel DH. Right diaphragmatic paralysis following orthotopic liver transplantation. J Okla State Med Assoc 1995; 88(4):149–153.

45. Paterson DL, Staplefeldt WH, Wagener MM, Gayowski T, Marino IR, Singh N. Intra-operative hypothermia is an independent risk factor for early cytomegalovirus infection in liver transplant recipients. Transplantation 1999; 67(8):1151–1155.

46. Shorr AF, Jackson WL. Transfusion practice and nosocomial infection: assessing the evidence. Curr Opin Crit Care 2005; 11(5):468–472.

47. Parker BM, Irefin SA, Sabharwal V, et al. Leukocyte reduction during orthotopic liver transplantation and postoperative outcome: a pilot study. J Clin Anesth 2004; 16(1):18–24.

48. Naka T, Wan L, Bellomo R, et al. Kidney failure associated with liver transplantation or liver failure: the impact of continuous veno-venous hemofiltration. Int J Artif Organs 2004; 27(11):949–955.

49. Maroto LC, Aguado JM, Carrascal Y, et al. Role of epicardial pacing wire cultures in the diagnosis of poststernotomy mediastinitis. Clin Infect Dis 1997; 24(3):419–421.

50. Paterson DL, Dominguez EA, Chang FY, Snydman DR, Singh N. Infective endocarditis in solid organ transplant recipients. Clin Infect Dis 1998; 26(3):689–694.

51. Mugnani G, Bergami M, Lazzarotto T, Bedani PL. Intestinal infection by cytomegalo-virus in kidney transplantation: diagnostic difficulty in the course of mycophenolate mofetil therapy. G Ital Nefrol 2002; 19(4):483–484.

52. Bouza E, Merino P, Muñoz P, Sánchez-Carrillo C, Yáñez J, Cortés C. Ocular tubercul-osis: a prospective study in a General Hospital. Medicine (Baltimore) 1997; 76:53–61.

53. Bouza E, Cobo-Soriano R, Rodríguez-Créixems M, Muñoz P, Suárez-Leoz M, Cortés C. A prospective search for ocular lesions in hospitalized patients with significant bacter-emia. Clin Infect Dis 2000; 30:306–312.

54. Chang FY, Singh N, Gayowski T, Drenning SD, Wagener MM, Marino IR. *Staphylo-coccus aureus* nasal colonization association with infections in liver transplant recipients. Transplanation 1998; 65(9):1169–1172.

55. Mermel LA, Maki DG. Bacterial pneumonia in solid organ transplantation. Semin Respir Infect 1990; 5(1):10–29.

56. Jensen WA, Rose RM, Hammer SM, et al. Pulmonary complications of orthotopic liver transplantation. Transplantation 1986; 42(6):484.

57. Jimenez-Jambrina M, Hernandez A, Cordero E, et al. Pneumonia after heart transplan-tation in the XXI century: a multicenter prospective study. In: 45th Interscience Confer-ence on Antimicrobial Agents and Chemotherapy, 2005 (K-1561/370).

58. Cisneros JM, Muñoz P, Torre-Cisneros J, et al. Pneumonia after heart transplantation: a multiinstitutional study. Clin Infect Dis 1998; 27:324–331.

59. Fraser TG, Zembower TR, Lynch P, et al. Cavitary Legionella pneumonia in a liver transplant recipient. Transpl Infect Dis 2004; 6(2):77–80.

60. Singh N, Gayowski T, Wagener M, Marino IR, Yu VL. Pulmonary infections in liver transplant recipients receiving tacrolimus. Changing pattern of microbial etiologies. Transplantation 1996; 61(3):396–401.

61. Nichols L, Strollo DC, Kusne S. Legionellosis in a lung transplant recipient obscured by cytomegalovirus infection and *Clostridium difficile* colitis. Transpl Infect Dis 2002; 4(1):41–45.

62. Horbach I, Fehrenbach FJ. Legionellosis in heart transplant recipients. Infection 1990; 18(6):361–363.

63. Gupta RK, Jain M, Garg R. *Pneumocystis carinii* pneumonia after renal transplantation. Indian J Pathol Microbiol 2004; 47(4):474–476.

64. Renoult E, Georges E, Biava MF, et al. Toxoplasmosis in kidney transplant recipients: report of six cases and review. Clin Infect Dis 1997; 24(4):625–634.

65. Chang GC, Wu CL, Pan SH, et al. The diagnosis of pneumonia in renal transplant recipients using invasive and noninvasive procedures. Chest 2004; 125(2):541–547.

66. Ampel NM, Wing EJ. Legionella infection in transplant patients. Semin Respir Infect 1990; 5(1):30–37.

67. Miller R, Burton NA, Karwande SV, Jones KW, Doty DB, Gay WA Jr. Early, aggressive open lung biopsy in heart transplant recipients. J Heart Transplant 1987; 6(2): 96–99.
68. Dowling JN, Pasculle AW, Frola FN, Zaphyr MK, Yee RB. Infections caused by Legionella micdadei and *Legionella pneumophila* among renal transplant recipients. J Infect Dis 1984; 149(5):703–713.
69. Singh N, Muder RR, Yu VL, Gayowski T. Legionella infection in liver transplant recipients: implications for management. Transplantation 1993; 56(6):1549–1551.
70. Ogunc G, Ozdemir T, Vural T, Suleymanlar G, Akaydin M, Karpuzoglu T. Legionnaires' disease following kidney transplantation. Mikrobiyol Bul 1993; 27(2):137–142.
71. La Scola B, Michel G, Raoult D. Isolation of *Legionella pneumophila* by centrifugation of shell vial cell cultures from multiple liver and lung abscesses. J Clin Microbiol 1999; 37(3):785–787.
72. Chaberny IF, Ziesing S, Gastmeier P. Legionella prevention in intensive care units. Anasthesiol Intensivmed Notfallmed Schmerzther 2004; 39(3):127–131.
73. Vonberg RP, Eckmanns T, Bruderek J, Ruden H, Gastmeier P. Use of terminal tap water filter systems for prevention of nosocomial legionellosis. J Hosp Infect 2005; 60(2):159–162.
74. Muñoz P, Rodriguez C, Bouza E. *Mycobacterium tuberculosis* infection in recipients of solid organ transplants. Clin Infect Dis 2005; 40(4):581–587.
75. Muñoz P, Palomo J, Muñoz R, Rodríguez-Creixéms M, Pelaez T, Bouza E. Tuberculosis in heart transplant recipients. Clin Infect Dis 1995; 21:398–402.
76. Paterson DL, Singh N, Gayowski T, Marino IR. Pulmonary nodules in liver transplant recipients. Medicine 1998; 77(1):50–58.
77. Aguado JM, Herrero JA, Gavalda J, et al. Clinical presentation and outcome of tuberculosis in kidney, liver, and heart transplant recipients in Spain. Spanish Transplantation Infection Study Group, GESITRA. Transplantation 1997; 63(9):1278–1286.
78. Muñoz P, Burillo A, Palomo J, Rodríguez-Creixéms M, Bouza E. *Rhodococcus equi* infection in transplant recipients: casereview of the literature. Transplantation 1997; 65:449–453.
79. Wiesmayr S, Stelzmueller I, Tabarelli W, et al. Nocardiosis following solid organ transplantation: a single-centre experience. Transpl Int 2005; 18(9):1048–1053.
80. Vigano SM, Edefonti A, Ferraresso M, et al. Successful medical treatment of multiple brain abscesses due to *Nocardia farcinica* in a paediatric renal transplant recipient. Pediatr Nephrol 2005; 20(8):1186–1188.
81. Queipo-Zaragoza JA, Broseta-Rico E, Alapont-Alacreu JM, Santos-Durantez M, Sanchez-Plumed J, Jimenez-Cruz JF. Nocardial infection in immunosuppressed kidney transplant recipients. Scand J Urol Nephrol 2004; 38(2):168–173.
82. Kahraman S, Genctoy G, Arici M, Cetinkaya Y, Altun B, Caglar S. Septic arthritis caused by *Nocardia asteroides* in a renal transplant recipient. Transplant Proc 2004; 36(5):1415–1418.
83. Nouza M, Prat V. Lung infection after kidney transplantation. I. Etiology, pathogenesis and clinical picture. Cas Lek Cesk 1990; 129(21):641–644.
84. Muñoz P, Burillo A, Bouza E. Mold infection in solid organ transplant patients. In: Bowden RA, Ljungman P, Paya C, eds. Transplant Infections. 2nd ed. Lippincott: Williams & Wilkins, 2003.
85. Gavaldà J, Len O, Rovira M, et al. Epidemiology of invasive fungal infections (IFI) in solid organ (SOT) and hematopoietic stem cell (HSCT) transplant recipients: a prospective study from Resitra. In: 45th Interscience Conference on Antimicrobial Agents and Chemotherapy, 2005 (M-990/461).
86. Dummer JS, Lazariashvilli N, Barnes J, Ninan M, Milstone AP. A survey of anti-fungal management in lung transplantation. J Heart Lung Transplant 2004; 23(12):1376–1381.
87. Monforte V, Roman A, Gavalda J, et al. Nebulized amphotericin B prophylaxis for Aspergillus infection in lung transplantation: study of risk factors. J Heart Lung Transplant 2001; 20(12):1274–1281.

88. Kramer MR, Denning DW, Marshall SE, et al. Ulcerative tracheobronchitis after lung transplantation. A new form of invasive aspergillosis. Am Rev Respir Dis 1991; 144(3 Pt 1):552–556.

89. Muñoz P, Palomo J, Guembe P, Rodriguez-Creixems M, Gijon P, Bouza E. Lung nodular lesions in heart transplant recipients. J Heart Lung Transplant 2000; 19(7): 660–667.

90. Muñoz P, Rodriguez C, Bouza E, et al. Risk factors of invasive aspergillosis after heart transplantation: protective role of oral itraconazole prophylaxis. Am J Transplant 2004; 4(4):636–643.

91. Singh N, Arnow PM, Bonham A, et al. Invasive aspergillosis in liver transplant recipients in the 1990s. Transplantation 1997; 64(5):716–720.

92. Singh N, Gayowski T, Wagener MM, Doyle H, Marino IR. Invasive fungal infections in liver transplant recipients receiving tacrolimus as the primary immunosuppressive agent. Clin Infect Dis 1997; 24(2):179–184.

93. Muñoz P, Burillo A, Bouza E. Environmental surveillance and other control measures in the prevention of nosocomial fungal infections. Clin Microbiol Infect 2001; 7(suppl 2):38–45.

94. Gavalda J, Len O, San Juan R, et al. Risk factors for invasive aspergillosis in solid-organ transplant recipients: a case-control study. Clin Infect Dis 2005; 41(1):52–59.

95. Paterson DL, Singh N. Invasive aspergillosis in transplant recipients. Medicine 1999; 78(2):123–138.

96. Husain S, Alexander BD, Muñoz P, et al. Opportunistic mycelial fungal infections in organ transplant recipients: emerging importance of non-Aspergillus mycelial fungi. Clin Infect Dis 2003; 37(2):221–229.

97. Husain S, Muñoz P, Forrest G, et al. Infections due to *Scedosporium apiospermum* and *Scedosporium prolificans* in transplant recipients: clinical characteristics and impact of antifungal agent therapy on outcome. Clin Infect Dis 2005; 40(1):89–99.

98. Singh N, Lortholary O, Alexander BD, et al. Antifungal management practices and evolution of infection in organ transplant recipients with *Cryptococcus neoformans* infection. Transplantation 2005; 80(8):1033–1039.

99. Singh N, Lortholary O, Alexander BD, et al. Allograft loss in renal transplant recipients with *Cryptococcus neoformans* associated immune reconstitution syndrome. Transplantation 2005; 80(8):1131–1133.

100. el-Ebiary M, Torres A, Fabregas N, et al. Significance of the isolation of Candida species from respiratory samples in critically ill, non-neutropenic patients. An immediate post-mortem histologic study. Am J Respir Crit Care Med 1997; 156(2 Pt 1):583–590.

101. Park KY, Park CH. Candida infection in a stent inserted for tracheal stenosis after heart lung transplantation. Ann Thorac Surg 2005; 79(3):1054–1056.

102. Palmer SM, Perfect JR, Howell DN, et al. Candidal anastomotic infection in lung transplant recipients: successful treatment with a combination of systemic and inhaled antifungal agents. J Heart Lung Transplant 1998; 17(10):1029–1033.

103. Grossi P, Farina C, Fiocchi R, Dalla Gasperina D. Prevalence and outcome of invasive fungal infections in 1,963 thoracic organ transplant recipients: a multicenter retrospective study. Italian. Study Group of Fungal Infections in Thoracic Organ Transplant Recipients. Transplantation 2000; 70(1):112–116.

104. Horvath J, Dummer S, Loyd J, Walker B, Merrill WH, Frist WH. Infection in the transplanted and native lung after single lung transplantation. Chest 1993; 104(3): 681–685.

105. Sun Q, Li L, Ji S, et al. Variation of CD4+ and CD8+ T lymphocytes as predictor of outcome in renal allograft recipients who developed acute respiratory distress syndrome caused by cytomegalovirus pneumonia. Transplant Proc 2005; 37(5):2118–2121.

106. Liebau P, Kuse E, Winkler M, et al. Management of herpes simplex virus type 1 pneumonia following liver transplantation. Infection 1996; 24(2):130–135.

107. Weiss RL, Colby TV, Spruance SL, Salmon VC, Hammond ME. Simultaneous cytomegalovirus and herpes simplex virus pneumonia. Arch Pathol Lab Med 1987; 111(3): 242–245.

108. Friedrichs N, Eis-Hubinger AM, Heim A, Platen E, Zhou H, Buettner R. Acute adenoviral infection of a graft by serotype 35 following renal transplantation. Pathol Res Pract 2003; 199(8):565–570.

109. Wright JJ, O'Driscoll G. Treatment of parainfluenza virus 3 pneumonia in a cardiac transplant recipient with intravenous ribavirin and methylprednisolone. J Heart Lung Transplant 2005; 24(3):343–346.

110. Kumar D, Humar A. Emerging viral infections in transplant recipients. Curr Opin Infect Dis 2005; 18(4):337–341.

111. Kumar D, Erdman D, Keshavjee S, et al. Clinical impact of community-acquired respiratory viruses on bronchiolitis obliterans after lung transplant. Am J Transplant 2005; 5(8):2031–2036.

112. Barton TD, Blumberg EA. Viral pneumonias other than cytomegalovirus in transplant recipients. Clin Chest Med 2005; 26(4):707–720, viii.

113. Slifkin M, Doron S, Snydman DR. Viral prophylaxis in organ transplant patients. Drugs 2004; 64(24):2763–2792.

114. Mazzone PJ, Mossad SB, Mawhorter SD, Mehta AC, Mauer JR. Cell-mediated immune response to influenza vaccination in lung transplant recipients. J Heart Lung Transplant 2004; 23(10):1175–1181.

115. Vilchez RA, McCurry K, Dauber J, et al. Influenza virus infection in adult solid organ transplant recipients. Am J Transplant 2002; 2(3):287–291.

116. Ison MG, Hayden FG. Viral infections in immunocompromised patients: what's new with respiratory viruses? Curr Opin Infect Dis 2002; 15(4):355–367.

117. Garbino J, Gerbase MW, Wunderli W, et al. Lower respiratory viral illnesses: improved diagnosis by molecular methods and clinical impact. Am J Respir Crit Care Med 2004; 170(11):1197–1203 (Epub 2004 Sep 10).

118. Haydar AA, Denton M, West A, Rees J, Goldsmith DJ. Sirolimus-induced pneumonitis: three cases and a review of the literature. Am J Transplant 2004; 4(1):137–139.

119. Singh N. Posttransplant fever in critically ill transplant recipients. Infectious Complications in transplant patients Kluwer Academic publishers 2000; N. Singh, JM Aguado editors. ISBN 0-7923-7972-1:113-132.

120. Ho MC, Wu YM, Hu RH, et al. Surgical complications and outcome of living related liver transplantation. Transplant Proc 2004; 36(8):2249–2251.

121. Rerknimitr R, Sherman S, Fogel EL, et al. Biliary tract complications after orthotopic liver transplantation with choledochocholedochostomy anastomosis: endoscopic findings and results of therapy. Gastrointest Endosc 2002; 55(2):224–231.

122. Piecuch J, Witkowski K. Biliary tract complications following 52 consecutive orthotopic liver transplants. Ann Transplant 2001; 6(1):36–38.

123. Testa G, Malago M, Broelseh CE. Complications of biliary tract in liver transplantation. World J Surg 2001; 25(10):1296–1299.

124. Elola-Olaso AM, Diaz JC, Gonzalez EM, et al. Preliminary study of choledochocholedochostomy without T tube in liver transplantation: a comparative study. Transplant Proc 2005; 37(9):3922–3923.

125. Stange BJ, Glanemann M, Nuessler NC, Settmacher U, Steinmuller T, Neuhaus P. Hepatic artery thrombosis after adult liver transplantation. Liver Transpl 2003; 9(6):612–620.

126. Tachopoulou OA, Vogt DP, Henderson JM, Baker M, Keys TF. Hepatic abscess after liver transplantation: 1990–2000. Transplantation 2003; 75(1):79–83.

127. Muñoz P, Menasalvas A, Bernaldo de Quiros JC, Desco M, Vallejo JL, Bouza E. Postsurgical mediastinitis: a case-control study. Clin Infect Dis 1997; 25(5):1060–1064.

128. Muñoz P. Management of urinary tract infections and lymphocele in renal transplant recipients. Clin Infect Dis 2001; 33(suppl 1):S53–S57.

129. Tolkoff Rubin NE, Rubin RH. Urinary tract infection in the immunocompromised host. Lessons from kidney transplantation and the AIDS epidemic. Infect Dis Clin North Am 1997; 11(3):707–717.

130. Kahan BD, Flechner SM, Lorber MI, Golden D, Conley S, Van Buren CT. Complications of cyclosporine-prednisone immunosuppression in 402 renal allograft recipients exclusively followed at a single center for from one to five years. Transplantation 1987; 43(2):197–204.

131. Ghasemian SM, Guleria AS, Khawand NY, Light JA. Diagnosis and management of the urologic complications of renal transplantation. Clin Transpl 1996; 10(2):218–223.

132. Peterson PK, Anderson RC. Infection in renal transplant recipients. Current approaches to diagnosis, therapy, and prevention. Am J Med 1986; 81(1A):2–10.

133. Kaplan B, Meier-Kriesche HU, Jacobs MG, et al. Prevalence of cytomegalovirus in the gastrointestinal tract of renal transplant recipients with persistent abdominal pain. Am J Kidney Dis 1999; 34(1):65–68.

134. Sarkio S, Halme L, Arola J, Salmela K, Lautenschlager I. Gastroduodenal cytomegalovirus infection is common in kidney transplantation patients. Scand J Gastroenterol 2005; 40(5):508–514.

135. Ponticelli C, Passerini P. Gastrointestinal complications in renal transplant recipients. Transpl Int 2005; 18(6):643–650.

136. Peter A, Telkes G, Varga M, Sarvary E, Kovalszky I. Endoscopic diagnosis of cytomegalovirus infection of upper gastrointestinal tract in solid organ transplant recipients: Hungarian single-center experience. Clin Transpl 2004; 18(5):580–584.

137. Boobes Y, Al Hakim M, Dastoor H, Bernieh B, Abdulkhalik S. Late cytomegalovirus disease with atypical presentation in renal transplant patients: case reports. Transplant Proc 2004; 36(6):1841–1843.

138. Sarmiento E, Fernandez-Yanez J, Muñoz P, et al. Hypogammaglobulinemia after heart transplantation: use of intravenous immunoglobulin replacement therapy in relapsing CMV disease. Int Immunopharmacol 2005; 5(1):97–101.

139. Muñoz P, Palomo J, Yanez J, Bouza E. Clinical microbiological case: a heart transplant recipient with diarrhea and abdominal pain. Recurring *C. difficile* infection. Clin Microbiol Infect 2001; 7(8):451–452, 458–459.

140. West M, Pirenne J, Chavers B, et al. *Clostridium difficile* colitis after kidney and kidney-pancreas transplantation. Clin Transpl 1999; 13(4):318–323.

141. Apaydin S, Altiparmak MR, Saribas S, Ozturk R. Prevalence of *Clostridium difficile* toxin in kidney transplant recipients. Scand J Infect Dis 1998; 30(5):542.

142. Nadir A, Wright HI, Naz-Nadir F, Cooper DK, Zuhdi N, Van Thiel DH. Atypical *Clostridium difficile* colitis in a heart transplant recipient. J Heart Lung Transplant 1995; 14(3):606–607.

143. Mistry B, Longo W, Solomon H, Garvin P. *Clostridium difficile* colitis requiring subtotal colectomy in a renal transplant recipient: a case report review of literature. Transplant Proc 1998; 30(7):3914.

144. Keven K, Basu A, Re L, et al. *Clostridium difficile* colitis in patients after kidney and pancreas-kidney transplantation. Transpl Infect Dis 2004; 6(1):10–14.

145. Schenk P, Madl C, Kramer L, et al. Pneumatosis intestinalis with *Clostridium difficile* colitis as a cause of acute abdomen after lung transplantation. Dig Dis Sci 1998; 43(11):2455–2458.

146. Lykavieris P, Fabre M, Pariente D, Lezeau YM, Debray D. *Clostridium difficile* colitis associated with inflammatory pseudotumor in a liver transplant recipient. Pediatr Transplant 2003; 7(1):76–79.

147. Bouza E, Muñoz P, Alonso R. Clinical manifestations, treatment and control of infections caused by *Clostridium difficile*. Clin Microbiol Infect 2005; 11(suppl 4):57–64.

148. Bouza E, Pelaez T, Alonso R, Catalan P, Muñoz P, Creixems MR. "Second-look" cytotoxicity: an evaluation of culture plus cytotoxin assay of *Clostridium difficile* isolates in the laboratory diagnosis of CDAD. J Hosp Infect 2001; 48(3):233–237.

149. Muñoz P, Bouza E, Cuenca-Estrella M, et al. *Saccharomyces cerevisiae* fungemia: an emerging infectious disease. Clin Infect Dis 2005; 40(11):1625–1634 (Epub 2005 Apr 25).

150. Ziring D, Tran R, Edelstein S, et al. Infectious enteritis after intestinal transplantation: incidence, timing, and outcome. Transplantation 2005; 79(6):702–709.

151. Ginsburg PM, Thuluvath PJ. Diarrhea in liver transplant recipients: etiology and management. Liver Transpl 2005; 11(8):881–890.

152. Singh N, Husain S. Infections of the central nervous system in transplant recipients. Transpl Infect Dis 2000; 2(3):101–111.

153. Singh N, Bonham A, Fukui M. Immunosuppressive-associated leukoencephalopathy in organ transplant recipients. Transplantation 2000; 69(4):467–472.

154. Ponticelli C, Campise MR. Neurological complications in kidney transplant recipients. J Nephrol 2005; 18(5):521–528.

155. Nash PJ, Avery RK, Tang WH, Starling RC, Taege AJ, Yamani MH. Encephalitis owing to human herpesvirus-6 after cardiac transplant. Am J Transplant 2004; 4(7):1200–1203.

156. Singh N, Paterson DL. Encephalitis caused by human herpesvirus-6 in transplant recipients: relevance of a novel neurotropic virus. Transplantation 2000; 69(12):2474–2479.

157. Razonable RR, Paya CV. The impact of human herpesvirus-6 and -7 infection on the outcome of liver transplantation. Liver Transpl 2002; 8(8):651–658.

158. Rogers J, Rohal S, Carrigan DR, et al. Human herpesvirus-6 in liver transplant recipients: role in pathogenesis of fungal infections, neurologic complications, and outcome. Transplantation 2000; 69(12):2566–2573.

159. Maschke M, Kastrup O, Diener HC. CNS manifestations of cytomegalovirus infections: diagnosis and treatment. CNS Drugs 2002; 16(5):303–315.

160. Gomez E, Melon S, Aguado S, et al. Herpes simplex virus encephalitis in a renal transplant patient: diagnosis by polymerase chain reaction detection of HSV DNA. Am J Kidney Dis 1997; 30(3):423–427.

161. Bamborschke S, Wullen T, Huber M, et al. Early diagnosis and successful treatment of acute cytomegalovirus encephalitis in a renal transplant recipient. J Neurol 1992; 239(4):205–208.

162. Wadei H, Alangaden GJ, Sillix DH, et al. West Nile virus encephalitis: an emerging disease in renal transplant recipients. Clin Transpl 2004; 18(6):753–758.

163. Kleinschmidt-DeMasters BK, Marder BA, Levi ME, et al. Naturally acquired West Nile virus encephalomyelitis in transplant recipients: clinical, laboratory, diagnostic, and neuropathological features. Arch Neurol 2004; 61(8):1210–1220.

164. DeSalvo D, Roy-Chaudhury P, Peddi R, et al. West Nile virus encephalitis in organ transplant recipients: another high-risk group for meningoencephalitis and death. Transplantation 2004; 77(3):466–469.

165. Ascher NL, Simmons RL, Marker S, Najarian JS. Listeria infection in transplant patients. Five cases and a review of the literature. Arch Surg 1978; 113(1):90–94.

166. Wiesmayr S, Tabarelli W, Stelzmueller I, et al. Listeria meningitis in transplant recipients. Wien Klin Wochenschr 2005; 117(5–6):229–233.

167. Limaye AP, Perkins JD, Kowdley KV. Listeria infection after liver transplantation: report of a case and review of the literature. Am J Gastroenterol 1998; 93(10):1942–1944.

168. Vargas V, Aleman C, de Torres I, et al. *Listeria monocytogenes*-associated acute hepatitis in a liver transplant recipient. Liver 1998; 18(3):213–215.

169. Mylonakis E, Hohmann EL, Calderwood SB. Central nervous system infection with *Listeria monocytogenes*. 33 years' experience at a general hospital and review of 776 episodes from the literature. Medicine (Baltimore) 1998; 77(5):313–336.

170. Husain S, Wagener MM, Singh N. *Cryptococcus neoformans* infection in organ transplant recipients: variables influencing clinical characteristics and outcome. Emerg Infect Dis 2001; 7(3):375–381.

171. Singh N, Gayowski T, Wagener MM, Marino IR. Clinical spectrum of invasive cryptococcosis in liver transplant recipients receiving tacrolimus. Clin Transpl 1997; 11(1):66–70.

172. Singh N, Rihs JD, Gayowski T, Yu VL. Cutaneous cryptococcosis mimicking bacterial cellulitis in a liver transplant recipient: case report and review in solid organ transplant recipients. Clin Transpl 1994; 8(4):365–368.

173. Rakvit A, Meyerrose G, Vidal AM, Kimbrough RC, Sarria JC. Cellulitis caused by *Cryptococcus neoformans* in a lung transplant recipient. J Heart Lung Transplant 2005; 24(5):642.

174. Gupta RK, Khan ZU, Nampoory MR, Mikhail MM, Johny KV. Cutaneous cryptococcosis in a diabetic renal transplant recipient. J Med Microbiol 2004; 53(Pt 5):445–449.

175. Baumgarten KL, Valentine VG, Garcia-Diaz JB. Primary cutaneous cryptococcosis in a lung transplant recipient. South Med J 2004; 97(7):692–695.

176. Basaran O, Emiroglu R, Arikan U, Karakayali H, Haberal M. Cryptococcal necrotizing fasciitis with multiple sites of involvement in the lower extremities. Dermatol Surg 2003; 29(11):1158–1160.

177. Utili R, Tripodi MF, Ragone E, et al. Hepatic cryptococcosis in a heart transplant recipient. Transpl Infect Dis 2004; 6(1):33–36.

178. Lee YA, Kim HJ, Lee TW, et al. First report of *Cryptococcus albidus*–induced disseminated cryptococcosis in a renal transplant recipient. Korean J Intern Med 2004; 19(1):53–57.

179. Simon DM, Levin S. Infectious complications of solid organ transplantations. Infect Dis Clin North Am 2001; 15(2):521–549.

180. Bonham CA, Dominguez EA, Fukui MB, et al. Central nervous system lesions in liver transplant recipients: prospective assessment of indications for biopsy and implications for management. Transplantation 1998; 66(12):1596–1604.

181. Torre-Cisneros J, Lopez OL, Kusne S, et al. CNS aspergillosis in organ transplantation: a clinicopathological study. J Neurol Neurosurg Psychiatr 1993; 56(2):188–193.

182. Baden LR, Katz JT, Franck L, et al. Successful toxoplasmosis prophylaxis after orthotopic cardiac transplantation with trimethoprim-sulfamethoxazole. Transplantation 2003; 75(3):339–343.

183. Wulf MW, van Crevel R, Portier R, et al. Toxoplasmosis after renal transplantation: implications of a missed diagnosis. J Clin Microbiol 2005; 43(7):3544–3547.

184. Conrath J, Mouly-Bandini A, Collart F, Ridings B. *Toxoplasma gondii* retinochoroiditis after cardiac transplantation. Graefes Arch Clin Exp Ophthalmol 2003; 241(4):334–338 (EPub 2003 Mar 22).

185. Wagner FM, Reichenspurner H, Uberfuhr P, Weiss M, Fingerle V, Reichart B. Toxoplasmosis after heart transplantation: diagnosis by endomyocardial biopsy. J Heart Lung Transplant 1994; 13(5):916–918.

186. Botterel F, Ichai P, Feray C, et al. Disseminated toxoplasmosis, resulting from infection of allograft, after orthotopic liver transplantation: usefulness of quantitative PCR. J Clin Microbiol 2002; 40(5):1648–1650.

187. Guitard J, Kamar N, Mouzin M, et al. Sulfadiazine-related obstructive urinary tract lithiasis: an unusual cause of acute renal failure after kidney transplantation. Clin Nephrol 2005; 63(5):405–407.

188. Arnold SJ, Kinney MC, McCormick MS, Dummer S, Scott MA. Disseminated toxoplasmosis. Unusual presentations in the immunocompromised host. Arch Pathol Lab Med 1997; 121(8):869–873.

189. Walker M, Zunt JR. Parasitic central nervous system infections in immunocompromised hosts. Clin Infect Dis. 2005; 40(7):1005–1015 (pub 2005 Mar 2).

190. Shin JH, Lee HK. Nocardial brain abscess in a renal transplant recipient. Clin Imaging 2003; 27(5):321–324.

191. Peraira JR, Segovia J, Fuentes R, et al. Pulmonary nocardiosis in heart transplant recipients: treatment and outcome. Transplant Proc 2003; 35(5):2006–2008.

192. Granel B, Serratrice J, Ene N, et al. Brain nocardiosis of good outcome occurring in a heart transplant recipient. Rev Med Intern 2003; 24(11):756–758.

193. Husain S, McCurry K, Dauber J, Singh N, Kusne S. Nocardia infection in lung transplant recipients. J Heart Lung Transplant 2002; 21(3):354–359.

194. Rodriguez C, Muñoz P, Rodriguez-Creixems M, Yañez JF, Palomo J, Bouza E. Blood-stream infections among heart transplant recipients. Transplantation 2006; 81(3):384–391.

195. Singh N, Gayowski T, Wagener MM, Marino IR. Predictors and outcome of early-versus late-onset major bacterial infections in liver transplant recipients receiving tacrolimus (FK506) as primary immunosuppression. Liver Transpl 2000; 6:54–61.

196. Singh N, Wagener MM, Obman A, Cacciarelli TV, de Vera ME, Gayowski T. Bacter-emias in liver transplant recipients: shift toward gram-negative bacteria as predominant pathogens. Liver Transpl 2004; 10(7):844–849.

197. Larson EL, Cimiotti JP, Haas J, et al. Gram-negative bacilli associated with catheter-associated and non-catheter-associated bloodstream infections and hand carriage by healthcare workers in neonatal intensive care units. Pediatr Crit Care Med 2005; 6(4): 457–461.

198. Harnett SJ, Allen KD, Macmillan RR. Critical care unit outbreak of *Serratia liquefaciens* from contaminated pressure monitoring equipment. J Hosp Infect 2001; 47(4):301–307.

199. Singh N, Gayowski T, Wagener MM, Marino IR. Bloodstream infections in liver trans-plant recipients receiving tacrolimus. Clin Transpl 1997; 11(4):275–281.

200. Singh N, Paterson DL, Gayowski T, Wagener MM, Marino IR. Predicting bacteremia and bacteremic mortality in liver transplant recipients. Liver Transpl 2000; 6(1):54–61.

201. Torgay A, Pirat A, Candan S, Zeyneloglu P, Arslan G, Haberal M. Internal jugular ver-sus subclavian vein catheterization for central venous catheterization in orthotopic liver transplantation. Transplant Proc 2005; 37(7):3171–3173.

202. Singh N, Squier C, Wannstedt C, Keyes L, Wagener MM, Cacciarelli TV. Impact of an aggressive infection control strategy on endemic *Staphylococcus aureus* infection in liver transplant recipients. Infect Control Hosp Epidemiol 2006; 27(2):122–126 (Epub 2006 Feb 8).

203. Sawyer RG, Crabtree TD, Gleason TG, Antevil JL, Pruett TL. Impact of solid organ transplantation and immunosuppression on fever, leukocytosis, and physiologic response during bacterial and fungal infections. Clin Transpl 1999; 13(3):260–265.

204. Cercenado E, Ena J, Rodríguez-Créixems M, Romero I, Bouza E. A conservative procedure for the diagnosis of catheter-related infections. Arch Intern Med 1990; 150: 1417–1420.

205. Muñoz P, de la Torre J, Bouza E, et al. Invasive aspergillosis in transplant recipients. A large multicentric study. In: 36th Interscience Conference of Antimicrobial Agents and Chemotherapy American Society for Microbiology, 1996.

206. Segall L, Moal MC, Doucet L, Kergoat N, Bourbigot B. Toxoplasmosis-associated hemophagocytic syndrome in renal transplantation. Transpl Int 2006; 19(1):78–80.

207. Roman CD, Habibian MR, Martin WH. Identification of an infected left ventricular assist device after cardiac transplant by indium-111 WBC scintigraphy. Clin Nucl Med 2005; 30(1):16–27.

208. Chang FY, Singh N, Gayowski T, Wagener MM, Marino IR. Fever in liver transplant recipients: changing spectrum of etiologic agents. Clin Infect Dis 1998; 26(1):59–65.

209. Toogood GJ, Roake JA, Morris PJ. The relationship between fever and acute rejection or infection following renal transplantation in the cyclosporin era. Clin Transpl 1994; 8(4):373–377.

210. von Muller L, Schliep C, Storck M, et al. Severe graft rejection, increased immunosup-pression, and active CMV infection in renal transplantation. J Med Virol 2006; 78(3): 394–399.

211. Toupance O, Bouedjoro-Camus MC, Carquin J, et al. Cytomegalovirus-related disease and risk of acute rejection in renal transplant recipients: a cohort study with case-control analyses. Transpl Int 2000; 13(6):413–419.

212. Heo JS, Park JW, Lee KW, et al. Posttransplantation lymphoproliferative disorder in pediatric liver transplantation. Transplant Proc 2004; 36(8):2307–2308.

213. Singh N, Gayowski T, Marino IR, Schlichtig R. Acute adrenal insufficiency in critically ill liver transplant recipients. Implications for diagnosis. Transplantation 1995; 59(12): 1744–1745.

214. Hummel M, Warnecke H, Schüler S, Luding K, Hetzer R. Risk of adrenal cortex insufficiency following heart transplantation. Klin Wochenschr 1991; 69(6):269–273.

215. Bromberg JS, Alfrey EJ, Barker CF, et al. Adrenal suppression and steroid supplementation in renal transplant recipients. Transplantation 1991; 51(2):385–390.

216. Bromberg JS, Baliga P, Cofer JB, Rajagopalan PR, Friedman RJ. Stress steroids are not required for patients receiving a renal allograft and undergoing operation. J Am Coll Surg 1995; 180(5):532–536.

217. Rodger RS, Watson MJ, Sellars L, Wilkinson R, Ward MK, Kerr DN. Hypothalamic-pituitary-adrenocortical suppression and recovery in renal transplant patients returning to maintenance dialysis. Q J Med 1986; 61(235):1039–1046.

218. Sever MS, Türkmen A, Yildiz A, Ecder T, Orhan Y. Fever in dialysis patients with recently rejected renal allografts. Int J Artif Organs 1998; 21(7):403–407.

219. Khan A, Ortiz J, Jacobson L, Reich D, Manzarbeitia C. Posttransplant lymphoproliferative disease presenting as adrenal insufficiency: case report. Exp Clin Transpl 2005; 3(1):341–344.

220. Dorschner L, Speich R, Ruschitzka F, Seebach JD, Gallino A. Everolimus-induced drug fever after heart transplantation. Transplantation 2004; 78(2):303–304.

221. Mourad G, Rostaing L, Legendre C, Garrigue V, Thervet E, Durand D. Sequential protocols using basiliximab versus antithymocyte globulins in renal-transplant patients receiving mycophenolate mofetil and steroids. Transplantation 2004; 78(4):584–590.

222. Khan SU, Salloum J, O'Donovan PB, et al. Acute pulmonary edema after lung transplantation: the pulmonary reimplantation response. Chest 1999; 116(1):187–194.

223. Husain S, Kwak EJ, Obman A, et al. Prospective assessment of Platelia Aspergillus galactomannan antigen for the diagnosis of invasive aspergillosis in lung transplant recipients. Am J Transplant 2004; 4(5):796–802.

224. Kwak EJ, Husain S, Obman A, et al. Efficacy of galactomannan antigen in the Platelia Aspergillus enzyme immunoassay for diagnosis of invasive aspergillosis in liver transplant recipients. J Clin Microbiol 2004; 42(1):435–438.

225. Fortun J, Martin-Davila P, Alvarez ME, et al. Aspergillus antigenemia sandwich-enzyme immunoassay test as a serodiagnostic method for invasive aspergillosis in liver transplant recipients. Transplantation 2001; 71(1):145–149.

226. Bouza E, Sousa D, Muñoz P, Rodriguez-Creixems M, Fron C, Lechuz JG. Bloodstream infections: a trial of the impact of different methods of reporting positive blood culture results. Clin Infect Dis 2004; 39(8):1161–1169 (Epub 2004 Sep 24).

227. Yao FY, Saab S, Bass NM, et al. Prediction of survival after liver retransplantation for late graft failure based on preoperative prognostic scores. Hepatology 2004; 39(1):230–238.

228. Pelletier SJ, Schaubel DE, Punch JD, Wolfe RA, Port FK, Merion RM. Hepatitis C is a risk factor for death after liver retransplantation. Liver Transpl 2005; 11(4):434–440.

229. Zilberberg MD, Epstein SK. Acute lung injury in the medical ICU: comorbid conditions, age, etiology, and hospital outcome. Am J Respir Crit Care Med 1998; 157(4 Pt 1):1159–1164.

230. Afessa B, Tefferi A, Hoagland HC, Letendre L, Peters SG. Outcome of recipients of bone marrow transplants who require intensive-care unit support [see comments]. Mayo Clin Proc 1992; 67(2):117–122.

231. Paz HL, Crilley P, Weinar M, Brodsky I. Outcome of patients requiring medical ICU admission following bone marrow transplantation. Chest 1993; 104(2):527–531.

232. Lebron Gallardo M, Herrera Gutierrez ME, Seller Perez G, Curiel Balsera E, Fernandez Ortega JF, Quesada Garcia G. Risk factors for renal dysfunction in the postoperative course of liver transplant. Liver Transpl 2004; 10(11):1379–1385.

233. Hosenpud JD, Bennett LE, Keck BM, Fiol B, Boucek MM, Novick RJ. The registry of the International Society for Heart and Lung Transplantation: fifteenth official report-1998. J Heart Lung Transplant 1998; 17:656–668.

234. Hadjiliadis D, Steele MP, Govert JA, Davis RD, Palmer SM. Outcome of lung transplant patients admitted to the medical ICU. Chest 2004; 125(3):1040–1045.
235. Sadaghdar H, Chelluri L, Bowles SA, Shapiro R. Outcome of renal transplant recipients in the ICU. Chest 1995; 107(5):1402–1405.
236. Biancofiore G, Bindi ML, Romanelli AM, Urbani L, Mosca F, Filipponi F. Stress-inducing factors in ICUs: what liver transplant recipients experience and what caregivers perceive. Liver Transpl 2005; 11(8):967–972.
237. Mandell MS, Lezotte D, Kam I, Zamudio S. Reduced use of intensive care after liver transplantation: influence of early extubation. Liver Transpl 2002; 8(8):676–681.
238. Krueger WA, Unertl KE. Selective decontamination of the digestive tract. Curr Opin Crit Care 2002; 8(2):139–144.

24

Infections in Asplenics in the Critical Care Unit

Jihad Slim and Leon G. Smith
Infectious Disease Division, Department of Medicine, Seton Hall P.G. School of Medicine, and St. Michael's Medical Center, Newark, New Jersey, U.S.A.

OVERVIEW

The terms postsplenectomy sepsis and overwhelming postsplenectomy infection (OPSI) are used to describe a clinical entity where an illness could evolve from good health to death within 24 hours, in the setting of a poorly functioning spleen.

In order to understand OPSI, a physician needs to be familiar with three concepts. The first is related to the high incidence of undiagnosed hyposplenism (1). Surgical splenectomy and sickle cell disease are two classical cases of easily recognizable defect, but congenital asplenia, coeliac disease, and alcoholism are some of the harder-to-recognize etiologies of a malfunctioning spleen. A simple albeit insensitive test for splenic function is the presence of Howell–Jolly bodies in the peripheral smear (2).

The second concept is that the clinical presentation is usually nonspecific, and patients rarely have an obvious focus of infection. Physicians need to have a high index of suspicion for OPSI; otherwise the diagnosis can be missed, and patients have more than 50% mortality rate from sepsis and discriminate intravascular coagulation (DIC) within a few hours of presentation (3).

Finally, the third concept is related to prevention of this entity by vaccines, antibiotic prophylaxis, education, and early empirical antibacterial therapy (4).

The question of why the spleen is so important has been heavily debated in the last century. Even though OPSI was well documented as early as 1952 in King and Schmacher's report in splenectomized infants younger than six months (5), it was not until the turn of this century that the medical community recognized the need to decrease splenic removal, mainly after trauma and in staging of lymphoma (6).

The spleen seems to function as the largest accumulation of lymphoid tissue in the body and thus has a variety of immune functions, some of which include removal of circulating organisms, production of opsonizing antibody, tuftsin synthesis or activation, and removal of senescent red blood cells (RBC) (7). Therefore, the presence in the peripheral smear of intraerythrocytic nuclear remnants called Howell–Jolly bodies is a measure of decreased splenic clearance (1). Although a more sensitive measure of splenic function is chromium-tagged heat damaged RBC clearance, it is more expensive and rarely used.

EPIDEMIOLOGY

It is difficult to define the scope of the problem because most people with hyposplenism are undiagnosed, and probably will never develop OPSI. In one study, reviewing over 100,000 peripheral blood smears, Howell–Jolly bodies were found in 0.5% of the samples (7).

Some of the most common reasons for malfunctioning of the spleen include surgical, or congenital asplenia (8), irradiation, infarction, infiltration (e.g., amyloidosis), granulomatous diseases (e.g., sarcoidosis), or cancer (primary, e.g., hemangiosarcoma, secondary, or lymphoma) (9). Hyposplenism has also been associated with advanced age (>70) (10), alcoholism (11), and a variety of autoimmune (12) and intestinal disorders (e.g., celiac disease) especially when splenomegaly is present (Table 1) (1,13). Moreover, the incidence of OPSI in postsurgical splenectomy is variable. In El-Alfy's study where 318 patients were followed for up to 17 years, 5.7% developed OPSI (14). Death rates have been reported to be 600 times greater than in the general population (5,15); but mortality is greatly dependent on patient's age, time elapsed since splenectomy, and underlying reason for hyposplenism; it varies from 38% to 69% (16–20). The yearly incidence has been estimated at 0.23% to 0.42% (16,21). In a review of the English literature from 1966 to 1996, the highest incidence of sepsis was 8.2% in younger patients with hemoglobinopathies, namely thalassemia major and sickle cell anemia (22). The incidence was 2.6% in another large cohort of patients splenectomized for hereditary spherocytosis (23); mortality in this setting was estimated at four to six cases per 10,000 patient-years (24).

Finally, another factor that makes those estimates very difficult to study is the fact that the majority of patients develop with passing time a hyperplasia of accessory spleens (25), which could restore some of their lost splenic function.

MICROBIOLOGY

Bacteria

Streptococcus pneumoniae is by far the most frequently reported pathogen causing OPSI (14–19), no specific serotype predominates, and penicillin resistance has been

Table 1 The Most Common Causes of Hyposplenism

Presumed mechanism	Conditions
Surgical removal	Trauma, ITP, hereditary spherocytosis
Congenital	Isolated congenital asplenia, or part of cardiopulmonary malformations
Atrophy	Sickle cell disease, irradiation, splenic artery occlusion
Infiltration	Amyloidosis, sarcoidosis, graft vs. host disease
Congestion	Portal hypertension
Autoimmune	Systemic lupus erythematosus, rheumatoid arthritis
Miscellaneous	Alcoholism, ulcerative colitis, celiac disease, elderly

Abbreviation: ITP, idiopathic thrombocytopenic purpura.

increasingly encountered in the last decade (26). Pneumococcus in the United States is rarely resistant to the respiratory fluoroquinolone, like gemifloxacin, moxifloxacin, gatifloxacin, and levofloxacin. No resistance to vancomycin, linezolid, and dapto-mycin has yet been reported (Table 2).

Haemophilus influenzae type b is classically the second most common pathogen isolated in patients with OPSI (27). Its incidence used to be 10 times less than Pneu-mococcus; it probably has decreased even more dramatically in the last 15 years since the universal use of conjugated HiB vaccine.

Capnocytophaga canimorsus (DF-2) is the classical zoonosis associated with OPSI; it is a gram-negative bacilli, part of the normal oral flora of dogs and cats. This organism is usually sensitive to penicillin, but can produce β-lactamase (28–30).

The fourth classical pathogen in this setting is *Neisseria meningitides* (27), but that is difficult to prove, because meningococcemia can lead to the same clinical picture as OPSI in patients with an intact spleen.

Other bacterial pathogens include Salmonella species (31), reported less fre-quently, usually reported in patients with other cell-mediated immune defect secondary to either the primary disease or its therapy. *Streptococcus suis* is another zoonosis asso-ciated with swine exposure (32,33). Other streptococci (32,34), staphylococcus, and gram-negative bacilli have been implicated in OPSI, but those are still less common, and their relationship to this syndrome is more difficult to establish. In a series of 26 bacteremic patients with *Bordetella holmesii*, 22 were hyposplenic; but those patients had a milder illness than classical OPSI, and none of them died (35). Other reports have found Human Granulocytic Ehrlichiosis to have a more severe, recurrent, and prolonged course in asplenic patients (36).

Parasites

Babesiosis is usually considered a mild illness in patients with normal spleen function. In hyposplenic patients it becomes a serious illness with increased mortality (37) and often requires therapy with clindamycin and quinine (38), or atovaquone and azithro-mycin, sometimes even exchange transfusion (39). Its epidemiology is often linked to Ixodes tick vector mainly from the coastal areas and islands of Massachusetts in the United States, and sometimes to blood transfusion.

Table 2 Pathogens Causing Infections in Hyposplenic Patients

Organisms	Features
Streptococcus pneumoniae	The most common cause of OPSI
Haemophilus influenzae type b	Incidence is decreasing
Capnocytophaga canimorsus	Exposure to dogs or cats
Meningococcus	Requires prophylaxis for close contacts
Streptococcus suis	Swine exposure
Bordetella holmesii	Cause prolonged febrile illness in asplenic patients
Human granulocytic ehrlichiosis	Morulae, intracellular inclusion within neutrophils
Babesiosis	Exposure to Ixodes ticks, or blood transfusion
Plasmodium species	Fulminant presentation of *Plasmodium vivax* or *P. malariae*
Other organisms	Salmonella, Staphylococcus spp., Streptococcus, *Escherichia coli*, Pseudomonas spp., VZV[a] . . .

[a]Varicella zoster virus reported mainly in patients with Hodgkin's lymphoma.
Abbreviations: OPSI, overwhelming postsplenectomy infection; VZV, varicella zoster virus.

Malaria theoretically would be more severe in asplenic patients, but *Plasmodium falciparum* infection course does not seem to be affected by splenectomy; on the other hand there are few case reports of fulminant *Plasmodium vivax* and *P. malariae* in asplenic patients (40).

CLINICAL PRESENTATION

Diagnosing OPSI is very difficult without a high index of suspicion, because in most instances the prodromal illness has a very short duration, 24 to 48 hours, and the symptoms are usually very nonspecific: low-grade fever with chills, myalgias, diarrhea, sometimes nausea, and pharyngitis (3). In most instances no site of infection can be found; within hours patient status can deteriorate and develop a picture of severe sepsis with disseminated intravascular coagulation and cardiovascular collapse with lactic acidosis (41). Ultimately if patients, survive this phase they may have purpura fulminans with symmetrical peripheral extremities gangrene necessitating multiple amputations (42).

In young children focal infections could be found, most often meningitis (43). In this setting it caries a grave prognosis. In a prospective study of *S. pneumoniae* infections in asplenic children in the United States, 26 episodes were observed in 22 children from eight hospitals over a six-year period, from 9/1993 to 8/1999; six deaths occurred, and five of them had meningitis (41).

In *C. canimorsus* infection, the port of entry secondary to a dog bite or a cat scratch could have formed an eschar, and that would be a clue for this infection. A peripheral smear can be very helpful to guide diagnosis: it will show the Howell–Jolly bodies, which should make physician consider hyposplenism, and it can even show the presence of bacteria, reflecting the enormous degree of bacteremia. Other techniques that would be helpful for diagnosing OPSI as well are acridine orange and Gram or Wright stain of the peripheral blood buffy coat showing the microorganisms. A peripheral smear would obviously make the diagnosis of babesiosis, showing the intraerythrocytic parasites, and often a high grade of parasitemia in this setting.

Differential Diagnosis

A variety of illnesses could be thought of in the prodromal phase of the illness. At this initial stage, before cardiovascular collapse, an astute physician would be able to think of OPSI only if the history brings up the hyposplenic state of the patient. A prior history of splenectomy would be an easy clue, but it would be important to elucidate all the other entities leading to hyposplenism, keeping in mind that known hyposplenic patients who have received their recommended vaccinations and are taking antibiotic prophylaxis are still at risk of OPSI (44,45).

Once hyposplenism is suspected—if the patient presents with rigors, chills, and fever, the patient should be promptly worked up and empirically treated for possible OPSI (46). Other helpful clues in the history regarding pathogens involved would be a dog or cat exposure for *C. canimorsus*, swine exposure for *S. suis*, and travel to endemic areas for babesiosis and malaria.

The physical examination before the severe sepsis phase is usually unrevealing. An abdominal scar suggesting a prior splenectomy could be a first clue. Rarely in an adult would one find a focal site of infection, but an eschar at the site of a dog bite that is a few days old would suggest Capnocytophaga as the culprit agent. In young children meningeal signs suggesting the diagnosis of meningitis could be the present-ing illness prior to cardiovascular collapse.

The laboratory findings are a combination of evidence of malfunctioning spleen and septic shock. An early clue could be the initial relatively normal platelet count in the presence of Howell–Jolly bodies, because asplenic patients have a relative thrombocytosis and early consumptive process will decrease the platelets. I cannot stress enough the importance of peripheral smear in this setting, because it can usually readily make the diagnosis of babesiosis but also could reveal the presence of bacteria. Blood cultures are usually positive at 24 hours or earlier, and other laboratory values pointing to severe sepsis will be present—hypoalbuminemia, lactic acidosis, renal insufficiency, prolonged thrombin time, decreased fibrinogen, and the presence of D-dimer.

Diagnosis

The presumptive clinical diagnosis should be made when a patient with known or suspected hyposplenism presents with fever, chills, and no localizing site for infec-tion. At this time blood cultures should be taken and antibiotics given without any delay. The peripheral smear should be examined for intraerythrocytic parasites, and a Gram or Wright stain of the smear looking for the presence of bacteria can be very helpful. Routine blood work and CXR need to be done, but would rarely help in establishing the diagnosis. Buffy coat smear is extremely valuable.

Antibiotics should be directed specifically against pneumococcus, but broader spectrum coverage should be considered until blood culture results are available.

Once severe sepsis has occurred the diagnosis could have been made; blood cultures could have been positive in the vast majority of cases. The prognosis at this stage is grave, and the management consists mainly of supportive care, plus adjusting antibiotics according to the susceptibility of the organism.

Therapy

S. pneumoniae is the most frequent pathogen isolated in the setting of OPSI. Early antibiotic therapy should cover this pathogen, keeping in mind the increasing preva-lence to penicillin resistance and the potential spread of fluoroquinolone resistance (2,47,48). As of the beginning of the 21st century, pneumococcus is still universally sus-ceptible to vancomycin, linezolid, daptomycin, and Quininipristin/Dalfopristin. Some authorities would suggest adding intravenous immunoglobulin in this setting (16).

H. influenzae type b and *C. canimorsus* (49) often produce β-lactamase; they are sensitive to third generation cephalosporins and to fluoroquinolones, as well as is meningococcus.

In summary the best choice of empirical antibiotic therapy when OPSI is suspected is vancomycin with a third generation cephalosporin such as ceftriaxone; if the patient is penicillin allergic, vancomycin with a fluoroquinolone (ciprofloxacin, levofloxacin, moxifloxacin, or gatifloxacin) is an adequate choice pending identifica-tion and susceptibility of the offending agent.

Another important aspect of the management of hyposplenic patients is pre-vention of future serious infections (46,50). There are four points to this end; they are well summarized in Castagnola's review paper (4):

1.   Administration of pneumococcal vaccine (PCV-7) every five years (51); its overall efficacy in preventing pneumococcal pneumonia is at best 70% (52).

Timing of the vaccine should ideally be two weeks prior to splenectomy. In cases where vaccination was not given prior to surgery, it seems that functional antibody response is better when vaccine is administered two weeks postsplenectomy as compared to the immediate postsurgical period (53).

Some authors suggest revaccinating every three years in this setting, because the antibody levels may decline more rapidly in asplenic patients (54–56). Another potential method to increase protection against pneumococcus would be a combined use of the heptavalent conjugated PCV-7 with the less immunogenic 23-valent pneumococcal vaccine (57).

Administration of Hib vaccine every five years is less well studied (58).

2. Lifelong antibiotic prophylaxis, based primarily on penicillin. This could be controversial, because Falletta et al. did not find an increased incidence of pneumococcal disease in sickle cell children who discontinued their prophylaxis compared to those who were still receiving it (59). This contrasts with Prophylaxis with oral penicillin on sickle cell anemia (PROPS I) study in 215 children with Hgb SS disease who were randomized to receive penicillin twice a day versus placebo. This study was terminated earlier than planned, because at eight months there was an 84% reduction in pneumococcal sepsis in the group receiving antibiotics (60). It seems that age is a determinant factor that may account for those differences between studies; children younger than five years have a 9.8/100 patient-years risk for pneumococcal bacteremia compared to 0.67/100 patient-years in older than five years when neither one is receiving antibiotic prophylaxis (61). Another caveat in long-term antibiotic prophylaxis has to do with patients' compliance, which when studied was demonstrated to be poor: 43% in Teach et al.'s study (62). It also could potentially lead to colonization with more resistant organisms.

Table 3 Suggested Checklist for Patients with Hyposplenism

	Date administered	Date of booster
Vaccines		
Polyvalent pneumococcal vaccine		Every 3–5 yr
Conjugated pneumococcal vaccine	a	
Haemophilus b conjugate vaccine		
Meningococcal C conjugate vaccine		
Inactivated influenza vaccine		Yearly
Live intranasal influenza vaccine	b	

	Dose	Dates
Chemoprophylaxis		
Penicillin V		
Amoxicillin		
Patient education		
Informed about types and risks of infection		
Given prescription for self-administered broad spectrum antibiotic, if medical assistance unavailable		
Medical alert bracelet or necklace		

[a]It may complement polyvalent pneumococcal vaccine.
[b]If indicated, it may be more immunogenic.

3. Delay of elective splenectomy, and tissue salvage in splenic trauma (63–69). Even though studies have shown improvement in humoral immune response after spleen autotransplantation (67), OPSI still occurs in the setting of partial splenectomy (70).

4. Finally, patient education about their illness would seem to be extremely important. A recent study of 318 splenectomized patients followed up through a 17-year period and found that patients with the best knowledge about OPSI had the lowest incidence of this disease (14). Yet most studies point to the lack of patient knowledge about their ailment, and failure of their physician to follow guidelines recommendations for their management (2,17,18,41,71–76).

Other recommendations include meningococcal A&C vaccine, avoidance of exposure to cats, and dogs, as well as measures to prevent insect exposures in endemic areas for babesia and malaria.

Some experts prescribe amoxicillin/clavulanic acid for self-administration with onset of any fever in patients with known hyposplenism (77).

A useful suggestion for improving awareness and management of patients with hyposplenism would be an alert bracelet and/or a card with boxes to be checked for all those prophylactic measures just mentioned (Table 3) (1,78).

REFERENCES

1. Brigden ML. Detection education and management of the asplenic or hyposplenic patient. Am Fam Physician 2001; 63:499–506.
2. Brigden ML, Pattullo AL. Prevention and management of overwhelming postsplenectomy infection—an update. Crit Care Med 1999; 27:836–842.
3. Styr B. Infection associated with asplenia: risks, mechanisms, and prevention. Am J Med 1990; 88:533N–542N.
4. Castagnola E, Fioredda F. Prevention of life-threatening infections due to encapsulated bacteria in children with hyposplenia or asplenia: a brief review of current recommendations for practical purposes. Eur J Haematol 2003; 71:319–326.
5. King H, Shumaker HB. Splenic studies I. Susceptibility to infection after splenectomy performed in infancy. Ann Surg 1952; 136:259.
6. Hansen K, Singer DB. Asplenic-hyposplenic overwhelming sepsis: postsplenectomy. Sepsis revisited. Pediatr Develop Pathol 2001; 4:105–121.
7. Sumaraju V, Smith LG, Smith SM. Infectious complications in asplenic hosts. Infect Dis Clin North Am 2001; 15:551–565.
8. Germing U, Pering C, Steiner S, et al. Congenital asplenia detected in a 60 year old patient with septicemia. Eur J Med Res 1999; 4:283–285.
9. Abrahamsen AF, Borge L, Holte H. Infection after splenectomy for Hodgkin's disease. Acta Oncol 1990; 29:167.
10. Markus HS, Toghill PJ. Impaired splenic function in elderly people. Age Aging 1991; 20:287.
11. Muller AF, Toghill PJ. Functional hyposplenism in alcoholic liver disease: a toxic effect of alcohol? Gut 1994; 35:679–682.
12. Germing U, Fischer R, Bauser U, et al. Pneumococcal septicemia in functional asplenia: first manifestation of systemic autoimmune disease? Z Rheum 1999; 58:31–34.
13. Doll DC, List AF, Yarbro JW. Functional hyposplenism. South Med J 1987; 80:999–1006.
14. El-Alfy MS, El-Sayed MH. Overwhelming postsplenectomy infection: Is quality of patient knowledge enough for prevention? Hematol J 2004; 5:77–80.

15. Lynch AM, Kapila R. Overwhelming postsplenectomy infection. Infect Dis Clin North Am 1996; 10:693–707.
16. Davidson RN, Wall RA. Prevention and management of infections in patients without a spleen. Clin Microbiol Infect 2001; 7:657–660.
17. Waghorn DJ. Overwhelming infection in asplenic patients: current best practice preventive measures are not being followed. J Clin Pathol 2001; 54:214–218.
18. Waghorn DJ, Mayon-White RT. A study of 42 episodes of overwhelming post-splenectomy infection: is current guidance for asplenic individuals being followed? J Infect 1997; 35: 289–294.
19. Lutwick LI. Life threatening infections in the asplenic or hyposplenic individual. Curr Clin Topics Infect Dis 2002; 22:78–96.
20. Deodhor HA, Marshall RJ, Barnes JN. Increased risk of sepsis after splenectomy. BMJ 1993; 307:1408–1409.
21. Cullingford GL, Watkins DN, Watts ADJ, et al. Severe late postsplenectomy infection. Br J Surg 1991; 78:716–721.
22. Bisharat N, Omari H, Lavi I, Raz R. Risk of infection and death among post-splenectomy patients. J Infect 2001; 43:182–186.
23. Schilling RF. Estimating the risk of sepsis after splenectomy in hereditary spherocytosis. Ann Intern Med 1995; 122:187–188.
24. Eber SW, Langendorfer CM, Ditzig M, et al. Frequency of very late sepsis after splenectomy for hereditary spherocytosis: impact of insufficient antibody response to pneumococcal infection. Ann Hematol 1999; 78:524–528.
25. Pearson HA, Johnson D, Smith KA, et al. Born-again spleen: return of splenic function after splenectomy for trauma. N Engl J Med 1978; 298(25):1389.
26. Machesky KK, Cushing RD. Overwhelming postsplenectomy infection in a patient with penicillin-resistant streptococcus pneumoniae. Arch Fam Med 1998; 7:178–180.
27. Spelman DW. Postsplenectomy overwhelming sepsis: reducing the risks. Med J Aust 1996; 164:648.
28. Hinrichs JH, Dunkelberg WE. DF-2 septicemia after splenectomy: epidemiology and immunologic response. South Med J 1980; 73:1638.
29. Mahrer S, Raik E. *Capnocytophaga canimorsus* septicemia associated with cat scratch. Pathology 1992; 24:194–196.
30. Kalb R, Kaplan MH, Tenebaum MJ, et al. Cutaneous infection at dog bite wounds associated with fulminant DF-2 septicemia. Am J Med 1985; 78:687–690.
31. Baccarani M, Fiacchini M, Galieni P, et al. Meningitis and septicemia in adults splenectomized for Hodgkin's disease. Scand J Haematol 1986; 36:492–498.
32. Gallagher F. Streptococcus infection and splenectomy. Lancet 2001; 357:1129–1130.
33. Francois B, Gissat V, Ploy MC, Vignon P. Recurrent septic shock due to streptococcus suis. J Clin Microbiol 1998; 36:2395.
34. Bar-Gil-Shitrit A, Raveh D, Yinnon A, Schlesinger Y. Overwhelming postsplenectomy infection caused by group B streptococcus: a case report and review of the literature. Infect Dis Clin Pract 2001; 10:42–44.
35. Shepard CW et al. *Bordetella holmesii* bacteremia: a newly recognized clinical entity among asplenic patients. Clin Infect Dis 2004; 38:799.
36. Rabinstein A, Tikhomirov V, Kaluta A, et al. Recurrent and prolonged fever in asplenic patients with human granulocytic ehrlichiosis. Quart J Med 2000; 93:198–201.
37. Hohenschild S. Babesiosis—a dangerous infection for splenectomized children and adults. Klin Paed 1999; 211:137–140.
38. Centers for disease control: clindamycin and quinine treatment for Babesia Microti infection. MMWR 1983; 32:65.
39. Rosner F, Zarrabi M, Benach JL, et al. Babesiosis in splenectomized adults. Review of 22 reported cases. Am J Med 1984; 76:696.
40. Looareesurwan S, Suntharasamai P, Webster HK, et al. Malaria in splenectomized patients: report of four cases and review. Clin Infect Dis 1993; 84:566.

41. Schutze GE, Mason EO Jr., Barson WJ, et al. Invasive pneumococcal infections in children with asplenia. Pediatr Infect Dis J 2002; 21:278–282.
42. Carpenter CT, Kaiser AB. Purpura fulminans in pneumococcal sepsis: case report and review. Scand J Infect Dis 1997; 29:479–483.
43. Holdsworth RJ, Irving AD, Cuschieri A. Postsplenectomy sepsis and its mortality rate: actual versus perceived risks. Br J Surg 1991; 78:1031–1038.
44. Klinge J, Hammersen G, Scharf J, et al. Overwhelming postsplenectomy infection with vaccine-type streptococcus pneumoniae in a 12-year old girl despite vaccination and antibiotic prophylaxis. Infection 1997; 25:368–371.
45. Abildgaard N, Nielsen JL. Pneumococcal septicemia and meningitis in vaccinated splenectomised adult patients. Scand J Infect Dis 1994; 26:615–617.
46. Davies JM, Barnes R, Milligan D. Update of guidelines for the prevention and treatment of infection in patients with an absent or dysfunctional spleen. Clin Med 2002; 2(5): 440–443.
47. Wang WC, Wong WY, Rogers ZR, et al. Antibiotic resistant pneumococcal infection in children with sickle cell disease in the US. J Pediatr Hematol Oncol 1996; 18:140.
48. Sakhalkar VS, Sarnaik SA, Asmar BI, et al. Prevalence of penicillin-nonsusceptible *Streptococcus pneumoniae* in nasopharyngeal cultures from patients with sickle cell disease. South Med J 2001; 94:401.
49. Roscoe DL, Zemcov SJV, Thornber D, et al. Antimicrobial susceptibilities and β-lactamase characterization of capnocytophaga species. Antimicrob Agents Chemother 1992; 36: 2197–2200.
50. British Committee for Standards in Haematology. Guidelines for the prevention and treatment of infection in patients with an absent or dysfunctional spleen. BMJ 1996; 312:430–434.
51. Advisory Committee on Immunization Practices. Prevent Pneumococcal Dis MMWR 1997; 46:1–24.
52. Shapiro ED, Berg AT, Austria R, et al. The protective efficacy of polyvalent pneumococcal polysaccharide vaccine. N Engl J Med 1991; 325(21):1453–1460.
53. Shatz DV, Schinsky MF, Pais LB, et al. Immune responses of splenectomized trauma patients to the 23-valent pneumococcal polysaccharide vaccine at 1 versus 7 versus 14 days after splenectomy. J Trauma 1998; 44:760–765.
54. Rutherford EJ, Livengood J, Higginbotham M, et al. Efficacy and safety of pneumococcal revaccination after splenectomy for trauma. J Trauma 1995; 39:448–452.
55. Hazelwood M, Kumararatne DS. The spleen. Who needs it anyway? Clin Exp Immunol 1992; 89:327–329.
56. Weintrub PS, Schiffman G, Addiego JE, et al. Long term follow up and booster immunization with polyvalent polysaccharide in patients with sickle cell anemia. J Paediatr 1984; 105: 261–263.
57. O'Brien KL, Swift AJ, Winkelstein JA, et al. Safety and immunogenicity of heptavalent pneumococcal vaccine conjugated to CRM(197) among infants with sickle cell disease. Pneumococcal conjugate vaccine study group. Pediatrics 2000; 106:965.
58. Li Volti S, Sciotti A, Fisichella M, et al. Immune responses to administration of a vaccine against haemophilus influenzae type B in splenectomized and non-splenectomized patients. J Infect 1999; 39:38–41.
59. Falletta JM, Woods GM, Verter JI, et al. Discontinuing penicillin prophylaxis in children with sickle cell anemia. J Pediatr 1995; 127:685–690.
60. Gaston MH, Verter JI, Woods G, et al. Prophylaxis with oral penicillin in children with sickle cell anemia. A randomized trial. N Engl J Med 1986; 314:1593.
61. Hord J, Byrd R, Stowe L, et al. *Streptococcus pneumoniae* sepsis and meningitis during the penicillin prophylaxis era in children with sickle cell disease. J Pediatr Hematol Oncol 2002; 24:470.
62. Teach SJ, Lillis KA, Grossi M. Compliance with penicillin prophylaxis in patients with sickle cell disease. Arch Pediatr Adolesc Med 1998; 152:274.

63. Pachter HL, Guth AA, Hofstetter SR, Spencer FC. Changing patterns in the management of splenic trauma: the impact of nonoperative management. Ann Surg 1998; 227:708–717.

64. Rose AT, Newman MI, Debelak J, et al. The incidence of splenectomy is decreasing: lessons learned from trauma experience. Am Surg 2000; 66:481–486.

65. Rozinov VM, Salel'ev SB, Keshishyan RA, et al. Organ-sparing treatment for closed spleen injuries in children. Clin Orthoped 1995; 320:34–39.

66. Mucha P. Changing attitudes toward the management of blunt splenic trauma in adults. Mayo Clin Proc 1986; 61:472.

67. Leemans R, Harms G, Rijkers GT, Timens W. Spleen autotransplantation provides restoration of functional splenic lymphoid compartments and improves the humoral immune response to pneumococcal polysaccharide vaccine. Clin Exp Immunol 1999; 117: 596–604.

68. Hoestra HJ, Tamminga RY, Timens W. Partial splenectomy in children: an alternative for splenectomy in the pathological staging of Hodgkin's disease. Ann Surg Oncol 1994; 1:480–486.

69. Bussel JH. Splenectomy-sparing strategies for the treatment and long-term maintenance of chronic idiopathic (immune) thrombocytopenic purpura. Sem Haematol 2000; 37(S1):1–4.

70. Svarch E, Nordet I, Gonzalez A. Overwhelming septicaemia in a patient with sickle cell/ beta thalassemia and partial splenectomy. Br J Haematol 1999; 104:930.

71. De Montalembert M, Lenoir G. Antibiotic prevention of pneumococcal infections in asplenic hosts: admission of insufficiency. Ann Hematol 2004; 83(1):18–21.

72. Kinnersley P, Wilkinson CE, Strinivason J. Pneumococcal vaccination after splenectomy: survey of hospital and primary care records. BMJ 1993; 307:1398–1399.

73. Brigden ML, Patullo A, Brown G. Pneumococcal vaccine administration associated with splenectomy: the need for improved education, documentation, and the use of a practical check-list. Am J Hematol 2000; 65:25–29.

74. Kind EA, Craft C, Fowles JB, McCoy CE. Pneumococcal vaccine administration associated with splenectomy: missed opportunities. Am J Infect Control 1998; 26:418–422.

75. Palejwala AA, Hong LY, King D. Doctors' knowledge of post-splenectomy prophylaxis. Int J Clin Pract 1997; 51:353–354.

76. Brigden ML, Pattullo A, Brown G. Practicing physician's knowledge and patterns of practice regarding the asplenic state: the need for improved education and a practical checklist. Can J Surg 2001; 44:210–216.

77. Finch RG, Read R. Lifelong penicillin may be ineffective. BMJ 1994; 308:132.

78. Mayon-White R. Protection for the asplenic patient. Prescribers J 1994; 34:165–170.

25
Infections in Burns

Steven E. Wolf and Basil A. Pruitt
*Division of Trauma and Emergency Surgery, Department of Surgery, University of Texas
Health Science Center, and Burn Center, United States Army Institute of Surgical
Research, San Antonio, Texas, U.S.A.*

Seung H. Kim
*Burn Center, United States Army Institute of Surgical Research, San Antonio,
Texas, U.S.A.*

INTRODUCTION

Over one million people are burned in the United States every year, most of whom
have minor injuries and are treated as outpatients. However, approximately 60,000
burns per year are serious to severe and require hospitalization. Roughly 3000 of these
patients die (1). Burns requiring hospitalization typically include burns of greater than
10% of the total body surface area (TBSA), and significant burns of the hands, face,
perineum, or feet.

Between 1971 and 1991, burn deaths from all causes decreased by 40%, with a
concomitant 12% decrease in deaths associated with inhalation injury (2). Since 1991,
burn deaths per capita have decreased another 25% according to Centers for Disease
Control (Fig. 1) (3). The graph in Figure 1 shows that burn deaths have been decreasing
by approximately 124 per year on a linear basis for the last 20 years ($r^2 = 0.99$), which
has been most pronounced in the African-American population. These improvements
were likely due primarily to effective prevention strategies resulting in fewer burns of
lesser severity, as well as significant progress in treatment techniques.

Improved patient care in the severely burned has undoubtedly improved survival.
Bull and Fisher first reported, in 1949, the expected 50% mortality rate for burn sizes in
several age groups (LA_{50}). They reported approximately one-half of children aged 0 to
14 with burns of 49% TBSA would die, 46% TBSA for patients aged 15 to 44, 27%
TBSA for those aged 45 to 64, and 10% TBSA for those 65 and older (4). These dismal
statistics have dramatically improved, with the latest reports indicating 50% mortality
for 98% TBSA burns in children 14 and under, and 75% TBSA burns in other young
age groups (5,6). Therefore, a healthy young patient with any size burn might be
expected to survive (7). The same cannot be said, however, for those aged 45 years or
more, where improvements have been much more modest, especially in the elderly (8).

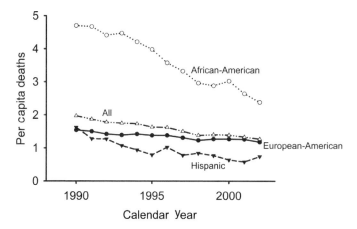

Figure 1 Per capita mortality from burns in the United States. The rate has been decreasing yearly at approximately 124 deaths/100,000 persons per year ($r = 0.99$).

Reasons for these dramatic improvements in mortality after massive burn that are related to treatment generally include better understanding of resuscitation, improvements in wound coverage, improved support of the hypermetabolic response to injury, enhanced treatment of inhalation injuries, and perhaps most importantly, control of infection.

Burn mortality can generally be divided into five causes:

1. Immolation and overwhelming damage at the site of injury, with relatively immediate death
2. Death in the first few hours/days due to overwhelming organ dysfunction associated with burn shock before infection can develop
3. Death due to medical error at some time during the hospital course
4. Development of progressive multiple organ failure later in the hospital course with or without infection, highlighted by the development of acute respiratory distress syndrome
5. Development of overwhelming infectious sepsis from the burn wound or other source in the days/weeks following the injury. This form is highlighted by cardiovascular collapse

The first cause is generally unavoidable, other than by preventing the injury in the first place. The second cause is unusual in modern burn centers with the advent of monitored resuscitation as advocated by Pruitt et al. (9) and Baxter and Shires (10). The third cause is minimized by good medical care, being rectified to some extent by the institution of local clinical guidelines, which are rapidly becoming the standard in intensive care units around the world. The last two are the most common causes of death for those who are treated at a burn center, and it is these two that are linked to the development of infection of the burn wound with microorganisms.

TREATMENT OF BURN WOUND TO CONTROL INFECTION

Two practices have revolutionized burn care to improve outcomes by decreasing invasive wound infections. Early excision and closure of the burn wound is one, which is essentially preventative by eliminating the eschar that harbors the microorganisms and by providing a further barrier to microorganism growth. The other is the timely and effective use of antimicrobials, both topical and systemic. The infected burn wound filled with invasive organisms is uncommon in most burn units due to the aggressive use of antibiotics and wound care techniques.

The mortality reduction in patients with extensive burns has been achieved principally by early excision and an aggressive surgical approach to deep wounds. Early removal of devitalized tissue prevents wound infections and decreases inflammation associated with the wound. In addition, it eliminates small colonized foci, which are a frequent source of transient bacteremia. Those transient bacteremias during surgical manipulations may prime immune cells to react in an exaggerated fashion to subsequent insults, leading to whole body inflammation—systemic inflammatory response syndrome (SIRS), and remote organ damage (multisystem organ failure). We recommend complete early excision of clearly full-thickness wounds within 48 hours of the injury, and coverage of the wound with autograft or allograft when autograft is not available. Within days, this treatment will provide a stable antimicrobial barrier to the development of wound infection. Barret and Herndon described a study in which they enrolled 20 subjects, 12 of whom underwent early excision (within 48 hours of injury) and eight underwent delayed excision (more than six days after injury). Quantitative cultures from the wound excision showed that early excision subjects had less than 10 bacteria/gram of tissue, while those who underwent delayed excision had more than 10^5 organisms, and three of these patients (37.5%) developed histologically proven burn wound infection compared to none in the early excision group (11). In another study from the same center, it was found that delayed excision was associated with a higher incidence of wound contamination, invasive wound infection, and sepsis with bacteremia compared to the early group when the rest of the hospitalization was considered (12). These two studies show that the best control of burn wound colonization and infection is obtained with early excision.

Before or after excision, control of microorganism growth is attained by the use of topical antibiotics. Available topical antibiotics can be divided into two classes: salves and soaks. Salves are generally applied directly to the wound with cotton dressings placed over them, and soaks are poured into cotton dressings on the wound. Each of these classes of antimicrobials has advantages and disadvantages. Salves may be applied once or twice a day, but may lose effectiveness in between dressing changes. More frequent dressing changes can result in shearing, with loss of grafts or underlying healing cells. Soaks will remain effective because antibiotic solution can be added without removing the dressing; however, the underlying skin can become macerated.

Topical antibiotic salves include 11.1% mafenide acetate (Sulfamylon), 1% silver sulfadiazine (Silvadene), polymyxin B, neomycin, bacitracin, mupirocin, and the antifungal agent nystatin (Table 1). No single agent is completely effective, and each has advantages and disadvantages. Silver sulfadiazine is the most commonly used. It has a broad spectrum of activity from its silver and sulfa moieties covering gram-positives, most gram-negatives, and some fungal forms. Some *Pseudomonas* species possess plasmid-mediated resistance. It is relatively painless upon application, has a high patient acceptance, and is easy to use. Occasionally, patients will complain of some burning sensation after it is applied, and a substantial number of patients will develop a transient leukopenia three to five days following its continued use. This leukopenia is generally harmless, and resolves with or without cessation of treatment. Mafenide acetate is another topical agent that also has a broad spectrum of activity through its sulfa moiety, particularly for resistant *Pseudomonas* and *Enterococcus* species. It also has the advantage of penetration of eschar, which is absent with silver sulfadiazine. Disadvantages include pain after

Table 1 Topical Antimicrobials Commonly Used in Burn Care

Antimicrobials	Advantages	Disadvantages
Salves		
Silver sulfadiazine (Silvadene® 1%)	Broad spectrum Relatively painless on application	Transient leukopenia Does not penetrate eschar May tattoo dermis with black flecks
Mafenide acetate (Sulfamylon® 11%)	Broad spectrum Penetration of eschar	Painful on application to partial thickness burns May cause an allergic rash Carbonic anhydrase activity
Polymyxin B/neomycin/bacitracin	Wide spectrum Painless on application Colorless, allowing direct inspection of the wound	Antimicrobial coverage less than alternatives
Mupirocin (Bactroban®)	Broad spectrum (especially *Staphylococcus* species)	Expensive
Nystatin	Broad antifungal coverage	May inactivate other antimicrobials (Sulfamylon)
Soaks		
Silver nitrate (0.5%)	Complete antimicrobial coverage Painless	Black staining when exposed to light Electrolyte leaching Methemoglobinemia
Mafenide acetate (Sulfamylon® 5%)	Same as salve	Same as salve
Sodium hypochlorite (Dakins' 0.05%)	Broad-spectrum coverage	Inactivated with protein contact Cytotoxic
Acetic acid	Broad-spectrum coverage (especially *Pseudomonas*)	Cytotoxic

application upon skin with sensation, such as in a second-degree wounds. It can also cause an allergic skin rash and has carbonic anhydrase inhibitory characteristics that can result in a metabolic acidosis when applied over large surfaces. For these reasons, mafenide sulfate is typically reserved for small full-thickness injuries, wounds with obvious bacterial overgrowth, or those full-thickness wounds that cannot be rapidly excised, such as in patients with concomitant devastating head injuries.

Petroleum-based antimicrobial ointments with polymyxin B, neomycin, and bacitracin are clear on application, are painless, and allow for easy wound observation. These agents are commonly used for treatment of facial burns, graft sites, healing donor sites, and small partial-thickness burns. Mupirocin is a relatively new petroleum-based ointment that has improved activity against gram-positive bacteria, particularly methicillin-resistant *Staphylococcus aureus* and selected gram-negative bacteria. Nystatin, either in a salve or powder form, can be applied to wounds to control fungal growth. Nystatin-containing ointments can be combined with other topical agents to potentially decrease colonization of both bacteria and fungi. The exception is the combination of nystatin and mafenide acetate because each will inactivate the other.

Available agents for application as a soak include 0.5% silver nitrate solution, 0.025% sodium hypochlorite (Dakins'), 5% acetic acid (Domburo's), and most recently 5% mafenide acetate solution. Silver nitrate has the advantage of painless application and virtually complete antimicrobial coverage. The disadvantages include its staining of surfaces to a dull gray or black when the solution dries. This can become problematic in deciphering wound depth during burn excisions and in keeping the patient and the patient's surroundings clean of the black staining with exposure to light. The solution is hypotonic as well, and continuous use can cause electrolyte leaching with rare methemoglobinemia as another complication. Dakins' solution is a basic solution with effectiveness against most microbes; however, it also has cytotoxic effects on the patients' wounds, thus inhibiting healing. Low concentrations of sodium hypochlorite have less cytotoxic effects while maintaining the antimicrobial effects in vitro. In addition, hypochlorite ion is inactivated by contact with protein, so the solution must be continually changed either with frequent application of new solution or continuous irrigation. The same is true for acetic acid solutions; however, this solution has been reported to be more effective against *Pseudomonas*, although this may only be a discoloration of pyocyanine released by this organism, without effect on its viability. Mafenide acetate soaks have the same characteristics as the mafenide acetate salve but are not recommended for the primary treatment of intact eschar.

It must be stated that all topical agents have been demonstrated to inhibit epithelialization of the wound to some extent, presumably due to toxicity of the agents to keratinocytes and/or fibroblasts, polymorphonuclear cells, and macrophages. Therefore, these agents should be used with this in mind. The alternative of wound infection occurring in an untreated wound, however, justifies the use of topical agents.

The use of perioperative systemic antimicrobials also has a role in decreasing burn wound sepsis until the burn wound is closed. Common organisms that must be considered when choosing a perioperative regimen include *Staphylococcus* and *Pseudomonas* species, which are prevalent in wounds. After massive excisions, gut flora are often found in the wounds, mandating consideration of these species as well, particularly *Klebsiella pneumoniae*. Perioperative antibiotics clearly benefit patients with injuries greater than 40% TBSA burns, as enumerated below.

The use of perioperative antibiotics has been linked to the development of multiply resistant strains of bacteria and fungus in several types of critical care units.

Considering this and other data, we recommend that systemic antibiotics be used short term (24 hours) routinely as perioperative treatment during excision and grafting, because the benefits outweigh the risks. We use a combination of vancomycin and amikacin for this purpose, covering the two most common pathogens on the burn wound in *Staphylococcus* and *Pseudomonas*. The preferred perioperative regimen included 1 g of vancomycin given intravenously one hour prior to surgery, and another 1 g, 12 hours after the surgical procedure, and a dose of amikacin (based on patient weight, age, and estimated creatinine clearance) given 30 minutes prior to surgery and again eight hours after surgery. Next, systemic antibiotics should be used for identified infections of the burn wound, pneumonia, etc., The antibiotics chosen should be directed presumptively at multiply resistant *Staphylococcus* and *Pseudomonas* and other gram-negatives.

The most common sources of sepsis are the wounds and/or the tracheobronchial trees; efforts to identify causative agents should be concentrated there. Another potential source, however, is the gastrointestinal tract, which is a natural reservoir for bacteria. Starvation and hypovolemia shunt blood from the splanchnic bed and promote mucosal atrophy and failure of the gut barrier. Early enteral feeding has been shown to reduce morbidity and potentially prevent failure of the gut barrier (13). At our institution, patients are fed immediately during resuscitation through a nasogastric tube. Early enteral feedings are tolerated in burn patients and preserve the mucosal integrity and may reduce the magnitude of the hypermetabolic response to injury. Support of the gut should accompany carefully monitored hemodynamic resuscitation.

Selective decontamination of the gut has been purported to be of use in preventing sepsis in the severely burned. de La Cal et al. showed a significant reduction in mortality in severe burns treated with selective gut decontamination, which was associated with a decreased incidence of pneumonia. This study analyzed 107 patients randomized to placebo or treatment (14). This is refuted by another smaller study, which showed no benefit to selective gut decontamination but only an increase in the incidence of diarrhea (15).

BURN WOUND INFECTION

Before the development of effective topical antibacterial chemotherapy, burn wound infections were the most common infections in burn patients, and invasive burn wound sepsis was the most common cause of death in patients who died in burn centers (16). Destruction of the blood vessels in the burned tissue renders it ischemic. The denatured protein comprising the eschar presents rich pabulum for microorganisms. Both these conditions conspire to make the burn wound a "locus minoris resistentiae" in the setting of burn-induced immunosuppression. Topical antimicrobial chemotherapy, achieved by the use of topical agents such as mafenide acetate, silver sulfadiazine, and silver nitrate soaks or silver impregnated materials, impedes colonization and reduces proliferation of bacteria and fungus on the burn wound. 11.1% mafenide acetate cream, which readily diffuses into eschar, can also control and even reduce the density of bacteria in a burn wound in which delayed initiation of topical antimicrobial therapy has permitted intraeschar proliferation of microorganisms. Control of the microbial density in the burn wound by topical therapy not only decreases the occurrence of burn wound infection per se but also permits burn wound excision to be carried out, with marked reduction in intraoperative bacteremia and endotoxemia. These two conditions formerly compromised the effectiveness of burn wound excision performed on a day other than the day of injury. The combined effect of topical therapy and early burn wound excision has decreased the incidence of invasive burn wound sepsis as the cause of death in patients at burn centers from 60% in the 1960s to only 6% in the 1980s. A historical study of the use of mafenide acetate in burned combatants during the Vietnam War demonstrated a 10% reduction in mortality in those with severe burns treated with mafenide versus those without topical treatment (17). In the past 14 years, invasive burn wound infection, both bacterial and fungal, has occurred in only 2.3% of 3876 patients admitted to the U.S. Army Burn Center in San Antonio (18), who were treated with early excision and topical/ systemic antibiotics as described above.

Organisms causing burn wound infections change over time and have anticipated, by approximately one decade, the predominant organisms now causing infections in other surgical ICUs. Prior to the availability of penicillin, beta hemolytic streptococcal infections were the most common infections in burn patients. Soon after penicillin became available, *Staphylococci* became the principal offenders. The subsequent development of antistaphylococcal agents resulted in the emergence of gram-negative organisms, principally *Pseudomonas aeruginosa*, as the predominant bacteria causing invasive burn wound infections. Topical burn wound antimicrobial therapy, early excision, and the availability of antibiotics effective against gram-negative organisms were associated with a recrudescence of staphylococcal infections in the late 1970s and 1980s, which has been followed by the reemergence of infections caused by gram-negative organisms in the past 15 years. During this time period, it was also noted that hospital costs and mortality increased in those patients with whom *Pseudomonas* organisms were isolated (19).

In the period 1991 to 2004, the fungi have become the predominant causative organisms of burn wound infection causing death; 72% of invasive burn wound infections in burn patients treated at the U.S. Army Burn Center were caused by fungi. In a very real sense, fungal burn wound infections represent a perverse manifestation of the success of current burn wound therapy; i.e., they occur relatively late (sixth or seventh week after burn) in patients with extensive burns who have undergone serial excision and grafting procedures with repeated perioperative broad-spectrum antibiotic coverage. This method of treatment provides an ecologic niche for the fungi in the residual open wounds. It was noted previously that with the introduction of topical mafenide acetate, wound infections caused by *Phycomycetes* and *Aspergillus* increased tenfold (20), and further measures such as patient isolation, wound excision, and other topical chemotherapy decreased bacterial infections dramatically, while having no effect on the fungi (21).

Of late, common isolates in the burn wound are those of *Acinetobacter* species, which are often resistant to available antibiotics. Currently at the U.S Army Burn Center, approximately 25% of the isolates from newly admitted patients are of this type. However, in no case were these organisms found to be invasive, and in those patients who died, infection with this organism was not found to be the most likely cause of death. Instead, it was invasive fungus or *K. pneumoniae*, which were deemed the likely cause of death in those who succumbed to burn wound infection. This is in congruence with the findings of Wong et al. in Singapore, who showed that acquisition of *Acinetobacter* was not associated with mortality. They did note, however, that acquisition of *Acinetobacter* was associated with the number of intravenous lines placed and length of hospital stay (22), thus increasing hospital costs (23). Of other historical note, the isolation of vancomycin-resistant *Enterococcus* species was common in burn centers in the 1990s, but again, these organisms were not found to cause invasive wound infection and were at best associative with burn death, which was much more likely to be due to other causes and other organisms.

Even though present-day burn wound care has significantly reduced the occurrence of invasive burn wound infections, those caused by fungi are more difficult to treat and are associated with a high mortality. The most common nonbacterial colonizers are *Candida* species, which, fortunately, seldom invade unburned tissues and rarely cross tissue planes. Isolation of this organism in two sites has been associated with longer wound healing and length of hospital stay, use of artificial dermis, and use of imipenem for bacterial infection (24). *Aspergillus* and *Fusarium* species, in that order, are the most common filamentous fungi that cause invasive burn wound infection, and these organisms may traverse tissue plains and invade unburned tissues (Fig. 2). The most aggressive fungi are the *Phycomycetes*, which produce ischemic necrosis as a consequence of the propensity of their broad nonseptate hyphae to invade and thrombose dermal and subdermal vessels. Rapidly progressing ischemic necrosis in an unexcised or even excised burn wound should alert the practitioner to the possibility of invasive phycomycotic infection as should proptosis of the globe of an eye. One should be particularly alert to the possibility of invasive phycomycotic infection in patients with persistent or recurrent acidosis.

Assessment of the microbial ecology in burn centers is common. The most recent data in the literature from burn wounds indicates that coagulase-negative *Staphylococcus* and *S. aureus* are the most common isolates on admission. In the following weeks, these organisms are superseded by *Pseudomonas*, indicating that these organisms are the most common found on burn wounds later in the course and are, therefore, the most likely organisms to cause infection (25). In another burn center, it was again found that late isolates are dominated by *Pseudomonas*, which was shown to be resistant to most antibiotics save amikacin and tetracycline (26).

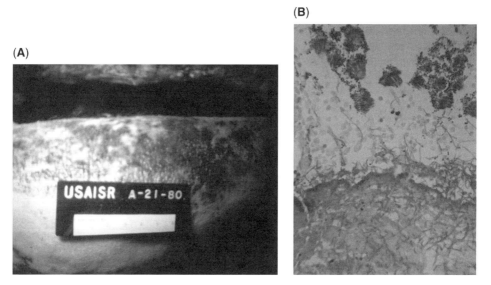

Figure 2 (**A**) Gross appearance and histologic finding of invasive *aspergillus* infection on the arm in a patient who succumbed to the infection. Note the discolored, dark, hemorrhagic appearance of the skin. (**B**) The histology shows clear evidence of hyphae down to viable tissue.

Diagnosis of Burn Wound Infection

It is essential to identify microbial invasion of the burn wound at the earliest possible time to prevent extensive microvascular involvement and hematogenous dissemination of the infecting organisms to remote tissues and organs. The entirety of the wound should be examined at the time of the daily wound cleansing to record any change in the appearance of the burn wound. The most frequent clinical sign of burn wound infection is the appearance of focal dark brown or black discoloration of the wound, but such change may occur as a consequence of focal hemorrhage into the wound due to minor local trauma (Fig. 3). The most reliable sign of burn wound infection is the conversion of an area of partial-thickness injury to full-thickness necrosis. Other clinical signs that should alert to the possibility of burn wound infection include unexpectedly rapid eschar separation, degeneration of a previously excised wound with neoeschar formation, hemorrhagic discoloration of the subeschar fat, and erythematous or violaceous discoloration of an edematous wound margin. Pathognomonic of invasive *Pseudomonas* infection are metastatic septic lesions in unburned tissue (*ecthyma gangrenosa*) (Fig. 4) and green discoloration of the subcutaneous fat by the pyocyanin produced by the invading organisms.

The appearance of any of those changes mandates immediate assessment of the microbial status of the burn wound. Because of the nature of the wound, bacteria and fungi will be found—some commensals and others opportunists. The mere presence of an organism, however, does not imply infection. It is only with invasion of organisms into the viable layer and thus gaining access to the bloodstream to release toxins and induce a severe inflammatory response that burn wound sepsis can occur. Surface swabs and even quantitative cultures, therefore, do not reliably differentiate colonization from invasion (27). Histologic examination of a biopsy specimen is the only means of accurately identifying and staging invasive burn wound infection (28).

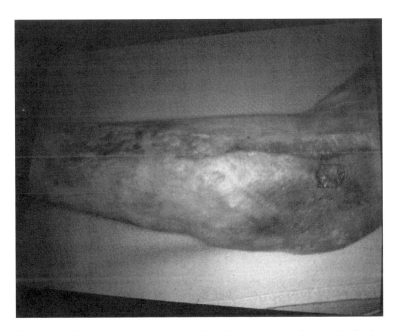

Figure 3   Gross appearance of invasive *Pseudomonas* infection in the burn wound. Note the discolored appearance that is distributed unevenly in the burn eschar.

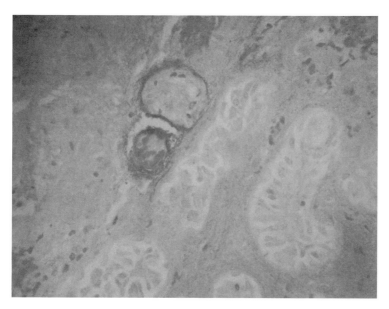

Figure 4 Ecthyma gangrenosum. Viable organisms are found "cuffed" around the vessel. This is hematogenous spread of the organism into the arterial tree, intimating bacteremia. Such lesions will be found throughout the body distant from the burn wound.

Using a scalpel, a 500 mg lenticular tissue sample is obtained from the area of the wound showing changes indicative of invasive infection. The biopsy must include not only eschar, but underlying, unburned subcutaneous tissues because the histologic diagnosis of invasive infection requires identification of microorganisms that have crossed the viable–nonviable tissue interface to take up residence and proliferate in viable tissue. The local anesthetic agent, if used, should be injected at the periphery of the biopsy site to avoid or minimize distortion of the tissue to be examined histologically. One-half of the biopsy specimen is processed for histologic examination to determine the depth of microbial penetration and identify microvascular invasion. The other half of the biopsy is quantitatively cultured to determine the specific microorganisms causing the invasive infection. The culture results are used to guide systemic antibiotic therapy.

The biopsy specimen is customarily prepared for histologic examination by a rapid section technique that affords diagnosis in three to four hours. Burn wound infection, if present, can then be staged on the basis of microbial density and depth of penetration to guide treatment. Alternatively, the specimen can be processed by frozen section technique, which yields a diagnosis within 30 minutes, but is associated with a 0.6% falsely positive diagnosis rate and a 3.6% falsely negative diagnosis rate (29). If the frozen section technique is utilized, permanent sections must be subsequently examined to confirm the frozen section diagnosis and exclude false negatives. The microbial status of the burn wound is classified according to the staging schema detailed in Table 2. In Stage I (colonization), the bacteria are limited to the surface and nonviable tissue of the eschar. Stage I consists of three subdivisions (A, B, and C) defined by the depth of eschar penetration and proliferation of microorganisms. Stage II (invasion) also consists of three subdivisions (A, B, and C) defined by the extent of invasion of microorganisms into nonviable tissue and involvement of lymphatics and microvasculature. Subsequent mortality increases as

Table 2 Histologic Staging of Microbial Status of the Burn Wound

Stage I: Colonization
  A. Superficial: microorganisms present only on burn wound surface
  B. Penetrating: variable depth of microbial penetration of eschar
  C. Proliferating: variable level of microbial proliferation of nonviable–viable tissue
     interface (subeschar space)
Stage II: Invasion
  A. Microinvasion: microorganisms present in viable tissue immediately subjacent to
     subeschar space
  B. Deep invasion: penetration of microorganisms to variable depth and expanse within
     viable subcutaneous tissue
  C. Microvascular involvement: microorganisms within small blood vessels and lymphatics
     (thrombosis of vessels is common)

the histologic staging increases from Stage IA to IIC, with a marked increase in mortality between Stage IC and IIA and a further increase with Stage IIB and IIC. Microvascular involvement connotes the likelihood of systemic spread and the development of burn wound sepsis, i.e., an invasive burn wound infection associated with systemic sepsis and progressive organ dysfunction.

A negative biopsy in association with progressive clinical deterioration mandates repeat biopsy from other areas of the wound showing changes indicative of infection. Successive biopsies that show progressive penetration and proliferation of microorganisms within the eschar indicate the need for emergency excision, or at the very least, a change in topical agent such as mafenide acetate for bacterial isolates, which can diffuse into the eschar and limit microbial proliferation. The high mortality associated with microvascular involvement and the recovery of positive blood cultures emphasizes the importance of early diagnosis prior to hematogenous dissemination of the invading microorganisms to remote tissues and organs or rapid proliferation locally with production of toxins.

An immediate change in wound care is called for if a diagnosis of invasive burn wound infection (Stage II) is made. Systemic antimicrobial therapy in full dosage should be initiated (amphotericin B or one of the newer agents in the case of fungal infections). The patient should be prepared for surgery and taken to the operating theater as soon as possible to excise the infected tissue, which, in the case of invasive fungal infection, may necessitate major amputation. Before excision of a wound harboring an invasive bacterial infection, one-half of the daily dose of a broad-spectrum penicillin (e.g., piperacillin tazobactam) should be suspended in 150 to 1000 mL of saline and injected by clysis into the subcutaneous tissues beneath the area of infection. A second clysis should be performed immediately before operation if more than six hours have elapsed from the initial clysis. The clysis therapy will prevent further proliferation of the invading organisms and reduce the number of viable bacteria and their metabolic by-products disseminated by operative manipulation of the infected tissue. In the case of invasive fungal infection, clotrimazole cream or powder should be applied to the infected area. Following excision of an area of invasive bacterial burn wound infection, the excised wound should be dressed with 5% mafenide acetate soaks. In the case of patients with fungal burn wound invasion, the excised wound should be covered with clotrimazole cream or powder. The patient should be returned to the operating room 24 to 48 hours later for thorough wound inspection and further excision of residual infected tissue, if necessary. That process is repeated until the infection is controlled and no further infected tissue is evident at the time of re-examination.

Successful treatment of patients with extensive burns involving the head and neck has been associated with an increased occurrence of superficial staphylococcal infections in healed and grafted wounds of the scalp and other hair-bearing areas. Those focal areas of suppuration have been termed "burn wound impetigo," which, if uncontrolled, can cause extensive epidermal lysis of the healed and grafted burns. Daily cleansing and twice-daily topical application of mupirocin ointment typically control the process and permit spontaneous healing of the superficial ulcerations. If not controlled with mupirocin, control may be obtained with frequent application or continuous irrigation with Dakins' (sodium hypochlorite) or Domburo's (acetic acid) solution.

Bacteremia

The topical antimicrobial chemotherapeutic agents commonly applied to burn wounds are bacteriostatic. They do not sterilize the burn wound but limit bacterial proliferation in the eschar and maintain microbial density at levels that do not overwhelm host defenses and invade viable tissue. Even so, manipulation of the wound by cleansing or surgical excision can result in bacteremia. In the 1970s, before widespread use of early excision, wound manipulation was associated with an overall 21% incidence of transient bacteremia (30). The incidence of bacteremia, which increased in proportion to the extent of burn and the vigor of the manipulation, provided the rationale for perioperative antibiotic administration as described above.

The previously noted decrease in invasive bacterial burn wound infection stimulated Mozingo et al. to reassess the incidence of bacteremia associated with burn wound cleansing and excision procedures. In 19 burn patients, those authors found only a 12.5% overall incidence of manipulation-induced bacteremia. The incidence of bacteremia was related to both the extent of burn and the time that had elapsed after the burn injury. Wound manipulation in patients with burns of less than 40% of the TBSA did not elicit bacteremia. In patients with more extensive burns, the incidence of bacteremia was 30% overall when wound manipulation occurred on or after the 10th postburn day and rose to 100% in patients whose burns involved more than 80% of the TBSA (31). These findings provide for omission of perioperative antibiotics for patients with burns of less than 40% of the TBSA, and for those with more extensive burns, who undergo excision prior to the 10th day after burn.

Bacteremia may also occur in association with uncontrolled infection in other sites. In a critically ill burn patient with life-threatening complications, recovery of multiple organisms from a single blood culture or different organisms from successive blood cultures indicate severe compromise of host resistance and should not be interpreted as contamination of the cultures. An antibiotic or antibiotics effective against all of the recovered organisms should be administered to such a patient at maximum dosage levels and the septic source of the blood-borne organisms should be identified and controlled. The comorbid effect of septicemia is organism specific. Historically, gram-negative septicemia and candidemia significantly increased mortality above that predicted on the basis of the extent of burn, but gram-positive septicemia had no demonstrable effect upon predicted mortality (32). Current techniques of wound care and improvements in general care of the burn patient have not only reduced the incidence of bacteremia but also significantly ameliorated the comorbid effect of gram-negative septicemia (33).

Sepsis

The diagnosis of sepsis on the basis of clinical criteria is made commonly in the severely burned, but, at times, a clear source from the burn wound, pneumonia, or bacteremia is not found. This is usually associated with progression of multiple organ failure in the absence of a source. In fact, investigators have shown that 17% of burned patients who develop sepsis associated with multiple organ failure will not have a preceding diagnosis of infection (34). In this condition, a thorough search should be made for an infectious source, including careful and repeated examination of the wound. Other potential sources include the urinary tract, endocarditis, catheter related sepsis, and meningitis. A perirectal abscess must also be considered. If a source is still not found, it is conceivable that the overwhelming signal of inflammation from the wound could be the cause. It must be emphasized that this is a diagnosis of exclusion, and even after the diagnosis is made, the search for a source of infection must continue. Oftentimes, these patients will be treated with presumptive wide-spectrum antibiotics. In this case, antifungal medications should be considered.

Of late, investigators have been in search of genetic markers that herald the development of sepsis, which could be related to the condition described above. Barber et al. recently described two single nucleotide polymorphisms in the DNA of patients who were more susceptible to the development of severe sepsis defined as signs of sepsis such as fever and high white blood cell count, and organ dysfunction or septic shock. The first, TLR4 + 896 G-allele, imparted a 1.8-fold increased risk of developing severe sepsis following burn relative to AA homozygotes. The second, tumor necrosis factor-alpha-308 A-allele, imparted a 1.7-fold increase in risk compared to GG homozygotes. However, these alleles were not associated with mortality (35). This early work signifies that slight genetic differences are likely to result in different responses to injury such as burn. Identification of these alleles may eventually assist practitioners in the care of these patients who are at risk and dictate different treatment.

Infections with Viruses

On occasion, fevers will develop in a burned patient, associated with herpetic lesions (herpes simplex virus-1), usually found in healed wounds, donor sites, or the face. This is characterized by the initial development of erythematous papules with or without a maculopapular erythematous rash that progress to vesicles and pustules. These lesions commonly rupture and develop crusts on the denuded base. Cytomegalovirus infections have also been reported in burned patients. The development of these lesions is thought to be reactivation of latent infection associated with burn-induced immunosuppression. Titers for antibodies to cytomegalovirus and herpes simplex virus type 1 may be found to increase, and intranuclear inclusion bodies in a biopsy from the lesion may also be found.

Excision is not required for the treatment of herpetic burn wound infections unless secondary invasive bacterial infection occurs in the herpetic ulcers. In fact, no changes in mortality or length of stay were found in those with viral infections and those without (36). Cutaneous ulcerations of herpetic infections should be treated with twice-a-day application of a 5% acyclovir ointment to decrease symptoms. Systemic herpes simplex virus-1 infections involving the liver, lung, adrenal gland, and bone marrow, though rare, are typically fatal and justify systemic acyclovir treatment. As noted above, rapidly expanding ischemic necrosis is characteristic of invasive phycomycotic infections and crusted, shallow, serrated lesions at the margin of a healing or recently healed partial-thickness burn, particularly in the nasolabial area, are typical of herpes simplex virus-1 infections. Identified viral infection is usually self-limited, but in severe cases, consideration can be given to systemic or topical treatment with acyclovir or ganciclovir.

Pneumonia

Pneumonia is now the most common infection in burned patients. The burn condition makes the patient fivefold more susceptible to the development of pneumonia because of mucociliary dysfunction associated with inhalation injury, atelectasis associated with mechanical ventilation, and impairment of innate immune responses (Fig. 5) (37). However, with better microbial control of the burn wound, the route of pulmonary infection has changed from hematogenous to airborne, and the predominant radiographic pattern has changed from nodular to bronchopneumonia (38). Nonetheless, some investigators still report a pneumonia rate of 48% in the severely burned treated in a burn center (39,40). Others have observed much lower rates (41–43).

The diagnosis of pneumonia in the burned patient is difficult, as the traditional harbingers of pneumonia of fever, high white blood cell count, and purulent sputum are common in the absence of infection in the severely burned, who have inflammation associated with the burn wounds. They are also often intubated for airway control for evidence of inhalation injury causing airway edema and unhealed wounds and purulence in the tracheobronchial tree. This provides a portal of entry for microbes into the airway. For this reason, we recommend that pneumonia in the severely burned be confirmed with the presence of three conditions: signs of systemic inflammation such as fever and high white blood cell count, radiographic evidence of pneumonia, and isolation of a pathogen on quantitative culture of a bronchoalveolar lavage specimen of 10 cc with greater than 10^4 organisms/cc of the return (44). Those patients with signs of sepsis and isolation of high colony counts of an organism on bronchoalveolar lavage without radiographic evidence of pneumonia are considered

(A)

(B)

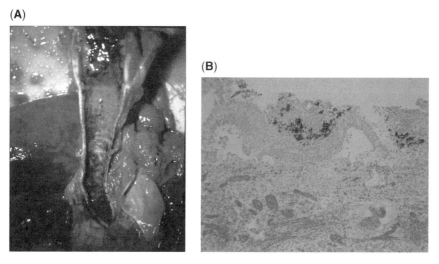

Figure 5 (**A**) Gross appearance and histology of inhalation injury. Note the denudation and hemorrhage in the trachea with erythema and soot. (**B**) The histologic appearance shows loss of epithelium and soot. The loss of the protective epithelium can lead to tracheobronchitis. Such findings are commonly found in the distal airways as well.

to have tracheobronchitis, which can become invasive with subsequent demise. These patients are then documented separately from those with pneumonia, but are treated similarly with systemic antibiotics directed at the predominant organism isolated on culture.

Organisms commonly encountered in the tracheobronchial tree include the gram-negatives, such as *Pseudomonas* and *Escherichia coli*, and, on occasion, the gram-positives such as *S. aureus*. When the diagnosis of pneumonia or tracheobronchitis is entertained, empiric antibiotic choice should include one that will cover both these types of organisms. We recommend piperacillin tazobactam and vancomycin given systemically until the isolates from the bronchoalveolar lavage are returned. The caveat to this is the finding of gram-negative organisms on routine surveillance cultures of the wound. Generally, microbes found on the wound do not reliably predict the causative agent of pneumonia, requiring separate microbial identification. This is certainly true for gram-positive organisms, but recent data from the U.S. Army Institute of Surgical Research indicates that identification of gram-negative organisms, particularly *Pseudomonas* and *Klebsiella* species on the wound of a patient with pneumonia, warrants specific presumptive antimicrobial coverage until the causative organism is determined. If sensitivities of the gram-negative bacteria on the wound are known, then antimicrobial therapy should, at the very least, include coverage of these.

Line Sepsis

As in other critically ill populations, the presence of indwelling catheters for infusion treatments provides a potential source of infection. Because of the relative frequency of bacteremia associated with treatment, relative immunosuppression, and the high concentrations of organisms on the skin often surrounding the access site for the intravascular device, line sepsis is common in the burned patient. Santucci et al. reported an incidence of 34 catheter-related bloodstream infections per 1000 central line days in burned patients (43). It has been well documented in other critically ill patients that the most likely portal of entry is the skin puncture site. Ramos et al. did show a significant reduction in catheter-related infection if the site of insertion was at least 25 cm from a burn wound (45). To date, no definitive prospective studies have been conducted to determine the true incidence of catheter-related infections related to the time of catheterization. For this reason, most burn centers have a policy to change catheter sites on a routine basis, every three to seven days until such information is available. Vigilant and scheduled replacement of intravascular devices presumably minimizes the incidence of catheter-related sepsis. The first can be done over a wire using sterile Seldinger technique, but the second change requires a new site. This protocol should be maintained as long as intravenous access is required. Whenever possible, peripheral veins should be used for cannulation even if the cannula is to pass through burned tissue. The saphenous vein, however, should be avoided because of the high risk of infectious thrombophlebitis. Should this complication occur in any peripheral vein, the entirety of the involved vein must be excised under general anesthesia with appropriate systemic therapy.

Other Infections

Aside from the burn wound infections, pneumonia, and catheter-related infections, burned patients are also susceptible to other infections similar to other critically ill patients (Table 3). The third most common site is the urinary tract because of the

Table 3 Infections in Burned Patients

Burn wound infection
Pneumonia
Catheter-related infection
Urinary tract infection
Sinusitis
Endocarditis
Infected thrombophlebitis
Infected chondritis of the burned ear

common presence of indwelling urethral catheters for monitoring of urine output. However, ascending infections and sepsis are uncommon because of the use of anti-biotics administered for prophylaxis and the treatment of other infections are com-monly concentrated in the urine and thereby reduce the risk of urinary tract infection. The exception to this is the development of fungiuria, most commonly from *Candida* species. When *Candida* species are found in the urine, systemic infec-tion should be considered, as the organisms may be filtered and sequestered in the tubules as a result of fungemia. The same holds true for the other fungi. For this rea-son, blood cultures are indicated in the presence of fungiuria to determine the source. If the infection is determined to be local, treatment with bladder irrigation of anti-fungals is indicated. Otherwise, systemic antifungal treatment should be initiated.

Because of the relative frequency of bacteremia/fungemia in the severely burned, sequestration of organisms around the heart valves can be found on occasion. In most large burn centers, at least one case per year of infectious endocarditis will be found on a search for a source of infection. In fact, about 1% of the severely burned develop this complication. The diagnosis is generally made by the persistent finding of pathogens in the blood in the presence of valvular vegetations found on echocardiography. This should generally be confirmed with transesophageal echo-cardiography if lesions are found on transthoracic echocardiography. If such a lesion is found, routine blood cultures should be performed to identify the offending organ-ism. Treatment should be long-term intravenous antibiotics (12 weeks) aimed at the isolate. In the presence of a hemodynamically significant valvular lesion, excision and valve replacement are indicated.

Sinusitis is a concern in burn patients because of the need for prolonged intubation of one or both nostrils with feeding tubes or an endotracheal tube (46). Headache, facial pain, or purulent discharge suggest this diagnosis. Computed tomo-graphy of the head and face is used to confirm the diagnosis. Treatment is generally focused on removal of the tubes, if possible, and topical decongestants. Sinus punc-ture for a specimen should be considered if the infection is thought to be life threatening, with systemic treatment of the isolate.

Meningitis is an uncommon infection in the burned patient but has been found in patients with deep scalp burns involving the calvarial bone and in those with indwelling intraventricular catheters for monitoring of intracranial pressures when there are concomitant head injuries. Only in these cases should this diagnosis be con-sidered, which can be confirmed with computed tomography of the head with intravenous contrast, or lumbar puncture. The diagnosis and treatment of meningitis is covered in depth in other chapters.

Lastly, an infection that is unique to burned patients is the development of infected chondritis of the ear cartilage. When the skin of the ear is damaged by a burn, this leaves a portal of entry for microorganisms to inhabit the cartilage of the ear, which is relatively privileged because of a lack of vascularization. This complication occurs two to three times per year in busy burn centers and can be minimized by the use of topical mafenide acetate cream for treatment of ear burns. This compound diffuses into the cartilage, making it a forbidding environment for bacteria. When the complication occurs, it is characterized by a red, painful, swollen ear that has been burned with open or recently healed wounds. Treatment is generally surgical with debridement of necrotic and infected cartilage. Adequate drainage of the area must take place with incisions along the outer edge of the pinna or posterior pinna to "bivalve" the ear if necessary. Following debridement, the wound should be treated with topical mafenide acetate cream.

SUMMARY

Infectious complications have decreased in the severely burned due to effective strategies for prevention and treatment. Nonetheless, infections in the severely burned are still common and can be lethal, particularly those in the burn wound and the lungs. Infections common to other critically ill patients are also seen in burned patients, which also require attention. Additional strategies to prevent and treat infections in burned patients are still needed and are being actively researched.

REFERENCES

1. Pruitt BA Jr., Goodwin CW, Mason AD Jr. Epidemiologic, demographic, and outcome characteristics of burn injury. In: Saunders WB, eds. Total Burn Care. London: D N Herndon, 2002:16–30.
2. Brigham PA, McLoughlin E. Burn incidence and medical care use in the United States: estimates, trends, and data sources. J Burn Care Rehabil 1996; 17:95–107.
3. www.cdc.gov/ncipc/wisqars
4. Bull JP, Fisher AJ. A study in mortality in a burn unit: standards for the evaluation for alternative methods of treatment. Ann Surg 1949; 130:160–173.
5. Herndon DN, et al. Determinants of mortality in pediatric patients with greater than 70% full-thickness total body surface area thermal injury treated by early total excision and grafting. J Trauma 1987; 27:208–212.
6. McDonald WS, Sharp CW, Deitch EA. Immediate enteral feeding in burn patients is safe and effective. Ann Surg 1991; 213:177–183.
7. Sheridan RL, Remensnyder JP, Schnitzer JJ, Schultz JT, Ryan DM, Thompkins RG. Current expectations for survival in pediatric burns. Arch Pediatr Adolesc Med 2000; 154:245–249.
8. Stassen NA, Lukan JK, Mizuguchi NN, Spain DA, Carrillo EH, Polk HC. Thermal injury in the elderly: when is comfort care the right choice? Am Surg 2001; 67:704–708.
9. Pruitt BA, Mason AD, Moncrief JA. Hemodynamic changes in the early post-burn patient: the influence of fluid administration and of a vasodilator (hydralazine). J Trauma 1971; 22:60–62.
10. Baxter CR, Shires T. Physiological response to crystalloid resuscitation of severe burns. Ann N Y Acad Sci 1968; 150:874–894.
11. Barret JP, Herndon DN. Effects of burn wound excision on bacterial colonization and invasion. Plast Reconstr Surg 2003; 111:744–750.
12. Xiao-Wu W, Herndon DN, Spies M, Sanford AP, Wolf SE. Effects of delayed wound excision and grafting in severely burned children. Arch Surg 2002; 137:1049–1054.

13. Gottschlich MM, Jenkins ME, Mayes T, Khory J, Kagan RJ, Warden GD. The 2002 clinical research award. An evaluation of the safety of early vs. delayed enteral support and effects on clinical, nutritional, and endocrine outcomes after severe burns. J Burn Care Rehabil 2002; 23:401–415.

14. de la Cal MA, et al. Survival benefit in critically ill burned patients receiving decontamination of the digestive tract: a randomized placebo-controlled, double-blind trial. Ann Surg 2005; 241:424–430.

15. Barret JP, Jeschke MG, Herndon DN. Selective decontamination of the digestive tract in severely burned pediatric patients. Burns 2001; 27:439–445.

16. Pruitt BA, Goodwin CW, Cioffi WG. Thermal injuries. In: Davis JH, Sheldon JH, eds. Surgery—a Problem Solving Approach. St Louis: Mosby-Year Book, 1995:643–719.

17. Brown TP, Cancio LC, McManus AT, Mason AD. Survival benefit conferred by topical antimicrobial preparations in burn patients: an historical perspective. J Trauma 2004; 56:863–866.

18. Pruitt BA Jr., McManus AT, Kim SH, Goodwin CW. Burn wound infections: current status. World J Surg 1998; 22:135–145.

19. Tredget EE, Shankowsky HA, Rennie R, Burrell RE, Logsetty S. Pseudomonas infections in the thermally injured patient. Burns 2004; 30:3–26.

20. Nash G, Foley FD, Goodwin MN, Bruck HM, Greenwald KA, Pruitt BA. Fungal burn wound infection. JAMA 1971; 215:1664–1666.

21. Becker WK, et al. Fungal burn wound infection—a ten-year experience. Arch Surg 1991; 126:44–48.

22. Wong TH, Tan BH, Ling ML, Song C. Multi-resistant acinetobacter baumannii on a burns unit–clinical risk factors and prognosis. Burns 2002; 28:349–357.

23. Wilson SJ, et al. Direct costs of multi-drug resistant acinetobacter baumannii in the burn unit of a public teaching hospital. Am J Infect Control 2004; 32:342–344.

24. Cochran A, Morris SE, Edelman LS, Saffle JR. Systemic candida infection in burn patients: a case-control study of management patterns and outcomes. Surg Infect (Larchmnt) 2002; 3:367–374.

25. Altoparlak U, Erol S, Akcay MN, Celebi F, Kadanali A. The time related changes of antimicrobial resistance patterns and predominant bacterial profiles of burn wounds and body flora of burned patients. Burns 2004; 30:660–664.

26. Estahbanati HK, Kashani PP, Ghanaatpisheh F. Frequency of pseudomonas aeruginosa serotypes in burn wound infections and their resistance to antibiotics. Burns 2002; 28:340–348.

27. Steer JA, Papini RP, Wilson AP, McGrouther DA, Parkhouse N. Quantitative microbiology in the management of burn patients. I. Correlation between quantitative and qualitative burn wound biopsy culture and surface alginate swab culture. Burns 1996; 22:173–176.

28. Pruitt BA Jr., McManus AT, Kim SH. Use of burn wound biopsies in the diagnosis and treatment of burn wound infection in die infektion beim brand verletzten. In: Lorenz S, Zellner PR, eds. Steinkopff Verlag Darmstadt. Darmstadt: Germany, 1993:55–63.

29. Kim SH, Hubbard GB, McManus WF, Mason AD, Pruitt BA. Frozen section technique to evaluate early burn wound biopsy: comparison with the rapid section technique. J Trauma 1985; 25:1134–1137.

30. Sasaki TM, Welch GW, Herndon DN, Kaplan JZ, Lindberg RB, Pruitt BA. Burn wound manipulation-induced bacteremia. J Trauma 1979; 19:46–48.

31. Mozingo DW, McManus AT, Kim SH, Pruitt BA. The incidence of bacteremia following burn wound manipulation in the early post-burn period. J Trauma 1997; 42:1006–1011.

32. Mason AD Jr., McManus AT, Pruitt BA Jr. Association of burn mortality and bacteremia: a 25-year review. Arch Surg 1986; 121:1027–1031.

33. Pruitt BA Jr., McManus AT, Kim SH. Burns. In: Gorbach SL, Bartlett JG, Blacklow NR, eds. 3rd ed. In: Infectious Diseases. Philadelphia: Lippincott Williams & Wilkins, 2004:860.

34. Fitzwater J, Purdue GF, Hunt JL, O'Keefe GE. The risk factors and time course of sepsis and organ dysfunction after burn trauma. J Trauma 2003; 54:959–966.

35. Barber RC, Aragaki CC, Rivera-Chavez FA, Purdue GF, Hunt JL, Horton JW. TLR4 and TNF polymorphisms are associated with an increased risk for severe sepsis following burn injury. J Med Genet 2004; 41:808–813.

36. Fidler PE, et al. Incidence, outcome, and long-term consequences of herpes simplex-virus type 1 reactivation presenting as a facial rash in intubated adult burn patients treated with acyclovir. J Trauma 2002; 53:86–89.

37. Shirani KZ, Pruitt BA, Mason AD. The influence of inhalation injury and pneumonia on burn mortality. Ann Surg 1987; 205:82–87.

38. Barillo DJ, McManus AT. Infection in burned patients. In: Cohen J, Powderly eds. Infectious Diseases 2nd ed. 2003.

39. deLa Cal MA, et al. Pneumonia in patients with severe burns: a classification according to the carrier state. Chest 2001; 119:1160–1165.

40. Rue LW III, Cioffi WG, Mason AD, McManus AT, Pruitt BA. Improved survival of burned patients with inhalation injury. Arch Surg 1993; 128:772–780.

41. Taneja N, Emmanuel R, Chari PS, Sharma M. A prospective study of hospital acquired infections in burn patients at a tertiary care referral centre in north India. Burns 2004; 30:665–669.

42. Geyik MF, Aldemir M, Hosoglu S, Tacyildiz HI. Epidemiology of burn units infections in children. Am J Infect Control 2003; 31:342–346.

43. Santucci SG, Gobara S, Santos CR, Fontana C, Levin AS. Infections in a burn intensive care unit: experience of seven years. J Hosp infect 2003; 53:6–13.

44. Wahl WL, Ahrns KS, Brandt MM, Rowe SA, Hemmila MR, Arbabi S. Bronchoalveolar lavage in diagnosis of ventilator-associated pneumonia in patients with burns. J Burn Care Rehabil 2005; 26:57–61.

45. Ramos GE, et al. Catheter infection risk related to the distance between insertion site and burned area. J Burn Care Rehabil 2002; 23:266–271.

46. McCormick JT, O'Mara MS, Wakefield W, Goldfarb IW, Slater H, Caushaj PF. Effect of diagnosis and treatment of sinusitis in critically ill burn victims. Burns 2003; 29:79–81.

26

Urosepsis in the Critical Care Unit

Burke A. Cunha

*Infectious Disease Division, Winthrop-University Hospital, Mineola, and
State University of New York School of Medicine, Stony Brook,
New York, U.S.A.*

INTRODUCTION

The most common cause of sepsis in patients admitted to the hospital for sepsis is urosepsis. Urosepsis may be defined as a urinary tract infection (UTI) that has seeded the bloodstream, accompanied by systemic symptoms. Urosepsis is also defined by demonstrating the same organisms cultured from urine and blood. Urosepsis may be community or nosocomially acquired. Community-acquired urosepsis occurs only under certain circumstances, i.e., in nonleukopenic, compromised hosts with preexisting renal disease or structural abnormalities of the urinary tract (UT). Nosocomial urosepsis may occur in normal as well as abnormal individuals with urologic manipulation (1).

UROSEPSIS

Community-Acquired

The organisms causing community-acquired UTI, i.e., *Escherichia coli*, *Proteus mirabilis, Klebsiella*, Enterococci (group D streptococci), group B streptococci, are the organisms isolated from blood and urine in urosepsis. Clinical scenarios that predispose urosepsis to occur are acute pyelonephritis, cystitis in nonleukopenic-compromised hosts [diabetes mellitus, systemic lupuserythromatosus (SLE), alcoholism, multiple myeloma, steroid therapy, etc.], those with unilateral/partial UT obstruction, preexisting renal disease, or renal/bladder calculi (Table 1). Bacteremia with systemic symptoms with or without hypotension may accompany any urosepsis. Febrile leukopenic-compromised hosts (e.g., cancer patients receiving chemotherapy) rarely have UTIs or develop urosepsis. Immune defects related to malignancy and/or chemotherapy do not diminish mucosal defenses, e.g., secretory IgA that protects against bacterial adherence to uroepithelial cells and UTI (2–8).

Nosocomial

Nosocomial urosepsis is caused by UT catheterization/instrumentation in nonleuko-penic hosts. Catheter-associated bacteriuria in the hospital does not result in

Table 1 Nosocomial Urosepsis and Urinary Tract Instrumentation

Organisms	Bacteriuria	Bacteremia	Bacteremia definitely associated with UT instrumentation
Escherichia coli	1007	72	9
Proteus	301	11	6
Klebsiella pneumoniae	243	29	4
Pseudomonas aeruginosa	296	31	1
Serratia marcescens	166	8	1
Enterococcus	181	20	4
Enterobacter	150	23	3
Citrobacter	15	2	2
Other bacteria	242	130	0
Total	2601	326	30
Conditions			Number of cases
Preexisting UT disease alone			23
Preexisting UT disease and Diabetes			4
Preexisting UT disease and cirrhosis			2
Preexisting UT disease, diabetes mellitus, cirrhosis			1
No preexisting UT disease			0
Total			30

Abbreviation: UT, urinary tract.
Source: Adapted from Ref. 2.

urosepsis in normal hosts. Bacteriuria will not result in bacteremia unless the patient has structural abnormalities of the genitourinary (GU) tract, i.e., congenital abnormalities of the collecting system, stone disease, or unilateral/bilateral obstruction due to intrinsic/extrinsic causes. Urologic instrumentation/procedures done in the presence of a UTI may result in bacteremia with systemic symptoms/hypotension. Urosepsis from urologic instrumentation/procedures may occur in normal or abnormal hosts (2,4,9,10).

Microorganisms associated with nosocomially acquired urosepsis are aerobic gram-negative bacilli or Enterococci. The most common pathogens are *E. coli* and *Klebsiella* or Enterococci. Less commonly, *Serratia, Enterobacter, Providencia, Citrobacter*, nonaeruginosa *Pseudomonas*, or *Pseudomonas aeruginosa* are potential nosocomial uropathogens related to GU instrumentation. Because the uropathogens causing community-acquired versus nosocomially acquired urosepsis are dissimilar, different therapeutic approaches are required for community and nosocomially acquired urosepsis (Table 2) (9–11).

Clinical Presentation

The clinical presentation of urosepsis is not different from sepsis from a non-GU source. Sepsis is the systemic manifestation of bacteremias with multiple organ involvement. The interaction between microorganisms and the host determines the systemic response rather than the origin of the infection. The clinical diagnostic

Table 2 Urosepsis: Community and Nosocomially Acquired

Type of UTI	Urosepsis		
	Common	Uncommon	Rare
Pyelonephritis: normal and abnormal hosts	+		
Cystitis: normal hosts			+
Cystitis: nonleukopenic-compromised hosts	+		
Prostatitis: normal and abnormal hosts		+	
Prostatic abscess	+		
Urinary tract instrumentation (TUR) with infected urine	+		
Urinary tract instrumentation (sterile urine)			+

Abbreviation: UTI, urinary tract infection.

approach is to identify systemic disorders or underlying UT abnormalities that predispose to urosepsis. A history of preexisting renal disease, repeated UTIs of the relapse variety, recent GU instrumentation, history of bladder/renal stones, or history of systemic illnesses (e.g., diabetes mellitus and SLE), indicate the basis of the patient's sepsis may be of UT origin, i.e., urosepsis (1,3–5).

Differential Diagnostic Considerations

The physical exam in urosepsis is unhelpful unless the patient has pyelonephritis, renal colic from stone disease or obstruction, or prostatitis. Gram stain and culture of the urine with urinalysis plus blood cultures are the definitive diagnostic tests. While blood cultures will not be available for some time, the Gram stain of the urine provides immediate microbiologic information regarding the likely cause of the patient's UTI/urosepsis.

Patients with acute pyelonephritis have pyuria and bacteriuria with CVA tenderness. Cystitis causing urosepsis always has one of the aforementioned underlying disorders that predisposes to urosepsis and has no localizing physical findings.

Nosocomial urosepsis is a relatively straightforward diagnosis when there has been recent urologic instrumentation because of the time relationships between the procedure and onset of urosepsis. The febrile/hypotensive patient in the critical care unit with an indwelling Foley catheter, with bacteria and pyuria, almost never has fever due to urosepsis unless the patient has diabetes mellitus or SLE, or is on steroids. Computed tomography/magnetic resonance imaging of the abdomen/GU tract may detect an intra-abdominal/pelvic infectious process likely to account for the fever Table 3 (1,4,5,9).

Patients presenting from the community with urosepsis may have stone or structural disease, acute prostatitis/prostatic abscess, or acute pyelonephritis. Acute pyelonephritis is diagnosed by the finding of a temperature of $\geq 102°F$ in a patient with CVA tenderness with renal origin, and by finding a uropathogen and white cells in the urine. In acute pyelonephritis, the Gram stain provides a presumptive, microbiologic diagnosis, which guides antibiotic selection. A Gram stain of the urine in acute pyelonephritis will reveal gram-positive cocci in pairs/chains, i.e., group B streptococci or group D streptococci. If the Gram stain of the urine shows gram-negative bacilli in acute pyelonephritis, they are aerobic gram-negative bacilli

Table 3 Catheter-associated Bacteriuria and Urosepsis

Clinical catheter setting	GU host factors	Risk of urosepsis	Preferred approach	Alternative approach
Indwelling [short-term] nonobstructed	Normal	Low	No antibiotics	Remove catheter as soon as possible
Indwelling (short- or long-term) obstructed	Normal	High	Correction of obstruction	Antibiotics should be administered until obstruction is relieved
Indwelling (long-term) nonobstructed				
Nonbacteremic	Normal	Low	No antibiotics	Chronic suppression
Bacteremic	Abnormal	High	Antibiotics for bacteremia	After acute therapy of urosepsis, chronic suppression
Indwelling [short- or long-term nonleukopenic compromised hosts] (SLE, DM, multiple myeloma, steroids, cirrhosis)	Abnormal	High	If possible, avoid catheter	Antibiotic prophylaxis

Abbreviations: GU, genitourinary; SLE, systemic lupus erythromatosus; DM, diabetes mellitus.

Table 4 Community-Acquired Urosepsis: Therapeutic Approach

Syndrome	Microorganisms	Urine Gram stain	Empiric coverage (Gram stain)	Empiric coverage (Gram stain not available)
Acute epididymitis elderly males	*Pseudomonas aeruginosa*	Gram-negative bacilli	Aminoglycoside Antipseudomonal penicillin Antipseudomonal 3rd generation cephalosporin Cefepime Aztreonam Meropenem	Aminoglycoside Antipseudomonal penicillin Antipseudomonal 3rd generation cephalosporin Antipseudomonal quinolone Meropenem
Acute prostatitis	Common coliforms	Gram-negative bacilli	Non-antipseudomonal 3rd generation cephalosporin Quinolone	Ampicillin + gentamicin Sulbactam/ampicillin Piperacillin + tazobactam Quinolone Meropenem
	Group D streptococci (enterococci)	Gram-positive cocci in pairs/chains	Ampicillin Vancomycin Meropenem	Ampicillin + gentamicin Piperacillin + tazobactam Quinolone Meropenem
Acute pyelonephritis	*E. coli* *Proteus mirabilis* *Klebsiella*	Gram-negative bacilli	Non-antipseudomonal 3rd generation cephalosporin Quinolone Cefepime Meropenem	Cefepime Aztreonam Piperacillin Quinolone

Table 5 Nosocomial Urosepsis: Therapeutic Approach

Syndrome	Microorganism	Urine Gram stain	Empiric coverage based on urine Gram stain
Post-urologic instrumentation/procedure	*Pseudomonas aeruginosa* *Enterobacter* species *Serratia* species *Stenotrophomonas maltophilia* *Burkholderia cepacia*	Slender/plump gram-negative bacilli	Meropenem Aminoglycosides Antipseudomonal penicillin/3rd generation cephalosporin Cefepime Aztreonam TMP-SMX Minocycline
Acute pyelonephritis	Group B streptococci Group D streptococci	Gram-positive cocci in pairs/ chains	Non-antipseudomonal 3rd generation cephalosporin Quinolone Meropenem
Catheter-associated bacteriuria / acute cystitis[a]	Group B streptococci	Gram-positive cocci in pairs/ chains or Gram-negative bacilli	Non-antipseudomonal 3rd generation cephalosporin
	Group D streptococci or aerobic gram-negative bacilli		Quinolone Meropenem

[a]Only in abnormal hosts with unilateral/bilateral UT obstruction, preexisting renal disease, or nonleukopenic compromised hosts (DM, SLE, cirrhosis, multiple myeloma, on steroids).

Abbreviation: TMP-SMX, trimethoprim-sulfamethoxazole.

because anaerobic gram-negative bacilli do not cause UTIs. Patients with acute prostatitis usually do not develop urosepsis, but urosepsis is a common sequelae of prostatic abscesses.

A difficult diagnosis in a septic patient without any localizing signs is prostatic abscess. "Fever everywhere, fever nowhere" traditionally has referred to an occult subdiaphragmatic abscess in a postoperative patient who became septic. Similarly, in a patient who has a history of prostatitis and no other IV line, GI/GU explanation for sepsis should be considered as having a prostatic abscess until proven otherwise. A transrectal ultrasound is the best way to make the diagnosis, which may require surgical drainage. Epididymitis in the elderly may occasionally present with urosepsis. The usual pathogens are aerobic gram-negative bacilli, especially *P. aeruginosa* (2,9–12).

ANTIMICROBIAL THERAPY

Antibiotic therapy of urosepsis depends on the likely pathogen to which it is related, whether it is a community- or nosocomially acquired infection. The causative microorganisms in community-acquired urosepsis are aerobic gram-negative bacilli or group B or D streptococci. The Gram stain of the urine rapidly differentiates between gram-positive cocci in pairs/chains from aerobic gram-negative bacilli. Further identification in the acute situation is not necessary to begin empiric therapy. Gram-positive cocci or group B or D streptococci, since *S. aureus*, i.e., gram-positive cocci in clusters, is not a uropathogen. *S. saprophyticus* is a uropathogen but does not cause urosepsis. In terms of gram-negative aerobic bacilli, it does not matter whether it is *E. coli*, *Proteus*, or *Klebsiella*, because coverage will be directed against all community-acquired uropathogens. With community-acquired urosepsis, the coverage is the same with the exception of epididymitis in the elderly, which is treated to include hospital-acquired aerobic gram-negative bacilli, e.g., *P. aeruginosa*. Any treatment that is effective against group D streptococci will also be effective against group B streptococci. (Table 4).

Nosocomial urosepsis is caused by aerobic gram-negative bacilli, based on the Gram stain or culture data from the urine or blood. Coverage should be directed against *P. aeruginosa*, which will cover all aerobic nosocomial uropathogens except the nonaeruginosa pseudomonads. If a nonaeruginosa *Pseudomonas* is isolated from the urine/blood, therapy should not be an aminoglycoside. Treatment of non-aeruginosa pseudomonad urosepsis should be with trimethoprim-sulfamethoxazole or a quinolone (12–17) (Table 5).

REFERENCES

1. Burke JP, Yeo TW. Nosocomial urinary tract infections. In: Mayhall CG, ed. Hospital Epidemiology and Infection Control. 3rd ed. Philadelphia, PA: Lippincott Williams & Wilkins, 2004:267–286.
2. Bryan CS, Reynold KL. Community-acquired bacteremic urinary tract infection: epidemiology and outcome. J Urol 1984; 132:490–493.
3. Holzheimer RG. Antibiotic induced endotoxin release and clinical sepsis: a review. J Chemother 2001; 1:159–172.

4. Wagenlehner FM, Naber KG. Hospital-acquired urinary tract infections. J Hosp Infect 2000; 46:171–181.

5. Paradisi F, Corti G, Mangani V. Urosepsis in the critical care unit. Crit Care Clin 1998; 1:165–180.

6. Anderson RU. Urinary tract infections in compromised hosts. Urol Clin North Am 1986; 13:727–734.

7. Measley RE Jr., Andriole VT. Bacterial urinary tract infections in diabetes. Infect Dis Clin North Am 1995; 9:25–51.

8. Patterson JE, Andriole VT. Bacterial urinary tract infections in diabetes. Infect Dis Clin North Am 1995; 9:25–51.

9. Bryan CS, Reynolds KL. Hospital-acquired bacteremic urinary tract infections epidemiology and outcome. J Urol 1984; 132:494–498.

10. Quintiliani R, Cunha BA, Klimek J, Maderazo EG. Bacteremia after manipulation of the urinary tract. The importance of pre-existing urinary tract disease and compromised host defenses. Postgrad Med 1978; 54:668–671.

11. Bahnson RR. Urosepsis. Urol Clin North Am 1986; 13:625–635.

12. Preheim LC. Complicated urinary tract infections. Am J Med 1985; 79:62–66.

13. Meares EM Jr. Current patterns in nosocomial urinary tract infections. Urology 1991; 37(suppl):9–12.

14. Stamm WE, Hooton TM. Management of urinary tract infections in adults. N Engl J Med 1993; 329:1328–1334.

15. Carson C, Naber KG. Role of fluoroquinolones in the treatment of serious bacterial urinary tract infections. Drugs 2004; 64:1359–1373.

16. Hendrickson JR. A cost-effective strategy for managing complicated urinary tract infections. J Crit Illness 1996; 11(suppl):S49.

17. Cunha BA. Antibiotic Essentials. (5th Ed) Royal Oak, MI: Physicians' Press, 2005.

27
Infections Related to Bioterrorism

David Schlossberg
Infectious Disease Section, Department of Medicine, Temple University School of Medicine, Philadelphia, Pennsylvania, U.S.A.

OVERVIEW

Introduction to the Clinical Problem

Epidemiology

Although bioterrorist agents can be acquired by inhalation, by ingestion, and by absorption through the skin, inhalation of an aerosolized agent is the most efficient mode of dissemination and is the one most likely to be employed by bioterrorists. Thus, many of the resultant illnesses will be respiratory or will be the form of infection resulting from inhalation of the offending agent.

While natural infection with most bioterrorist agents can be suspected on the basis of geographic or behavioral exposure, such clues will not help assess a bioterrorist attack. In fact, the converse is true in that infection outside an endemic area would suggest intentional spread of disease, as with plague in the Northeast United States. Additional clues include deviation from the usual epidemiology, such as multiple patient clusters of botulism, and infection without the usual vector, for example, Eastern equine encephalitis without local mosquitos. Unusual progression of illness also provides grounds for suspicion, as in fulminant pneumonia in healthy young patients or smallpox masquerading as varicella with uncharacteristic (for varicella) prominence in the extremities.

MICROBIOLOGY

The major pathogens or diseases most likely to present in the critical care setting are those designated as Category A by the Centers for Disease Control and Prevention (CDC) (Table 1). This categorization reflects the relative ease of dissemination, the high mortality rate, and the need for special public health action to avoid panic in the general population.

A longer secondary list of potential bioterrorism-related diseases would include CDC Category B agents (which have a lower mortality than Category A and are more difficult to disseminate), a variety of chemical agents, and acute radiation sickness.

Table 1 Centers for Disease Control and
Prevention Category A

Anthrax
Smallpox
Plague
Tularemia
Botulism
Hemorrhagic fever viruses

This list includes Q fever, brucellosis, glanders, Venezuelan equine encephalitis (VEE), Eastern Equine Encephalitis (EEE), Western equine encephalitis (WEE), foodborne or waterborne pathogens, melioidosis, typhus, psittacosis, toxins [nerve agents, ricin, mycotoxins, epsilon toxin, Staph enterotoxin B (SEB), cyanide, phosgene, and vesicants], and acute radiation exposure. Some of these latter agents/diseases are not likely to be encountered in the critical care setting, e.g., brucellosis and most foodborne pathogens. Others are not infectious agents per se but are included in the table of differential diagnosis because they can mimic infectious diseases.

CDC Category C is the third-highest priority among potential bioterrorist agents; this category includes emerging pathogens such as Nipah virus, tickborne encephalitis viruses, and multidrug resistant *Mycobacterium tuberculosis*. These infections will not be discussed further.

CLINICAL PRESENTATION

Anthrax is caused by the gram-positive bacillus *Bacillus anthracis*, which persists in soil as a spore. Exposure to contaminated soil infects animals, and humans become infected via contact with infected animals or their products. Direct contact with these animals causes cutaneous anthrax, a syndrome of a painless papule progressing to necrotic ulceration with surrounding edema and regional adenopathy. More rarely, ingestion of infected meat produces pharyngeal or gastrointestinal anthrax, with abdominal pain and bloody diarrhea.

However, the type of anthrax most likely to be encountered in the critical care setting is the one best suited for bioterrorist use—inhalational anthrax. This form is spread by aerosol dissemination of spores, which are then inhaled. Those inhaled spores that are not phagocytized by lung macrophages reach mediastinal lymph nodes and germinate into vegetative *B. anthracis*, producing edema toxin and lethal toxin. After several days, a nonspecific illness develops, characterized by fever, headache, nonproductive cough, and myalgias, and, a few days later, the patient is in extremis, with high fever and respiratory compromise from edema of the neck and mediastinum. Some patients develop pulmonary infiltrates, but these are due to hemorrhage and necrosis, not pneumonia; the pathophysiologic process is a fulminant mediastinitis, with hemorrhage and necrosis. If pleural effusions develop, they, too, are hemorrhagic (Fig. 1). Progression to confusion and seizures suggests a complicating anthrax meningitis, which is usually hemorrhagic, producing the "cardinal's cap" (Fig. 2).

Inhalational anthrax resembles many other illnesses, so that the differential diagnosis is extensive. The early flu-like illness may be mistaken for influenza and other respiratory viruses and the various other etiologies of atypical pneumonia. Once mediastinal involvement supervenes, the differential diagnosis should also include tuberculosis, histoplasmosis, tularemia, malignancy, and aortic aneurysm (3–5).

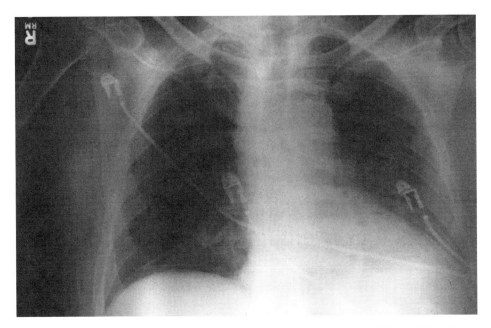

Figure 1 Inhalational anthrax: widened superior mediastinum and possible small left pleural effusion. *Source*: From Ref. 1.

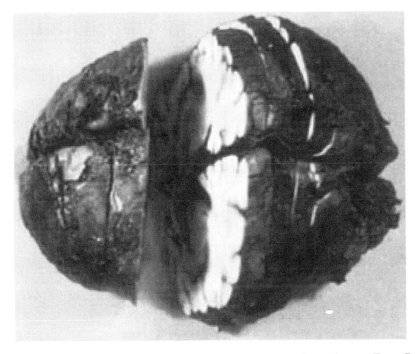

Figure 2 Cardinal's cap: hemorrhagic meningitis in anthrax. *Source*: From Ref. 2.

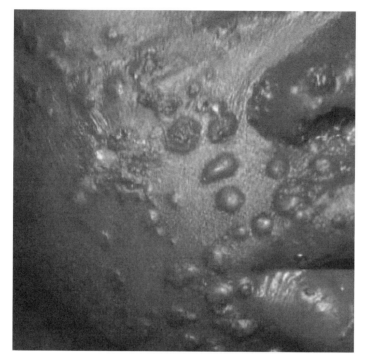

Figure 3 Smallpox lesions. *Source*: From Ref. 2.

In smallpox, a nonspecific febrile prodrome is followed by the characteristic rash (Fig. 3) on the face and limbs, which then spreads to the trunk. The lesions begin as papules and then evolve into pustules. Smallpox lesions differ from those of varicella: they are round and deep, appear at the same time and therefore are all of the same size and in the same stage of development and are most numerous on the face and extremities—not the trunk. Smallpox scabs—unlike those of varicella—harbor live virus and may transmit disease. Complications of ordinary smallpox, or variola major, include encephalitis, pneumonia, cellulitis, arthritis, and destructive keratoconjunctivitis. A hemorrhagic form of smallpox, seen in pregnant patients, progresses to widespread ecchymoses and is usually fatal. In the malignant form of smallpox, the lesions coalesce without ever progressing to pustules; this form is also generally fatal (6).

Plague is caused by the gram-negative bacillus *Yersinia pestis*. It is traditionally spread to man by fleas that have fed on infected animals, by direct contact with infected animals, or by inhaling infectious droplets from patients with pneumonic plague. However, bioterrorists would most likely spread plague via aerosol, producing pneumonic plague, which is the form least commonly acquired naturally. The resultant pulmonary infection is characterized by pulmonary infiltrates, which often cavitate, and by cough productive of bloody sputum. Many victims also develop gastrointestinal signs and symptoms, including abdominal pain, vomiting, and diarrhea. If plague is spread by infected fleas, typical buboes (inflamed lymph nodes draining the inoculation site) may form, with resultant fever and chills. Some patients progress to septicemic plague if the organism enters the bloodstream; this syndrome resembles meningococcemia, with petechiae and purpura, disseminated intravascular coagulation (DIC), and acral necrosis. Bloodstream invasion may then be complicated by plague meningitis (7,8).

Tularemia, caused by *Francisella tularensis*, infects a huge variety of small animals, and it spreads to man by direct contact with infected animals or via arthropod vectors. The most frequent form of naturally acquired tularemia is ulceroglandular, a combination of cutaneous inoculation and regional adenopathy. If the inoculation site is not evident, a glandular form may result, and, if the inoculation is in the conjunctiva, an oculoglandular syndrome develops, with eye inflammation and cervical or preauricular adenopathy. A typhoidal form resembles typhoid fever, with abdominal pain, headache, fever, and cough. Ingestion of *F. tularensis* results in stomatitis and pharyngitis.

Pneumonic tularemia may be primary or secondary: primary from inhalation, e.g., in people exposed to sick animals or to laboratory specimens, and secondary from infection elsewhere in the body with bacteremic spread to the lungs. The resultant pulmonary syndrome is distinctive, with bronchiolitis, pneumonitis, pleural effusions, and hilar adenopathy. Because terrorists would most likely use airborne spread (less likely than contaminating the water supply), patients encountered in the intensive care unit would probably have tularemic pneumonia. Tularemia should be suspected as a cause of severe pneumonia in patients with characteristic complications of hilar adenopathy on Chest X-ray (CXR), rash (erythema nodosum, maculopapular or vesicular eruptions), relative bradycardia, enteritis, appendicitis, or meningitis (9).

Clostridium botulinum and, less commonly, *C. baratii* and *C. butyricum* produce a family of neurotoxins; some of these toxins, types A, B, C, and F, cause disease in humans by blocking acetylcholine release at the neuromuscular junction, with resultant flaccid paralysis called botulism. Botulism can be acquired by ingestion of preformed toxin or spores, or by infection of wounds with toxin-producing clostridia. Worldwide, most naturally acquired cases of botulism result from ingestion of preformed toxin in food that has not been preserved properly. In the United States, the most common form of botulism is infant botulism, attributed to ingestion of spores in honey or soil. The spores then germinate and elaborate the botulinum toxin. However, adequate heating inactivates the toxin, as does chlorine, so that contamination of the food or water supply would be an unlikely route of bioterrorist attack. On the other hand, the toxin can be aerosolized, and this is the most likely form of bioterrorist use of botulinum toxin.

Classic signs and symptoms of botulism are symmetric cranial nerve involvement, with blurred vision, diplopia, dysphagia, and dysarthria. Descending paralysis supervenes, often with respiratory distress. Autonomic dysfunction is common, with hypertension or hypotension and tachycardia. Patients are typically afebrile and not toxic appearing. If the toxin is foodborne, nausea, vomiting, and diarrhea may herald the neurologic illness. Inhalational disease is less well defined in humans (10,11).

The viral hemorrhagic fevers (VHFs) are infections caused by four groups of viruses: filoviruses, arenaviruses, bunyaviruses, and flaviviruses. The best-known representatives of each of these virus families are listed in Table 2. Most of these viruses are transmitted by arthropods, by exposure to infected rodents, or by aerosolization of the virus from the infected rodents' excreta; however, there are exceptions, and no vector has yet been identified for Ebola. This capacity to spread by aerosol suggests airborne spread as the most likely route of bioterrorist attack, although Dengue is less likely to be used by bioterrorists, because it requires reexposure to the Dengue virus to produce the severe form, dengue hemorrhagic fever, and it is not easily spread by aerosol.

The illnesses that result from infection with the hemorrhagic fever viruses involve many organ systems, with a wide array of clinical complications. Thus,

Table 2 Hemorrhagic Fever Viruses

Representative viruses	Location	Usual vector	Virus family
Ebola	Africa	Unknown	Filovirus
Marburg	Africa	Unknown	Filovirus
Lassa fever	West Africa	Rodents	Arenavirus
New World hemorrhagic fevers (include Machupo virus in Bolivia, Sabia virus in Brazil, Junin virus in Argentina, Guanarito virus in Venezuela, and Whitewater Arroyo virus in California)	North and South America	Rodents	Arenavirus
Hantavirus (include Hantaan virus and Sin Nombre virus)	Worldwide	Rodents	Bunyavirus
Rift Valley fever	Africa, Middle East	Mosquitos	Bunyavirus
Dengue	Worldwide	Mosquitos	Flavivirus
Yellow fever	Africa, Latin America	Mosquitos	Flavivirus
Kyasanur Forest disease	India	Ticks	Flavivirus

patients may develop various combinations of fever, prostration, headache, abdominal pain, myalgias, encephalitis, rash, arthralgias, and renal failure. However, the common denominator is an acutely ill patient with fever and toxicity, often complicated by a bleeding diathesis. The hemorrhagic phenomena may take the form of hematuria, gastrointestinal bleeding, conjunctival hemorrhage, and petechiae, and all the VHF can be complicated by DIC. Adult respiratory distress syndrome may complicate infection with Hantavirus pulmonary syndrome, New World hemorrhagic fevers, and some flaviviral infections (11,12).

Q Fever is caused by *Coxiella burnetii*. Its bioterrorist potential derives from its ability to infect men with only a single organism and its transmissibility—unlike other rickettsiae—via aerosol. The illness produced is nonspecific, with fever, myalgias, cough, headache, and chest pain, with some patients progressing to pneumonia or hepatitis. Chest X ray may demonstrate hilar adenopathy and pleural effusions in addition to infiltrates. Many patients develop neurologic complications, including encephalitis, cerebellitis, and cranial nerve involvement.

Viral encephalitides (Venezuelan equine encephalitis, Eastern equine encephalitis, and Western equine encephalitis) are spread to man from animal hosts via mosquitos. However, these viruses are highly infectious by aerosol, are relatively stable, and replicate to substantial numbers under laboratory conditions, so that bioterrorist use is possible. The encephalitis produced is frequently complicated by ataxia, cranial nerve palsies, and seizures, with mortality ranging from less than 0.5% for VEE to 50% with EEE. Because there is no person-to-person spread, human cases without a local mosquito vector would be suspicious, as would disease in healthy young adults, because most victims of these viruses are children or adults over the age of 50.

Glanders is a bacterial infection of horses, mules, and donkeys caused by *Burkholderia mallei*. Bioterrorists would probably spread antibiotic resistant strains of this organism by aerosol. Cutaneous inoculation produces localized infection, which may disseminate via the bloodstream, producing a papulopustular rash and generalized abscesses and pneumonia. This form of glanders is usually fatal. If spread by aerosol, pneumonia would result directly. Glanders is contagious, and strict infection control is essential.

Melioidosis is caused by the gram-negative bacterium *Burkholderia pseudomallei*. It may be spread by cutaneous inoculation and probably by ingestion and inhalation. When septicemia develops, a rapidly fatal course is seen in half the victims, often accompanied by a characteristic pustular rash. Necrotizing pneumonia and visceral and subcutaneous abscesses are known complications.

Rickettsia prowazekii is the cause of typhus, usually spread to man by lice and occasionally by flying squirrels. The classic presentation includes fever, chills, and headache in association with the characteristic rash: a macular eruption beginning in the axillae, and then becoming petechial. The rash then spreads to the trunk and extremities, sparing face, palms, and soles. Concern for bioterrorist use of *R. prowazekii* centers on the likelihood of engineering strains resistant to currently available antimicrobials.

Psittacosis, from infection with *Chlamydophila* (Chlamydia) *psittaci*, causes systemic infection that is often complicated by atypical pneumonia. Fever and headache are common, and epistaxis and splenomegaly in a patient with atypical pneumonia should raise this diagnostic possibility.

Clostridium perfringens types B and D produce Epsilon Toxin. The most likely bioterrorist use of this toxin would be via aerosolization rather than through the food supply, and manifestations in men, extrapolated from observations in animals, would probably result in pulmonary edema (13).

SEB is a superantigen polypeptide produced by staphylococci. SEB usually causes food poisoning but also may produce (along with toxic shock syndrome toxin-1) the staphylococcal toxic shock syndrome. SEB can also be spread by aerosol, resulting in nausea and vomiting, fever, and shortness of breath (14,15).

DIFFERENTIAL DIAGNOSTIC CONSIDERATIONS

Table 3 presents the major clinical syndromes produced by bioterrorist agents (16–21). These syndromes are grouped by clinical presentation, with the realization that some presentations may be atypical and misleading. The table lists the bioterrorist agents considered most likely to be employed in an attack and most likely to result in admission to a critical care unit. Common causes of these syndromes, i.e., those not due to bioterrorism, are statistically more likely and should always be suspected first. However, bioterrorist agents should be part of the differential diagnosis, especially in patients with critical illness.

DIAGNOSIS

In general, the greatest diagnostic hurdle regarding bioterrorist agents is failure to consider these diseases in the first place. Once that barrier is overcome, most of the agents can be proven or strongly suspected. Much of the bacteriology should be carried out in specialized laboratories at an appropriate level of expertise. Advice regarding obtaining and handling specimens is available from local and state Health Departments and the CDC in Atlanta, Georgia.

The diagnosis of inhalational anthrax is suspected clinically on the basis of toxicity, mediastinal involvement, hemorrhagic meningitis, and hemorrhagic pleural

Table 3 Clinical Presentations of Bioterrorist-Related Diseases Encountered in the Critical Care Setting

Syndrome	Etiology	Comments
Encephalitis/seizures	VEE, EEE, WEE	Suspect anthrax with bloody CSF; Acute Radiation Syndrome often accompanied by nausea, vomiting, and diarrhea, with erythema and hair loss. Nerve agents have typical additional symptoms, e.g., blurred vision, rhinorrhea, salivation, bronchospasm; cyanide causes dyspnea, seizures, and coma and should be considered in acyanotic patients who appear hypoxic and have smell of bitter almonds on their breath or in gastric washings
	Anthrax	
	Nerve agents (organophosphates, e.g., sarin, tabun, soman, cyclosarin, VX)	
	Cyanide	
	Radiation	
Rash and fever	Plague, typhus (acral gangrene); smallpox, melioidosis, glanders, vesicants, mycotoxins (vesicopustular rash); petechiae (typhus); bleeding diathesis (HFVs, hemorrhagic smallpox)	Vesicants, or blistering agents (e.g., mustard) cause skin burn and blistering, with respiratory distress if inhaled; mycotoxins (e.g., yellow rain) cause skin blistering and gangrene, nausea and vomiting and GI hemorrhage
Fulminant pneumonia	Plague, tularemia, anthrax, Q fever, glanders, melioidosis, ricin	Clues: bloody sputum in plague, hilar adenopathy in tularemia and Q fever, mediastinal widening in anthrax. Ricin may cause purulent mediastinitis, mimicking anthrax, in association with necrotizing pneumonia and pulmonary edema; it also produces gastroenteritis with GI hemorrhage, fever, hepatic necrosis
Noncardiac respiratory distress, with or without pulmonary edema	HFVs (hantavirus pulmonary syndrome, some flaviviruses, some New World hemorrhagic fevers), Staph enterotoxin B, cyanide, pulmonary toxicants (e.g., chlorine, phosgene, and diphosgene), epsilon toxin, vesicants (e.g., mustard)	Phosgene and other pulmonary toxicants (chlorine, diphosgene) cause laryngeal edema and wheezing, with ARDS developing after a characteristic delay of 48 hr; cyanide causes dyspnea, seizures, and coma and should be considered in acyanotic patients who appear hypoxic and have smell of bitter almonds on their breath or in gastric washings; vesicants, or blistering agents (e.g., mustard) cause skin burn and blistering, with respiratory distress if inhaled

Widened mediastinum in acutely ill patient	Anthrax, tularemia, ricin, Q fever	Anthrax causes hemorrhagic mediastinal adenitis; tularemia and Q fever have associated adenopathy; ricin may cause purulent mediastinitis, mimicking anthrax, in association with necrotizing pneumonia and pulmonary edema; a clue to ricin poisoning would be associated gastrointestinal hemorrhage and hepatic necrosis
Paralysis	Botulism, nerve agents (organophosphates, e.g., sarin, tabun, soman, cyclosarin, VX)	Nerve agents have typical associated findings, e.g., blurred vision, rhinorrhea, salivation, and bronchospasm
Gastroenteritis	Salmonella, Shigella, and other foodborne pathogens; Staph enterotoxin B; radiation; nerve agents (organophosphates, e.g., sarin, tabun, soman, cyclosarin, VX); ricin; mycotoxins	Nerve agents have typical associated findings, e.g., blurred vision, rhinorrhea, salivation, and bronchospasm; GI hemorrhage seen with intestinal anthrax, colitis due to *Escherichia coli* and Shigella, ricin, and mycotoxins. Acute Radiation Syndrome often associated with erythema and hair loss accompanying severe nausea, vomiting, and diarrhea. Diarrhea may be seen as a nonspecific complication of many diseases with major manifestations in other organ systems, e.g., melioidosis, typhus and ricin poisoning

Abbreviations: HFVs, hemorrhagic fever viruses; CSF, cerebrospinal fluid; GI, gastrointestinal; ARDS, adult respiratory distress syndrome; VEE, Venezuelan equine encephalitis; EEE, Eastern equine encephalitis; WEE, Western equine encephalitis.

effusion. Definitive diagnosis requires microbiologic confirmation: cerebrospinal fluid, skin lesions, and peripheral blood (buffy coat smears) demonstrate broad, gram-positive bacilli on Gram stain; these specimens should also be cultured, but only in a level B laboratory of the Laboratory Response Network for Bioterrorism. Because, as described above, inhalational anthrax produces mediastinitis but not pneumonitis, culture and Gram stain of sputum are not likely to be positive. Immunohistochemical staining and polymerase chain reaction (PCR) are available through the CDC.

Smallpox is suspected by the characteristic rash. It is diagnosed by serology, PCR, or immunohistochemical studies to detect specific antigen, and by culture, which should be taken by a health care worker who has been vaccinated, using mask and gloves. Consultation should be undertaken immediately with the CDC or local Health Department, and specimens should be evaluated at a biologic safety level 4 laboratory. Electron microscopy of vesicular fluid is not specific, as it identifies orthopoxvirus but cannot specify variola.

Plague is diagnosed by cultures of clinical specimens, including sputum, blood, and lymph node aspirate if a bubo is present. Laboratory personnel should be alerted, because plague can be contracted in the laboratory, and cultures should be performed under biolevel safety two conditions. On Gram stain, the typical safety pins are seen, gram-negative bacilli with bipolar staining. The CDC and local Health Department may be able to provide specialized testing with PCR and direct fluorescent antibody, and a rapid diagnostic test for bedside testing is under development.

Tularemic pneumonia should be suspected in a patient with pneumonia, hilar adenopathy, and pleural effusion. The organism can be cultured from blood, pharynx, sputum, gastric washings, and lesions of the skin or conjunctiva; small gram-negative coccobacilli are seen on Gram stain, and may be visible on smears of the peripheral blood (Fig. 4). The laboratory should be alerted, because cultures require special media and should be held for at least 10 days, and because tularemia can be contracted in the laboratory. PCR and immunohistochemical stains can be performed if available, but serology is not helpful in the acute infection, because it cross reacts, rises late, persists for years, and may be attenuated by antibiotic administration.

Botulism should be suspected in any patient with a combination of cranial nerve disturbances and paralysis, particularly if there are also gastrointestinal symptoms and if clusters of such cases are reported. Diagnosis is made by assay of toxin in serum, stool, vomitus, gastric aspirate, and implicated foodstuffs. If aerosol dissemination is suspected, swabs of the nasal mucosa should also be assayed. Electromyography (EMG) is suggestive, though not diagnostic, with normal motor conduction and sensory nerve amplitudes, decreased evoked muscle action potential, and the characteristic facilitation following rapid repetitive nerve stimulation.

To establish a diagnosis of the hemorrhagic fever viruses, diagnostic specimens should be sent to specialized laboratories, those which operate at biosafety level 4. At these sites, PCR, serologies, and viral isolation can be performed (Fig. 5).

The diagnosis of Q fever can be established serologically, by immunologic stains and PCR of tissue, and by culture, although laboratory workers may be secondarily infected by aerosols. Psittacosis is also best diagnosed by serology, as culture is dangerous for laboratory personnel.

Viral encephalitides, glanders, and melioidosis are diagnosed by cultures of appropriate specimens and serologic testing. Typhus is diagnosed by serology or by detection of rickettsiae in tissue biopsies, either by PCR or by direct staining.

SEB is diagnosed by ELISA of blood and body secretions, and Epsilon Toxin is detectable by ELISA and PCR of clinical specimens.

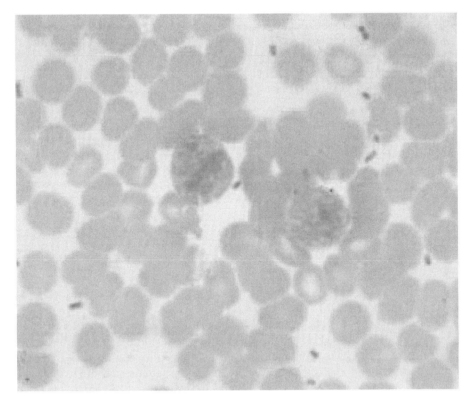

Figure 4 Giemsa stain of peripheral blood smear showing *Francisella tularensis*. *Source*: From Ref. 2.

THERAPY

Nonspecific Therapy

Nonspecific therapy must address not only therapeutic modalities directed at the patient, but also the possible contagious nature of certain agents of bioterrorism. Those agents most capable of person-to-person spread, and recommended

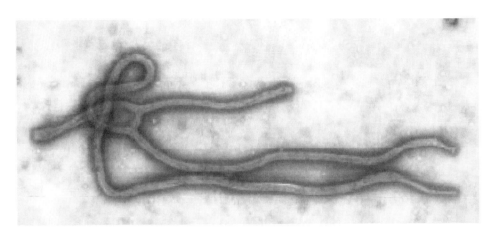

Figure 5 Electron micrograph of Ebola virus. *Source*: From Ref. 2.

Table 4 Bioterrorist Agents Capable of Person-to-Person Spread

Disease	Prophylaxis (v. text)
Smallpox	Vaccine for contacts within 4 days
Pneumonic plague	Doxycycline or ciprofloxacin for 7 days
Some hemorrhagic fever viruses: Lassa fever, New World hemorrhagic fevers, hantaviruses (rare), Ebola and Marburg	None recommended if asymptomatic; treat with ribavirin if contact of arenavirus, bunyavirus or unknown VHF becomes ill within 21 days of exposure
Q fever (rare)	Tetracyclines or macrolides may be effective late in incubation period
Glanders	None recommended
Some foodborne pathogens, e.g., Shigella	None recommended

Abbreviation: VHFs, viral hemorrhagic fevers.

prophylaxis for contacts, are listed in Table 4. Table 5 summarizes basic principles of patient precautions and isolation and indicates appropriate procedures for the major agents of bioterrorism (12,22–24).

An additional nonspecific aspect of patient management is proper and timely notification of authorities when a bioterrorist attack is suspected. The local health department should be notified immediately, both to facilitate diagnosis of the individual patient through the proper laboratories and to initiate the coordinated efforts of local, state, and national authorities necessary to investigate and control a bioterrorist attack. In general, the local health department will then ensure notification of local law enforcement agencies, the FBI, the state health department, and the CDC in Atlanta, Georgia (25).

Specific Therapy

Specific recommendations for each infectious agent are listed below. Off-label uses of antimicrobials are recommended frequently in the treatment of agents of bioterrorism, as the benefits are often thought to outweigh the risks. Nevertheless, the critical care physician should be aware of approved indications of antimicrobials as well as their toxicity and drug interactions.

Clearly, no one agent or regimen can cover all diagnostic possibilities in the critical care setting, and, as noted, not all bioterrorist agents are treatable. Nevertheless, it is notable that most treatable pneumonias likely to result from bioterrorism (plague, tularemia, anthrax, Q fever, glanders, and melioidosis) show some degree of susceptibility to doxycycline. Thus, if bioterrorism is a possible cause of a patient's severe pneumonia, and no specific etiology is suspected or proven, it would be reasonable to include doxycycline in the initial treatment regimen.

Anthrax: Nonantimicrobial treatment of anthrax has included administration of corticosteroids (for severe mediastinal edema or meningitis), angiotensin-converting enzyme inhibitors, and calcium channel blockers. Antisera from patients who were vaccinated against *B. anthracis* have been administered to patients, and large pleural effusions should be drained.

Antimicrobial treatment of anthrax should assume resistance to penicillin and doxycycline until susceptibility testing can be performed; this precaution results from

Table 5 Patient Precautions and Isolation

	Standard precautions: gown, mask, and eye protection during procedures likely to cause splashes of body fluids; gloves when touching patient or body fluids	Airborne precautions: single room with negative air-pressure ventilation; if air not exhausted externally, should have HEPA filtration. Respiratory protective device, e.g., N95 respirator while in patient's room	Droplet precautions: mask and eye protection if within 3 ft of patient	Contact precautions: gown and gloves when entering room
Anthrax	X			
Glanders	X			
Melioidosis	X	X		
Pneumonic plague	X		X	
Tularemia	X			
Q fever	X			
Smallpox	X	X (also—regular mask on pt)		X
VEE	X			
Viral encephalitis	X			
VHF	X	X	X	X
Toxins: botulism, ricin, mycotoxins, staphylococcus enterotoxin B	X			

Abbreviations: VHF, viral hemorrhagic fever; VEE, Venezuelan equine encephalitis; HEPA, high efficiency particulate absorbing.

the known strains of anthrax that have been engineered to be resistant to both penicillin and doxycycline, in addition to the β-lactamase production by some strains of
B. anthracis. Thus, initial presumptive therapy for inhalational anthrax should
include IV ciprofloxacin (adults: 400 mg q12 hours IV or 500 mg q12 hours PO; children: 10 mg/kg q12 hours IV, max 400 mg/dose or 15 mg/kg q12 hours PO, max
500 mg/dose) plus one to two additional antimicrobials from the list of rifampin,
vancomycin, penicillin, ampicillin, chloramphenicol, imipenem, clindamycin, and
clarithromycin. Some feel that clindamycin offers the advantage of inhibiting production of the toxins, which cause much of the morbidity in anthrax. If resistance
to doxycycline is not proven or suspected, this agent may be used with or instead
of ciprofloxacin (adults 100 mg q12 hours IV and PO; children: 100 mg q12 hours
PO and IV if weight >45 kg, and 2.2 mg/kg q12 hours PO and IV if weight <45 kg).
Oral therapy can be used after a clinical response, and treatment can be undertaken
with amoxicillin in infants, children, and women who are pregnant or breastfeeding,
as long as the strain is not resistant to penicillin.

Controversy surrounds the duration of therapy. Three recommendations are
suggested by various authorities: (i) 60 days of antimicrobials, (ii) 100 days of
antimicrobials (anthrax spores have been shown to survive in mediastinal nodes
of monkeys for 100 days after exposure), or (iii) 100 days of antimicrobial therapy
plus three doses of anthrax vaccine (because monkeys that were protected after exposure by both antimicrobials and vaccine were resistant to reinfection, while those
protected by antimicrobials alone were not) (3–5,26).

Smallpox: If feasible, patients should be in a negative-pressure room or one
with high-efficiency particulate air filtration; contact precautions should be
instituted, with masks, gowns and gloves, and the patient should wear a mask. Management is supportive, although ribavirin and cidofovir are active in vitro and
cidofovir may be considered in severe cases. Postexposure prophylaxis with smallpox
vaccine is recommended for those exposed to variola via a sick patient or terrorist
attack. Vaccination will prevent disease in many and death in most vaccinees if given
within four days of exposure; some degree of protection may be seen even if vaccination is performed up to 10 days following exposure. In the critical care setting,
vaccination should be given to exposed health care workers, laboratory personnel
handling specimens, and others who contact the patient's clothes (e.g., laundry
workers). Because smallpox has caused infection via airborne spread throughout a
hospital, vaccination of all patients and workers in the hospital should be considered
if there are multiple patients admitted with smallpox, e.g., following a bioterrorist
attack. Detailed accounts of the vaccination process and vaccine reactions are
beyond the scope of this paper and have been reviewed elsewhere (6,27,28).

Plague: Although streptomycin is the historic standard for plague therapy, gentamicin is more readily available and can be administered once daily, although it is
not approved by the Food and Drug Administration for treatment of plague.
Central nervous system involvement is probably best treated with chloramphenicol,
though this agent should be avoided in children younger than two years. Alternatives
include doxycycline and ciprofloxacin, which can be utilized PO when the patient
has improved, to complete 10 days of therapy. Medical personnel exposed to patients
with pneumonic plague should receive antibiotic prophylaxis with PO doxycycline
or ciprofloxacin for seven days. Pneumonic plague is transmissible by respiratory
droplets, actually a form of contact spread. Thus, those in contact with the patient
should employ eye protection, masks, gloves, and gowns until the patient has
received 48 hours of effective treatment.

Doses of antimicrobials are as follows: for gentamicin (IM or IV)—adults, 5 mg/kg once daily, or 1.7 mg/kg three times daily following a 2 mg/kg loading dose; for children, 2.5 mg/kg three times daily. For doxycycline, the adult IV dose is 100 mg twice daily or 200 mg once daily, and the PO dose is 100 mg twice daily. Children: if >45 kg, give adult doses; if <45 kg, 2.2 mg/kg IV twice daily, with a maximum of 200 mg/day; oral dose is the same as the IV dose. For ciprofloxacin, adults take 400 mg IV or 500 mg PO twice daily, and children take 15 mg/kg IV twice daily and 20 mg/kg PO twice daily. If chloramphenicol is used, the dose is 25 mg/kg four times daily IV or PO for both adults and children (older than two years). The concentration of chloramphenicol should be kept between 5 and 20 µg/mL to reduce the likelihood of bone marrow suppression, and daily dosages of 4 g are the maximum for children. Children younger than two years should not receive chloramphenicol (8).

Tularemia: Treatment of tularemia is best undertaken with parenteral gentamicin (10 days), with doxycycline (14–21 days) and ciprofloxacin (10 days) as alternatives; PO doxycycline or ciprofloxacin may be used after patient improvement. This represents off-label uses for gentamicin and ciprofloxacin, but strains of *F. tularensis* resistant to streptomycin and tetracyclines have been developed in the laboratory.

Doses of antimicrobials are as follows: Gentamicin—IM/IV—adults, 5 mg/kg/day, children, 2.5 mg/kg tid; doxycycline IV/PO—adults 100 mg bid, children <45 kg, 2.2 mg/kg bid; if >45 kg, as per adults; ciprofloxacin IV—adults, 400 mg bid, children, 15 mg/kg bid, with a maximum of 1 g/day; ciprofloxacin PO, adults 500 mg bid, children, 15 mg/kg bid (9).

Botulism: Supportive treatment is essential and often requires mechanical ventilation. Equine antitoxin in bivalent (AB) and monovalent (E) forms are available from the CDC for all states except Alaska and California, which supply their own antitoxins. Botulism immune globulins are available from California for the treatment of infant botulism types A and B ("BIG"), and additional immune globulins under investigation include a human pentavalent (ABCDE) and an equine heptavalent (A to G) preparation. Antibiotic therapy is used only for wound botulism; it may actually be detrimental in intestinal botulism, by releasing additional toxin following massive killing of clostridia (10).

Viral hemorrhagic fevers: Ribavirin may demonstrate a therapeutic effect in Lassa fever, New World hemorrhagic fevers, some hantaviral infections, and Rift Valley fever. Thus, ribavirin therapy should be considered for any suspected VHF if the etiology is unknown, if the etiology is proven to be an arenavirus or bunyavirus, and for contacts of arenavirus and bunyavirus patients who become ill within three weeks, because person-to-person spread is possible with Lassa fever, New World hemorrhagic fevers, and (rarely) with hantaviruses. For the treatment of Rift Valley fever, interferon alpha has also been recommended. Although ribavirin is contraindicated in pregnancy and is approved only in aerosolized form for children (for respiratory syncytial virus), the benefits may outweigh the risks if a pregnant or young patient has a proven or suspected infection due to arenavirus or bunyavirus.

Specific therapy is not available for Ebola virus, but extreme caution must be taken with patients infected with this agent, because filoviruses are readily transmitted person-to-person; in fact, filoviruses are present not only in blood, body secretions, seminal fluid, and tissues, but may even be demonstrable in sweat and therefore may be transmissible by contact with a victim's intact skin. Strict airborne and barrier precautions should be instituted (Table 4) (11,12,29,30).

The treatment of Q fever is tetracycline or doxycycline for one week after defervescence. Prophylaxis with tetracyclines or macrolides late in the incubation period may prevent disease, but person-to-person spread is rare.

Viral encephalitides have no specific therapy; treatment is supportive. There is no person-to-person spread.

Glanders is susceptible in vitro to many antimicrobials, including doxycycline, ciprofloxacin, ceftazidime, and imipenem, and the combination of trimethoprim plus sulfonamides appears efficacious in vivo on the basis of limited data. Glanders is contagious; so part of patient management must include appropriate isolation.

Melioidosis in its severe forms requires prolonged treatment, e.g., six months or more. A variety of regimens have been recommended, including ceftazidime, imipenem, and piperacillin/tazobactam. Recent observations suggest resistance to Trimethoprim/Sulfamethoxazole (TMP/SMX). Doxycycline and amoxicillin/clavulanate may be adequate for disease of only moderate severity.

Typhus: It is treated with doxycycline until patients are afebrile for 72 hours. Chloramphenicol is the alternative therapy. One of the bioterroristic threats of typhus is the prospect of strains engineered to be resistant to current antimicrobials.

Psittacosis is treated with tetracycline or doxycycline for 10 to 21 days; patients who cannot take tetracyclines should be treated with erythromycin.

With no specific therapy, only supportive treatment is available for the viral encephalitides, Epsilon toxin, and SEB; intravenous immune globulin has been recommended for SEB, but its use is not established.

CONCLUSION

Care for victims of bioterrorism in the critical care setting is complex. The initial challenge is inclusion of bioterrorist agents in the differential diagnosis. Then, in addition to diagnosis and management of the individual patient, additional issues

Table 6 Useful Telephone Numbers and Web Sites

Telephone numbers
CDC Emergency Response Hotline (24 hr): 770–488–7100; CDC Bioterrorism Preparedness and Response Program questions: 404–639–0385
Botulism: CDC 404–639–2206 (after hours 2888)
  California Department of Health (Infant Botulism): 510–540–2646
Smallpox: CDC Clinician Information Line for Smallpox and Smallpox Vaccination: (877) 554–4625
Core web sites
Centers for Disease Control—many links; covers clinical, lab, preparedness and control, emergency response, http://www.bt.cdc.gov/
IDSA—extensive clinical, with slide sets; info on detection and notification, http://www.idsociety.org/BT/ToC.htm
Listing of State Public Health Laboratories, http://www.aphl.org/Public_Health_Labs/index.cfm
Listing of State Public Health Agencies, http://www.statepublichealth.org/index.php
U.S. Army http://www.usamriid.army.mil
Smallpox: www.cdc.gov/smallpox

Abbreviations: CDC, Centers for Disease Control and Prevention; IDSA, Infectious Disease Society of America; BT, bioterrorism.

include effective isolation of patients, proper handling of specimens, management of contacts, and notification of legal and public health authorities. In addition to consultation with infectious disease and infection control colleagues in the hospital, and collaboration with the local health department, further information is available from the emergency telephone numbers and Web sites listed in Table 6.

REFERENCES

1. CDC: www.cdc.gov/ncidod/EID/vol7no6/jerniganG1.htm.
2. CDC: Morbidity and Mortality Weekly Report (MMWR) 2004; 53(RR-8).
3. Swartz MN. Recognition and management of anthrax—an update. N Engl J Med 2001; 345:1621–1626.
4. Inglesby TV, O'Toole T, Henderson DA, et al. Anthrax as a biological weapon, 2002. JAMA 2002; 288:2236–2252.
5. Bell DM, Kozarsky PE, Stephens DS. Clinical issues in the prophylaxis, diagnosis and treatment of anthrax. Available at: http://www.cdc.gov/ncidod/Emerging Infectious Diseases (EID)/vol8no2/01–0521.htm.
6. Breman JG, Henderson DA. Diagnosis and management of smallpox. N Engl J Med 2002; 346:1300–1308.
7. Mandell GL, Bennett JE, Dolin R. Principles and Practice of Infectious Disease. Philadelphia: Churchill Livingstone, 2004.
8. Inglesby TV, Dennis DT, Henderson DA, et al. Plague as a biological weapon. JAMA 2000; 283:2281–2290.
9. Dennis DT, Inglesby TV, Henderson DA, et al. For the Working Group on Civilian Biodefense Tularemia as a Biological Weapon: Medical and Public Health Management. JAMA 2001; 285:2763–2773.
10. Arnon SS, Schechter R, Inglesby TV, et al. For the Working Group on Civilian Biodefense. Botulinum Toxin as a Biological Weapon: Medical and Public Health Management. JAMA 2001; 285:1059–1070.
11. Office of the Surgeon General, Department of the Army. Textbook of Military Medicine: Medical Aspects of Chemical and Biological Warfare. Available at: http://www.vnh.org/MedAspChemBioWar.
12. Borio L, Inglesby TV, Peters CJ, et al. For the Working Group on Civilian Biodefense Hemorrhagic Fever Viruses as Biological Weapons: Medical and Public Health Management. JAMA 2002; 287:2391–2405.
13. Iowa State University Center for Food Security and Public Health. Available at: http://www.vetmed.iastate.edu/services/institutes/cfsph/AboutUs.html.
14. Gilbert DN, Moellering RC, Sande MA. The Sanford Guide to Antimicrobial Therapy. 33rd ed. Hyde Park, VT: Antimicrobial Therapy, Inc., 2003.
15. Greenfield RA, Brown BR, Hutchins JB, et al. Microbiological, biological and chemical weapons of warfare and terrorism. Am J Med Sci 2002; 323:326–339.
16. Schlossberg D. Medical Interventions for Bioterrorism and Emerging Infections. Newtown, PA: Handbooks in Health Care, 2004.
17. CDC classification at http://www.bt.cdc.gov/agent/agentlistchem-category.asp.
18. Lee EC. Clinical manifestations of sarin nerve gas exposure. JAMA 2003:290.
19. The Medical Letter on Drugs and Therapeutics 2002; 44:1–4.
20. Ford MD, Delaney KA, Ling LJ, Erickson T. Clinical Toxicology. Philadelphia: WB Saunders Co., 2001.
21. CDC: www.bt.cdc.gov/agent/ricin.
22. CDC: http://www.bt.cdc.gov/.
23. Report of the Committee of Infectious Diseases: Red Book. 26th ed. American Academy of Pediatrics, 2003.
24. www.lcs.mgh.harvard.edu/bioterrorism.

25. Biological and chemical terrorism: strategic plan for preparedness and response recommendations of the CDC Strategic Planning Workgroup. MMWR 2000; 49(RR-4).
26. Bartlett JG, Inglesby TV, Borio L. Management of anthrax. CID 2002; 35:851–858.
27. Henderson DA, Inglesby TV, Bartlett JG, et al. Smallpox as a biological weapon. In: Henderson DA, Inglesby TV, O'Toole, eds. Bioterrorism: Guidelines for Medical and Public Health Management. Chicago: AMA Press, 2002.
28. Morbidity and Mortality Weekly Report (MMWR) 2003; 52(RR04):1–28.
29. Morbidity and Mortality Weekly Report (MMWR) 2000; 49:709–711.
30. The Medical Letter on Drugs and Therapeutics 2001; 43:87–89.

28

Antibiotic Dosing in Hepatic/Renal Insufficiency

Damary C. Torres
College of Pharmacy and Allied Health Professions, St. John's University, Jamaica, and Winthrop-University Hospital, Mineola, New York, U.S.A.

Donna Sym
College of Pharmacy and Allied Health Professions, St. John's University, and North Shore University Hospital, Jamaica, New York, U.S.A.

April Correll
Winthrop-University Hospital, Mineola, New York, U.S.A.

INTRODUCTION

Dosing of antibiotics in organ dysfunction can be problematic. One must weigh the risks of overdose, which can range from nausea to seizures, against the risk of underdose, which can lead to resistance and treatment failure. Additionally, the level of organ dysfunction of the kidneys and/or the liver and the status of the patient are also critical factors. When a patient is receiving hemodialysis (HD), peritoneal dialysis (PD), or continuous renal replacement therapy (CRRT), clearance of the drug changes and dosing must be adjusted for each of these modalities. This chapter will elucidate some of the dosing and administration issues of antimicrobials in patients with renal or hepatic failure and those undergoing the different types of renal replacement therapy.

ANTIBIOTIC DOSING IN HEPATIC FAILURE

Liver disease can affect both the metabolism and the disposition of drugs (1). The half-life of an antibiotic excreted by the liver may be prolonged if there is significant hepatic insufficiency. However, there is no definitive laboratory test to determine hepatic insufficiency comparable to the serum creatinine for renal insufficiency. One can look at a patient's albumin, prolonged prothrombin time, level of abdominal ascites, and encephalopathy. These can be graded, and the patient can be assigned to a Child-Pugh class, which will determine mild, moderate, or severe hepatic disease. Unfortunately there are minimal recommendations for dose adjustment of antibiotics based on the Child-Pugh class (2). It is difficult to predict specific dose adjustments, but it should be realized that a dosing change may be necessary, and drug levels may need monitoring. A small number of studies were conducted, which focused on patients with varying degrees of cirrhosis, and recommendations were made regarding antibiotic dosing; however, these data cannot be extrapolated to all or various forms of liver disease.

There are two types of liver disease that can impact the hepatic metabolism of drugs: chronic liver disease and acute hepatitis. Chronic liver disease is often secondary to alcohol abuse and chronic viral hepatitis. It typically involves irreversible, chronic hepatocyte damage resulting in a decrease in blood flow to healthy hepatic cells and/or a decrease in hepatocyte function, i.e., cytochrome P450 (CYP450) system. Chronic liver disease has a large impact on alterations in drug disposition. If there is a high degree of portal blood flow shunting, drugs with high extraction ratios will be predominantly affected. These drugs can also have increased oral bioavailability because there may be a decrease in the first pass effect. This will result in higher plasma concentrations, a prolonged pharmacologic effect, and potential toxic side effects. Drugs that exhibit high protein binding (>90%) can have increased volumes of distribution due to hypoalbuminemia or ascites, resulting in a prolonged half-life and elimination. This situation can occur with chloramphenicol.

Severe chronic liver disease can also impact the kidneys. There is a decrease in renal blood flow and glomerular filtration, and elimination of drugs that are renally eliminated will be impaired (1). This scenario can be seen with aminoglycosides. Concomitant liver disease can result in increased risk of nephrotoxicity. It is best not to use aminoglycoside in patients with hepatorenal syndrome or patients with prothrombin time prolongation due to underlying liver disease. Leukopenia can be seen in patients with underlying liver disease treated with β-lactam antibiotics. This can be the result of increased antibiotic levels, causing bone marrow suppression. Drugs that are excreted or detoxified by the liver will have increased levels in patients with hepatic dysfunction. For example, chloramphenicol and clindamycin should have dose reductions to avoid toxicity (2). Drugs affected by oxidative metabolism are more sensitive to hepatic dysfunction compared to drugs that are primarily conjugated (1). In acute hepatitis, hepatocyte damage can be mild and transient or it can develop into chronic and severe disease. There can be changes in drug distribution, which will depend on the severity of the disease.

Certain drugs can also alter the liver metabolism of numerous and various drugs by enzymatic induction or inhibition of the CYP450 system. Inducers are drugs that increase hepatic drug clearance by increasing hepatic extraction ratio and/or hepatic blood flow. This can result in decreased drug levels and therapeutic failures. Rifampin is an example of an enzymatic inducer, which can result in subtherapeutic levels of drugs metabolized by CYP450 if given concomitantly. Induction can be detected within two days after starting rifampin, and it is often necessary to increase the dose of drugs given in combination. However, it is important to remember to decrease the dose if the inducing agent is discontinued. Inhibitors are drugs that decrease metabolism of other agents resulting in increased levels and toxicity. Inhibition can be competitive or noncompetitive. The inhibitor acts as an alternate substrate for the enzyme in competitive inhibition or the inhibitor can inactivate the enzyme in noncompetitive inhibition. Chloramphenicol inhibits CYP450 in a noncompetitive manner, and effects are noted within 24 hours of a single dose. It can inhibit the metabolism of tolbutamide in diabetics. Ciprofloxacin by an unknown mechanism decreases the clearance of theophylline by 25%. Other examples of inhibitors of drug metabolism are sulfisoxazole, isoniazid, and metronidazole (1).

In conclusion, patients with liver disease are more likely to experience adverse effects than patients with normal hepatic function. There is little information about the pharmacodynamics of drugs in this patient population, and dosing recommendations are broad and nonspecific. As a general dosing guideline, patients with chronic active hepatitis or cirrhosis should start with half the usual dose of a drug if it is eliminated by oxidative metabolism. Future studies are necessary to evaluate hepatic dysfunction and the dosing of numerous drugs (1).

ANTIBIOTIC DOSING IN RENAL INSUFFICIENCY AND FAILURE

The correct dosing of drugs is important to provide a therapeutic effect as well as to avoid potential side effects and toxicities. The following section will review why critically ill patients are prone to renal insufficiency, some basic pharmacokinetic principles, and why dosing changes for certain drugs are necessary.

Assessment of Renal Function

Determination of renal function is important and necessary when determining the dosing of drugs. The current standard for determining a patient's renal function is the Cockcroft–Gault equation (3):

$$CrCl = [(140 - \text{age in years}) \times \text{IBW in kg}] / [\text{SrCr in mg/dL} \times 72] \times 0.85 \text{ for females} \quad (1)$$

where CrCl is creatinine clearance, IBW-ideal body weight, and SrCr is serum creatinine. Although this equation appears simple to use, we must keep in mind how specific patient parameters may alter its accuracy. When using the Cockcroft–Gault equation, it is important to remember that IBW and not total weight is used to calculate clearance. Because creatinine is a metabolic by-product of muscle, its concentration is directly related to a person's muscle mass only. Fat and extra fluid weight should not be used when calculating clearance. Using an obese person's total weight will cause this equation to overestimate their actual clearance; so the actual body weight should be used (4). Similarly, if IBW is used for emaciated patients IBW, the equation will overestimate patient clearance. Another factor that may need to be adjusted for is the actual serum creatinine level. It has been established that the elderly and emaciated populations tend to have a smaller muscle mass and therefore a smaller creatinine production. This decreased production results in a low level of serum creatinine, which does not correctly correspond to its renal elimination (2). Because this level is considered to be inaccurate, many clinicians will adjust this population's creatinine levels from less than 1 mg/dL to 1 mg/dL. Serum creatinine levels are also altered by many other variables such as diet, muscle degradation, drugs, and patient's overall health. For these reasons, serum creatinine levels, which are unstable and changing, cannot be relied upon to calculate the clearance (5).

The original study by Cockcroft and Gault included 534 patients from the Queens Mary Veterans Home (3). Over 96% of these subjects were male and 29 of the subjects were rejected, because two measured serum creatinine levels differed by more than 20%. From this large group, patients were rejected from entering the smaller study group if their 24-hour creatinine excretion differed by more than 20%, if 24-hour creatinine excretion was less than 10 mg/kg, and if records were inadequate. The ages of the men in the study group ranged from 18 to 92 years, with most patients between the ages of 50 to 59 years old. The mean serum creatinine for men in group II ranged from 0.99 to 1.39 mg/100 mL. The patients in the Cockcroft and Gault study are much different than those seen in the critical care unit. Most critically ill patients do not have stable serum creatinine and due to renal insufficiency may excrete less than 10 mg/kg of creatinine/day. The Cockcroft–Gault equation can therefore not be relied upon to correctly predict clearance in the renal-insufficient population.

In the critically ill population other factors must be used for the estimation of renal function instead of the Cockcroft–Gault equation. One way of determining if the kidneys are functional is to look at the patient's urine output. If the patient is not producing any urine, and urinary obstruction is ruled out, it can be assumed the patient does not have adequate filtration of the blood and thus renal insufficiency (5). Another way of assessing renal function is by looking at the patient's serum electrolytes (6). Impaired renal function causes a rise in serum potassium, magnesium, and phosphorus. Drugs that are dependent on renal clearance will also have an increase in serum levels with impaired renal function. High serum levels of vancomycin, aminoglycosides, procainamide, and theophylline are a few drugs that may indicate renal impairment. Cystatin C is another method that is being studied to evaluate renal function in critically ill patients. Although still being studied, it is believed that cystatin C measurements can show even small changes in renal filtration even where the Cockcroft–Gault equation could not (5,7).

Factors Affecting Renal Function in the Critically Ill

In addition to the adjustment of weight and laboratory serum creatinine values, there are other factors that may affect patients' renal function in the critically ill population. Hypotension in the critically ill is very common due to blood loss and sepsis. Approximately 25% of cardiac output is directed to the kidneys, and a decrease will causes a direct drop in renal pressure (7). Because filtration in the kidney is pressure dependent, a decrease in pressure will inhibit the ability of the kidney to filter out solutes as well as drugs (6). Another factor that may affect the function of the kidneys is concomitantly administered drugs. Critically ill patients normally require the use of many different pharmaceutical agents in order to help them survive. Some of these agents may cause direct harm, thus decreasing the kidneys' ability to function properly. Drugs commonly used in the intensive care unit (ICU), which can cause renal insufficiency, are listed in Table 1.

Pharmacokinetic Principles

Loading Dose

Loading doses, if applicable, are considered an important part of antibiotic therapy. It is important that critically ill patients, especially those suffering from sepsis, achieve adequate blood concentrations of antibiotic quickly. Many times patients with renal insufficiency have had a loading dose withheld due to concerns about causing unwanted toxicity. In reality, the loading dose administered is not influenced by renal function but instead by the patient's volume of distribution. The following equation shows parameters, which affect loading dose (5).

$$\text{Loading dose} = V_d \times \text{conc} \tag{2}$$

where conc is the blood concentration desired after the loading dose and V_d is the volume of distribution for that drug. The concentration of the loading dose is

Table 1   Drugs Which Can Cause Renal Insufficiency

Prerenal azotemia	ACE inhibitors
	Cyclosporine
	NSAIDs
Proximal tubular injury	Aminoglycosides
	Radiocontrast agents
	Foscarnet
Medullary thick ascending limb injury	Amphotericin
	Cyclosporine
	Radiocontrast agents
Intratubule obstruction	Acyclovir
	Sulfadiazine
Allergic interstitial nephritis	Acyclovir
	Aminoglycosides
	Beta-lactams
	Ciprofloxacin
	Furosemide
	Glyburide
	Phenytoin
	Thiazides
Acute tubular necrosis	Amphotericin
	Contrast dye
Post-renal failure (obstruction)	Sulfonamides

Abbreviations: ACE, angiotensin converting enzyme; NSAIDs, nonsteroidal anti-inflammatory drugs.
Source: From Refs. 6 and 7.

therefore not in any way dependent on the patients ability to clear that drug; so the normal loading dose is considered acceptable. However, dose adjustments for loading doses may be necessary in certain patient populations. Those patients suffering from extensive third spacing of fluid, ascites, or edema may require a higher loading dose than a patient with normal fluid balance (8,9). In contrast, a patient who is suffering from severe dehydration will have a smaller volume and therefore may require a smaller loading dose to achieve a desired blood concentration.

Subsequent Doses

In order to determine why doses need to be adjusted in renal insufficiency, it is important to understand some basic pharmacokinetic principles. The desired outcome of antibiotic administration is to obtain a serum drug concentration that is considered therapeutic, while not exceeding a concentration that may cause toxicity. This fine balance can be described by the following equation (4):

$$\text{Conc avg} = \frac{\text{Dose administered}/\tau}{\text{Clearance}} \tag{3}$$

where conc avg is the desired steady-state blood concentration, τ represents the dosing interval of the drug, and the dose administered is normally expressed as total dose over 24 hours. This concludes that if the dose administered is too large for the patient's clearance, or if the clearance of the patient is reduced, than the drug concentration will rise. The opposite is also true, if the dose administered is small or the clearance is increased, the serum concentration will decline. This equation is very basic, and many drugs have their own parameters by which to calculate the actual dose for a patient's particular clearance. Specific drugs will not be discussed here, but their equations can be found in various references. It is necessary to estimate to the best of our ability a patient's approximate clearance, so we can administer the appropriate amount of a drug.

Half-Life: Effects on the Dosing Interval

Half-life is the time required for the total amount of drug in the body to be decreases by one-half. The following equation is used to determine half-life (4):

$$T_{1/2} = 0.693 \times (V_d)/Cl \tag{4}$$

where $T_{1/2}$ is the half-life, V_d is the volume of distribution, and Cl is the clearance of the drug. This equation shows us that the half-life is dependent on two patient variables, the patient's volume of distribution (V_d) and the patient's clearance. If a critically ill patient has an increase in volume due to ascites or edema, the half-life will subsequently increase and it will take longer for the drug concentration to be reduced by half. The more important factor associated with half-life is the clearance. As the patient's clearance is compromised, the half-life will be extended. This extended half-life in the renal-insufficient population requires the clinician to extend the dosing interval. The excretion of some drugs is independent of renal function, and, therefore, changes in dosing are not necessary in renally compromised patients. Table 2 gives examples of drugs that do not require renal dosing.

Antibiotic Categories: An Overview

Aminoglycosides

Aminoglycosides are a viable option for the treatment of infections in the critically ill population when appropriate. Unfortunately, many patients in the ICU have existing renal failure, and clinicians are hesitant to use these nephrotoxic drugs in fear that they will worsen the patients' already compromised renal function. However, with appropriate monitoring of serum peaks and troughs and corresponding dosage adjustments, this should not be a concern, and the ability to monitor these drugs makes them a good choice in patients with renal insufficiency or failure. The clinician may use these levels and modify their patient's therapy to gain the best possible outcome while avoiding toxicity.

The currently available aminoglycosides include gentamycin, tobramycin, and amikacin, all of which are cleared renally. An advantage of using an aminoglycoside

Table 2 Antibiotics that Are Not Renally Eliminated

Amphotericin
Ceftriaxone
Chloramphenicol
Clindamycin
Doxycycline
Macrolide antibiotics (azithromycin, clarithromycin,
  and erythromycin)
Minocycline
Moxifloxacin
Nafcillin
Oxacillin

Source: From Refs. 8 and 19.

is its postantibiotic effect (PAE). PAE means the bacteria will continue to die and prevent bacteria regrowth hours after drug concentrations decline. A meta-analysis preformed by Hatala et al. showed that there was no difference in cure rates with once daily dosing, and overall toxicity was reduced, and others confirmed these results (10,11). This high peak followed by a drug-free interval is believed to be beneficial for the kidney rather than smaller more frequent doses.

Vancomycin

Due to the possibility of resistant organisms, vancomycin is a common antimicrobial used in the ICU setting. Vancomycin's main pathway of elimination is via the kidney, and, therefore, caution must be taken when it is prescribed. In patients with normal renal function, the normal elimination half-life is four to eight hours, but in patients with renal failure, the half-life is prolonged for days or even weeks (4,12). Unlike aminoglycosides, vancomycin does not exhibit a concentration-dependent killing of bacteria, but it must remain above the minimal inhibitory concentration (MIC) in order to sustain this effect (13). Serum levels may be drawn for vancomycin, and it is therefore an easy drug to adjust in critically ill patients. As with other antibiotics, a decrease in the first dose is not necessary, but subsequent doses of vancomycin should be decreased or, a single full dose may be administered every few days. An important note about vancomycin is it has no oral bioavailability, so it cannot be given orally to treat a systemic infection (4).

Beta-Lactams

The beta-lactam antibiotics include the penicillins, cephalosporins, and carbapenems. Most beta-lactams are dependent on the kidneys for their excretion through passive and active transport (14). Because many critically ill patients have renal impairment, the dose and/or dosing interval of these agents must be adjusted. These drugs, like vancomycin, are not concentration dependent, but are dependent on the overall time their concentration remains above the MIC (13). As beta-lactams exhibit a limited PAE, they cannot be administered by a high once daily dose, and are usually dosed between two and six times daily, depending on the agent.

Some studies have shown an advantage in using beta-lactams by continuous infusion. A continuous infusion administers a set dose over a 24-hour period, thus preventing serum levels from dropping below the MIC (15,16). By constantly keeping serum concentrations above the MIC, it is believed that drug failures in severe or resistant infections will be reduced. As with traditional bolus dosing, a full-loading dose should be administered prior to the start of the continuous infusion in order to quickly achieve a level above the MIC. Another advantage of this regimen is the prevention of the peak and valley effect seen with traditional dosing. Prevention of this may help alleviate side effects seen with high drug concentrations. The amount of drug infused may also be adjusted daily if laboratory reports show changes in MIC. A pharmacoeconomic advantage is a decrease in overall drug administered per day, which may be offset by increases in monitoring due to unfamiliarity with this type of dosing (15).

Fluoroquinolones

The fluoroquinolone antibiotics are dependent on their serum concentrations or peak MIC but also their 24-hour AUC-area under the curve:MIC ratio. In their dosing, it is therefore important to achieve a high peak concentration and maintain that concentration over a 24-hour period (13). The AUC:MIC is especially important for resistant bacteria. In these cases, it is important to keep the drug concentration above the MIC throughout the entire dosing interval (17,18). Many of the third and fourth-generation fluoroquinolones have the ability to maintain their MIC:AUC ratio with once daily dosing. Most of the fluoroquinolone antibiotics are dependent on renal excretion and therefore will require adjustments in their dose or dosing interval. The exception is moxifloxacin, which is partially dependent on hepatic metabolism and does not require an adjustment (19).

Antifungals

Fungal infections in the ICU are almost inevitable for those patients who have been receiving long-term antibiotics. In the past, the drug of choice for most fungal infections was amphotericin B. Although this drug has been proven efficacious, its renal and other adverse effects are undesirable in those with already impaired renal function. The new liposomal encapsulation of amphotericin B reduces toxicity, although the mechanism of this decreased toxicity is not known (17). It is believed that encapsulation in phospholipids results in decreased interaction with cellular membranes and therefore decreases the insult on the kidneys. Fluconazole has also proven to be as efficacious as amphotericin in the treatment of noninvasive candidiasis infection (17). The advantage of fluconazole is the absence of renal toxicity, although its dose must still be adjusted in renal insufficiency (20). As with renally eliminated antibiotics, a loading dose of fluconazole should be administered before a dose reduction is implemented.

Caspofungin is another antifungal increasingly used in the critically ill patient due to its lack of renal toxicity and because it does not need adjustment in renal insufficiency. It should also be noted that caspofungin utilizes a large bolus dose in order to reach peak serum levels quickly (21). The newest antifungal available, voriconazole, has shown not to be nephrotoxic and, in fact, is mostly metabolized by the liver's CYP450 system. Unfortunately, its intravenous (IV) use is limited in patients with renal failure due to the accumulation of the solubilizing excipient, SBECD, which is found in the parenteral formulation (22,23).

Antivirals

Viruses can also cause infections in critically ill patients. The use of antiviral medications in the critically ill population is limited because of the lack of available IV preparations. Currently, the only IV antiviral available for the treatment of herpes simplex virus is acyclovir. The main route of elimination for acyclovir is renal, and, therefore, it must be dosed accordingly. Many studies have shown that acyclovir can actually cause renal insufficiency by intratubular precipitation in dehydrated and oliguric patients (24). The best way to prevent renal insult with this drug is to make sure that patients are adequately hydrated during therapy.

Ganciclovir is an antiviral agent which is used to treat cytomegalovirus, especially in organ transplant patients. Ganciclovir's use in critically ill patients is not widespread, but when used, it does require adjustment for renal insufficiency. Like acyclovir, it also has the potential to cause renal toxicity, so adequate hydration of patients is recommended to prevent further renal complications (24).

Miscellaneous Agents

Metronidazole is an antibiotic commonly used for parasitic as well as certain bacterial infections. Its dose does not require a reduction except for those patients whose CrCl is less that 10 mL/min. Metronidazole is commonly used as a once-daily dose of

1 g, especially in the renally insufficient population. Although metronidazole does not exhibit PAE, its half-life in renal insufficiency is extended, thus allowing for serum concentrations to remain therapeutic for extended periods of time (25).

Conclusion

The consideration of a drug's excretion is extremely important in the critically ill patient. We must not assume that the appearance of normal serum creatinine level indicates a patient's kidneys are functioning properly. Other ways of evaluating renal function must be used to determine the patients present renal function such as urine output and serum electrolytes. When this estimation is made, we must then select the appropriate dose or dosing interval for drugs that are dependent upon renal excretion. A careful selection of dosing will optimize antibiotic effects while preventing serious dose-related outcomes.

ANTIBIOTIC DOSING IN INTERMITTANT RENAL REPLACEMENT THERAPY

The overall incidence rate of end-stage renal disease (ESRD) has increased each year since 1980, with an incidence rate of 333 per million in 2002 (26). Treatment options available can include HD and PD commonly as continuous ambulatory PD (CAPD). The choice between HD and CAPD can be determined by a patient's age, size, lifestyle, ability to perform self-care, and vascular access. While HD continues to be the most common therapy for ESRD (>90%), CAPD is usually favored in patients with unstable cardiac disease and younger, smaller (<80 kg) patients who prefer a more flexible schedule and have the manual dexterity to perform dialysate exchanges (4,27).

Hemodialysis

The purpose of dialysis is to correct electrolyte disturbances and to remove drugs, toxins, and excess water from the body. It is an artificial process where a patient's anticoagulated blood and dialysis fluid (an electrolyte solution) flow through a dialyzer (pseudokidney) on opposite sides of a semipermeable membrane (4,27).

Dialyzer

A hemodialyzer is a semipermeable membrane that allows water and some solutes to pass. It is a plastic device consisting of various types of dialysis membranes arranged in two types of configurations: flat plate (or parallel plate) and hollow fiber. The flat plate dialyzer is made up of sandwiched sheets of membrane. Blood and dialysate circulate between these alternating sheets; however this type of dialyzer is not commonly used. The hollow-fiber dialyzer has thousands of capillary tubes the length of the dialyzer. Blood flows in the tubes, and the dialysate flows outside the tubes in the remaining space in the dialyzer. This type of dialyzer is most commonly used in the United States. The types of dialysis membranes include conventional (cellulose), semisynthetic (cellulose acetate), and synthetic (polysulfone, polymethylmethacrylate, and polyacrylonitrile). These membranes differ in biocompatibility, surface area, and pore size. Synthetic membranes are more biocompatible, whereas cellulose membranes can result in a complement response and cytokine release. This can cause symptoms of fever, hypotension, and platelet activation in some patients, especially those who are critically ill. Conventional and semisynthetic dialyzers have smaller pores than synthetic dialyzers; therefore, drug clearance decreases for these dialyzers as molecular size or weight increases. As a result, synthetic dialyzers such as polysulfone membranes are most commonly used in the United States. The majority of dialysis centers in the United States reuse hemodialyzers due to expense, but also reuse reduces anaphylactoid reactions to membranes and complement activation. Strict cleansing and sterilization reprocess procedures are utilized (4,27).

Dialysate

Dialysates are composed of the following electrolytes, which are present in a standard range: sodium, potassium, calcium, magnesium, chloride, and bicarbonate. It is then added to purified water and prior to delivery is heated to 37°C (4,27).

Transport Process

Solutes are removed from the blood by diffusion and convection. In the diffusion process, toxins are removed from the blood by diffusing down their concentration gradients into the dialysate. In order to maximize the concentration gradient of toxin exposure to the membrane, blood and dialysate flow in opposite directions. If equilibrium is reached, the net movement of toxins is zero; however, for most substances equilibrium is not achieved. This may be the result of the rapid flow rates of blood and dialysate or large molecular size of solutes (4,27). In convection, plasma water is removed from blood by ultrafiltration. This water also carries solute into the dialysate (4,27). "Dialysance" is the terminology used to describe the process of drug removal from the dialysis machine. It is also referred to as dialysis clearance and is the amount of blood completely cleared of the drug (in mL/min) and is defined by the equation:

$$Cl_D = [Q(C_a - C_v)]/C_a \tag{5}$$

C_a = drug concentration in arterial blood (blood entering machine), C_v = drug concentration in venous blood (blood leaving kidney machine), Q = rate of blood flow to kidney machine, and Cl_D is dialysance (28,29).

Characteristics that Impact Removal by HD

The efficiency of drug removal is determined by the following factors: the characteristics of the membrane, blood and dialysate flow rates through the dialyzer, and the properties of the drug. It is important to know the specifics of these factors in order to evaluate the dialyzability of drugs. Many published HD dosing guidelines are based on older dialyzer membranes and can underestimate the removal of drugs compared to newer membranes. It is suggested that hemodialyzer clearance must enhance total body clearance by 30% to be significant, and this parameter is used to determine the need for supplemental antibiotic dosing after HD (4,27,29,30).

Dialyzer Characteristics.   The surface area and type of dialyzer membrane will impact the ability to dialyze a drug. Large-pore membranes, i.e., polysulfone and polyacrylonitrile are able to clear larger-sized molecules (500–1500 Da) and have greater permeability to water and are termed "high-flux." It is this type of membrane that is able to remove as much as 50% of a vancomycin dose. Large-surface area membranes are able to clear large quantities of small molecules and are termed "high-efficiency." Increase in dialysate flow rate maintains the concentration gradient across the membrane and increasing blood flow rate (Q_b) allows more drug to reach the dialyzer membrane for removal (4,27,29,30).

Drug Characteristics. Certain characteristics can determine if a drug is likely or unlikely to be dialyzed. These characteristics include molecular weight, hydrophilicity, protein binding, volume of distribution (V_d), and the dialysis clearance in relation to total elimination of the drug. Drugs weighing less than 500 Da are removed by HD, whereas drugs greater than 500 Da are inadequately dialyzed by low-flux dialysis. Lipid-soluble drugs are not easily removed in contrast to water-soluble drugs, which are rapidly removed by the dialysate. Only the free unbound drug is able to cross the dialysis membrane. Therefore, drugs that are highly protein bound are not easily removed. Typically, drugs which are greater than 90% bound to plasma proteins will have minimal removal by dialysis procedures. For example, oxacillin (molecular size = 458 Da) is 94% protein bound, and less than 5% is removed by conventional HD. Alternately, azlocillin (molecular size 461 Da) is only 30% protein bound, and up to 50% is removed by HD. Both drugs have a molecular size that is dialyzable; however, the protein binding of oxacillin hinders HD removal. Drugs with large V_d (>2 L/kg) are less concentrated in the blood and are not readily dialyzable. In contrast, drugs with small V_d (0.7–1 L/kg) are more concentrated in the blood and are therefore available to be removed by dialysis as long as they are not highly protein bound. For example, aminoglycosides and cephalosporins have small V_d and are removed by HD. Also, drugs concentrated in tissues are less likely to be dialyzed (29–32).

Redistribution Phenomenon. One can expect an increase or rebound in plasma concentration after dialysis, if the rate of transport of drug from plasma during dialysis is greater than the rate of transport from the peripheral compartment into the central compartment. This is also seen if the tissue clearance, is decreased during HD. This can cause an overestimation of dialysis clearance, typically if only one pre- and postdialysis serum concentration is obtained. Rebound has been observed with vancomycin, tobramycin, gentamicin, and netilmicin. The concentration of tobramycin increased by 7% within 10 minutes after dialysis, with a maximum increase of 18.3% seen at 1.7 hours. A gentamicin rebound of 25.7% was noted one hour after dialysis (32). Rebound of vancomycin plasma concentrations has been observed for three to six hours after high-flux HD. Therefore, it is necessary to wait anywhere from two to six hours after dialysis to draw blood to determine drug levels (33).

Pharmacodynamics of Antibiotics. Pharmacodynamics describes the relationship between measurements of drug exposure in serum, tissues, and body fluids and the pharmacologic and toxic effects of the drug. Antibiotics have two types of kill characteristics: concentration-dependent and time-dependent killing. In concentration-dependent killing, the rate and extent of bactericidal action increases with increasing drug concentration. Here the goal is to maximize the concentration of the antibiotic. Antibiotics that exhibit this type of kill characteristic are fluoroquinolones and aminoglycosides. Their efficacy can be predicted by measuring AUC/MIC and Peak/MIC (also termed Cmax/MIC) ratios, respectively. AUC/MIC is the ratio of the total exposure of drug to the MIC of the infecting organism and Cmax/MIC is the ratio of highest concentration attained in a dosing interval to the MIC. For example, aminoglycosides eradicate gram-negative organisms best when they achieve peak concentrations (C_{max}) that are 10 to 12 times above the MIC (34). This concept led to the single daily dosing of aminoglycosides. A large study by Nicolau et al. dosed aminoglycosides at 7 mg/kg if the CrCl was greater than 60 mL/min (35). At a CrCl of 40 to 59 mL/min, the same dose was used, but the dosing interval was widened to 36 hours, and at a clearance of 20 to 39 mL/min the dosing interval was increased to 48 hours. These dosing regimens achieved adequate peaks and troughs that were undetectable. Aminoglycosides are greatly affected by dialysis; therefore, knowledge of the patient's volume of distribution (V_d) and dialysis clearance is necessary to dose appropriately to achieve an adequate peak (36). The pharmacokinetic model for dosing in HD patients is to give a single dose at the conclusion of a dialysis session. A significant amount of drug is lost between dialysis sessions and during dialysis, and this postdialysis dose returns the drug level to the targeted peak concentration. The postdialysis replacement dose can be calculated by the following equation:

Postdialysis replacement dose
$$= (V)(C_{ss}\text{peak})(1 - [(e^{-(\text{Cl}_{pat})(t_1)})(e-^{(\text{cl}_{pat}+\text{Cl}_{dial})})/V(T_d)]) \tag{6}$$

where t_1 is the interdialysis period or time from peak concentration to the beginning of dialysis.

T_d is the dialysis period, Cl_{pat} is the clearance of the patient, Cl_{dial} is the clearance of dialysis, V is the volume of distribution, and C_{ss} peak is the desired peak concentration (4).

In regard to fluoroquinolones, the AUC/MIC ratio of greater than 125 is the desired target for eradication of gram-negative organisms, and an AUC/MIC ratio of greater than 30 is the desired target for eradication of gram-positive organisms. Renally excreted fluoroquinolones are dose adjusted in HD patients by increasing the dosing interval. Concentration-dependent killing antibiotics commonly exhibit a PAE. This is described as the persistent inhibitory effect on an organism that results from drug exposure after the drug has been completely removed. There is a delay before microorganisms recover and reenter a log growth period (34).

The theory of time-dependent killing explains that the extent of microbial killing is dependent on the "duration" of exposure of the drug to the bacteria at the site of infection (time > MIC). Antibiotics which exhibit this type of kill characteristic are beta-lactams, macrolides, clindamycin, glycopeptides, tetracyclines, and trimethoprim. The concentration of drug does not have to remain above the MIC for the entire dosing interval to achieve sufficient antimicrobial effect (e.g., T>MIC for 30% to 50% of dosing interval is often adequate), but for maximal killing, the concentration should exceed the MIC for 90% to 100% of the dosing interval (34,37). Beta-lactams that are renally excreted commonly have their dose reduced and the dosing interval extended in HD patients. Many are significantly removed by HD, and maintenance doses should be administered immediately after HD. If more aggressive therapy is necessary, a dose prior to HD followed by a dose post-HD may be warranted (30). Vancomycin, a glycopeptide antibiotic, is not significantly removed by standard high-efficiency HD, but is removed by high-flux HD. Typically HD patients are started with a dose of 19 mg/kg, and are redosed when the level is 15 mg/L. The estimated residual vancomycin clearance is 3 to 4 mL/70 kg/min, and high-flux HD has been reported to remove 17% of vancomycin over two hours. The initial peak concentration can be calculated by the following equation:

$$C = (S)(F)(\text{Loading Dose})/V \tag{7}$$

where $S = 1$, $F = 1$, $V =$ volume of distribution. The predialysis concentration can be calculated by the following equation:

$$C_2 = C(e^{-kt}) \tag{8}$$

where $K = Cl/V_d$ (Cl is the estimated residual clearance in L/hr), t (hours) is time from dose given to HD session. And the postdialysis concentration is calculated with the following equation:

$$C_{postdialysis} = C_2(0.83) \qquad (9)$$

Because high-flux HD removes 17% of drug, the postdialysis plasma concentration will be 83% of the predialysis concentration. Any intrinsic clearance during HD is minimal and is ignored (4). In summary, the dosing interval is widened for time-dependent killing antibiotics in order to allow the patient more time to clear the drug. Because many are removed by HD, a supplemental dose is given after dialysis to assure the concentration of the drug is maintained above the MIC of the organism.

Peritoneal Dialysis

CAPD is a commonly utilized type of PD. The elimination of drug occurs by its transfer across the peritoneal membrane from plasma to dialysate (38). About 1 to 3 L of dialysate solution is instilled in the peritoneal cavity via a surgically placed catheter. It will dwell there for three to eight hours and is then drained and replaced by new dialysate solution. There are typically three exchanges during the day, and a fourth overnight exchange resulting in fluid removal totaling approximately 1300 mL. As the dialysate dwells in the peritoneal cavity, toxins are removed by diffusion down a concentration gradient. Because the dialysate fluid remains in the peritoneal cavity for hours, equilibrium is achieved and the concentration gradient is decreased resulting in a decrease in the elimination rate of substances. CAPD must occur continually in order to achieve adequate removal of substances. This is different than HD where there is a constant perfusion of fresh dialysate throughout the session resulting in a consistently high concentration gradient. Convection also plays a role in the removal of water and substances. The amount of fluid removal can be controlled by the osmotic pressure of the dialysate. The electrolyte composition includes sodium, chloride, calcium, magnesium, and lactate and is at physiologic levels, and dextrose concentrations vary (i.e., 1.5%, 2.5%, and 4.25%). Higher dextrose concentrations result in larger amounts of fluid removal. As discussed in HD, the efficiency of drug removal is determined by the characteristics of the dialysate membrane, blood and dialysate flow rates, and the properties of the drug (4,27). In CAPD, the dialysate flow rate is the determining factor and can be increased by increasing the number of exchanges per day and also by increasing the volume of dialysate used per exchange. The membrane is the living peritoneal membrane, and the Q_b is dependent on cardiac output, and these components are not readily altered (39). The residual clearance of the patient will contribute to the removal of drug also. If the patient's residual clearance is substantially greater than the CAPD clearance then the drug will not be cleared significantly by CAPD. As a rule, if the maximum CAPD clearance is less than 25% of the patient's residual clearance, no drug dose adjustment is necessary upon initiation or discontinuation of CAPD. As previously discussed, drugs equilibrate into the dialysate fluid and are removed with the exchange of this fluid. This removal is based on the assumption that drugs equilibrate, and this assumption is most likely correct for low molecular weight (<500 Da) drugs. Larger drugs may not equilibrate during the average six-hour dwell time and therefore are removed to a lesser degree. As mentioned before, only unbound drug can be removed; therefore, highly protein-bound drugs are minimally removed by CAPD. Aminoglycosides have a low molecular weight with low protein binding and are removed by CAPD. Alternatively, vancomycin, although low in protein binding, is a large molecule. Peritonitis will increase the transfer of drug across the peritoneal membrane and systemic absorption of intraperitoneally administered drugs (39).

ANTIBIOTIC DOSING IN CRRT

HD is done intermittently over a period of two to four hours. During this period, the estimated CrCl of the patient is between 150 to 160 mL/min, but when not on HD, the patient with renal failure has a CrCl of less than 10 mL/min (40). The dramatic change in volume status caused by the rapid depletion of intravascular volume can lead to hemodynamic instability that a critically ill patient may not be able to tolerate. Additionally, this may cause further ischemic damage to the kidneys, which can prolong the time to recovery of renal function (41–47). It is also difficult to achieve fluid and acid–base balance (41).

PD may also not be the best choice for critically ill patients. While it is slower and gentler than HD, surgery is required to place the catheter in the abdomen, which may delay the PD, and some patients may not be surgical candidates at the moment when they most need renal replacement therapy. Additionally, critically ill patients may have poor blood flow to the abdomen, which can compromise the efficacy of PD, and the large-volume exchanges may impair respiratory function. The slow rate of fluid and toxin exchange in PD makes it inappropriate for patients who require rapid or significant correction of volume or metabolic abnormalities (41,48).

CRRT is advantageous in many critically ill patients, because it allows for slower fluid and electrolyte exchange and metabolic product removal, which will not significantly compromise hemodynamic status. Additionally, this method allows for precise fluid and metabolic control, removes cytokines which can be detrimental, and allows for unlimited nutritional support (49–54). These advantages can all lead to improved patient outcomes over traditional HD or PD. In studies, these advantages have not translated into a survival advantage except in select patient populations (41). Disadvantages of CRRT include the need for careful supervision by trained and experienced personnel, and for anticoagulation, which may be a problem for patients with certain hematological disorders, surgical patients, or other patients who are at high risk for bleeding. Bleeding rates in one study were 8.4% (55). Other complications include excess fluid removal and associated hemodynamic compromise, hypotension, filter clotting, electrolyte abnormalities, lactic acidosis, access malfunction, infection and sepsis, and allergic reactions (55,56).

The causes of acute renal failure in critically ill patients as discussed previously can be varied, but the goals are always to maintain fluid and electrolyte, acid–base and solute homeostasis; prevent further renal injury; promote healing and renal function recovery; and permit administration of supportive care measures, such as nutrition. These goals are easier to achieve with CRRT than with HD or PD. CRRT is best for patients who are hemodynamically unstable, catabolic, or fluid overloaded, while HD should be reserved for more stable patients (41).

There are different types of CRRT that vary according to the membrane used, the type of vascular access, and the mechanism for solute and fluid removal. The pressure driving the dialysis can be from the patient himself in arteriovenous systems or from an external peristaltic pump in venovenous systems (41). Patients who are critically ill may not be candidates for an arteriovenous system due to their compromised hemodynamic status, and so a venovenous system, which can maintain a constant blood flow of 100 to 200 mL/min, may be preferred (41,51). There are also problems with arterial vascular access, so venous access is more commonly employed (41,50,57–61).

Continuous Renal Replacement Therapy

Fluid and solute removal can be done through diffusion, as is done in HD where molecules diffuse from an area of high concentration to an area of low concentration, and efficiency is determined by blood flow, concentration, and countercurrent flow rate of the dialysate, as well as the porosity and surface area of the dialysis membrane, as described above. In CRRT, this can be thought of as continuous HD and depending on the source of the driving pressure, the systems can be termed "continuous arteriovenous hemodialysis" (CAVHD) or continuous venovenous hemodialysis (CVVHD). Fluid and solute removal is more commonly achieved through hemofiltration, which uses convection. Convection is the solvent drag or the transport of molecules across a membrane following a liquid, so that both the liquid and the molecules are removed in equal amounts, and efficiency is determined by blood flow, filtration rate, the surface area of the filter, and the sieving coefficient (SC). The SC is the ratio of drug concentration in the filtrate to simultaneous drug concentration in the arterial blood and is usually estimated by the protein binding of a drug. For example, a drug that is 70% protein bound would have a SC of 0.3. The hemofilters used typically have large pore size that allows the passage of medium-sized molecules including proteins and cytokines. The cytokines removed are proinflammatory mediators (e.g., tumor necrosis factor-α), which, along with interleukins 6, 8, 10, and others, play a role in the pathogenesis of septic shock syndrome; therefore, hemofiltration may help prevent septic shock and multiorgan failure, irrespective of renal function (41,51,62). Hemofiltration can be thought of as glomerular filtration without tubular reabsorption or secretion. Depending on the source of the driving pressure, the systems can be termed "continuous arteriovenous hemofiltration" (CAVH) or "continuous venovenous hemofiltration" (CVVH). Finally, hemodiafiltration is a combination of both HD and hemofiltration and is the most efficient system. The two systems can be run concurrently or sequentially and depending on the source of pressure would be termed "continuous arteriovenous hemodiafiltration" or continuous venovenous hemodiafiltration (CVVHDF) (41,63). These abbreviations had not been consistent, but, in 1996, Bellomo et al. proposed this nomenclature, which has been adopted by most clinicians (64). While the abbreviations used to describe the systems include the word "continuous," the system is not always run 24 hours per day. It is usually run as patients require it and can tolerate it. These fluctuation in drug clearance rates when CRRT is on or off may affecte drug dosing

The factors that affect drug clearance in CRRT can be divided into mechanical factors and drug factors. Mechanical factors include Q_b, the type of membrane, the surface area of the membrane, the transmembrane pressure, and the pore size of the membrane. Drug factors include molecular weight, protein binding, volume of distribution, tissue binding, drug charge, and intrinsic renal clearance (41,48,51, 63,65–67).

The membrane surface area is usually between 0.25 to 2 m^2, but will decline over days because of blood clots and fibrin deposition on the membrane. It is not possible to measure the decline in surface area. Some drugs and substances such as aminoglycosides and tumor necrosis factor-α can adhere to the membrane, in particular, the AN69 membranes. At a later point in time, the drug can be displaced from the membrane, increasing serum levels without new administration of the drug (67).

The transmembrane pressure is the difference between the hydrostatic and oncotic pressures across the membrane. It can be increased by several factors including increasing blood flow, increasing countercurrent dialysate flow rate, applying negative pressure to the dialysate or ultrafiltrate compartment, or changing the concentration of dialysate. With arteriovenous systems the Q_b is 80 to 100 mL/min, which equals an ultrafiltration rate (UFR) or glomerular filtration rate (GFR) of 10 to 15 mL/min, but with venovenous systems, the Q_b is 125 to 150 mL/min, which equals a UFR or GFR of 20 to 30 mL/min. When these are combined in hemodiafiltration, the GFR is 30 to 50 mL/min. Therefore, the clinician can assume a GFR of 10 to 50 mL/min when dosing drugs (67).

The pore size can vary dramatically between products and the type of CRRT used. The high-flux membranes used in CAVHD and CVVHD allow molecules of 5000 to 20,000 Da to pass, and the membranes used in CAVH and CVVH allow molecules of 20,000 to 50,000 Da to pass. Clinicians should determine which membrane is used in institution, so they may determine which drugs will pass through (41,51,63).

Smaller molecules pass through membranes most easily, but with the larger-membrane pores and especially with the high blood flow seen with external pumps, medium-sized molecules can also be removed and molecular size becomes a less important issue. With diffusion, as is done in arteriovenous systems, larger-molecular-weight drugs take longer time to diffuse, but in the more commonly used venovenous systems with blood pumping, more blood is processed more quickly, minimizing the effect of molecular weight. Additionally, most drugs have a molecular weight of less than 1500 Da, so this is an issue for only select drugs (67).

Protein binding will prohibit passage through the membrane, so only drugs with a low-protein binding, i.e., less than 80%, will pass through. In some patients with acute illness, serum concentrations of albumin may decrease as α₁-acid glycoprotein levels increase. While this would increase the free levels of albumin-bound drugs, it would decrease the free levels of drugs bound to α₁-acid glycoprotein. Also, the binding affinity of drugs for albumin may be altered by uremia, pH, hyperbilirubinemia, displacement by other drugs, heparin, free fatty acids, and other parameters. These changes may affect the level of protein binding and even drugs that are normally highly protein bound can pass through the membrane. Using published tables of protein-binding percentages, which are determined in healthy people with normal renal function, may not be accurate in patients with acute renal failure who are critically ill (41,42). Because anionic molecules such as albumin do not pass through the membrane, they may retard the passage of cationic molecules such as aminoglycosides. This may partially explain the discrepancy between the level of protein binding of 10% for aminoglycosides with an expected SC of 0.9 and the actual SC of 0.81. A SC of 1 indicates free passage. This is called the Gibbs–Donnan effect (40,48,67). In CVVH and CVVHDF, drug removal is not linear and the SC may not completely reflect current drug removal from the body (48).

The volume of distribution and availability in the systemic circulation can significantly impact drug removal. Drugs with a large volume of distribution have a strong affinity for tissue and so are only available in the systemic circulation in small amounts. An example is digoxin, where serum levels are measured in nanograms, but tissue concentrations would be measured in milligrams. Therefore, removal of the drug will be slow. Because the human body consists of approximately 67% water, a drug that is well distributed to all fluid compartments would have a volume of distribution of 0.7 L/kg, so a drug with a larger volume of distribution would not be efficiently removed by CRRT or other types of renal replacement therapy, although with continuous dialysis or filtration, there is more time for movement between the tissue and vascular compartments, so the drug will be removed over time. The larger the volume of distribution, the less efficiently the drug will be removed by any form of renal replacement therapy (41,67).

The metabolic pathway of the drug can impact the clearance. In intermittent HD, only drugs in which the GFR constitutes more than 30% of the total clearance are considered significant. CRRT is more efficient, but unless the CRRT dose is very high, drugs that are not at least 30% renally eliminated will not be efficiently removed by CRRT. It is also important to consider the patient's residual renal function, which may be difficult to estimate. Serum creatinine-blood urea nitrogen, (BUN), and urine output may not be accurate reflections due to the delay between changing renal function and these parameters. As discussed previously, mathematical equations may not accurately reflect a patient's renal function in the setting of rapidly changing serum creatinine levels (41,48,51,66,67). Drugs that are not renally eliminated are usually not significantly affected by CRRT, but total body clearance can be modestly increased. For example, in someone with normal renal function, 60% of a ceftriaxone dose is renally eliminated and 40% is hepatically eliminated. De Clari determined that in patients undergoing CVVH, the hemofiltration concentration was 11% of the serum concentration (68). This may be important when treating infections caused by organisms that are only intermediately sensitive to the antibiotic in question, and even a small decrease in serum levels can compromise the efficacy of the drug. To determine the clearance of a drug in a convection system such as CVVH, multiply the SC times the UFR, which is available for many antimicrobials. If the SC is not available, the unbound fraction of the drug can be used. Alternatively, the clinician can measure levels in the total volume of dialysate or ultrafiltrate and measure several serum levels, but this is obviously cumbersome and impractical in most situations (41).

Recommendations

There are many issues to be considered when dosing drugs in patients who are receiving a form of renal replacement therapy. However, based on the parameters of each type of renal replacement therapy and the pharmacokinetics of antimicrobials, therapy for a patient can be individualized (Table 3). Some general principles can be used to guide the clinician's decision. Before making any adjustments, the clinician should determine which type of renal replacement therapy is being used, and the individual parameters including frequency, flow rate, filter, and others; if the patient has any residual renal function; the status of other organ function; patient fluid status; drug factors including volume of distribution, protein binding, molecular weight, and active fraction eliminated renally; and what drugs must be administered so that dosage adjustments can be made and the SCs determined. As data changes, further adjustments will be needed (41).

For drugs in which loading doses are recommended, the loading dose can be administered regardless of the renal replacement therapy used. The clinician should take caution and evaluate the patient's other pharmacokinetic parameters, including the volume of distribution, which may require a dose adjustment. Whenever possible,

Table 3 Factors Affecting Dosage Recommendations in Renal Replacement Therapy

Drug factors	Patient factors	Renal replacement factors
Ability to use local therapy	Residual renal function	Membrane used
Ability to monitor serum levels	Other organ function	Type of therapy
Intrinsic metabolic pathway	Fluid status	Frequency of therapy
Drug charge		Ultrafiltration rate
Protein binding		
Volume of distribution		
Loading dose		
Therapeutic index of drug		

Abbreviation: UFR, ultrafiltration rate.
Source: From Ref. 66.

local therapy should be used, for example, the use of oral vancomycin or metronidazole for *Clostridium difficile* colitis or bladder irrigation for candidial urinary tract infections.

Drugs that can be routinely monitored through serum levels, including aminoglycosides and vancomycin, are preferred so that the dose can be titrated for each individual patient using the appropriate pharmacokinetic equations. For drugs that are not routinely monitored, several challenges exist. If the patient is underdosed, it may lead to resistant organisms and therapeutic failure, especially if it is an intermediately resistant organism that would require a higher MIC (48). In the case of overdose, the risk of toxicity will depend on the antimicrobial in question. For example, the fluoroquinolones can cause seizures at high doses, while the beta-lactams have a much higher therapeutic index (48,67). Therefore, it is a careful balance between therapeutic failure and unacceptable toxicity.

In HD and PD, more information exists regarding dose adjustments for antimicrobials. These recommendations address when to give the dose (before or after dialysis) and the adjusted dose and frequency. However, in CRRT, there is often only limited information. Typically, CRRT provides an artificial clearance of approximately 10 to 50 mL/min and one can follow the dosage recommendations in the product information, literature, or antimicrobial-dosing handbooks for this CrCl range. Because CRRT is usually done in patients whose renal function will eventually start to improve, it is important to consider the residual renal function also, especially as they begin to recover (66,67). Drugs that are more than 30% eliminated by GFR and that can pass through the membrane will require supplemental doses in renal replacement therapy (67).

Kroh et al. developed a formula to determine a dose for patients undergoing CRRT (69). First, a factor (*p*) for dosage adjustment must be determined by the following equation:

$$p = Qx + (UFR \times SC)/CL \tag{10}$$

where Qx is any remaining elimination capacity of the body, UFR is the ultrafiltration rate, SC is the sieving coefficient and CL is the total clearance in someone with normal renal function. The adjusted dose is then calculated by this equation:

$$D = p \times Do \tag{11}$$

where Do is the dose for an otherwise health person. Other investigators have proposed similar equations, which can be used when there is no information in the literature regarding dose adjustments in these patients.

Due to the variability in patients' clinical status, the various combinations of renal replacement therapy, and the low number of clinical trials, it is challenging to make broad recommendations. Clinicians should evaluate patients individually and apply the principles above to determine the most appropriate dose and schedule for the patient. Additionally, close monitoring of the patient will be critical to ensure efficacy without untoward toxicity.

CONCLUSION

In summary, dosing of antimicrobial agents in patients with organ dysfunction involves many issues and considerations. Patients are unique, and each case must be considered individually using the information above to make appropriate decisions to cure or control infections while limiting toxicity to patients.

REFERENCES

1. Brouwer KLR, Dukes GE, Powell JR. Influence of liver function on drug disposition. In: Evans WE, Schentag JJ, Jusko W, eds. Applied Pharmacokinetics: Principles of Therapeutic Drug Monitoring. 3rd ed. Vancouver, WA: Lippincott, Williams & Wilkins, 1992:6-1–6-59.
2. Reese RE, Betts RF. Antibiotic use. A practical approach to infectious disease. 4th ed. Boston, MA: Little, Brown and Company, 1996:1059–1093.
3. Cockcroft D, Gault M. Prediction of creatinine clearance from serum creatinine. Nephron 1976; 16:31.
4. Winter ME. Basic Clinical Pharmacokinetics. 4th ed. Baltimore, Maryland: Lippincott, Williams & Wilkins, 2004.
5. Comstock TJ. Renal Dialysis. In: Koda-Kimble MA, Young LY, Kradjan WA, Guglielmo BJ, eds. Applied Therapeutics The Clinical Use of Drugs. 8th ed. Baltimore, Maryland: Lippincott, Williams & Wilkins, 2005:33-1–33-14.
6. Mueller B. Acute renal failure. In: DePiro J, et al. eds. Pharmacotherapy: A Pathophysiologic Approach. Stamford, CT: Appelton & Lange, 1999:706–732.
7. Kapadia N. Special issues in the patient with renal failure. Crit Care Clin 2003; 19:233–251.
8. Livornese L. Use of antibacterial agents in renal failure. Infect Dis Clin North Am 2001; 15:983–1102.
9. Sampliner R, Perner D, Ponll R, et al. Influence of ascitis on tobramycin pharmacokinetics. J Clin Pharmacol 1984; 24:43–46.
10. Barza M et al. Single or multiple daily doses of aminoglycosides: a meta analysis. BMJ 1996; 312:338–345.
11. Hatala R et al. One daily aminoglycoside dosing in immunocompetent adults: a meta-analysis. Ann Intern Med 1996; 124:717–725.
12. Garaud J et al. Vancomycin pharmacokinetics in critically ill patients. J Antimicrob Chemother 1984; 14(suppl):53–57.
13. Goldberg J. Optimizing antimicrobial dosing in the critically ill. Curr Opin Crit Care 2002; 8:435–440.
14. Reginald F. Drug therapy individualization for patients with renal insufficiency. In: DePiro J et al, eds. Pharmacotherapy: A Pathophysiologic Approach. Stamford, CT: Appelton & Lange, 1999:872–889.

15. Macgowan A. Continuous infusion of B-lactams antibiotics. Clin Pharmacokinetics 1999; 35:391–402.
16. Bernard E et al. Is there rationale for the continuous infusion of cefepime? A multi-disciplinary approach. Clin Microbiol Infection 2003; 9:339–349.
17. Ambrose P et al. Infections in critical care: antibiotics in the critical care unit. Crit Care Clin 1998; 2:283–309.
18. Owens R. Antibiotic therapy: clinical use of the fluoroquinolones. Med Clin of North Amer 2000; 84:1447–1469.
19. Micromedex. Moxifloxacin monograph. Accessed May 25, 2005.
20. Micromedex. Fluconazole monograph. Accessed May 25, 2005.
21. McGee W et al. Successful treatment of *candida krusei* infection with caspofungin acetate: a new antifungal agent. Crit Care Med 2003; 31:1577–1578.
22. Jeu L et al. Voriconazole. Clin Ther 2003; 25:1321–1381.
23. Johnson L. Voriconazole: a new triazole antifungal agent. Clin Infect Dis 2003; 36(5): 630–637.
24. Izzedine H. Antiviral drug-induced nephrotoxicity. Am J Kidney Dis 2005; 45:804–817.
25. Micromedex. Metronidazole monograph. Accessed May 25, 2005.
26. http://www.usrds.org (accessed May 2005).
27. Singh AK, Brenner BM. Dialysis in the treatment of renal failure. Kasper DL, Fauci AS, Longo DL, Braunwald E, Hauser SL, Jameson, JL, eds. Harrison's Principles of Internal Medicine, 16th ed. New York: McGraw-Hill, 2005:1663–1667.
28. Sargel L, Yu ABC. Dosage adjustment in renal disease. Applied Biopharmaceutics and Pharmacokinetics. 3rd ed. Norwalk, CT: Appelton and Lange, 1993:435–463.
29. Lam YWF, Banerji S, Hatfield C, et al. Principles of drug administration in renal insufficiency. Clin Pharmacokinet 1997; 32(1):30–57.
30. St. Peter WL, Redic-Kill KA, Halstenson CE. Clinical pharmacokinetics of antibiotics in patients with impaired renal function. Clin Pharmacokinet 1992; 22(3):169–210.
31. Brater DC, Hall SD. Disposition and dose requirements of drugs in renal insufficiency. In: Selden DW, Giebisch G, eds. The Kidney: Physiology and Pathophysiology. 3rd ed. Baltimore, MD: Lippincott, Williams & Wilkins, 2000:2923–2940.
32. Matzke GR, Millakin SP. Influence of renal function and dialysis on drug disposition. In: Evans WE, Schentag JJ, Jusko W, eds. Applied Pharmacokinetics: Principles of Therapeutic Drug Monitoring. 3rd ed. Vancouver, WA: Lippincott, Williams & Wilkins, 1992:8-1–8-49.
33. Launay-Vacher V, Izzedine H, Mercadal L, et al. Clinical review: use of vancomycin in haemodialysis patients. Critical Care 2002; 6:313–316.
34. Craig WA. Pharmacodynamics of antimicrobials: General concepts and applications. In: Nightingale CH, Murakaw T, Ambrose PG, eds. Antimicrobial Pharmacodynamics in Theory and Clinical Practice, New York: Marcel Dekker, 2002:1–22.
35. Nicolau DP, Freeman C, Belliveau PP, et al. Experience with once-daily aminoglycoside program administered to 2184 adult agents. Antimicrob Agents Chemother 1995; 39: 650–655.
36. Pinder M, Bellomo R, Lipman J. Pharmacological principles of antibiotic prescription in the critically ill. Anesth Intensive Care 2002; 30:134–144.
37. Drusano GL. Antimicrobial pharmacodynamics: critical interactions of "bug and drug". Nat Rev Microbiol 2004; 2:289–300.
38. Taylor CA, Abdel-Rahman E, Zimmerman SW, et al. Clinical pharmacokinetics during continuous ambulatory peritoneal dialysis. Clin Pharmcokinet 1996; 31(4):293–308.
39. Ronco C, Clark W. Factors affecting hemodialysis and peritoneal dialysis efficiency. Seminars in Dialysis 2001; 14:257–262.
40. Tam VH, Lomaestro BM. Drug dosing in patients undergoing continuous renal replacement therapy. The New York Health-system Pharmacist 2001; 20(3):10–14.
41. Joy MS, Matzke GR, Armstrong DK, et al. A primer on continuous renal replacement therapy for critically ill patients. 1998; 32:362–375.

42. Bressolle F, Kinowski J, de la Coussaye JE, et al. Clinical pharmacokinetics during continuous haemofiltration. Clin Pharmacokin 1994; 26:457–471.

43. Burchardi H. Hemofiltration. In: Vincent JL, eds. Update in Intensive Care and Emergency Medicine. New York: Springer-Verlag, 1989:340–347.

44. Gernomous R, Schneider N. Continuous arteriovenous hemodialysis: a new modality for the treatment of acute renal failure. Trans Am Soc Artific Intern Organs 1984; 30:610–613.

45. Golper TA. Continuous arteriovenous hemofiltration in acute renal failure. Am J Kidney Dis 1985; 6:373–386.

46. Golper TA, Bennett WM. Drug removal by continuous arteriovenous hemofiltration: a review of evidence in poisoned patients. Med Tox Adv Drug Exper 1988; 3:341–349.

47. Kaplan AA, Longnecker RE, Folkert YW. Continuous arteriovenous hemofiltration: a repost of six months experience. Ann Intern Med 1984; 93:124–126.

48. Cotterill S. Antimicrobial prescribing in patients of hemofiltration. J Antimicrob Chemother 1995; 36:773–780.

49. Grootendorst AF, Bouman CSC, Hoeben KNH, et al. The role of continuous renal replacement therapy in sepsis and multiorgan failure. AM J Kid Dis 1996; 29(suppl 3):S50–S57.

50. Tominaga G, Ingegno M, Ceraldi C, et al. Vascular complications continuous arteriovenous hemofiltration in trauma patients. J Trauma 1993; 35:285–289.

51. Thadhani R, Pascual M, Bonventre JV, et al. Acute renal failure. N Engl J Med 1996; 334:1448–1460.

52. Bellomo R, Tipping P, Boyce N. Continuous venovenous hemofiltration with dialysis removes cytokines form the circulation of septic patients. Crit Care Med 1993; 21:522–526.

53. Bellomo R. Continuous hemofiltration as blood purification in sepsis. New Horiz 1995; 3:732–737.

54. Bellomo R, Mehta R. Acute renal replacement therapy in the intensive care unit: now and tomorrow. New Horiz 1995; 3:760–767.

55. Ronco C. Continuous renal replacement therapies in the treatment of acute renal failure in intensive care patients: part 2. Clinical indication and prescriptions. Nephrol Dial Transplant 1994; 9(suppl 4):201–209.

56. Ronco C, Bellomo R. Complications with continuous renal replacement therapy. Am J Kid Dis 1996; 28(suppl 3):100–104.

57. Manns M, Sigler MH, Teehan BP. Continuous renal replacement therapies: an update. Am J Kidney Dis 1998; 32(2):185–207.

58. Bellomo R, Parkin G, Love J, et al. A prospective comparative study of continuous arteriovenous hemofiltration and continuous venovenous hemodiafiltration in critically ill patients. Am J Kidney Dis 1993; 21:400–404.

59. Bellomo R. Choosing a therapeutic modality: hemofiltration versus hemodialysis versus hemodiafiltration. Semin Dial 1996; 9:88–92.

60. Uldall R. Vascular access for continuous renal replacement therapy. Semin Dial 1998; 9:93–97.

61. Golper TA, Jacobs AA. Pumps utilized during continuous renal replacement therapy. Semin Dial 1996; 9:119–124.

62. Moreno L, Heyka RJ, Paganini EP. Continuous renal replacement therapy: cost considerations and reimbursement. Semin Dial 1996; 9:209–214.

63. Forni LG, Hilton PJ. Continuous hemofiltration in the treatment of acute renal failure. N Engl J Med 1997; 336(18):1303–1309.

64. Bellomo R, Ronco C, Mehta RL. Nomenclature for continuous renal replacement therapies. Am J Kidney Dis 1996; 28(suppl 3):52–57.

65. Bickley SK. Drug dosing during continuous arteriovenous hemofiltration. Clin Pharm 1998; 7:198–206.

66. Schetz M, Ferdinande P, van der Berghe G, et al. Pharmacokinetics of continuous renal replacement therapy. Intensiv Care Med 1995; 21:612–620.

67. Golper TA, Marx MA. Drug dosing adjustments during continuous renal replacement therapies. Kid Intl 1998; 53(suppl 66):S-165–S-168.
68. De Clari F. Ceftriaxone pharmacokinetics during continuous arteriovenous hemofiltration. J Antimicrob Chemother 1991; 27:294–396.
69. Kroh UF, Dehne M, El Abed K, et al. Drug dosing during continuous hemofiltration: pharmacokinetics and practical implications. In: Sieberth, et al., eds. Continuous Hemofiltration, Contributions to Nephrol 1991; 93:127–130.

29
Adverse Reactions to Antibiotics

Eric V. Granowitz and Richard B. Brown
Division of Infectious Disease, Baystate Medical Center and Tufts University School of Medicine, Springfield, Massachusetts, U.S.A.

INTRODUCTION

Each year many patients are hospitalized with adverse drug reactions. Life-threatening reactions include arrhythmias, hepatotoxicity, acute renal failure, and antiretroviral therapy–induced lactic acidosis. In addition, 6% to 7% of hospitalized patients experience a serious adverse drug reaction (1). Approximately 5% of serious inpatient reactions are fatal, making hospital-related adverse drug reactions responsible for approximately 100,000 deaths in the United States annually. The elderly are at especially high risk of reactions (2). Many of these reactions result in intensive care unit (ICU) admission.

More than 70% of ICU patients receive antibiotics for therapy or prophylaxis, with much of this use being empiric and over half of the recipients receiving multiple agents (3,4). The clinical presentation of an adverse drug reaction may be very different in an ICU patient than in a healthier individual because of both the severity of the ICU patient's illness (which often requires that the patient be heavily sedated and paralyzed) and the multiple therapies that patient often requires. Therefore, attributing a particular adverse reaction to a specific antibiotic can be extremely difficult, may involve several factors operating in unison, and can tax the minds of the brightest clinicians.

Adverse reactions associated with drug use include allergies, toxicities, and side effects. Allergy implies that the reaction is due to an immunological state characterized by hypersensitivity to a drug (5). Many are IgE-mediated and occur soon after drug administration. Examples of IgE-mediated type 1 hypersensitivity reactions include bronchospasm, hypotension, and early-onset urticaria. Non–IgE-mediated reactions include acute interstitial nephritis, hemolytic anemia, erythema multiforme, Stevens–Johnson syndrome, toxic epidermal necrolysis, and serum sickness. Toxicity implies the administration of drugs in quantities exceeding those capable of being physiologically "managed" by the host, and is generally due to excessive dosing and/or impaired drug metabolism. Examples of toxicity caused by excessive dosing include penicillin-related neurotoxicity (e.g., twitching and seizures) and the toxicities caused by aminoglycosides. Decreased drug metabolism or clearance may be due to impaired hepatic or renal function. For example, penicillin G neurotoxicity may be precipitated by aminoglycoside-induced renal failure. Side effects reflect the large number of adverse reactions that are neither immunologically mediated nor related to toxic levels of the drug. An example is the dyspepsia often noted with erythromycin.

This chapter will describe some of the adverse reactions to antibiotics that occur in ICU patients. We will concentrate on those agents likely to be employed in the critical care situation, but will not attempt to be encyclopedic. In Table 1, we summarize and prioritize the most common antibiotic-related adverse reactions seen in the ICU. This chapter does not attempt to address drug interactions, antibiotic dosing, or issues specific to pregnant or pediatric patients.

ANAPHYLAXIS

Anaphylaxis is commonly used to refer to acute hypersensitivity reactions that can result in immediate urticaria, laryngospasm, bronchospasm, hypotension, and occasionally death. In the critical care setting, these reactions may be masked by underlying conditions or other therapies. While anaphylaxis can be precipitated by antigen–antibody complexes, it is usually IgE mediated. The binding of antibiotic epitopes to specific preformed IgE antibodies on the surface of mast cells results in the release of histamine and other mediators that lead to the aforementioned clinical presentations. β-Lactams are more often associated with these reactions than other antimicrobials. Best data exist for penicillin where the risk of anaphylaxis is about 0.01% (6). Death occurs in 1 of every 100,000 courses of this agent (5). Conversely, only 10% to 20% of patients who claim to have an allergy to penicillin are truly allergic as determined by skin testing (7). Patients with a history of atopy are not predisposed to anaphylaxis. Fifty percent of patients with a positive skin test will have an immediate reaction when challenged with penicillins (8). Approximately 10% of patients who test positive to penicillin will experience an allergic reaction (only rarely anaphylaxis) when given a cephalosporin (8,9). The incidence of carbapenem cross-reactivity with penicillin may be even higher (10,11). Administering aztreonam is safe in patients with a history of anaphylaxis to all β-lactams except ceftazidime (5).

NEPHROTOXICITY

Acute renal failure is common in ICU patients and is associated with a risk of mortality of greater than 60% (12). Numerous agents used in the ICU are capable of affecting renal function. Mechanisms include decreased glomerular filtration, acute tubular necrosis, interstitial nephritis, and crystallization of the drug within the tubules. With regard to antibiotics, the aminoglycosides and amphotericins are the prototypical classes associated with acute renal failure; however, other agents including β-lactams and sulfonamides have been implicated. As with other antibiotic-associated adverse reactions, the likelihood of nephrotoxicity from antimicrobials is greater in patients with conditions or medications that can independently cause this complication. Therefore, the clinician must have a firm knowledge of the ICU patient's condition and medications to best manage nephrotoxicity.

Gentamicin, tobramycin, and amikacin are the aminoglycosides that are used most often. Traditionally, these drugs were used to treat infections caused by aerobic gram-negative bacilli. When treating these organisms with multiple daily doses of

Table 1 Frequency and Severity of Adverse Reactions to Antibiotics

	Penicillins	Cephalosporins	Monobactams	Carbapenems	Aminoglycosides	Tetracyclines	Chloramphenicol	Rifamycins	Metronidazole	Macrolides/Azalide	Clindamycin	Glycopeptides	Streptogramins	Lipopeptides (daptomycin)	Oxazolidinones	Sulfonamides and trimethoprim	Quinolones	Nitrofurantoin	Amphotericins	Triazoles	Caspofungin	Flucytosine	Acyclovir	Ganciclovir
Anaphylaxis	IIIB	IIIB	IB	IIIB	IB	IB	IB	IB	IB	IB	IB	IIB	IB		IB	IIB	IB	IB	IB	IB	IB	IB	IB	IB
Nephrotoxicity	IIB	IIB		IIB	IIIB			IB				IIA				IIA	IIA		IIIB				IIB	IIIB
Anemia	IIA	IIA		IIA	IIA		IIIB								IIIA	IIB			IIA			IIIB		
Leukopenia	IIB	IIB	IIB	IIB			IIIB				IIA	IIA	IIA		IIA	IIB			IIA			IIIB		IIIB
Thrombocytopenia	IIB	IIB	IIB	IIB			IIIB	IIB				IIIA			IIIB	IIB			IIA			IIB		IIIB
Coagulopathy (other than thrombocytopenia)																								
Dermatological toxicity (excluding phlebitis)	IIIB	IIIB		IIIB		IIA		IIA				IIIA				IIIB				IIA				
Neurotoxicity	IB			IB	IIIB	IIA			IIA	IIIB					IIB	IB	IIIA			?				
Cardiotoxicity										IIIB		IB			IB		IIB		IB					
Hepatotoxicity	IIIA	IIA		IIA		IIA		IIIB	IIA	IIA	IIA		IIA			IIA	IIA	IIB	IIA	IIA		IIB		
Musculoskeletal toxicity													IIIB	IIIA			IIA							
Electrolyte abnormalities	IIB			IIA												IB			IIIB					
Fever	IIIA	IIIA	IIIB											IIB	IIB	IIIA			IIIB	IIA				
Diarrhea	IIIB	IIIB	IIB	IIIB		IIB	IIB	IIB		IIB	IIIB		IIB	IIB	IIB	IIB	IIB	IIB						IIIB

Note: The *relative* frequencies at which different antibiotics cause a specific adverse reaction (e.g., anaphylaxis) are rated as I (least frequent), II, or III (most frequent). The severity of the reaction are rated as A (mild or moderate) or B (severe) based upon published reports and the authors' opinions. Cells are left blank if reactions are infrequent and usually mild and ? indicates visual disturbance due to voriconazole is common, but it is unclear if the mechanism is due to neurological dysfunction.

gentamicin, the goal was to achieve peak levels of 4 to 10 μg/mL and trough levels of 1 to 2 μg/mL. Use of aminoglycosides has declined in the last 30 years, because other agents with broad gram-negative coverage (e.g., antipseudomonal penicillins, advanced generation cephalosporins, and fluoroquinolones) have become available. Gentamicin is now most commonly used for "synergy" against serious infections caused by enterococci, viridans streptococci, and staphylococci. When treating gram-positive cocci, the goal of gentamicin dosing is to achieve a peak of 3 μg/mL and a trough of less than 1 μg/mL. Using lower doses reduces the risk of aminoglycoside-related toxicities.

Aminoglycoside-induced nephrotoxicity occurs in 7% to more than 25% of patients who receive selected compounds from within this class (13). It generally results from impairment of tubular function and, when severe, can cause acute tubular necrosis. A major study suggests that gentamicin (26%) is more nephrotoxic than tobramycin (12%) when relatively small changes in serum creatinine are employed as a gauge of renal function (13). Employing this criterion, nephrotoxicity is generally noted between 6 and 10 days after starting an aminoglycoside. However, other investigations have challenged this conclusion (14). Aminoglycoside-induced acute tubular necrosis is generally nonoliguric and completely reversible. However, occasional patients require temporary dialysis and the rare patient requires permanent dialysis.

Cost of aminoglycoside-induced nephrotoxicity may be substantial. One study demonstrated that nephrotoxicity resulted in an average of 2.7 additional hospital days, including 1.5 additional ICU days (15). Factors that contribute to aminoglycoside-induced nephrotoxicity include dose, duration of treatment, and use of other tubular toxins (16). Elevation of trough aminoglycoside levels has also been implicated (14). Although numerous dosing nomograms have been employed to calculate optimal doses of these agents, even patients with peak and trough levels within recommended ranges can develop nephrotoxicity.

Meta-analyses have demonstrated that in immunocompetent adults, a single daily dose of an aminoglycoside is effective for infections caused by gram-negative bacilli (employing bacteriologic cure as an end point) and is less toxic than the traditional multiple daily doses (17,18). Therefore, for non-neutropenic patients with normal renal function who have infections caused by gram-negative bacilli, it is preferable to give a 5-mg/kg dose of gentamicin or tobramycin once daily (19).

Until recently, amphotericin B was the drug of choice for severe fungal infections due to *Candida* or *Aspergillus*. Additionally, this agent is also used for cryptococcal meningitis, an AIDS-associated illness that occasionally requires treatment in an ICU. Amphotericin B can affect the renal tubules, renal blood flow, or glomerular function; renal dysfunction is seen in at least 60% to 80% of patients who receive this drug (20). However, return to prior renal function generally occurs, and few patients suffer serious long-term renal sequelae. Rarely, irreversible renal failure is noted when the agent is used in high doses for prolonged periods (21). Risk factors for amphotericin B toxicity include abnormal baseline renal function, daily and total drug dose, and concurrent use of other nephrotoxic agents (e.g., aminoglycosides and diuretics) (20,22). However, some studies have not found that other drugs enhance amphotericin B-induced nephrotoxicity (23). Reversing sodium depletion and optimizing volume status prior to infusing the drug can decrease the risk of amphotericin B-induced nephrotoxicity (20,24).

In 1995, liposomal preparations of amphotericin B became available. These preparations are associated with a substantially decreased risk of nephrotoxicity compared with the parent compound (25,26). Typical doses of the liposomal preparation are up to 5 mg/kg/day. Nephrotoxicity with newer broad-spectrum antifungals such as voriconazole and caspofungin is very rare. The importance of the reduced risk of nephrotoxicity of these new agents needs to be weighed against the substantially increased acquisition costs compared with those of amphotericin B.

β-Lactams, fluoroquinolones, sulfonamides, and rifampin can occasionally cause interstitial nephritis. Although classically associated with methicillin (27,28), interstitial nephritis has been noted with numerous other β-lactams (29–32). It is thought to be an allergic reaction and, when seen, generally follows prolonged and/or high-dose therapy. There are no data demonstrating that underlying renal dysfunction predisposes β-lactam–treated patients to interstitial nephritis if dosage adjustments are made (32). Historically, renal failure was believed to be acute in onset and associated with fever, chills, rash, and arthralgias. However, more recent data suggest that antibiotic-induced interstitial nephritis should be suspected in any patient on a potentially offending agent, who develops acute renal dysfunction (29). Urinary eosinophilia supports the diagnosis, but is present in less than half of the patients. Conclusive documentation of this disease requires renal biopsy. Discontinuation of the offending agent generally reverses the process and permanent sequelae are unusual.

Sulfonamides and acyclovir can crystallize in the renal tubules causing acute renal failure. Sulfonamides can also block tubular secretion of creatinine; this causes the serum creatinine to rise but glomerular filtration rate is unchanged. Patients on rifampin often develop orange-colored urine of no clinical consequence.

HEMATOLOGICAL ADVERSE REACTIONS

Anemia

Linezolid (33–35), amphotericin B, chloramphenicol, and ganciclovir cause anemia by suppressing erythropoiesis. Chloramphenicol (infrequently employed in the United States) frequently causes a reversible anemia that is much more common if circulating drug concentrations exceed the recommended range. In approximately 1 of every 25,000 recipients, chloramphenicol causes an idiosyncratic irreversible aplastic anemia (36). β-Lactams, nitrofurantoin, and rarely aminoglycosides can cause hemolytic anemia. Patients who are glucose 6-phosphate dehydrogenase–deficient are predisposed to sulfonamide and doxycycline-induced hemolytic anemia.

Leukopenia

Leukopenia and/or agranulocytosis may occur with the use of many antibiotics and is generally reversible, but can result in serious infections. An additive phenomenon can occur when antibiotics capable of causing these phenomena are used together with other agents or in conditions that can also suppress bone marrow function. Anti-infectives that can cause neutropenia or agranulocytosis include trimethoprim–sulfamethoxazole (37,38), most β-lactams (38–42), vancomycin (43–45), macrolides, clindamycin, chloramphenicol, flucytosine, and amphotericin B. The risk of agranulocytosis with trimethoprim–sulfamethoxazole is greater than the risk with a sulfonamide alone.

Severe neutropenia develops in 5% to 15% of recipients of β-lactams (42,46). Duration of therapy more than 10 days, high doses of medication, and severe hepatic dysfunction predispose patients to this condition (46,47). Likelihood of neutropenia is less than 1% when shorter courses of β-lactams are used in patients with normal liver function (45). Methicillin and nafcillin were traditionally the most common offenders (39–41). Only rare patients develop infection as a result of this decrease in functioning leukocytes. High-dose β-lactams can also prolong cancer chemotherapy–induced neutropenia in patients being treated for fever. Vancomycin-induced neutropenia is uncommon and generally occurs only after more than two weeks of intravenous treatment, as is used in patients with infective endocarditis or osteomyelitis (44,45). The etiology does not appear to be direct bone marrow toxicity, but rather peripheral destruction or sequestration of circulating myelocytes. Prompt reversal of the neutropenia generally occurs after vancomycin is discontinued.

Thrombocytopenia

Thrombocytopenia related to antibiotic use may result from either immune-mediated peripheral destruction of platelets or a decrease in the number of megakaryocytes (48). The oxazolidinone linezolid is the most likely antimicrobial to cause platelet destruction (33–35). In one study, linezolid-induced thrombocytopenia occurred in 2% of patients receiving two weeks of therapy or less, 5% of those receiving two to four weeks of therapy, and 7% in those receiving more than 4 weeks of the drug (34). Sulfonamides, vancomycin, rifampin, and rarely β-lactams (including penicillin, ampicillin, methicillin, cefamandole, cefazolin, and cefoxitin) have also been reported to cause platelet destruction (42). Prompt recognition and removal of the offending agent is the appropriate therapy. Marrow-induced thrombocytopenia is commonly noted with chloramphenicol, is usually dose related, and, if not associated with aplastic anemia, is reversible with discontinuation of the drug.

Coagulation

A relationship between antibiotics and coagulation factors has been recognized for many years, and anecdotal reports of clinical bleeding associated with the use of these products have existed for decades (8,49). Historically, the problem has been confounded by numerous other patient variables that could, in their own right, be associated with bleeding. Examples include malnutrition, renal or hepatic failure, malignancy, and medications. Clinical bleeding after admission to an ICU is often encountered and has been identified as a significant cause of mortality. Best data suggest that 10% to 11% of patients experience this complication after admission to an ICU. Most commonly documented bleeding sites are the upper gastrointestinal (GI) tract (35%), urinary tract (25%), and skin/wound (16%). Events associated with bleeding include mechanical ventilation, medications (e.g., heparin and coumadin), malnutrition, and underlying disease such as renal and hepatic failure (50,51). Moxalactam, a third-generation cephalosporin released in the early 1980s and now defunct in the United States, was associated with this adverse reaction to an appreciable degree (52–54).

Following this observation, numerous other studies were performed to evaluate the role of antibiotics in clinical bleeding. Table 2 depicts mechanisms by which antibiotics cause bleeding, and the products most often implicated (48). Although many studies have found an association between antibiotics and clinical bleeding, in complex patients with multiple underlying diseases and on multiple medications, a causative role may only be identified by in-depth, statistically validated

Table 2 Mechanisms for Antibiotic-Associated Bleeding

Mechanism	Antibiotics implicated
Bone marrow suppression	Chloramphenicol
Immunologic platelet destruction	Rifampin, sulfonamides, cephalothin, penicillin G[a], tetracycline, and streptomycin[a]
Potentiation of warfarin	Rifampin, metronidazole, chloramphenicol, and other broad-spectrum agents[a]
Antagonism of prothrombin	Moxalactam, cefoperazone, cefamandole, cefmenoxime, cefoxitin[a], and cefazolin[a]
Dysfunctional platelet aggregation	Penicillin G, carbenicillin, ticarcillin, piperacillin, and moxalactam

[a]Rarely reported.
Source: Adapted from Ref. 48.

investigations, and products not commonly recognized as a cause of bleeding may be implicated (55).

Dysfunctional platelet aggregation, an important mechanism by which selected antibiotics may cause bleeding, is mostly noted with penicillins. It was reported in the 1970s as an important complication of the use of carbenicillin (56). Among penicillins, it is most likely to be noted with penicillin G and advanced-generation penicillins (57). The problem is dose related, may be exacerbated by renal failure, and is additive to other factors seen in critically ill patients that could, in their own right, be associated with dysfunctional platelet aggregation (57,58). Most commonly, the reason for dysfunctional platelet aggregation is that carboxyl groups on the acyl side chain block binding sites located on the platelet surface, resulting in the inability of platelet agonists such as adenosine diphosphate (ADP) to effect aggregation (57). This process is best identified by performing a template bleeding time, and will be missed if only prothrombin time international normalized ratio (INR) and partial thromboplastin time (PTT) are measured. It should be suspected in patients with bleeding not accounted for by abnormalities in INR or PTT, and often presents as diffuse oozing from sites of cutaneous trauma (tracheostomy, intravenous and arterial lines, etc.) that cannot be easily controlled by direct pressure.

Probably, the most common reason for antibiotic-associated bleeding in the ICU is prolongation of the INR. Historically, antibiotics associated with INR prolongation include cefamandole, moxalactam, and cefoperazone (52–54,59,60). Other less commonly implicated antibiotics are cefotetan and cefmetazole (61). All of these products contain an N-methyl thiotetrazole (NMTT) ring attached to the third position of the six-membered dihydrothiazine molecule. NMTT can interfere with prothrombin synthesis within the hepatocyte through competitive inhibition (62,63) and, in malnourished or vitamin K–depleted patients, can cause INR prolongation and occasional clinically evident bleeding. Alternatively, the major impact of many agents may be through an alteration of normal GI flora (64). In the experience of the authors, most of this bleeding is from the upper GI tract. Prophylactic administration of vitamin K to patients at risk may be protective when agents containing the NMTT ring need to be administered. The usual dose of vitamin K is 10 to 20 mg once or twice weekly. Other cephalosporins such as cefoxitin may also cause clinical bleeding. In a large prospective investigation of the relationship between antibiotics and clinical bleeding in complex, hospitalized patients, moxalactam and cefoxitin were the only antibiotics that could be statistically implicated (55). Etiology for this relationship is unclear, but may involve other side chains or a direct effect on GI flora (65). In patients with INR prolongation and especially clinical bleeding associated with such a prolongation, the possibility of a relationship to antibiotics should be carefully explored.

In summary, many antibiotics may be associated with laboratory abnormalities of coagulation and occasional clinical bleeding that can be life threatening. In critically ill patients, antibiotic administration may be one of many factors that can cause bleeding. A combination of underlying disease, antibiotics, and other medications occasionally results in this complication. The INR, PTT, and template bleeding times are valuable tools to assess the risk and mechanism for bleeding and point the clinician toward possible causes and remedies. In complex patients with multiple underlying diseases and medication needs, antibiotic choices may be occasionally determined by their potential for causing bleeding.

DERMATOLOGICAL TOXICITY

Rashes are common in ICU patients and present as a highly variable group of conditions with implications ranging from innocuous to life-threatening. The problem is complicated because skin abnormalities in ICU patients can be caused by disease, pressure, and medications. Identification of an offending agent may be difficult because of the large number of medications received by the ICU patient and difficulties in temporally associating the rash with initiation of any single agent. The critically ill patient may prove especially enigmatic because of difficulties in clinical evaluation. Factors that should lead the clinician to suspect a serious drug reaction include facial edema, urticaria, mucosal involvement, palpable or extensive purpura, blisters, fever, or lymphadenopathy (66). The presence of significant eosinophilia is associated with more severe disease. Virtually any antimicrobial agent may cause a rash (only rarely pathognomonic), but this problem appears to occur more commonly with β-lactams, sulfonamides, and vancomycin. Discontinuation of the offending agent is usually the most important initial strategy. In the setting of a severe reaction, rechallenge with the presumed offending agent is generally contraindicated.

Maculopapular eruptions associated with antibiotics are especially common. Generally, onset is at least five days after starting the offending agent. The rash usually becomes generalized and is often pruritic. Other medications that cause maculopapular rashes include hydantoins, barbiturates, and selected antiarrhythmics (66). Differential diagnosis includes viral exanthems and milia. Clinical presentation may be altered in patients with thrombocytopenia or other coagulopathies, where hemorrhage into the skin may modify the appearance of the rash. The pathogenesis of most maculopapular rashes is unknown, and not clearly associated with definite immunologic mechanisms (5). In some instances, the likely offending agent can be continued and the rash will stabilize or disappear. In patients with penicillin-induced mild-to-moderate maculopapular rashes, it is generally safe to use cephalosporins. If the rash is severe or associated with mucosal lesions or exfoliation, the offending agent should almost always be discontinued.

Stevens–Johnson syndrome represents erythema multiforme with mucosal involvement. Some clinicians claim that it is a distinct entity (66). The most commonly implicated antibiotics are the aminopenicillins and sulfonamides. Onset is typically one to three weeks after starting the offending agent. Clinically, symmetrical target lesions are often associated with maculopapular and urticarial plaques and, sometimes, vesicular lesions. The presence of the latter portends severe disease (66). Stevens–Johnson syndrome can involve mucosae of the eyes, mouth, entire GI tract, and the genitourinary tract. Up to 25% of cases may be restricted to the oral mucosa. Constitutional symptoms are usually present. Mortality is up to 5%. Diagnosis can be proven by skin biopsy with immunofluorescent staining; this should be performed in questionable cases. Determining the etiology of the rash may be difficult because numerous infections (for which the offending antibiotic may have been prescribed) can cause a similar rash. Examples include pneumococcal, mycoplasmal, and staphylococcal infections. The presence of Stevens–Johnson syndrome should trigger a thorough evaluation of the patient's medications and discontinuation of likely offenders. It can evolve into toxic epidermal necrolysis; mortality of this condition is 30% (66). Although the benefits of corticosteroid therapy are unproven, these products are often employed in treatment.

"Red man" ("redneck") syndrome is a transient reaction to vancomycin characterized by flushing of the head and neck typically beginning within an hour of the start of an infusion. Pruritus, and occasionally angioedema, can occur (67). Severe cases have been associated with hypotension, chest pain, and rarely, severe cardiac toxicity and death (68). Incidence may be as high as 47% in patients and is substantially higher in human volunteers (69). One study documented a dose-related increase in circulating histamine concentrations that correlated with the severity of the reaction (70). The problem is more frequently associated with rapid administration (i.e., within 30 minutes) and with larger doses. Histamine antagonists may abort the syndrome in patients who require vancomycin and who continue to have red man syndrome despite slow administration of the drug (67,71).

A particularly difficult problem in the ICU is differentiating between septic and drug-induced (chemical) phlebitis. Both may be associated with redness, heat, and tenderness at the intravenous site. Therapy for the former is removal of the catheter and appropriate antibacterial agents, while the latter is treated with catheter removal and moist heat. Presence of lymphangitic streaking or purulent drainage from the catheter site generally indicates infection. The offending organism can frequently be characterized by a Gram stain of purulent drainage. A "cord" in the absence of the above-mentioned findings is most likely due to chemical phlebitis. Antibiotics most likely to cause phlebitis include potassium penicillin, cephalosporins, vancomycin, streptogramins, and amphotericin B.

NEUROTOXICITY

Ototoxicity

Drug-induced ototoxicity in the ICU can result in hearing loss or vestibular dysfunction. The severity of underlying illness of ICU patients and the use of sedatives or paralyzing agents may make it impossible to diagnose these complications. Although routine otologic testing of some hospitalized patients receiving potentially ototoxic drugs has been promulgated (72), in practice such testing is not routinely employed. Therefore, the clinician must recognize the circumstances that could result in ototoxicity and take steps to decrease its likelihood. Macrolides/azalides and aminoglycosides are the agents most likely to be associated with cranial nerve VIII dysfunction.

In the ICU, erythromycin and azithromycin are commonly used to treat community-acquired pneumonia. They can cause bilateral hearing loss and/or labyrinthine dysfunction that are generally reversible within two weeks of discontinuing the agent (73–75). However, permanent hearing loss or vertigo can occur (76–78). These complications are dose related, and usually occur in the presence of renal and/or hepatic dysfunction (76). Most reported causes have occurred with the use of 4 g of erythromycin daily (73). A prospective study in patients with pneumonia documented sensorineural hearing loss in approximately 25% of patients treated with this dose, while no patients who received lesser doses or control agents developed this condition (73).

Aminoglycosides can cause ototoxicity or vestibular dysfunction, which may be permanent. Risk is approximately 10% to 22% (13,79), and toxicity, for reasons stated above, may be extremely difficult to identify in the ICU patient. Factors associated with aminoglycoside-induced cranial nerve VIII dysfunction include dose, dosing frequency, duration of treatment, baseline creatinine clearance, anemia, fever, advanced age, and concomitant use of other ototoxic agents (79–81). Cumulative dose is important and the clinician should therefore be wary of administering repeated courses of aminoglycosides.

In the past, vancomycin has been rarely associated with sensorineural hearing loss (82). Hearing loss was permanent if vancomycin was not promptly discontinued. Likelihood of ototoxicity was increased in the presence of renal dysfunction or when vancomycin was administered with an aminoglycoside (83). Some studies noted an association between serum concentrations more than 30 μg/mL and ototoxicity (84). Over the past 30 years, the purity of vancomycin has improved dramatically; current data do not allow a determination of whether ototoxicity is still caused by the antibiotic itself or was due to impurities in older preparations.

Other Neurotoxicity

Antibiotics can also occasionally cause peripheral nerve or acute central nervous system (CNS) dysfunction (e.g., seizures and abnormal mentation). Most peripheral neuropathies occur with prolonged administration of selected antibiotics (e.g., peripheral neuropathy associated with metronidazole), a situation not likely to occur in ICU patients. This will not be further discussed.

Hallucinations, twitching, and seizures can be caused by penicillin, imipenem/cilastatin, ciprofloxacin, and rarely other β-lactam antibiotics (85,86). The mechanism for the seizures is unknown; however, it has been hypothesized that β-lactams interfere with the inhibitory neurotransmitter function of γ-aminobutyric acid (85). Although more commonly noted following direct CNS administration, intravenous aqueous penicillin G may cause CNS toxicity when given intravenously in amounts exceeding 20 to 50 million units/day to normal-size adults (85). Other data suggest that the risk of seizure with older β-lactams occurs only with serum levels more than 250 μg/mL or with doses greater than 25 g/day. Patients with abnormal renal function, hyponatremia, or preexisting CNS lesions may experience neurotoxicity at lower doses.

Imipenem/cilastatin is an extremely broad-spectrum antibiotic commonly used in the ICU. The maximum recommended dose in adults with normal renal function is 4 g/day. Seizures occur more regularly with this agent than with other β-lactams. Initial human data found the incidence of seizures to be 0.9% to 2.0% (87,88). Post-marketing assessments place this percentage at 0.1% to 0.15% (88). Animal studies confirm that neurotoxicity with imipenem/cilastatin may be noted at substantially lower blood levels than with other β-lactams (86). Our practice has been to virtually never employ imipenem/cilastatin in doses more than 2 g/day unless treating *Pseudomonas aeruginosa* infections. Seizures have not been noted in almost two decades of regular use.

Fluoroquinolones are broad-spectrum agents active against gram-negative bacilli that do not have the significant ototoxic or nephrotoxic potential of the aminoglycosides. However, CNS adverse effects include headache, and seizures have been reported in 1% to 4% of patients receiving these agents (89). Hallucinations, slurred speech, and confusion have also been noted; these generally resolve rapidly once the offending agent is discontinued. Presence of underlying CNS disorders may predispose to neurotoxicity. Interactions with theophylline may allow clinical presentations at lower doses (89–91). Patients on serotonin reuptake inhibitors who are given linezolid can develop serotonin syndrome characterized by agitation, neuromuscular hyperactivity, elevated fever, hypotension, and even death (92,93).

Neuromuscular blockade has been reported with most aminoglycosides (85). Clinical presentation is that of acute paralysis and apnea that develops soon after drug administration. Amikacin, gentamicin, and tobramycin are less likely to be associated with this syndrome than neomycin, kanamycin, and streptomycin (85). Risk may be increased when aminoglycosides are employed in conjunction with other neuromuscular blocking agents or with anesthesia. Due to this potential toxicity, aminoglycosides should be avoided in patients with myasthenia gravis. Therapy includes administration of intravenous calcium and discontinuation of the offending agent.

Minocycline can cause vertigo. Trimethoprim–sulfamethoxazole use can precipitate aseptic meningitis. Approximately, one-third of patients receiving voriconazole experience transient visual changes usually with the first dose. The mechanism of this reaction is unknown; neurotoxicity or a direct effect on the retina is possible. No irreversible visual sequelae have been described.

CARDIOTOXICITY

Erythromycin use prolongs cardiac depolarization. A recent cohort study of patients receiving oral erythromycin found a twofold increased risk of sudden death in patients receiving this drug (94). While the cohort did not examine ICU patients, the results force us to reconsider whether the use of erythromycin is appropriate in these patients who are at especially high risk of developing life-threatening arrhythmias. QT-interval prolongation has also been seen in patients on fluoroquinolones. Risks may be additive with other medications (e.g., amiodarone) capable of prolonging the QT interval.

Myocardial depression, hypotension, and sudden death have been reported with vancomycin use, generally in the setting of rapid administration in the perioperative period (68,95–97). Some of these effects may be due to vancomycin-induced histamine release resulting in vasodilatation; others are probably due to a direct negative inotropic effect (97). Similarly, rapid administration of amphotericin B has been associated with ventricular fibrillation and asystole, especially in patients with renal dysfunction (23). The mechanism may be release of intracellular K^+ with resultant hyperkalemia. Amphotericins and pentamidine infusions can also precipitate hypotension.

HEPATOTOXICITY

Liver-function test abnormalities are common in ICU patients. Sepsis, severe hypoxemia, congestive heart failure, and primary hepatobiliary disease are the usual causes. Abnormalities are generally classified as predominantly hepatitis, cholestasis, or mixed. Rifampin commonly causes hepatitis, which is occasionally severe. Semisynthetic penicillins are frequent causes of hepatotoxicity, especially when combined with clavulanic acid. Cephalosporins, imipenem–cilastatin, tetracyclines, macrolides, sulfonamides, quinolones, clindamycin, chloramphenicol, streptogramins, nitrofurantoin, azoles, and ganciclovir can all cause hepatotoxicity (98). Prolonged courses of high-dose ceftriaxone can cause both hepatitis and cholestasis by promoting biliary sludge formation.

MUSCULOSKELETAL TOXICITY

Streptogramins can cause patients to experience severe arthralgias and myalgias. Daptomycin use is associated with elevations in creatinine phosphokinase of uncertain clinical consequence.

ELECTROLYTE ABNORMALITIES

Amphotericin B can cause clinically significant hypokalemia, hypomagnesemia, and renal tubular acidosis. Electrolyte abnormalities must be anticipated with replenishment of the appropriate electrolyte to prevent future problems.

Aqueous penicillin G is generally administered as the potassium salt (1.7 MEq K^+ per million units of penicillin). With doses of more than 20 million U/day, patients (especially those with renal failure) may develop clinically important hyperkalemia. A sodium preparation of aqueous penicillin G is manufactured and should be employed when the risk of hyperkalemia is significant.

Fluconazole can cause hypokalemia. Although employed infrequently, ticarcillin disodium should be used carefully in patients requiring salt restriction. Pentamidine use is associated with potentially life-threatening hyperkalemia and hypoglycemia.

FEVER

Best available data suggest that up to one-third of hospitalized patients will experience fevers (99) that are commonly noninfectious (100,101). Although nosocomial fever prolongs length of stay, it is not a predictor of mortality (100). Management of nosocomial fever remains controversial. Most authorities recommend antibiotic restraint in stable patients pending the results of a thorough evaluation for the cause of the fever. However, empiric antibiotics should be started promptly in most patients in whom fever is associated with significant immunosuppression (e.g., asplenia and neutropenia) or hemodynamic instability (102). Many ICU patients are difficult to examine thoroughly because of tubes, lines, and other acute-care paraphernalia, and clinical clues ordinarily obtained by history may not be available because of intubation, sedation, coma, or other circumstances that interfere with patient communication. Numerous medications have been associated with fever; intramuscular administration may also result in temperature rise (103). Most cases are not associated with hypersensitivity reactions. Among antibiotics, β-lactams, sulfonamides, and the amphotericins most commonly cause fever. Sulfonamide-induced fever is especially common in HIV-infected patients. In contrast, fluoroquinolones and aminoglycosides are unusual causes of drug-related fever. In the opinion of the authors, neither the degree nor characteristics of the fever help define its cause. Fever of both infectious and noninfectious etiologies may be high-grade, intermittent, or recurrent (104). Rigors may occasionally be noted with noninfectious causes of fever and serve only to define the rate of temperature rise.

Diagnosis of drug fever is made on the basis of a strong clinical suspicion, excluding other causes, and resolution of fever following discontinuation of the offending agent. A clinical "pearl" is that the patient frequently appears better than the physician would suspect after seeing the fever curve. The presence of rash and/or eosinophilia also favors this diagnosis. Resolution of fever after the offending agent is discontinued can take days, because it depends upon the rate of the agent's metabolism.

ANTIBIOTIC-ASSOCIATED DIARRHEA AND COLITIS

Since antibiotics first became available, it has been recognized that these products can cause diarrhea. In the ICU, additional causes of diarrhea include nutritional supplementation, other medications, underlying diseases, and ischemic bowel. In addition to being a nuisance, antibiotic-associated diarrhea can result in fluid and electrolyte disturbances, blood loss, and, when associated with colitis, occasional bowel perforation and death. Early recognition of antibiotic-associated diarrhea is important because prompt treatment can often minimize morbidity and prevent the rare fatality.

The relationship between antibiotic administration, diarrhea, and the presence of *Clostridium difficile* in the colon was first reported in the late 1970s (105,106). Antibiotic use changes the colonic flora allowing the overgrowth of *C. difficile*. This organism then causes diarrhea by releasing toxins A and B, which promote epithelial cell apoptosis, inflammation, and secretion of fluid into the colon. *C. difficile* is currently the most common identifiable cause of nosocomial diarrhea. However, no more than 25% of all cases of antibiotic-associated diarrhea are caused by this organism (107). Rates vary dramatically among hospitals and within different areas of the same institution ranging from less than 1 in 1000 admissions to more than 30 per 1000 discharges (108).

Although virtually all antibiotics have been implicated, the most common causes of *C. difficile* diarrhea are ampicillin or amoxicillin, cephalosporins, and clindamycin (109–112). Because they are inactive against most colonic anaerobes, aminoglycosides, and trimethoprim–sulfamethoxazole are less likely to cause *C. difficile* diarrhea. Nosocomial acquisition of this organism is the most likely reason for patients to harbor it (113,114). Hospital sources of *C. difficile* include hands of personnel, inanimate environmental surfaces, and asymptomatic patient carriers (110,111). In addition to antibiotic use, risk factors for acquisition include cancer chemotherapy, severity of illness, and duration of hospitalization. For all of these reasons, the ICU is an important site of antibiotic-associated diarrhea and colitis.

The clinical presentation of antibiotic-associated colitis is highly variable, ranging from asymptomatic carriage to septic shock. Secondary bacteremia has been reported (115). In adults, diarrhea is the most common symptom. Time of onset of diarrhea is variable, and may be noted weeks after a course of antibiotic has been completed. Most commonly, diarrhea begins within the first week of antibiotic administration. More severe cases are associated with the presence of pseudomembranous colitis. Unusual presentations of this disease include acute abdominal pain, fever, or leukocytosis with minimal or no diarrhea (116). On occasion, the presenting feature may be intestinal perforation or septic shock (117).

In the critical care setting, diagnosis of antibiotic-associated diarrhea, pseudomembranous colitis, and toxic megacolon is complicated by numerous factors. Adequate history and physical examination may be unobtainable because of patient sedation, coma, or medical paralysis. Similarly, critically ill patients may have numerous other reasons for diarrhea, abdominal pain, fever, or leukocytosis. Investigations have demonstrated that the following clinical predictors can be used to help identify *C. difficile* colitis: onset of diarrhea more than 6 days after initiation of antibiotics, hospital stay more than 15 days, fecal leukocytes on microscopy, and the presence of semiformed (as opposed to watery) stools (118). Validation of this model in the critical care setting is needed.

Antibiotic-associated diarrhea and colitis should be suspected in all ICU patients who have received antimicrobial agents and who present with diarrhea and/or abdominal pain and tenderness. Their role in severe abdominal events should be suspected; in patients with abdominal pain, workup for *C. difficile* colitis should ideally be performed prior to abdominal surgery. Diagnosis is usually made by the less-sensitive (~67%) rapid enzyme immunoassay or a more sensitive (~90%) but slower tissue culture assay (119). The finding of pseudomembranes on sigmoidoscopy is also diagnostic and can negate the need for exploratory laparotomy.

Optimal therapy of *C. difficile* diarrhea/colitis depends to a large extent on clinical presentation, severity of disease, and need for ongoing antimicrobial therapy. Antiperistaltic agents should be avoided (120). If feasible, the offending antibiotic should be discontinued. In mild cases this may suffice, and specific antibiotic therapy for *C. difficile* may be unnecessary. In many instances, however, patients in the ICU require ongoing antibiotic therapy. When antibiotics are indicated, the offender can be replaced by an agent less likely to be associated with this condition (121).

Oral metronidazole is the agent of choice for most patients sick enough to require treatment (110,111,121). Metronidazole is recommended for initial therapy because it is far less expensive than oral vancomycin and less likely to promote colonization with vancomycin-resistant enterococci. A prospective investigation comparing oral metronidazole and vancomycin found no significant differences in either rate of improvement, relapse, or recurrent colonization with *C. difficile* (122). Metronidazole is the only agent that may be efficacious parenterally (123); vancomycin given intravenously is not secreted into the gut. Metronidazole therefore plays a preeminent role in critically ill patients when problems with GI absorption preclude oral or nasogastric treatments. In especially severe cases, patients can be treated with the combination of high-dose intravenous metronidazole and nasogastric or rectal infusions of vancomycin. Although therapy with other agents administered per rectum has been promulgated, this approach has not been compared directly to other standard regimens.

ANTIBIOTIC-RESISTANT SUPERINFECTIONS

In the ICU, the use of antibiotics can predispose recipients to colonization and infection with methicillin-resistant *Staphylococcus aureus*, vancomycin-resistant Enterococcus (*mostly Enterococcus faecium*), multidrug-resistant gram-negative bacilli, and fungi. Detailed discussion of these superinfections is beyond the scope of this chapter.

SUMMARY

Antibiotics are commonly used in the ICU. Adverse effects are regularly encountered and must be anticipated. The problem is complicated by the multiplicity of medications and underlying conditions in most ICU patients that affect the presentation and management of adverse reactions. When possible, the intensivist should employ the fewest number of antibiotics necessary, choosing those least likely to cause adverse reactions.

ACKNOWLEDGEMENT

The authors are grateful to Pauline Blair for her excellent assistance in preparing this chapter.

REFERENCES

1. Lazarou J, Pomeranz BH, Corey PH. Incidence of adverse drug reactions in hospitalized patients: A meta-analysis of prospective studies. JAMA 1998; 279:1200–1205.
2. Faulkner CM, Cox HL, Williamson JC. Unique aspects of antimicrobial use in older adults. Clin Infect Dis 2005; 40:997–1004.
3. Roder BL, Nielsen SL, Magnussen P, et al. Antibiotic usage in an intensive care unit in a Danish university hospital. J Antimicrob Chemother 1993; 32:633–642.
4. Vincent JL, Bihari DJ, Suter PM, et al. The prevalence of nosocomial infections in intensive care units in Europe. JAMA 1995; 274:639–644.
5. Saxon A, Beall GN, Rohr AS, et al. Immediate hypersensitivity reactions to beta-lactam antibiotics. Ann Intern Med 1987; 107:204–215.
6. Idsoe O, Guthe T, Wilcox RR, et al. Nature and extent of penicillin side-reactions with particular reference to fatalities from anaphylactic shock. Bull WHO 1968; 38:159–188.
7. Salkind AR, Cuddy PG, Foxworth JW. Is this patient allergic to penicillin? An evidence-based analysis of the likelihood of penicillin allergy. JAMA 2001; 19:2498–2505.
8. Park MA, Li, JTC. Diagnosis and management of penicillin allergy. Mayo Clin Proc 2005; 80:405–410.
9. Petz LD. Immunologic cross-reactivity between penicillins and cephalosporins: a review. Infect Dis 1978; 137:S74–S79.
10. Saxon A, Adelman DC, Patel A, et al. Imipenem cross-reactivity with penicillin in humans. J Allergy Clin Immunol 1988; 82:213–217.
11. Prescott WA Jr., DePestel DD, Ellis JJ, et al. Incidence of carbapenem-associated allergic-type reactions among patients with versus patients without a reported penicillin allergy. Clin Infect Dis 2004; 38:1102–1107.
12. Sponsel IIT, Anderson RJ. Acute renal failure. In: Parillo JF, Bone RC, eds. Critical Care Medicine: Principles of Diagnosis and Management. St. Louis: Mosby, 1995: 1035–1058.

13. Smith CR, Lipsky JJ, Laskin OL, et al. Double-blind comparison of the nephrotoxicity and auditory toxicity of gentamicin and tobramycin. N Engl J Med 1980; 302:1106–1109.

14. Matzke GR, Lucarotti RL, Shapiro HS. Controlled comparison of gentamicin and tobramycin nephrotoxicity. Am J Nephrol 1983; 3:11–17.

15. Eisenberg JM, Loffer H, Glick HA, et al. What is the cost of nephrotoxicity associated with aminoglycosides? Ann Intern Med 1987; 107:900–909.

16. Sawyers CL, Moore RD, Lerner SA, et al. A model for predicting nephrotoxicity in patients treated with aminoglycosides. J Infect Dis 1986; 153:1062–1068.

17. Hatala R, Dinh T, Cook DJ. Once-daily aminoglycoside dosing in immunocompetent adults: a meta-analysis. Ann Intern Med 1996; 124:717–725.

18. Barza, M, Ioannidis JP, Capelleri, JC. Single or multiple daily doses of aminoglycosides: a meta-analysis. BMJ 1996; 312:338–344.

19. Prins JM, Buller HR, Kuijper EJ, et al. Once versus thrice daily gentamicin in patients with serious infections. Lancet 1993; 341:335–346.

20. Gallis HA, Drew RH, Pickard WW. Amphotericin B: 30 years of clinical experience. Rev Infect Dis 1990; 12:308–329.

21. Takacs FJ, Tomkiewicz ZM, Merrill JP. Amphotericin B nephrotoxicity with irreversible renal failure. Arch Intern Med 1963; 59:716–724.

22. Fisher MA, Talbot GH, Maislin G, et al. Risk factors for amphotericin B-associated nephrotoxicity. Am J Med 1989; 87:547–552.

23. Clements JS, Peacock JE. Amphotericin B revisited: reassessment of nephrotoxicity. Am J Med 1990; 88(suppl 5):22N–27N.

24. Heidemann HT, Gerkens JF, Spickard WA, et al. Amphotericin B nephrotoxicity in humans decreased by salt repletion. Am J Med 1983; 75:476–481.

25. Wiebe VJ, DeGRegorio MW. Liposome-encapsulated amphotericin B: a promising treatment for disseminated fungal infections. Rev Infect Dis 1988; 10:1097–1099.

26. Gates C, Pinney RJ. Amphotericin B and its delivery by liposomal and lipid formulations. J Clin Pharm Ther 1993; 18:147–153.

27. Baldwin DS, Levine BB, McCluskey RT, et al. Renal failure and interstitial nephritis due to penicillin and methicillin. N Engl J Med 1968; 279:1245–1252.

28. Galpin JE, Shinaberger JH, Stanley TM, et al. Acute interstitial nephritis due to methicillin. Am J Med 1978; 65:756–765.

29. Linton AL, Clark WF, Driedger AA, et al. Acute interstitial nephritis due to drugs. Arch Intern Med 1980; 93:735–741.

30. Roselle GA, Clyne DH, Kauffman CA. Carbenicillin nephrotoxicity. South Med J 1978; 71:84–86.

31. Burton JR, Lichtenstein NS, Colvin RB, et al. Acute renal failure during cephalothin therapy. JAMA 1974; 229:679–682.

32. Manian FA, Stone WJ, Alford RH. Adverse antibiotic effects associated with renal insufficiency. Rev Infect Dis 1990; 12:236–249.

33. Green SL, Maddox JC, Huttenbach ED. Linezolid and reversible myelosuppression. JAMA 2001; 285:1291.

34. Birmingham MC, Rayner CR, Meagher AK, et al. Linezolid for the treatment of multidrug resistant, Gram-positive infections: experience from a compassionate-use program. Clin Infect Dis 2003; 36:159–168.

35. Bernstein WB, Trotta RF, Rector JT, et al. Mechanisms for linezolid-induced anemia and thrombocytopenia. Ann Pharmacother 2003; 37:517–520.

36. Wallerstein RO, Condit PK, Kasper CK, et al. Statewide study of chloramphenicol therapy and fatal aplastic anemia. JAMA 1969; 208:2045–2050.

37. Anonymous. Anti-infective drug use in relation to the risk of agranulocytosis and aplastic anemia. A report from the International Agranulocytosis and Aplastic Anemia Study. Arch Intern Med 1989; 149:1036–1040.

38. Andres E, Maloisel F. Antibiotic-induced agranulocytosis: a monocentric study of 21 cases. Arch Intern Med 2001; 161:2610.

39. Markowitz SM, Rothkopf M, Holden FD, et al. Nafcillin-induced agranulocytosis. JAMA 1975; 232:1150–1151.

40. Sandberg M, Tuazon CU, Sheagren JN. Neutropenia probably resulting from nafcillin. JAMA 1975; 232:1152–1154.

41. Neftel KA, Hauser SP, Muller MR. Inhibition of granulopoiesis in vivo and in vitro by β-lactam antibiotics. J Infect Dis 1985; 152:90–98.

42. Bang NU, Kammer RB. Hematologic complications associated with β-lactam antibiotics. Rev Infect Dis 1983; 5(suppl 2):S380–S393.

43. West BC. Vancomycin-induced neutropenia. South Med J 1981; 74:1255–1256.

44. Kaufman CA, Severance PJ, Silva J Jr., et al. Neutropenia associated with vancomycin therapy. South Med J 1982; 75:1131–1133.

45. Kesarwala HH, Rahill WJ, Amaram N. Vancomycin-induced neutropenia. Lancet 1981; 1:1423.

46. Olaison L, Belin L, Hogevik H, et al. Incidence of β-lactam-induced delayed hypersensitivity and neutropenia during treatment of infective endocarditis. Arch Intern Med 1999; 159:607–615.

47. Singh N, Yu VL, Mieles LA, et al. β-lactam antibiotic-induced leukopenia in severe hepatic dysfunction: risk factors and implications for dosing patients with liver disease. Am J Med 1993; 94:251–256.

48. Brown RB, Sands M, Ryczak M. Bleeding as a side effect on antibiotics. Infect Med 1987; 4:386–392.

49. Natelson EA, Brown CH III, Bradshaw MW, et al. Influence of cephalosporin antibiotics on blood coagulation and platelet function. Antimicrob Agents Chemother 1976; 9: 91–93.

50. Brown RB, Klar J, Teres D, et al. Prospective study of clinical bleeding in intensive care unit patients. Crit Care Med 1988; 16:1171–1176.

51. Pinco GF, Gallus AS, Hirsh J. Unexpected vitamin K deficiency in hospitalized patients. CMA J 1973; 109:880–883.

52. Panwalker AP, Rosenfeld J. Hemorrhage, diarrhea and superinfection associated with the use of moxalactam. J Infect Dis 1983; 147:171–172.

53. Weitekamp MR, Aber RC. Prolonged bleeding time and bleeding diathesis associated with moxalactam administration. JAMA 1983; 249:69–71.

54. Baxter JG, Marble DA, Whitfield LR, et al. Clinical risk factors for prolonged PT/PTT in abdominal sepsis patients treated with moxalactam or tobramycin plus clindamycin. Ann Surg 1985; 201:96–102.

55. Brown RB, Klar J, Lemeshow S, et al. Enhanced bleeding with cefoxitin or moxalactam. Statistical analysis within a defined population of 1493 patients. Arch Intern Med 1986; 146:2159–2164.

56. Brown CH III, Natelson EA, Bradshaw MW, et al. The hemostatic defect produced by carbenicillin. N Engl J Med 1974; 291:265–270.

57. Fass RJ, Copelan EA, Brandt JT, et al. Platelet-induced bleeding caused by broad-spectrum antibiotics. J Infect Dis 1987; 155:1242–1248.

58. Malpass TW, Harker LA. Acquired disorders of platelet function. Semin Hematol 1980; 17:242–258.

59. Bertino JS, Kozak AJ, Reese RE, et al. Hypoprothrombinemia associated with cefamandole use in a rural teaching hospital. Arch Intern Med 1986; 146:1125–1128.

60. Shenkenberg TD, Mackowiak PA, Smith JW. Coagulopathy and hemorrhage associated with cefoperazone therapy in a patient with renal failure. South Med J 1985; 78: 488–489.

61. Kline SS, Mauro VF, Forney RB, et al. Cefotetan-induced disulfuram-type reactions and hypoprothrombinemia. Antimicrob Agents Chemother 1987; 31:1328–1331.

62. Lipsky JJ. N-methyl thio-tetrazole inhibition of the gamma carboxylation of glutamic acid: possible mechanism for antibiotic-associated hypoprothrombinemia. Lancet 1983; 2:192–193.

63. Mackie IJ, Walshek, Cohen H, et al. Effects of N-methyl-thiotetrazole cephalosporin on haemostasis in patients with reduced serum vitamin K_1 concentrations. J Clin Path 1986; 39:1245–1249.

64. Bang NU, Tessler SS, Heidenreich RO, et al. Effects of moxalactam on blood coagulation and platelet function. Rev Infect Dis 1982; 4(suppl):S546–S554.

65. Shevchuk YM, Conly JM. Antibiotic-associated hypoprothrombinemia: a review of prospective studies, 1966 to 1988. Rev Infect Dis 1990; 6:1109–1126.

66. Roujeau JC, Stern RS. Severe adverse cutaneous reactions to drugs. N Engl J Med 1994; 331:1272–1285.

67. Wallace MR, Mascola JR, Oldfield EC III. Red man syndrome: incidence, etiology, and prophylaxis. J Infect Dis 1991; 164:1180–1185.

68. Glicklich D, Figura I. Vancomycin and cardiac arrest. Ann Intern Med 1984; 101: 880–881.

69. O'Sullivan TL, Ruffing MJ, Lamp KC, et al. Prospective evaluation of red man syndrome in patients receiving vancomycin. J Infect Dis 1993; 168:773–776.

70. Polk RE, Healy DP, Schwartz LB, et al. Vancomycin and the red-man syndrome: pharmacodynamics of histamine release. J Infect Dis 1988; 157:502–507.

71. Sahai J, Healy DP, Garris R, et al. Influence of antihistamine pretreatment on vancomycin-induced red-man syndrome. J Infect Dis 1989; 160:876–881.

72. Fausti SA, Henry JA, Schaffer HI, et al. High-frequency audiometric monitoring for early detection of aminoglycoside ototoxicity. J Infect Dis 1992; 165:1026–1032.

73. Swanson DJ, Sung RF, Fine MJ, et al. Erythromycin ototoxicity: prospective assessment with serum concentrations and audiograms in a study of patients with pneumonia. Am J Med 1992; 92:61–69.

74. Wallace MR, Miller LK, Nguyen MT, et al. Ototoxicity with azithromycin. Lancet 1994; 343:241.

75. Lo SH, Kotabe S, Mitsunaga L. Azithromycin-induced hearing loss. Case report. Am J Health Sys Pharm 1999; 56:380–383.

76. Umstead GS, Neumann KH. Erythromycin ototoxicity and acute psychotic reaction in cancer patients with hepatic dysfunction. Arch Intern Med 1986; 146:897–899.

77. Agusti C, Ferran F, Gea J, et al. Ototoxic reaction to erythromycin. Arch Intern Med 1991; 151:380.

78. Ress BD, Gross EM. Irreversible sensorineural hearing loss as a result of azithromycin ototoxicity. A case report. Ann Otol Rhinol Laryngol 2000; 109:435–437.

79. Moore RD, Smith CR, Leitman PS. Risk factors for the development of auditory toxicity in patients receiving aminoglycosides. J Infect Dis 1984; 149:23–30.

80. Gatell JM, Ferran F, Araujo V, et al. Univariate and multivariate analyses of risk factors predisposing to auditory toxicity in patients receiving aminoglycosides. Antimicrob Agents Chemother 1987; 31:1383–1387.

81. Fee WE Jr. Gentamicin and tobramycin: comparison of ototoxiciy. Rev Infect Dis 1983; 5(suppl 2):S304–S313.

82. Farber BF, Moellering RC Jr. Retrospective study of the toxicity of preparations of vancomycin from 1974 to 1981. Antimicrob Agents Chemother 1983; 23:138–141.

83. Hermans PE, Wilhelm MP. Vancomycin. Mayo Clin Proc 1987; 62:901–905.

84. Cook FV, Farrar WE. Vancomycin revisited. Arch Intern Med 1978; 88:813–818.

85. Snavely SR, Hodges GR. The neurotoxicity of antibacterial agents. Arch Intern Med 1984; 101:92–104.

86. Eng RHK, Munsif AN, Nangco BG, et al. Seizure propensity with imipenem. Arch Intern Med 1989; 149:1881–1883.

87. Barza M. Imipenem: first of a new class of beta-lactam antibiotics. Ann Intern Med 1985; 103:552–559.

88. File TM, Tan JS. Recommendations for using imipenem-cilastatin–the most broad spectrum antibiotic. Hosp Form 1987; 22:534–542.

89. Hooper DC, Wolfson JS. Fluoroquinolone antimicrobial agents. N Engl J Med 1991; 324: 384–394.

90. Neu HC. Use of fluoroquinolones. Infect Dis Clin Pract 1992; 1:1–10.

91. Radandt JM, Marchbands CR, Dudley MN. Interactions of fluoroquinolones with other drugs: mechanisms, variability, clinical significance, and management. Clin Infect Dis 1992; 14:272–284.

92. Lavery SR, Ravi H, McDaniel WW, et al. Linezolid and serotonin syndrome. Psychosomatics 2001; 42:432–434.

93. Gillman PK. Linezolid and serotonin toxicity. Clin Infect Dis 2003; 37:1274–1275.

94. Ray WA, Murray KT, Meredith S, et al. Oral erythromycin and the risk of sudden death from cardiac causes. N Engl J Med 2004; 351:1089–1096.

95. Dajee H, Laks H, Miller J, et al. Profound hypotension from rapid administration of vancomycin during cardiac operation. J Thoracic Cardiovascul Surg 1984; 87: 145–146.

96. Mayhew JF, Deutsch S. Cardiac arrest following administration of vancomycin. Can Anaesthesiol Soc J 1985; 32:65–66.

97. Southorn PA, Plevak DJ, Wright AJ, et al. Adverse effects of vancomycin administered in the perioperative period. Mayo Clin Proc 1986; 61:721–724.

98. Brown SJ, Desmond PV. Hepatotoxicity of antimicrobial agents. Semin Liver Dis 2002; 22:157–167.

99. Cunha BA, Shea KW. Fever in the intensive care unit. Infect Dis Clin North Am 1996; 10:185–209.

100. Arbo MJ, Fine MJ, Hanusa BH, et al. Fever of nosocomial origin: etiology, risk factors, and outcomes. Am J Med 1993; 95:505–512.

101. McGowan JE, Rose RC, Jacobs NF, et al. Fever in hospitalized patients. Am J Med 1987; 82:580–586.

102. DiNubile MJ. Acute fevers of unknown origin. A plea for restraint. Arch Intern Med 1993; 153:2525–2526.

103. Semel JD. Fever associated with repeated intramuscular injections of analgesics. Rev Infect Dis 1986; 8:68–72.

104. Mellors JW, Horwitz RI, Harvey MR, et al. A simple index to identify occult bacterial infection in adults with acute unexplained fever. Arch Intern Med 1987; 147:666–671.

105. Larsen HE, Parry JV, Price AB, et al. Underdescribed toxin in pseudomembranous colitis. Br Med J 1977; 1:1246–1248.

106. Bartlett JG, Chang TW, Gurwith M, et al. Antibiotic-associated pseudomembranous colitis due to toxin-producing clostridia. N Engl J Med 1978; 298:531–534.

107. Bartlett JG. Antibiotic-associated diarrhea. Infect Clin Dis Pract 1992; 16:1–5.

108. Samore MH, Degirolami PC, Tlucko A, et al. *Clostridium difficile* colonization and diarrhea at a tertiary care hospital. Clin Infect Dis 1994; 18:181–187.

109. Nelson DE, Auerbach SB, Baltch Al, et al. Epidemic *Clostridium difficile*-associated diarrhea: role of second and third generation cephalosporins. Infect Cont Hosp Epidemiol 1994; 15:88–94.

110. Kelly CP, Pothoulakis C, LaMont JT. *Clostridium difficile* colitis. N Engl J Med 1994; 330:257–262.

111. Bartlett JG. Antibiotic-associated diarrhea. Clin Infect Dis 1992; 15:573–581.

112. Watanakunakorn PA, Watanakunakoarn C, Hazy J. Risk factors associated with *Clostridium difficile* diarrhea in hospitalized adult patients: a case-control study—sucralfate ingestion is not a negative risk factor. Infect Control Hosp Epidemiol 1996; 17:232–235.

113. McFarland LV, Schwartz DM, Stamm WE. Risk factors for *C. difficile* carriage and *C. difficile*-associated diarrhea in a cohort of hospitalized patients. J Infect Dis 1990; 162:678–684.

114. McFarland LV, Mulligan ME, Kwok RYY, et al. Nosocomial acquisition of *Clostridium difficile* infection. N Engl J Med 1989; 320:204–210.

115. Wolf LE, Gorbach SL, Granowitz EV. Extraintestinal *Clostridium difficile*: 10 years' experience at a tertiary-care hospital. Mayo Clin Proc 1998; 73:943–947.
116. Wanahita A, Goldsmith E, Marino BJ, et al. *Clostridium difficile* infection in patients with unexplained leukocytosis. Am J Med 2003; 115:543–546.
117. Triadafilopoulos G, Hallstone AE. Acute abdomen as the first presentation of pseudomembranous colitis. Gastroenterology 1991; 101:685–691.
118. Manabe YC, Vinetz JM, Moore RC, et al. *Clostridium difficile* colitis: an efficient clinical approach to diagnosis. Ann Intern Med 1995; 123:835–840.
119. Fekety R. Guidelines for the diagnosis and management of *Clostridium difficile*-associated diarrhea and colitis. Am J Gastroenterol 1997; 92:739–750.
120. Bartlett JG. Treating antibiotic-associated diarrhea and colitis in the ICU. J Crit Illness 1995; 10:30–36.
121. Gerding DN, Johnson S, Peterson LR, et al. *Clostridium difficile*-associated diarrhea and colitis. Infect Cont Hosp Epidemiol 1995; 16:459–477.
122. Wenisch C, Parschalk B, Hasenhundl M, et al. Comparison of vancomycin, teicoplanin, metronidazole, and fusidic acid for the treatment of *Clostridium difficile*-associated diarrhea. Clin Infect Dis 1996; 22:813–818.
123. Bolton RP, Culshaw MA. Faecal metronidazole concentrations during oral and intravenous therapy for antibiotic associated colitis due to *Clostridium difficile*. Gut 1986; 27: 1169–1172.

30

Antibiotic Kinetics in the Febrile Multiple System Trauma Patient

Donald E. Fry

Department of Surgery, University of New Mexico School of Medicine, Albuquerque, New Mexico, U.S.A.

INTRODUCTION

In no place throughout clinical medicine is the role of antibiotics more important than in the severely injured patient. Judicious and appropriate antibiotics are important for preventive indications when the traumatized patient requires a surgical procedure. Specific antibiotic therapy is necessary when infectious complications occur at the site of injury. Nosocomial infections occur at numerous locations during critical care management and during the prolonged convalescence of these patients and require antimicrobial chemotherapy. In the patient with an injury-severity score >30, antibiotics are employed frequently during the hospitalization and the emergence of resistant and unusual pathogens make the appropriate management of the infectious complications in these patients a formidable challenge.

The principles in the utilization of antibiotics for different indications in the trauma patient have become established over the last several decades. For preventive indications, the antibiotic should be given immediately prior (<60 min) to the skin incision. The antibiotic should be able to act against the likely pathogens to be encountered in the procedure. Prolonged preventive antibiotics administered after the procedure do not benefit the patient and should be stopped within 24 hours of the procedure. Infections that occur at the site of traumatic injury require antibiotic therapy against the clinically suspected and the culture-documented pathogens, in conjunction with aggressive surgical drainage and debridement of the primary focus of infection. Because of the impact of the critical care unit, hospital microflora, and antecedent antibiotic treatment, nosocomial infections will notoriously be secondary to resistant organisms and must have susceptible evidence to guide choices of treatment.

While the above principles in the use of antibiotics are generally accepted, infection continues to be the major cause of death for injured patients without severe head injury who survive the initial 48 hours following the insult. The reasons for deaths due to infections in the face of optimum antibiotic utilization are; (i) the magnitude of contamination exceeds the capacity of the host and therapy to control,

(ii) profound immunosuppression is associated with the injury, and (iii) antimicrobial resistance produces an array of pathogens that become very elusive to treatment.

Another consideration that should be contemplated is whether the pathophysiologic changes of the severely injured patient create a clinical scenario where conventional antibiotic strategies may fail. Failure may have inappropriate dosing as a contributing factor, because the conventional dosing strategies that are employed with the utilization of systemic antibiotics are inadequate. This chapter will detail the systemic changes that are the result of the systemic activation of the human inflammatory cascade, and also why these changes require a reassessment of antibiotic dosing strategies in febrile multiple trauma patients.

NORMAL PHARMACOKINETICS OF ANTIBIOTICS

The study of the biological processes which ultimately determine antibiotic concentration at the effector site is referred to as pharmacokinetics. The biological processes that comprise pharmacokinetics include absorption, volume of distribution, biotransformation, and drug excretion. For antibiotics, the quantitative evaluation of each of these components is used to design the dose and the treatment interval that will be employed for clinical trials and subsequent use of the drug. The clear objective of pharmacokinetic assessment is to provide antibiotic concentrations that will ensure activity against the likely pathogens that are consistent with quantitative susceptibility information. A second objective is to maintain antibiotic concentrations within nontoxic limits. In the process of drug development, antibiotics are studied in healthy, normal volunteers. Even in the phase 3 prospective, randomized trials, the severity of illness that is evaluated with a new antibiotic product is not extreme. It is a fact that phase 3 trials of peritonitis customarily study perforative appendicitis patients. The studies are geared to have few if any deaths, and obviously, the studies are aimed at having no differences in the clinical outcomes. Only when new antibiotics are approved for use is there a meaningful trial of the drug in a critically ill population.

Absorption of antibiotics that will be used in the multiple injury trauma patient will be nearly 100% since all are given intravenously. This results in rapid distribution of the drug throughout the body water compartments to which it will have access. Intramuscular antibiotic administration would generally not be prudent in the trauma patient because severe soft tissue injury, shock, and expanded interstitial water volume would make systemic uptake less dependable. Oral antibiotics generally do not have a place in trauma patients during hospitalization because many will have nasogastric tubes in place or may have postinjury gastrointestinal ileus. The favorable bioavailability of quinolones, linezolid, and perhaps others that are in development may result in some reevaluation of the use of oral antibiotics in hospitalized trauma patients. Utilization of the gastrointestinal tract for nutritional support has been very effective in many trauma patients, and the intestinal tract may evolve as a route for the administration of antibiotics.

The distribution of the antibiotic after administration becomes a critically important issue. Each antibiotic has a unique volume of body water that it accesses following intravenous administration. The physiochemical properties of the drug, which govern the distribution in the patient, include the electrical charge of the molecule in solution, its solubility, its movement through cell membranes of different tissues, its lipophobic or lipophilic character, and whether metabolism is a requirement for elimination from the body. The distribution of the drug in body water is further modified by its degree of protein binding, because highly bound drugs will functionally be restricted in the extracellular water volume.

Unique features of the patient will also affect the distribution of the antibiotic and accordingly its concentration in serum. Cardiac output, regional blood flow, and the volumes of intravenous fluids that are administered will change elimination and distribution. The route of drug elimination may be adversely affected by either preexisting or acquired abnormalities of renal or hepatic function. Disease processes affecting protein concentrations in plasma will particularly impact the drug that is highly protein bound.

In Figure 1, the concentrations of a hypothetical antibiotic in the serum of a patient are illustrated after intravenous administration. A rapid peak concentration is achieved, which is largely dictated by the rate of infusion. The distribution of the drug throughout the various compartments and tissues that are accessed result in an equilibrium concentration, and from that point the elimination of the drug proceeds in a consistent fashion. A semi-logarithm plot is used for the concentration at each time point and this yields a linear configuration to the elimination plot. Extrapolation of the semi-logarithm elimination plot to time-zero permits calculation of the volume of distribution (V_d) of the drug in this specific set of clinical circumstances. The volume of distribution equals the total dose of drug given (D) divided by the

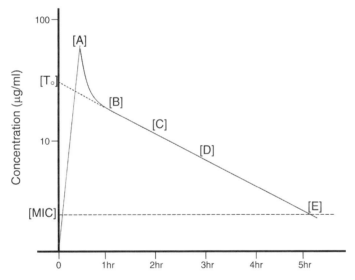

Figure 1 Illustrates the clearance curve of a theoretical antibiotic. The ordinate is the antibiotic concentration expressed in $\log_{10}$. The abscissa is time in hours. *A*, represents the peak concentration after intravenous administration. *B*, represents the maximum concentration after full equilibration of the antibiotic with all body water compartments to which that drug has access. *C*, is the concentration of the antibiotic after one $T_{1/2}$. *D*, is the concentration after the second $T_{1/2}$. *E* is the time intercept when the concentration of the drug reaches the MIC for the target organism that would be treated with the antibiotic being studied. T_o is the extrapolated concentration of the drug assuming full equilibration of the entire administered dose and without any elimination. From T_o and the dose of administration, the V_d can be calculated. V_d is a theoretical calculation that can be influenced by factors other than the actual body water of drug distribution. Thus, this calculated variable may actually be greater than total body water (>0.6 L/kg). *Abbreviation*: MIC, minimum inhibitory concentration.

time-zero theoretical concentration $[T_0]$, or $D/[T_0] = V_d$. Thus, 1 g of an antibiotic ($1 \times 10^6\,\mu g$) with an extrapolated $[T_0] = 50\,\mu g/mL$ results in a $V_d = 20,000\,m$, or 20 L. In an 80 kg patient, this would customarily be expressed as 0.25 L/kg.

The linear configuration of drug elimination over time permits the calculation of the biological elimination half-life ($T_{1/2}$). The $T_{1/2}$ is the period of time required for the equilibrated plasma concentration of the drug to decline by 50%. The expectation is that the plasma concentration reflects the dynamic processes of equilibration of the central pool (i.e., plasma) with the multiple different pools and compartments in which the drug is present. Antibiotics are generally considered to have a single $T_{1/2}$ that describes elimination of the drug, but some may have a second $T_{1/2}$ that describes clearance at low concentrations.

Knowledge of the V_d and $T_{1/2}$ allows the design of dosage and dosage intervals for the antibiotic. If our theoretical drug in Figure 1 was deemed to have toxicity at concentrations above 80 µg /mL, then it would be desirable to have the concentration below that threshold for the treatment interval. Furthermore, the treatment interval between individual doses requires an understanding of the rate at which concentrations of the drug decline and the minimum inhibitory concentration (MIC) of the drug against the likely pathogens that would be encountered. If the MIC for likely pathogens was 5 µg/mL, and the $T_{1/2}$ of our drug was two hours, then four $T_{1/2}$ would give a drug plasma concentration of 6.25 µg/mL which remains above the target MIC. Thus, a rational configuration of the use of this drug would be a 1 g dose that was repeated every eight hours. This theoretical design obviously assumes that maintenance of the drug concentration must be above the MIC at all time intervals. The postantibiotic effect is seen where certain antibiotics (e.g., aminoglycosides) bind irreversibly to bacterial cell targets (e.g., ribosomes), and the action of the antibiotic persists after the therapeutic concentration is no longer present. Antibiotics with a significant postantibiotic effect can have treatment intervals that are greater than would be predicted by the above model. Nevertheless, the above strategy is generally used for the design of the therapeutic application of drugs in clinical trials. The design is derived from studies conducted in healthy volunteers and clinical trials are generally performed in patients without critical illness.

Biotransformation is the process by which the parent drug molecule is metabolized following infusion. Some antibiotics require biotransformation to exhibit antimicrobial activity (e.g., clindamycin), and others will have metabolism result in inactivity of the drug, while still others may have both the parent drug and the metabolite with retained biological activity (e.g., cefotaxime).

Biotransformation may occur via a number of pathways, although, hepatic metabolism is most common. Biotransformation may occur within the gastrointestinal tract, the kidney epithelium, the lungs, and even within the plasma itself. Hepatic biotransformation may result in the metabolite being released within the blood, resulting commonly in attenuation of action and facilitation of elimination via the kidney. Hepatic metabolism may result in the inactivated metabolite being eliminated within the bile.

Clearly, abnormalities within the organ responsible for biotransformation will affect the process. Intrinsic hepatic disease from cirrhosis will alter hepatic biotransformation. The cytochrome P-450 system requires molecular oxygen; therefore, poor perfusion or oxygenation of the liver from any cause will impact hepatic metabolism of specific drugs. Cytochrome P-450 may be induced by other drugs or be competitively inhibited. Drug interaction becomes yet another variable to influence concentration.

Excretion of the antibiotic occurs with or without biotransformation. Some drugs are eliminated unchanged by the kidney into the urine, or excreted by the liver into the bile. The rate of elimination of the unchanged drug directly affects the $T_{1/2}$. Excretion of unchanged drug via the biliary tract, which in turn can be reabsorbed, may create an enterohepatic circulation that results in prolonged drug presence in the patient. When either the intact drug or metabolic product is dependent on a specific organ system for elimination, intrinsic disease becomes an important variable in the overall pharmacokinetic profile.

PATHOPHYSIOLOGY OF INJURY AND FEVER

The extreme model to characterize abnormal pharmacokinetics for any drug used in patient care would be in the febrile, multiple system injury patient. Extensive torso and extremity injuries result in soft tissue injuries that activate the human systemic inflammatory response. This requires extensive volume resuscitation for maintenance of intravascular volume and tissue perfusion. Extensive tissue injury results in tissue contamination. Blunt chest trauma requires intubation and prolonged ventilator support. The injuries lead to prolonged incapacitation and recumbence. The patients are immunosuppressed from the extensive injuries, transfusions, and protein-calorie malnutrition. Infection becomes the second wave of activation of systemic inflammation. Infection becomes a complication at the sites of injury, at the surgical sites of therapeutic interventions, and as nosocomial complications at sites remote from the injuries. Fever and hypermetabolism are common and add an additional compounding variable at a time when antimicrobial treatment is most important in the patient's outcome. Antibiotics are invariably used in the febrile, multiple injured patient, but they are dosed and redosed using the model of healthy volunteers initially employed in the development of the drug. Are antibiotics dosed in accordance with the pathophysiologic changes of the injury and febrile state?

Extensive tissue injury and invasive soft tissue infection share the common consequence of activating local and systemic inflammatory pathways. The initiator events of human inflammation include the activation of; (i) the coagulation cascade, (ii) platelets, (iii) mast cells, (iv) the bradykinin pathway, and (v) the complement cascade. The immediate consequence of the activation of these five initiator events is the vasoactive phase of acute inflammation. The release of both nitric oxide–dependent (bradykinin) and –independent (histamine) pathways result in relaxation of vascular smooth muscle, vasodilation of the microcirculation, increased vascular capacitance, increased vascular permeability, and extensive movement of plasma proteins and fluid into the interstitial space (i.e., edema). The expansion of intravascular capacitance and the loss of oncotic pressure mean that the V_d for many drugs will be expanded. Shock, injury and altered tissue perfusion have been associated with the loss of membrane polarization, and the shift of sodium and water into the intracellular space. At a theoretical level, there is abundant reason to anticipate that the conventional dosing of antibiotics may be inadequate in these circumstances (Fig. 2).

The vascular changes of activation of the inflammatory cascade also result in the relaxation of arteriolar smooth muscle and a reduction in systemic vascular resistance. The reduction in systemic vascular resistance becomes a functional reduction in left ventricular afterload, which combined with an appropriate preload resuscitation of the severely injured patient leads to an increase in cardiac index. The hyperdynamic circulation of the multiple trauma patients leads to the "flow" phase of the post-resuscitative patient. Increased perfusion of the kidney and liver results in acceleration of excretory functions and potential enhancement of drug elimination. It can be

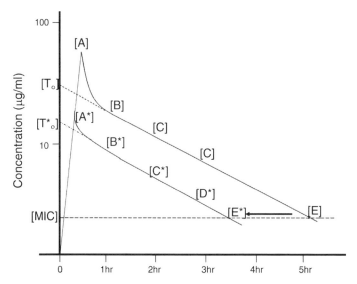

Figure 2 The influence upon the clearance curve of the theoretical antibiotic in Figure 1 of an increase in extracellular and/or intracellular water in a trauma patient that has fever secondary to invasive infection. The peak concentration A^* and the equilibrated peak concentration B^* are less than those concentrations observed under normal circumstances. The $T_o{}^*$ is reduced because of the increase in V_d. In this model, the $T_{1/2}$ has not changed, but the time point where the drug concentration E^* intercepts the MIC is 1.5 hours earlier (illustrated by the *arrow*) than would ordinarily be the case (E). *Abbreviation*: MIC, minimum inhibitory concentration.

anticipated that $T_{1/2}$ will be reduced. Subsequent organ failure from the ravages of sustained sepsis results in impairment of drug elimination and prolongation of $T_{1/2}$.

Severe injury results in the infiltration of the soft tissues with neutrophils and monocytes as part of the phagocytic phase of the inflammatory response. Proinflammatory cytokine signals are released from the phagocytic cells, from activated mast cells, and from other cell populations. The circulation of these proinflammatory signals leads to a febrile response with or without infection. The febrile response is associated with systemic hypermetabolism, and autonomic and neuroendocrine changes that further amplify the systemic dyshomeostasis. Proinflammatory signaling upregulates the synthesis of acute phase reactants and downregulates the synthesis of albumen, which further impacts the restoration of oncotic pressure and predictable drug pharmacokinetics. The summed effects of injury, fever, and the sequela of systemic inflammation result in pathophysiologic alterations (Table 1) that compromise the effectiveness of antibiotic therapy because of suboptimal dosing.

CLINICAL DATA

The discussion to this point has focused upon the theoretical effects which the pathophysiologic changes of multiple injury, fever, and systemic inflammation will have on antibiotic pharmacokinetics. A review of the literature identifies a paucity of clinical studies in this patient population, despite the fact that antibiotics are used for a wide array of indications in these patients. The effects of pathophysiologic changes upon antibiotic therapy will be cited among studies of critically ill patients in the intensive care unit, and not exclusively in multiple trauma patients.

Table 1 Pathophysiologic Changes of the Systemic Inflammatory Response that is Triggered by Injury, Fever, and Sepsis

Pathophysiologic change	Theoretical pharmacokinetic effect
Increase in extracellular water	Increased volume of distribution; reduced peak concentration; reduction in AUC
Increased intracellular water	Increased volume of distribution; reduced peak concentration; reduction in AUC
Change in vascular permeability	Reduction in serum proteins; adverse effects upon highly protein bound drugs.
Elevated cardiac output	Increased hepatic and renal perfusion; reduction in biological elimination half-life
Reduction in vascular resistance	Reduced hepatic and renal perfusion, reduced drug clearance
Systemic inflammatory response syndrome	Endothelial damage, reduced microcirculatory flow, hepatic and renal dysfunction and increased half-life and drug clearance

Note: Each of the pathophysiologic parameters has a theoretical impact upon antibiotic pharmacokinetics.
Abbreviation: AUC, area under the curve.

Preventive Antibiotics in the Injured Patient

Preventive antibiotics have been used for over 30 years in trauma patients (1). The recognized principles of preoperative administration of an antibiotic with activity against the likely pathogens to be encountered have been the hallmark of utilization in this setting. However, trauma patients have blood loss and large volumes of resuscitation in the period of time leading up to, and during, the operative intervention. Sequestration of the resuscitation volume into injured tissue results, and the obligatory expansion of the extracellular water volume contribute to a vastly expanded V_d. Should antibiotic doses be modified in this clinical setting?

Ericsson et al. (2) studied penetrating abdominal trauma patients with a regimen of preventive antibiotics that employed clindamycin and amikacin. In a limited number of preliminary study patients, they noted that conventional doses of 7.5 mg/kg amikacin given preoperative resulted in suboptimal peak serum concentrations (13.5–18.0 μg/mL) compared to effective therapeutic peak concentrations (25–28 μg/mL) at 30 minutes after infusion when 11 mg/kg of the drug was administered.

The explanation for the lower antibiotic concentrations in the conventional dosing regimen was found in the larger V_d and short $T_{1/2}$ that were seen in the trauma patients compared to normal controls. In a study of eight patients who averaged 37 years of age and had normal creatinines, each received between 6.7 to 11 mg/kg of amikacin. The measured V_d was 20.9 L compared to the estimated normal of 14.3 L. The $T_{1/2}$ was measured at 1.9 hours and the estimated normal $T_{1/2}$ for amikacin was 3.3 hours. Subsequent studies of an additional 28 trauma patients confirmed the impact of the increased V_d and the increased elimination rates of the drug in adversely affecting preventive antibiotic concentrations (3).

A prospective study examined the wound and intraabdominal infection rates of penetrating abdominal trauma patients who received different doses of amikacin (2). The data are illustrated in Table 2. Significantly, higher doses of amikacin resulted in statistically reduced infection rates in all patients studied. Subgroup analysis indicated that lower infection rates were identified in patients with high volume blood loss

Table 2 The Differences in Clinical Outcomes of Infection when 7.5 mg/kg of Amikacin is Compared to 10 mg/kg of Amikacin in Trauma Patients with Penetrating Abdominal Trauma

Patient characteristic	7.5 mg/kg (%)	≥10 mg/kg (%)	p	Comment
All patients	21/87 (24)	5/63 (8)	<0.01	The dose does matter!
No colon injury	12/57 (21)	1/48 (2)	<0.005	Small inoculum responds well to preventive drug
Colon injury	9/30 (30)	4/15 (27)	N.S.[a]	Large inoculum eliminates effectiveness
Blood loss >6 L	16/43 (37)	3/27 (11)	<0.02	Loss of antibiotic?
ISS[b] >20	11/32 (34)	1/18 (6)	<0.025	Large dose is necessary for large injuries
ISS[b] <20	10/55 (18)	4/45 (9)	N.S.[a]	May have been a type-2 statistical error

[a]Not significant.
[b]Injury severity score.

and in patients with injury severity scores >20. No improvement in infection rates was seen in patients when colon injury was present, indicating that high inocula of surgical site contamination cannot likely be overcome by preventive antibiotics. This observed uncertainty about antibiotic pharmacokinetics in the setting of blood loss and injury have led to some experimental investigation in the use of continuous infusion of antibiotics as a means to overcome the problem. Another strategy has been to simply not use potentially toxic agents like the aminoglycosides, but rather choose β-lactam alternatives where toxicity concerns are minimized and larger doses can be safely utilized.

The data which evaluates other antibiotics in preventive indications in trauma patients is very limited. Rosemurgy et al. (4) studied ceftizoxime in 53 celiotomies of trauma patients who received a conventional dose of preoperative antibiotic. They identified lower antibiotic concentrations is selected patients in the recovery room, and found that lower postoperative antibiotic concentrations was predictive of postoperative infections. They identified blood loss, extensive intraoperative resuscitation, and expanded V_d as likely causes for reduced postoperative antibiotic concentrations and recommended consideration of increased preoperative dose of preventive antibiotics.

Aminoglycosides

The aminoglycosides, more than any antibiotic group, have been studied most extensively in the setting of critical illness. Nephro- and ototoxicity have been the driving issues that have stimulated pharmacokinetic studies of the aminoglycosides. However, the data indicate that perhaps more patients have been underdosed than have received toxic levels of these antibiotics. Given that gentamicin and the other aminoglycosides have been demonstrated to have highly variable pharmacokinetics even with patients who appear to have normal kidney function (5), it is not surprising that physiologic changes of trauma and clinical fever will further compound an already difficult situation.

Niemiec et al. (6) studied 100 trauma and other surgical patients in the surgical intensive care unit. All study patients received at least one aminoglycoside with the majority receiving gentamicin or tobramycin. The V_d increased approximately 50% greater than normal for this population with one patient demonstrating a threefold increase. The $T_{1/2}$ was highly variable with a range from 1.6 to 63 hours. $T_{1/2}$ increased with age. Using individual patient pharmacokinetic parameters, adjustments in gentamicin doses ranged from 1.4 to 15.5 mg/kg/day for these patients. In similar studies by Reid et al. (7), both gentamicin and tobramycin were found to require dramatic increases in dosing in the intensive care unit patients, largely due to the increased V_d that was observed. In this latter study, drug elimination rates were strongly influenced by the patient's serum creatinine as a marker of clinical renal function. Despite larger doses that were required, doses of the aminoglycosides were given less frequently with patients having a creatinine above 1 mg/dL.

Summer et al. (8) studied 22 sepsis/septic shock patients following the administration of intravenous tobramycin at 2 mg/kg. They identified 59% of patients that had blood concentration of the antibiotic that was significantly below expected concentrations. The expanded V_d was considered to be responsible for the low blood concentrations.

Dasta and Armstrong (9) studied aminoglycoside pharmacokinetics in 181 critically ill patients in a surgical intensive care unit. The V_d was identified at 0.36 L/kg which was 60% to 70% above expected normal. The $T_{1/2}$ was highly variable with a range of 1.1 to 69.3 hours. Additional studies have validated that the observations of increased V_d and highly variable $T_{1/2}$ are applicable to all of the aminoglycosides in trauma (10) and intensive care unit patients (11).

Understanding these changes of aminoglycosides under circumstances of trauma, fever, and critical illness should lead to pharmacokinetic dosing and changes in the management of these patients. Zaske et al. (12) reported improved survival in burn patients undergoing dosing changes to address the pharmacokinetic changes. Once-daily dosing of aminoglycosides has become very common at present, but again the pharmacokinetic observations have demonstrated that conventional doses will be inadequate, especially for the younger trauma patient with normal renal function.

Vancomycin

Like the aminoglycosides, the pharmacokinetics of vancomycin is highly variable among patients with normal renal function (13). Reid et al. (7) studied the pharmacokinetics of vancomycin in infected surgical intensive care unit patients. They assumed and documented that the V_d of vancomycin was essentially that of total body water, i.e., 0.6 L/kg. While the linear regression for V_d for vancomycin did cluster about the 0.6 L/kg, the variability was quite high with an R^2 for the relationship only being 0.15. In selected cases, the V_d was so high that it actually exceeded the theoretical maximum of 1.0 L/kg reflecting probable tissue binding the antibiotic. Pharmacokinetic dosing required a 20% increase in the predicted dose of vancomycin, but a 50% increase in the interval between doses which reflected a longer $T_{1/2}$ than expected.

Vancomycin pharmacodynamics in burn patients have been noted to be quite variable. Rybak et al. (14) noted that V_d was quite variable, but only averaged about 10% more than control patients or intravenous drug abusers. Vancomycin clearance was 143 mL/min in the burn patient which was more than twice as great as that seen in control patients (68 mL/min). Vancomycin patients required larger and more frequent doses of the drug to achieve satisfactory peaks and troughs during therapy. The hyper-dynamic circulation of the burn patient with normal kidney function was thought to be the basis for accelerated drug clearance. Garrelts and Peterie (15) made similar observations with respect to a reduced $T_{1/2}$ in burn patients receiving vancomycin.

β-Lactam Antibiotics

Studies of the cephalosporin antibiotics have been limited as many of the commonly used drugs (e.g., cefazolin) have not been studied in trauma or febrile states. Virtually all have been in the third-generation group of cephalosporins. Van Dalen and Vree (16) studied V_d and $T_{1/2}$ in critically ill patients after the administration of ceftriaxone, the most commonly employed third-generation cephalosporin. They identified that the pharmacokinetics patterns were very similar to aminoglycosides with an expanded V_d and wide interpatient variability in $T_{1/2}$. They concluded that unique nomograms needed to be developed to permit dosing of ceftriaxone that was consistent with each patient's unique severity of disease profile. Yet another study demonstrated similar findings with a 90% increase in V_d and drug clearance was increased in patients with normal renal function (17). Patients with diminished renal function demonstrated a very prolonged $T_{1/2}$ and posed a serious problem of potential drug accumulation.

Hanes et al. (18) studied ceftazidime in critically ill trauma patients. They identified that the V_d increased from 0.21 ± 0.03 L/kg in healthy volunteers to 0.32 ± 0.14 L/kg in the trauma patients. It was felt that the large dose of the antibiotic (2 g every eight hours) overcame the pharmacokinetic changes in that only 8% of patients had subtherapeutic serum concentrations beneath the MIC. Dailly et al. (19) studied ceftazidime in burn patients who were not in the acute postinjury phase, noted an increased V_d, and also identified lower clearance of the drug. They suggested that the expanded V_d could serve as a reservoir for the drug and result in slow return to the circulation, which would explain the reduced clearance. Gomez et al. (20) noted a significantly increased V_d and an increased $T_{1/2}$, but antibiotic clearance and bioavailability (i.e., "area under the curve") were not changed. Angus et al. (21) studied intermittent versus continuous infusion of ceftazidime in septic patients and concluded that every eight hours dosing of the drug left the patient at-risk for subtherapeutic concentrations because of the increased V_d. They concluded that continuous infusion would prove to use less total drug and would insure reliable therapeutic drug concentrations.

Cefepime is a commonly used antibiotic especially later in the trauma patient's course when fever and nosocomial infection are significant issues. Bonapace et al. (22) studied 12 patients with burns (average of 36% total body surface) with suspected or documented infection and found a reduction in concentrations due to increased V_d and that doses of 1 g every eight hours, and 2 g every 12 hours resulted in blood concentrations above the MICs of organisms likely to be targeted by this drug. Lipman et al. (23) studied 10 patients who were critically ill with sepsis and found that 80% of trough levels were beneath the MIC_{50} for *Pseudomonas aeruginosa*. Kieft et al. (24) studied cefopime in patients with the septic syndrome and identified nearly a doubling of the V_d and a prolonged $T_{1/2}$. They indicated that 2 g every 12 hours still resulted in adequate trough concentrations for expected MICs of pathogens, and also noted a widely variable pharmacokinetic profile in their patients, especially in the elderly.

The pharmacokinetics of aztreonam were studied in 28 critically ill, mostly trauma patients, with gram-negative infections (25). The V_d was nearly doubled over anticipated values for this study population. The patients were a relatively young group (age = 35 years) and received 2 g of aztreonam every six hours. Trough levels were above the MICs of likely pathogens, despite the increase in V_d. The larger dose of aztreonam was the likely reason that adverse effects were not seen from the increase in V_d. McKindley et al. (26) similarly identified increased V_d in trauma patients with pneumonia, and also identified prolongation of the $T_{1/2}$.

Carbapenems

The carbapenem group of antibiotics is commonly used to treat infected trauma patients, especially with hospital-acquired bacteria. The data with imipenem has been quite variable. Boucher et al. (27) found that average V_d was comparable to controls in patients with burns, but did note the highly variable observations in the burn group. Dailly et al. (28) noted increased V_d and increased imipenem clearance rates in burn patients. McKindley et al. (26) also noted increased V_d and significantly lower plasma concentrations in trauma patients with pneumonia, while Belzberg et al. (29) noted very unpredictable V_d and $T_{1/2}$ in critically ill patients and that very high V_d and low serum concentrations may contribute to treatment failures in this population of patients. Fish et al. (30) made the unique observation of the efficient clearance of imipenem by continuous venovenous hemofiltration and have indicated that this variable in addition to pharmacokinetic changes may be an additional reason to increase antibiotic administration. Similar pharmacokinetic observations were made with meropenem (31). V_d and $T_{1/2}$ tended to be similar to normal adult measurements in surgical patients with intraabdominal infection and other surgical infections.

Quinolones

While specific data in the trauma patient are not available, the quinolone group of antibiotics appear to follow a different pattern of pharmacokinetic change in the critically ill patient and can be anticipated to have a different pattern in the injured patient as well. Lipman et al. (32) studied 18 critically ill patients for several days into the patients' treatment with ciprofloxacin. While normal volunteers will have a $V_d = 1.8$ L/kg and a $T_{1/2} = 4$–5 hours, adverse changes were not seen in severely infected patients treated with ciprofloxacin. The V_d was 1.2–1.4 L/kg and $T_{1/2}$ was 3.2 to 3.9 hours. Peak and trough concentrations did not appear to be influenced by the septic state. These observations with ciprofloxacin were confirmed in patients with intraabdominal infection (33).

Studies with levofloxacin in patients with critical illness (34) and with ventilator-associated pneumonia (35) have similarly demonstrated no adverse changes in pharmacokinetic profiles. The observation that the quinolone group of antibiotics has very large V_d that exceeds total body water means that increases in extracellular water volume have little impact. This potentially constitutes an advantage for this group of antibiotics in the febrile, critically ill patient, and perhaps in the trauma patient as well.

Linezolid

A significant number of reports have identified treatment failures for both methicillin-sensitive and methicillin-resistant *Staphylococcus aureus* (MRSA) infections from treatment with vancomycin (36–39). This has led to considerable interest in the identification of alternative antibiotic treatment for both community-associated and hospital-acquired Staphylococcal infections. Linezolid is the first of a new class of oxazolidinone antibiotics that appears to have a particular role in the treatment of MRSA infections. The V_d of this drug in patients and normal volunteers has been at 0.6–1.0 L/kg, which like the quinolones is a V_d that exceeds total body water. $T_{1/2}$ of four to seven hours has been reported. Whitehouse et al. (40) reported linezolid pharmacokinetics on 28 patients with gram-positive infections in the intensive care unit. They found a $V_d = 0.63$ L/kg and $T_{1/2} = 2.6$ hours. Trough concentrations were adequate for the treatment of susceptible organisms. Of note, no modification was necessary for either renal or hepatic dysfunction. The combined observations of the quinolones and linezolid suggests that antibiotics with V_d that exceed total body water are less likely to be adversely affected by physiologic changes of injury, critical illness, and sepsis.

SUMMARY

The actual number of studies that have examined the febrile, multiple trauma patient are only a few, and conclusions about pharmacokinetic changes in this population must be extrapolated at this time from studies of intensive care unit patients, septic patients, burn patients and others with critical illness. More clinical studies are needed in this area. However, it is clear that antibiotic concentrations are adversely affected for most drugs as the injured and septic patient progressively accumulates "third space" volume. The quinolones and perhaps linezolid are exceptions. Clearance of antibiotics appears to be highly variable and clearly is influenced by drug concentration changes, cardiac output changes, their influence upon kidney and liver perfusion, and their effect upon the intrinsic coexistent dysfunction of the kidney or liver. For most antibiotics used in the multiple trauma patients, it is likely that they are underdosed and that inadequate antibiotic administration contributes to both treatment failures and to emerging patterns of antimicrobial resistance. More studies of antibiotic pharmacokinetics in the multisystem injured patient are necessary.

REFERENCES

1. Fullen WD, Hunt J, Altemeier WA. Prophylactic antibiotics in penetrating wounds of the abdomen. J Trauma 1972; 12:282.
2. Ericsson CD, Fischer RP, Rowlands BJ, et al. Prophylactic antibiotics in trauma: the hazards of underdosing. J Trauma 1989; 29:1356–1361.
3. Reed RL, Ericcson CD, Wu A, et al. The pharmacokinetics of prophylactic antibiotics in trauma. J Trauma 1992; 32:21–27.
4. Rosemurgy AS, Dillon KR, Kurto, et al. Ceftizoxime use in trauma celiotomy: pharmacokinetics and patient outcomes. J Clin Pharmacol 1995; 35:1046–1051.
5. Zaske DE, Cipolle RJ, Rotschafer, et al. Gentamicin pharmacokinetics in 1,640 patients: method for control of serum concentrations. Antimicrob Agents Chemother 1982; 21:407–411.
6. Niemiec PW, Allo MD, Miller CF. Effect of altered volume of distribution on aminoglycoside levels in patients in surgical intensive care. Arch Surg 1987; 122:207–211.
7. Reid RL, Wu AH, Miller-Crotchett P, et al. Pharmacokinetic monitoring of nephrotoxic antibiotics in surgical intensive care patients. J Trauma 1989; 29:1462–1470.

8. Summer WR, Michael JR, Lipsky JJ. Initial aminoglycoside levels in the critically ill. Crit Care Med 1983; 11(12):948–950.

9. Dasta JF, Armstrong DK. Variability in aminoglycoside pharmacokinetics in critically ill surgical patients. Crit Care Med 1988; 16:327.

10. Townsend PL, Fink MP, Stein KL, Murphy SG. Aminoglycoside pharmacokinetics: dosage requirements and nephrotoxicity in trauma patients. Crit Care Med 1989; 17: 154–157.

11. Fernandez de Gatta MM, Mendez ME, Romano S, et al. Pharmacokinetics of amikacin in intensive care unit patients. J Clin Pharm Ther 1996; 21:417–421.

12. Zaske DE, Bootman JL, Solem LB, Strate RG. Increased burn patient survival with indi-vidualized dosages of gentaminin. Surgery 1982; 91:142–149.

13. Rotschafer JC, Crossley K, Zaske DE, et al. Pharmacokinetics of vancomycin: observa-tions in 28 patients and dosage recommendations. Antimicrob Agents Chemother 1982; 22:391–394.

14. Rybak MJ, Albrecht LM, Berman JR, et al. Vancomycin pharmacokinetics in burn patients and intravenous drug abusers. Antimicrob Agents Chmother 1990; 34:792–795.

15. Garrelts JC, Peterie JC. Altered vancomycin dose versus serum concentration relationship in burn patients. Clin Pharmacol Ther 1988; 44:9–13.

16. Van Dalen R, Vree TB. Pharmacokinetics of antibiotics in critically ill patients. Intensive Care Med 1990; 16(suppl 3):S235–S238.

17. Joynt GM, Lipman J, Gomersall CD, et al. The pharmacokinetics of once-daily dosing of ceftriaxone in critically ill patients. J Antimicrob Chemother 2001; 47:421–429.

18. Hanes SD, Wood GC, Herring V, et al. Intermittant and continuous ceftazidime infusion for critically ill trauma patients. Am J Surg 2000; 179:436–440.

19. Dailly E, Pannier M, Jolliet P, Bourin M. Population pharmacokinetics of ceftazidime in burn patients. Br J Clin Pharmacol 2003; 56:629–634.

20. Gomez CMH, Cordingly JJ, Palazzo MGA. Altered pharmacokinetics of ceftazidime in critically ill patients. Antimicrob Agents Chemother 1999; 43:1798–1802.

21. Angus BJ, Smith MD, Suputtamongkol Y, et al. Pharmacokinetic-pharmacodynamic evaluation of ceftazidime continuous infusion versus intermittent bolus injection in septi-caemic melioidosis. Br J Clin Pharmacol 2000; 49:445–452.

22. Bonapace CR, White RL, Friedrich LV, et al. Pharmacokinetics of cefepime in patients with thermal burn injury. Antimicrob Agents Chemother 1999; 43:2848–2854.

23. Lipman J, Wallis SC, Rickard C. Low plasma cefepime levels in critically ill septic patients: pharmacokinetic modeling indicates improved troughs with revised dosing. Antimicrob Agents Chemother 1999; 43:2559–2561.

24. Kieft H, Hoepelman AIM, Knupp CA, et al. Pharmacokinetics of cefepime in patients with the sepsis syndrome. J Antimicrob Chemother 1993; 32(suppl B):117–122.

25. Cornwell EE, Belzberg H, Berne TV, et al. Pharmacokinetics of aztreonam in critically ill surgical patients. Am J Health-Syst Pharm 1997; 54:537–540.

26. McKindley DS, Boucher BA, Hess MM, et al. Pharmacokinetics of aztreonam and imipe-nem in critically ill patients with pneumonia. Pharmacotherapy 1996; 16:924–931.

27. Boucher BA, Hickerson WL, Kuhl DA, et al. Imipenem pharmacokinetics in patients with burns. Clin Pharmacol Ther 1990; 48:130–137.

28. Dailly E, Kergueris MF, Pannier M, et al. Population pharmacokinetics of imipenem in burn patients. Fundam Clin Pharmacol 2003; 17:645–650.

29. Belzberg H, Zhu J, Cornwell EE, et al. Imipenem levels are not predictable in the critically ill patient. J Tauma 2004; 56:111–117.

30. Fish DN, Teitelbaum I, Abraham E. Pharmacokinetics and pharmacodynamics of imipe-nem during continuous renal replacement therapy in critically ill patients. Antimicrob Agents Chemother 2005; 49:2421–2428.

31. Hurst M, Lamb HM. Meropenem: a review of its use in patients in intensive care. Drugs 2000; 59:653–680.

32. Lipman J, Scribante J, Gous AGS, et al. Pharmacokinetic profiles of high-dose intravenous ciprofloxacin in severe sepsis. Antimicrob Agents Chemother 1998; 42:2235–2239.
33. Gous A, Lipman J, Scribante J, et al. Fluid shifts have no influence on ciprofloxacin pharmacokinetics in intensive care patients with intra-abdominal sepsis. Int J Antimicrob Agents 2005; 26:50–55.
34. Rebuck JA, Fish DN, Abraham E. Pharmacokinetics of intravenous and oral levofloxacin in critically ill adults in a medical intensive care unit. Pharmacotherapy 2002; 22: 1216–1225.
35. Pea F, Di Qual E, Cusenza A, et al. Pharmacokinetics and pharmacodynamics of intravenous levofloxacin in patients with early-onset ventilator-associated pneumonia. Clin Pharmacokinet 2003; 42:589–598.
36. Gonzalez C, Rubio M, Romero-Vivas J, et al. Bacteremic pneumonia due to *Staphylococcus aureus*: a comparison of disease caused by methicillin-resistant and methicillin-susceptible organisms. Clin Infect Dis 1999; 29:1171–1177.
37. Chang FY, Peacock JE Jr., Musher DM, et al. *Staphylococcus aureus* bacteremia: recurrence and the impact of antibiotic treatment in a prospective multicenter study. Medicine 2003; 82:333–339.
38. Wunderink RG, Rello J, Cammarata SK, et al. Linezolid versus vancomycin: analysis of two double-blind studies of patients with methicillin-resistant *Staphylococcus aureus* nosocomial pneumonia. Chest 2003; 124:1789–1797.
39. Weigelt J, Itani K, Stevens D, et al. Linezolid versus vancomycin in treatment of complicated skin and soft tissue infections. Antimicrob Agents Chemother 2005; 49:2260–2266.
40. Whitehouse T, Cepeda JA, Shulman R, et al. Pharmacokinetic studies of linezolid and teicoplanin in the critically ill. J Antimicrob Chemother 2005; 55:333–340.

31

Antibiotic Selection and Control of Resistance in the Critical Care Unit

Burke A. Cunha

Infectious Disease Division, Winthrop-University Hospital, Mineola, and
State University of New York School of Medicine,
Stony Brook, New York, U.S.A.

INTRODUCTION

Overview of Antimicrobial Therapy in the CCU

Early empiric antimicrobial therapy is essential in the critical care unit (CCU) because in many cases a specific diagnosis is not possible at the outset. For antimicrobial therapy to be effective, the patient has to have an infectious disease that is amenable to antimicrobial therapy, and the therapy should be administered as soon as possible to achieve maximum therapeutic effect. Antimicrobial therapy should be directed at the most likely pathogens involved in the infectious process, which derive from the flora of the focus of infection. It is obvious that antimicrobial therapy should be administered as soon as possible to critically ill patients to achieve maximum therapeutic benefit. There are many infectious processes that require surgical intervention in addition to appropriate antimicrobial therapy. Surgical intervention is the primary therapeutic intervention when the patient's infectious disease process is based on the obstruction or perforation of a viscus, an abscess, or infected associated material, i.e., central intravenous (IV) line, shunts, biliary or urethral stents, etc. In all of these situations, antimicrobial therapy is adjunctive, and removal of an infected device, relief of obstruction, correction of perforation, or abscess drainage should not be delayed with the expectation that antimicrobial therapy alone can bring the infection under control (1,2).

ANTIBIOTIC SELECTION IN THE CCU

Perspective on Antibiotic Therapy in the CCU

Antimicrobial therapy is usually administered intravenously initially to achieve rapid onset of effect. Oral therapy may be used in some cases in the intensive care unit if the process is not so acute that therapeutic blood levels achievable one hour after oral therapy would be critical to the patient. In selecting an antibiotic to be administered intravenously or orally, the clinician should take into account five different factors.

Of prime importance is selecting an antibiotic with the appropriate spectrum relative to the site of infection. If the spectrum is inappropriate, nothing else matters, and suboptimal therapy in terms of spectrum is not much better than no therapy at all. The second consideration relates to pharmacokinetic (PK) or pharmacodynamic (PD) considerations. PK/PD parameters have to do with selecting the optimal dose and dosing frequency for the antibiotic selected. The most important consideration related to PK/PD factors is the patient's functional hepatic and renal capacity. PK/PD considerations are also important in hosts with situations that would change the volume of distribution (V_d), e.g., ascites, burns, etc., or relate to a difficult-to-penetrate tissue, e.g., prostate and central nervous system (CNS). The next factor that should be taken into account in selecting antimicrobial therapy is that of antimicrobial resistance.

Resistance potential of the antibiotic selected is often overlooked. Resistance potential of an antibiotic is important because even though an antibiotic with a high resistance potential that is selected may save the patient, it may cause long-lasting and widespread resistance problems in the CCU and subsequently in the hospital. The next consideration the clinician must take into account is the safety profile of the antimicrobial being considered. Side effects may be considered as common and minor, or infrequent but serious. Given a choice, the clinician should opt for the antimicrobial with the best safety profile. If this is not possible, then selecting an antimicrobial with a common but unimportant side effect is obviously preferable to selecting one with a rare but serious potential adverse effect. With antibiotic selection, cost is a factor outside of the CCU. The expense of a hospital stay in the CCU setting outweighs any cost differentials between antimicrobial regimens in the seriously ill patient in the CCU (2–7).

Factors in Antibiotic Selection

Antimicrobial Spectrum

Selecting an antibiotic with appropriate spectrum is the critical determination in selecting an antimicrobial for empiric therapy in the CCU setting. Each organ system has a "normal flora," which becomes the pathogenic flora when host defenses are disrupted or breached. It is usually possible by history taking, physical examination, and routine laboratory/radiologic tests to localize the site of infection to an anatomical location. The commonest sites for sepsis in the CCU are intravascular gastrointestinal (GI) tract or genitourinary (GU) tract (1–3).

Antibiotic Selection Based on the Site of Infection. The predictable pathogens related to central IV-line infections are derivatives of skin pathogens, i.e., *Staphylococcus aureus*, *Staphylococcus epidermidis*, coagulase-negative staphylococci, enterococci, or aerobic gram-negative bacilli. Uropathogens associated with nosocomial urosepsis include *Pseudomonas aeruginosa*, enterococci, and nonfermentative gram-negative aerobic bacilli. With community-acquired urosepsis, the common coliforms or enterococci are the most likely pathogens to be taken into account in selecting empiric therapy for urosepsis. For intra-abdominal or pelvic sepsis, the organisms are related to the site of infection in the GI tract. Excluding the biliary tract, whose pathogens are *Klebsiella*, *E. coli*, or enterococci, infections of the liver, distal small bowel, colon, or pelvis are due to *Bacteroides fragilis* and aerobic coliform bacilli (1,3).

Bacteriostatic or Bactericidal. It does not matter if the antibiotic selected is bacteriostatic or bactericidal. Both bacteriostatic and bactericidal antibiotics kill at the same rate. Bactericidal antibiotics have only been shown to have potential advantage in febrile neutropenia, CNS infections, and bacterial endocarditis, and even in these situations, there are exceptions in each category (1,8).

Appropriate vs. Excessive Spectrum.   Empiric antimicrobial therapy for criti-cally ill patients in the CCU should have an appropriate but not excessive spectrum of activity. Because empiric antimicrobial therapy is based on coverage of the most likely pathogens, which is a function of the anatomical location of the site of infec-tion, there is no need for excessively broad coverage. There is also no advantage in narrowing the coverage after specific pathogens are identified later during hospitali-zation, if the drug chosen initially was optimal (1,9,10).

PK/PD Considerations.   For most critically ill patients in the CCU, PK/PD considerations are as important as spectrum. Clearly, the usually recommended dose is preferred, and underdosing could have an adverse effect on the patient in terms of resistance or therapeutic failure (1,4).

Intravenous vs. Oral Dosing.   The full recommended usual doses of antibiotics administered intravenously are the preferred mode of administration for most patients. Alternately, depending upon the PK attributes of the drug, some antibiotics may be administered intramuscularly, if the patient is not in shock. Even critically ill patients in the CCU have normal or near-normal GI absorption, permitting the administration of antibiotics via nasogastric (NG) tubes. Giving patients in the CCU setting antibiotics via an NG tube is acceptable, if achieving therapeutic blood levels in one hour versus 30 minutes is a critical consideration. Critically ill patients absorb efficiently through the proximal GI track, but not through intramuscularly administered antibiotics. Clearly, only certain antibiotics are available for IV admin-istration, which limits the antibiotic selection to those agents available in pill or cap-sule form, which can be crushed/solubilized and administered via the nasogastric tube. The majority of patients in the CCU with non-CNS infections do well with optimal dosing/dosing interval administered in an appropriate fashion (1,11).

CNS Infection and CSF Penetration.   In certain situations, PK/PD factors are important in the selection of an antimicrobial agent, i.e., CNS infections. Patients in the CCU for meningitis or brain abscess should be treated with an antibiotic with first, an appropriate spectrum, and second, that penetrates the CNS with normal or high dose. Clinicians should be familiar with the CNS penetrance of various antibiotics in terms of achievable cerebrospinal fluid (CSF) concentrations in relationship to simultaneous serum levels. Some antibiotics, even in the presence of inflammation, do not achieve therapeutic concentration in the CSF and should obviously not be used for CNS infections. Other agents, e.g., meropenem 2 g (IV) q8h = meningeal dose ver-sus 1 g (IV) q8h = usual dose; cefepime 2 g (IV) q8h = meningeal dose versus 2 g (IV) q12h = usual dose, can be administered at "meningeal doses," which permit therapeu-tic CNS penetration.

Certain antibiotics penetrate the CSF in the presence or absence of meningeal inflammation. For this reason, they achieve therapeutic CNS/CSF concentrations even with normal dosing, i.e., chloramphenicol, TMP-SMX, doxycycline, minocycline, metronidazole, and acyclovir. Other antibiotics may require not only meningeal dosing but also intrathecal (IT) dosing to achieve adequate CSF levels, e.g., vancomycin (30–60 mg/kg/day (IV) ± IT dose 20 mg/day versus usual dosing (15 mg/kg/day) (1,11).

Dosing in Renal or Hepatic Insufficiency.   Dosing recommendations are usually for adult patients with normal hepatic and renal function. There are no good tests of hepatic function as exist for renal function, i.e., serum creatinine or creatinine clearance. If empiric antimicrobial therapy is selected with a drug that is primarily hepatically eliminated, and given to a patient with severe liver disease, there are two therapeutic options. The clinician can either decrease the dose of the drug by half per day, or use an alternate renally eliminated antibiotic with the same spectrum of activity. In patients with renal insufficiency or renal failure, the initial dose given is the same as in patients with intact renal function. In patients with renal insufficiency, it is the maintenance dose and not the initial dose, which must be decreased in proportion to the creatinine clearance. For example, the usual dose of vancomycin for non-CNS infections is 1 g (IV) q12h (15 mg/kg/day). In patients with renal insufficiency, beginning empiric treatment with vancomycin intravenously, an initial 1 g dose should be given, which is the usual dose in patients with normal renal function. The subsequent dose depends on the degree of renal insufficiency as determined by the creatinine clearance. Because vancomycin's elimination is directly proportional to the GFR as measured by the creatinine clearance, vancomycin dosage should be decreased in proportion to the patient's renal function. In decreasing the maintenance dose of renally eliminated drugs in renal insufficiency, the dose may be decreased for mild renal insufficiency, the interval may be increased in moderate renal insufficiency and in severe renal insufficiency, the dose or interval should be decreased (1,12–16).

Dosing in Renal Failure on Hemodialysis or Peritoneal Dialysis. The protein binding (percent) and V_d in addition to the peak serum concentrations and molecular size are the primary determinants of dialyzability. Traditionally, patients on hepatically eliminated antibiotics are not dialyzable and the doses do not need to be decreased in renal failure and a postdialysis dose does not have to be administered. In patients with renal insufficiency being given renally eliminated antibiotics, the daily dose should be decreased in direct proportion to the renal dysfunction. The PK parameters determine whether a posthemodialysis (HD) or postperitoneal dialysis (PD) supplementary dose needs to be given. In such cases, the dosing between the dialyses should be based on the patient's renal insufficiency or creatinine clearance. In addition, whenever dialysis occurs, a post-HD or -PD dose needs to be given (1,12,13).

Other Dosing Considerations. Other situations where PK/PD factors need to be taken into account are in burn patients and in those with massive ascites. Most antibiotics do not penetrate into well-encapsulated abscesses. The treatment for well-encapsulated abscesses is antimicrobial therapy appropriate for the location of the abscess, and if found early may still be in the phlegmon stage before the abscess becomes encapsulated. Before the phlegmon stage, antibiotics may penetrate into the area and sterilize/contain the infectious process. Once the abscess is well formed and surrounded by a thick wall, antimicrobial therapy is suppressive or adjunctive, but percutaneous or surgical drainage will be needed for a cure (17–20).

Antibiotic Resistance Potential

Overview of Resistance. The antibiotics selected for empiric therapy in the CCU should take into account the resistance potential of the antibiotic. While the initial goal is to control the infection in the individual patient, the long-term goal of therapy is to minimize the emergence of resistance in the CCU environment by careful antibiotic selection. Antibiotic resistance may occur on the basis of clonal spread or may be induced by certain antimicrobials. The clonal spread of resistance can be interrupted by effective infection control measures. Clonally spread resistance of the same strain is not a function of antibiotic use. Antibiotic resistance, which is related to antibiotic use, occurs with all antibiotic classes, but only certain antibiotics within each class are responsible for the resistance problems associated with each class. Volume of antibiotic used per se does not cause resistance problems unless the antibiotic being used has a high resistance potential. Antibiotics with a low resistance potential can be used with great intensity over long periods of time and not result in problems with antimicrobial resistance (2,4,21,22).

Low vs. High Resistance Potential Antibiotics. Using third-generation cephalosporins as an example, there are five third-generation cephalosporin antibiotics that have been in widespread use worldwide. Descriptions of resistance related to third-generation cephalosporins either consider the class as a group, which is incorrect, or correctly analyze the contribution of each member as related to the resistance attributes of the group. Given the large body of literature on resistance among third-generation cephalosporins, a careful analysis reveals that there has been no clinically significant resistance to cefotaxime, ceftizoxime, cefoperazone, or ceftriaxone over the last several decades. The only third-generation cephalosporin associated with resistance problems has been and continues to be ceftazidime. Therefore, it can be said that all of the third-generation cephalosporins have a low resistance potential except ceftazidime, which should be viewed as having a high resistance potential. The resistance associated with ceftazidime is primarily related to *Pseudomonas aeruginosa* and to a lesser extent *Klebsiella* and *Enterobacter* species. In the CCU setting, unless there is no other antibiotic available besides ceftazidime, clinicians should opt for another cephalosporin with anti–*P. aeruginosa* activity, e.g., cefoperazone, or the fourth-generation cephalosporin, cefepime; alternately, the clinician could opt for a monobactam with antipseudomonal activity, e.g., aztreonam, a carbapenem with anti–*P. aeruginosa* activity, i.e., meropenem, an aminoglycoside, e.g., amikacin, or polymyxin B. All other things being equal, try to avoid using antibiotics with a high resistance potential (23–25).

Ceftazidime has the other unfortunate attribute of increasing the prevalence of methicillin resistant *Staphyloccus aureus* (MRSA) in institutions where it is used extensively. Alternate therapy for *P. aeruginosa* has been described, (vide supra). Other alternatives in the CCU for *S. pneumoniae* with a low resistance potential include "respiratory quinolones," i.e., levofloxacin, moxifloxacin, gatifloxacin, or cefepime, meropenem, ertapenem, etc. Imipenem is another commonly used antibiotic in the CCU setting with a high resistance potential, i.e., *P. aeruginosa*. With respect to *P. aeruginosa*, there are other alternatives to use empirically or specifically in treating *P. aeruginosa* infections. If a carbapenem for anti–*P. aeruginosa* use is selected, then meropenem is the preferred choice. Imipenem, shares with ceftazidime the propensity for increasing MRSA prevalence (20,26–32).

Although antibiotics may be considered as having a high or low resistance potential with respect to selected organisms, it does not mean that the individual use of such agents will invariably result in resistance. It does mean that low resistance antibiotics used in high volume over long periods of time are exceedingly unlikely to develop resistance problems, if other factors are kept constant. Antibiotics with a high resistance potential are likely to develop resistance problems, even if used in low volume for either short or long periods of time. Because the therapeutic armamentarium is so extensive at the present time, it is almost always possible to opt for a low resistance potential antibiotic (1,4).

Antibiotic Side Effects

Overview of Antibiotic Side Effects in the CCU. Patients who are critically ill in the CCU do not need superimposed problems of antibiotic adverse effects added to their already serious problems. As with antimicrobial resistance, if the choice is between agents where the only difference has to do with safety profile, then the clinician should opt for the agent with the superior safety profile. The application of the safety profile to the patient profile also needs to be taken into consideration.

For example, it makes little sense to avoid using drugs that are potentially nephrotoxic in a patient with no renal function on HD. It would also make no sense to treat a patient who had ischemic colitis with a drug that could cause *C. difficile* colitis, e.g., clindamycin. These two situations aside, the clinician should select a drug that has a good safety profile. In situations where clinicians must choose between an antibiotic with a common but mild side effect and one with an infrequent but potentially serious side effect, the clinician should obviously opt for the lesser of two evils. The commonest related side effects in CCU patients include antibiotic-associated diarrhea, chemical phlebitis related to IV therapy, seizures, and drug hypersensitivity reactions (33).

Anaphylaxis and Nonanaphylactoid Reactions. Allergic history will determine the likelihood of the patient having a reaction to penicillin. The clinician should determine, if possible, if the reaction to penicillin is anaphylactoid or nonanaphylactoid. Patients who have had nonanaphylactoid reactions to penicillin may safely be given β-lactam antibiotics. If an allergic reaction occurs in such patients, the reaction will be of the same type and order of magnitude as had occurred previously, e.g., rash or drug fever. Patients who have had anaphylactic reactions to penicillins should be given drugs, which are antigenically unrelated to β-lactams. Ideal drugs to treat patients with anaphylactic or nonanaphylactic allergies to β-lactams are the monobactams and carbapenems. It is a common clinical misconception that because carbapenems bear structural similarity to β-lactam antibiotics, they are antigenically similar, which they are not. If a patient has anaphylactic reaction to penicillin or β-lactam, then carbapenems, particularly meropenem, may be used with confidence and safety without risk of cross reactions (6,34–36).

Phlebitis. Antimicrobials that have been associated with venous phlebitis should not be used in preference to those not associated with phlebitis problems. Commonly, chemical phlebitis is related to administering the antimicrobial too quickly or in an inadequate volume, and is not related to the drug per se (1,11).

***C. difficile* Diarrhea or Colitis.** *C. difficile* diarrhea is the commonest cause of nosocomial diarrhea. In the CCU, the commonest cause of hospital-acquired diarrhea is overzealous enteral feeds, not *C. difficile*. *C. difficile* diarrhea is common in the CCU, as is *C. difficile* colitis. Patients in the CCU who develop diarrhea should be considered as having *C. difficile* diarrhea until proven otherwise, and placed on appropriate precautions and treated with an anti–*C. difficile* diarrhea agent pending *C. difficile* stool toxin testing. If the patient is subsequently found not to have *C. difficile* diarrhea, the anti-*C. difficile* antibiotic may be discontinued. If the patient has diarrhea due to the enteral feed, this may be demonstrated by decreasing greatly or stopping the enteral feed for 24 hours. If the patient's diarrhea is due to the enteral feed, it will decrease or stop when the enteral feed is cut back or stopped. The high hourly volume of the enteral feed may be at fault, or the patient may need to be switched to an alternate enteral feed preparation to solve the problem. Patients with *C. difficile* colitis almost always follow inadequately recognized or treated *C. difficile* diarrhea. *C. difficile* colitis may be suspected in patients with *C. difficile* diarrhea, if the diarrhea abruptly stops, the patient suddenly develops a temperature of $\geq 102°F$, or the patient develops otherwise unexplained acute abdominal pain. Antibiotics are not equal in their *C. difficile* diarrhea potential. As with antibiotic resistance, individual agents rather than certain classes predispose to *C. difficile* diarrhea or colitis. Clindamycin and β-lactam antibiotics and, to a lesser extent, the quinolones are the common causes of *C. difficile* diarrhea among antibiotics that would be used in the CCU setting. Certain antibiotics are rarely, if ever, associated with *C. difficile* diarrhea or colitis, i.e., carbapenems, doxycycline, minocycline, aztreonam, amino-glycosides, TMP-SMX, and polymyxin B (18,19,37).

Seizures. Seizures are caused by many drugs, but by relatively few antibiotics used in the CCU setting. The most common causes of seizures in CCU patients related to antimicrobial therapy are imipenem and ciprofloxacin. Ciprofloxacin among the quinolones is unique in its seizure potential. Among the carbapenems, imipenem but not meropenem has been associated with seizures. With both cipro-floxacin and imipenem, seizure likelihood is increased in renal insufficiency. Other things being equal, clinicians should select other agents besides ciprofloxacin or imi-penem in patients with renal failure, or history of a seizure disorder. Ciprofloxacin and imipenem may also cause seizures in patients with normal renal function, but the incidence is lower than in those with renal insufficiency (1,11,18,19).

Antibiotic Cost

Antibiotic cost is of importance to the institution. Antibiotic cost includes the acqui-sition cost of the antibiotic, the administration cost of the antibiotic, as well as indir-ect costs, e.g., monitoring and therapeutic failure. Because the costs of being in a CCU exceed any small difference in the total cost of antibiotics among patients, antibiotic cost in the CCU is the least important factor in antibiotic selection. As mentioned previously, the most important determinants of antibiotic selection in the CCU are spectrum, safety profile, and resistance potential, and cost is a tertiary consideration (2,6).

Other Considerations in Antibiotic Selection

Antibiotic Inhibition of Endotoxin or Cytokine Activity. In treating sepsis from a GI or GU source, consideration should be given to selecting an antibiotic that minimizes endotoxins or cytokine release. Aerobic gram-negative bacilli, the major pathogens in sepsis originating from the GI or GU tract, release endotoxins or cytokines, which mediate end-organ damage. Release of endotoxins or cytokines is maximal during cell death. Most antibiotics have no effect on endotoxin release because gram-negative bacilli are destroyed by the antibiotic, but some have an inhibitory effect on endotoxins or cytokine release. The advantage in selecting an antibiotic with the appropriate spectrum, that in addition has endotoxin or cyto-kine inhibiting properties, is clearly advantageous.

The commonly used antibiotics that are active against gram-negative bacilli, which have no effect/intensify endotoxin/cytokine release from dying cells during therapy, are the β-lactam class of antimicrobials. Of the antibiotics studied, the ones that have been shown to inhibit endotoxin or cytokine release are the carbapenems. Imipenem and meropenem have been shown to not only effectively kill gram-negative bacilli, but also to effectively minimize endotoxin or cytokine release from dying cells, because the endotoxin- or cytokine-inhibiting properties of carbapenems are another indication of their dissimilarity to β-lactams, which they resemble structurally. In situations where multiorgan dysfunction or shock emanating from a focus of infection in the GI or GU tract is present, carbapenems, e.g., meropenem, has the dual advantage of a high degree of effectiveness, and in addition a potent inhibitory effect on endotoxin or cytokine release. The inhibition of endotoxin or cytokine release should minimize or prevent further end-organ dysfunction (Table 1) (11,36).

Table 1 Factors in Antibiotic Selection in the Critical Care Unit

Antimicrobial spectrum
  Appropriate for the site of infection
  No need/advantage in changing to a narrower spectrum antibiotic if the isolated strain was
    sensitive to the initial empiric antibiotic selected

Pharmacokinetic/pharmacodynamic considerations
  Use full recommended dose for CCU infections
  Underdosing may be associated with therapeutic failure/resistance
  Select an antibiotic pharmacokinetically suited for special dosing situations, e.g., CNS
    infections, select an agent that penetrates the CNS/CSF at the usual dose, e.g.,
    chloramphenicol, TMP-SMX, ceftriaxone; or use "meningeal doses" with antibiotics
    that require higher doses for therapeutic CSF levels, e.g., "meningeal doses" of
    meropenem 2 g (IV) q8h, or cefepime 2 g (IV) q8h

Resistance potential
  Preferentially use "low resistance" potential antibiotics
    3rd generation cephalosporins (except ceftazidime)
    4th generation cephalosporins (cefepime)
    Respiratory quinolones
    Doxycycline/minocycline (except tetracycline)
    Meropenem
    Ertapenem
    Aztreonam
    Amikacin (not gentamicin/tobramycin)
    Daptomycin linezoid
    Polymyxin B
    tigacycline
  Preferentially use antibiotics that do not increase incidence/prevalence of MRSA/VRE
    Vancomycin (VRE)
    Ceftazidime (MRSA)
    Ciprofloxacin (MRSA)
    Imipenem (MRSA)
  Combination therapy does not usually prevent resistance
    Exceptions include combination antituberculosis therapy, aminoglycoside/
      antipseudomonal penicillin combinations, and amphotericin B and 5 flucytosine.
    Combining a "high resistance" potential antibiotic with a "low resistance" potential
      antibiotic will not eliminate the resistance potential of the "low resistance" antibiotic
      component of therapy, e.g., ceftazidime (high resistance potential) plus amikacin (low
      resistance potential), ceftazidime will still induce *Pseudomonas aeruginosa* resistance
  Narrowing antibiotic spectrum does not prevent resistance

Safety profile
  Preferentially select antibiotics with infrequent/mild adverse events (meropenem,
    ertapenem, daptomycin, tigacycline, polymyxin B)
  Avoid antibiotics associated with seizures or *Clostridium difficile* diarrhea
    Imipenem (seizures)
    Ciprofloxacin (seizures)
    β-lactams (*C. difficile*)
  Treat penicillin-allergic patients (nonanaphylactic) reactions with cephalosporins
  Treat penicillin-allergic patients anaphylactic reactions (anaphylaxis, liver,
    hypotension, laryngospasm, or bronchospasm) with meropenem or another non
    β-lactam antibiotic, e.g., tigacycline
Antibiotic costs to hospital
  Cost is a relatively minor consideration in the CCU

(Continued)

Table 1 Factors in Antibiotic Selection in the Critical Care Unit (*Continued*)

Preferentially use monotherapy instead of combination therapy whenever possible

Avoid antibiotics that increase indirect costs, i.e., those that require monitoring, cause phlebitis, cause resistance, ↑MRSA/VRE, prevalence *C. difficile* diarrhea/colitis, or that are unlikely to be effective for the infection being treated, i.e., little/moderate vs. a high degree of activity against the pathogen(s) being tested

Endotoxin/cytokine inhibitors

Preferentially use antibiotics that inhibit/decrease endotoxin/cytokine release to treat infections due to gram-negative bacilli with multi-organ dysfunction

Meropenem

Respiratory quinolones

Avoid if possible antibiotics that increase endotoxin/cytokine reactions that may increase end-organ dysfunction

β-Lactams

Abbreviations: CCU, critical care unit; CNS, central nervous system; CNF, cerebrospinal fluid; MRSA, methicillin resistant *Staphylococcus aureus*; VRE, vancomycin resistant enterococci; TMP-SMX, trimethoprim sulfamethoxazole.

CONTROL OF RESISTANCE IN THE CCU

Overview of Acquired Antibiotic Resistance

Antibiotic resistance in the CCU may involve a wide variety of organisms, but of greatest concern is resistance among aerobic, nonfermentative gram-negative bacilli. Nonfermentative gram-negative bacilli, i.e., *Klebsiella* species, *Enterobacter* species, *Serratia* species, *P. aeruginosa*, and *Acinetobacter* species. Even when these organisms are sensitive to antibiotics, the problem is they are sensitive to a relatively limited number of antibiotics versus other gram-negative or gram-positive organisms excluding MRSA and Vancomycin resistant enterococci (VRE). If these nonfermentative aerobic gram-negative bacilli become resistant, there are even fewer drugs available that are effective against resistant strains. With gram-positive organisms in the CCU, i.e., MRSA and VRE, there are more therapeutic options available to treat these organisms (21,22,37–39).

Before therapy is considered to treat highly resistant or multiresistant organisms in the CCU, careful consideration must be given to the role of the organism in the clinical context of the patient. Culture or recovery of the gram-negative and gram-positive organisms mentioned from various body sites in the great majority of cases represents colonization rather than infection. As a general principle, colonization should not be treated (1,18,19,40).

Antimicrobial resistance to antibiotics occurs by point mutation, which may or may not be induced by antimicrobial therapy. The spread of resistant organisms may be due to clonal spread or may be due to continued pressure by certain antibiotics inducing resistance in certain organisms. Antimicrobial resistance may be termed natural or acquired. Natural resistance refers to the spectrum beyond the usual activity of a given antibiotic. Acquired resistance refers to an organism that is ordinarily or has previously been susceptible to an antibiotic, but subsequently becomes resistant to it. Acquired resistance may be further divided into "relative resistance" or "high-grade resistance." Relative resistance can usually be overcome by increasing the dose of the antibiotic to achieve concentrations above the increased MICs of the organisms.

High-grade resistance may be overcome by high levels of antimicrobials, but absolute resistance cannot be overcome by increasing the dose of the antibiotic. Antimicrobial resistance to a particular antibiotic usually is confined to one or two organisms in its usual spectrum of activity. Ceftazidime, for example, is known to induce resistance with *P. aeruginosa* but remains highly active against most other aerobic gram-negative bacilli. Antibiotic resistance may be mediated via several mechanisms. Resistance may be due to the inability of the antibiotic to penetrate into the organism via porin channels. Resistance may also be mediated by enzymes, e.g., β-lactamases that inactivate the antibiotic by disrupting the rings of β-lactam antibiotics. There are several different and new β-lactamases that have been described that inactivate β-lactams. Not uncommonly encountered are extended spectrum β-lactamases (ESBLs) that are potent inhibitors of β-lactamase, and are highly resistant to many antibiotics. Other antibiotics interfere with a variety of intracellular activities, i.e., DNA-gyrase inhibitors with quinolones, ribosomal inhibitors with macrolides or tetracyclines. Mechanisms, however, do not explain the differences in antibiotic resistance potential among different classes of antibiotics. Enzyme inactivation is also the primary mechanism of aminoglycoside resistance affecting intracellular enzymes. Alterations in penicillin-binding proteins are another mechanism of antimicrobial resistance (18,19,23,37).

Of the antibiotics that cause acquired antimicrobial resistance, the commonality of mechanisms in an antibiotic class does not explain why one or two agents in a class are associated with resistance while the others are not. Ceftazidime, for example, is unique among the third-generation cephalosporins in being associated with *P. aeruginosa* resistance whereas other members of the class are not. Literature referring to third-generation cephalosporin resistance usually lumps members of this class together, which is misleading and incorrect. Studies relating to third-generation cephalosporin resistance that analyze each individual member of a class, i.e., cefotaxime, ceftizoxime, cefoperazone, ceftriaxone, and ceftazidime invariably show that ceftazidime is the sole agent responsible for the resistance among third-generation cephalosporins. A mechanistic approach does not explain why there is *P. aeruginosa* resistance problems with imipenem, but not with meropenem. In every antibiotic class, there are single members associated with resistance while the rest of the class can be used in high volume for extended periods of time without inducing any appreciable resistance. The approach to the control of resistance in the CCU depends on preventing resistance as a consequence of therapy, and containing its spread within the unit and in the hospital. Antibiotic usage should be selective, and clinicians should be aware of the resistance potential of antibiotics. In addition to their effective spectrum, antibiotics should be considered as having a high or low resistance potential. Other things being equal, the clinicians should select the antibiotic between two drugs with a similar spectrum, and select the one with a lower resistance rather than a higher resistance potential. The use of selective antimicrobial therapy, appropriate versus excessive, and more importantly, the exclusive utilization of antibiotics with a low resistance potential will minimize resistance problems in a CCU, and subsequently in the institution. If resistance problems are present in the CCU, changes in formulary/prescribing habits, as well as effective infection control measures will be needed to halt the spread of infection and eliminate the resistance problem. The substitution of antibiotics with a low resistance potential on formulary for those with a high resistance potential is the fundamental step in preventing as well as minimizing existing resistance problems (Table 2) (37,41,42).

Several unsuccessful strategies have been tried in the CCU setting to minimize resistance and include CCU formularies and antibiotic cycling in the CCU. These approaches are ineffective and have failed because they do not utilize the key

Table 2 Resistance Terminology

Natural resistance
Beyond the usual spectrum of an antibiotic. Example: ~25% of *Streptococcus pneumoniae* are
   naturally resistant to macrolides
Acquired resistance
Microbial resistance to a previously sensitive organism. Example: ampicillin-resistant
   Hemophilus influenzae
Intermediate/relative resistance
Widespread increase in MIC_{90} of organisms over time. Organisms still susceptible to
   antibiotic at achievable serum/tissue concentrations
Intermediate susceptibility/resistance is concentration sensitive because antibiotic
   susceptibility is concentration dependent. Example: penicillin-resistant *S. pneumoniae*
High-level/absolute resistance
Sudden increase in MIC_{90} of an isolate during therapy
   High-grade resistance cannot be overcome by an increasing antibiotic concentration even
      with higher than usual clinical doses. Example: gentamicin-resistant *Pseudomonas
         aeruginosa*
Use antibiotics active against highly resistant strains. Example: moxifloxacin or levofloxacin
   for penicillin-resistant *S. pneumoniae*
Class susceptibility testing
Tetracycline-resistant *S. pneumoniae* are *sensitive* to doxycycline (including most penicillin-
   resistant strains)
Antibiotic resistance class terminology
Because antibiotic resistance is agent specific, it is misleading to label antibiotic resistance as
   class phenomenon. Examples: Ceftazidime-resistant *P. aeruginosa* not 3rd generation
   cephalosporin resistant, Imipenem-resistant *P. aeruginosa* not carbapenem-resistant
   Class susceptibility testing is useful for most antibiotics, but specific antibiotic testing often
   shows differences

---

determinant of resistance, i.e., the resistance potential of the antibiotic in their approaches. Treatment should be reserved for treating bona fide infection due to these organisms (43–50).

   Although colonization precedes infection, treatment of colonizing organisms does not eliminate the colonization and predisposes to colonization by highly resistant organisms. Resistant organisms may be introduced into the CCU via a colonized patient from another part of the hospital or from the community.

The Relationship Between Antibiotic Use in the CCU and Resistance

In the intensive care setting, antibiotic use is intense, and multiple antibiotics are given because the patient's clinical situation is desperate and a specific diagnosis has not been confirmed permitting more selective therapy. Commonly in practice, antibiotics are added to "cover" organisms in the sputum, the urine, and wounds, which have no clinical relevance. Colonization of respiratory secretions in the CCU is the rule, not the exception. Unless potential pathogens acting as colonizers recovered from respiratory secretions can be shown to be the causative agent of tracheal bronchitis or nosocomial pneumonia, they should be ignored from a thera-peutic standpoint. If antibiotics with a "high resistance potential" are used to "cover" colonizing organisms particularly in respiratory secretions, then the stage is set for the transition from sensitive colonizing organisms to resistant colonizing organisms. If the patient subsequently develops an infection, it will be with a highly resistant or multiresistant organism because of unnecessary antecedent antimicrobial therapy. Although colonizing organisms should not be treated when recovered from their usual sites of colonization, treatment with a low resistance potential antibiotic is less egregious, and although unnecessary, at least will not predispose to subsequent resistance. The best clinical approach is to appreciate that the organism represents colonization and not infection, and not treat it at all, but contain its spread within the CCU with effective infection control containment measures (1,9,10,40).

Empiric antimicrobial therapy is necessarily broad, but the use of multiple antibiotics with duplicating or excessive coverage against the purported pathogen is unnecessary. Polypharmacy with broad-spectrum antibiotics can predispose to an increased incidence of drug side effects, drug–drug interactions, and promote the emergence of gram-positive resistant organisms, e.g., MRSA and VRE. As a general concept, "antibiotic tonnage" is a predictor of subsequent colonization with MRSA or VRE; however, MRSA is much more likely to be selected out from the normal flora by the use of antibiotics that predispose to MRSA colonization, i.e., ceftazidime, ciprofloxacin, and imipenem. The use of other antibiotics in each of these classes regardless of volume does not predispose to MRSA colonization. IV vancomycin is the single antibiotic that is most likely to predispose to subsequent colonization by VRE organisms. The unlimited use of other anti-MRSA antibiotics, i.e., daptomycin, linezolid, quinupristin, or dalfopristin does not predispose to VRE colonization. The clinical principle to minimize the emergence of gram-negative and gram-positive organisms in the CCU is to preferentially use antibiotics with a "low resistant potential" in preference to those in the same class with a "high resistance potential" (1,11,18,19,50).

In the CCU setting, antibiotics with a low resistance potential, which are most useful because of their spectrum and activity against aerobic gram-positive pathogens, include meropenem, cefepime, aztreonam, amikacin, third-generation cephalosporins (excluding ceftazidime), quinolones (excluding ciprofloxacin), and second-generation cephalosporins (excluding cefamandole), doxycycline/minocycline (excluding tetracycline), and polymyxin B. The antibiotics that predispose to *P. aeruginosa* resistance include ciprofloxacin, ceftazidime, and imipenem. ESBLs may be induced by the use of ceftazidime, in particular. Empiric treatment for ESBL-producing strains of *Klebsiella*, *Enterobacter*, or *E. coli* is with a carbapenem (1,18,19,37).

Against gram-positive organisms excluding *Streptococcus pneumoniae*, antibiotics that predispose to MRSA colonization include ciprofloxacin, ceftazidime, and imipenem. Against MRSA, the antibiotics that do not predispose to MRSA when being used to treat MSSA or gram-positive organisms include daptomycin, linezolid, quinupristin-dalfopristin, or minocycline. The antibiotic most likely to result in an increase in prevalence but not resistance of VRE is parenteral (not oral) vancomycin. As mentioned previously, excluding these specific examples, the nonselective use of multiple antibiotics may predispose to MRSA or VRE because the antibiotic being used does not have anti–MRSA/VRE activity. Empiric treatment with antibiotics that have activity against or do not predispose to such organisms will not result in subsequent colonization or infection with gram-positive or gram-negative organisms independent of the volume used (1,11,18,19).

Resistance Control in the CCU

The single most important concept to limit resistance among gram-positive and gram-negative organisms in the CCU is the selective use of antimicrobial agents with a "low resistance potential." To prevent spread of existing resistance problems, effective infection control measures should be combined with substituting/preferentially using antibiotics with a "low resistance potential" in place of those with a "high resistance potential," which are responsible for the problem. If resistance problems are viewed in this context, it is apparent what constitutes effective and ineffective methods to control resistance in the CCU (Table 3) (30,48–50).

Table 3 Antibiotic Resistance

Key concepts
Antibiotic resistance is agent specific
  Antibiotic resistance is not related to antibiotic class, or duration of use

Antibiotic (agent-specific) resistance occurs early, not late
  If antibiotic resistance to a specific antibiotic develops, it occurs early, within 2 years of
    general use
  Antibiotics demonstrating resistance early, high resistance potential antibiotics, will have
    resistance problems as long as the antibiotic is used
  Antibiotics that do not develop resistance problems within 2 years of use, low resistance
    potential antibiotics, do not develop resistance later, even after prolonged/high volume use
Control strategies
Successful resistance preventative strategies
  Eliminate antibiotics from animal feeds
  Restricted hospital formulary (controlled usage of antibiotics with high resistance
    potential)

Unsuccessful resistance preventative strategies
  Rotating formularies
  Special/rotating CCU/ICU formularies
  Restricting certain antibiotic classes (3rd generation cephalosporins, quinolones)
  "Reserving" antibiotics for future use
  Combination therapy to avoid resistance[a]
    antibiotic de-escalation

Successful antibiotic resistance control strategies
  Effective infection control measures
    Microbial surveillance to detect resistance problems early
    Rapid implementation of infection control precautions to limit/contain spread of clonal
      resistance
Hospital formulary
  Restricted hospital formulary (strictly controlled usage of antibiotics with high resistance
    potential)
  Unrestricted use of antibiotics with a low resistance potential
CCU prescriber
  Preferentially use low resistance potential antibiotics instead of high resistance potential
    antibiotics with the same spectrum

Abbreviations: CCU, critical care unit; ICU, intensive care unit.
Source: with few exceptions (antipseudomonal penicillins and aminoglycosides, HIV therapy, anti-TB therapy) combining antibiotics (a low resistance at high resistance potential antibiotic or two high resistance potential antibiotics)

Ineffective measures include nonselective limiting of antimicrobial volume. Volume is only indirectly related to VRE colonization but not resistance per se. Special CCU formularies also are ineffective because they do not address the fundamental problem of considering antibiotics as having a high or low resistance potential. The limited CCU formulary also does not take into account the problem of the introduction of patients from the community/hospital with resistant organisms, patients outside of the CCU/hospital, and the transfer of patients outside of the CCU into the hospital/community with newly acquired resistant organisms (48–50).

Antibiotic cycling is another unproven and potentially dangerous maneuver. Antibiotic cycling ignores the critical importance of the resistance potential of the antibiotics being cycled. Cycling of low resistance antibiotics is prone to failure and will cause more resistance and not even control the existing resistance problems. If high and low resistance antibiotics are cycled without appreciating the difference in their resistance potential, then the potential good of the low resistance antibiotics is negated by the subsequent cycling of antibiotics with a high resistance potential. If clinicians in the CCU are preferentially using antibiotics with a low resistance potential, there is no reason for or potential benefit from antibiotic cycling (43,44,50).

Effective Antibiotic Resistance Measures in the CCU

The infection control measures aside, from an antibiotic usage standpoint, the two most critical factors in controlling antibiotic resistance are a selective antibiotic formulary and selective antibiotic use in the CCU that substitutes low resistance potential antibiotics for those with the same spectrum that are of a high resistance potential in each antibiotic class. If an institution has existing resistance problems in the CCU, then first, formulary substitution should be made, allowing the unrestricted use of low-resistant potential antibiotics, and highly restrict or eliminate their high resistance potential counterparts. A change in formulary, if not negated by a separate CCU formulary, can then be implemented by physicians prescribing low resistance antibiotics preferentially in the CCU setting. These two factors operating in concert with effective infection control measures will prevent, minimize, and/or reverse resistance problems in the CCU (5,37,41,48–50).

REFERENCES

1. Cunha BA. Antibiotic Essentials (5th Ed). Royal Oak, MI: Physicians Press, 2006.
2. Cunha BA. Factors in antibiotic selection for the seriously-ill hospitalized patients. Antibiot Clin 2003; 7(S2):19–24.
3. Cunha BA. Factors in antibiotic formulary selection: antibiotic spectrum (part I). Pharm Ther 2003; 28:396–399.
4. Cunha BA. Factors in antibiotic formulary selection: pharmacokinetics/pharmacodynamic factors (part II). Pharm Ther 2003; 28:468–470.
5. Cunha BA. Factors in antibiotic formulary selection: antibiotic resistance (part III). Pharm Ther 2003; 28:524–527.
6. Cunha BA. Factors in antibiotic formulary selection: antibiotic adverse effects (part IV). Pharm Ther 2003; 28:594–596.
7. Cunha BA. Factors in antibiotic formulary selection: antibiotic costs (part V). Pharm Ther 2003; 28:662–665.
8. Pankey GA, Sabath LD. Clinical relevance of bacteriostatic versus bactericidal mechanisms of action in the treatment of gram-positive bacterial infections. Clin Infect Dis 2004; 38:864–870.

9. Cunha BA. Intensive care, not intensive antibiotics. Heart Lung 1994; 23:361–362.

10. Ambrose PG, Owens RC Jr., Quintiliani R, et al. Antibiotic use in the critical care unit. Crit Care Clin 1998; 14:283–308.

11. Kucers A, Crowe S, Grayson ML, et al., eds. The Use of Antibiotics: A Clinical Review of Antibacterial, Antifungal, and Antiviral Drugs. 5th ed. Oxford: Butterworth-Heinemann, 1997.

12. Anderson RJ, Schrier RW, eds. Clinical Use of Drugs in Patients with Kidney and Liver Disease. Philadelphia, WB: Saunders Company, 1981.

13. Bennett WM, Aronoff GR, Golper TA, et al., eds. Drug Prescribing in Renal Failure. 2nd ed. Philadelphia: American College of Physicians, 2000.

14. Moellering RC Jr. Monitoring serum vancomycin levels: climbing the mountain because it is there? Clin Infect Dis 1994; 18:544–546.

15. Cunha BA, Deglin J, Chow M, et al. Pharmacokinetics of vancomycin in patients undergoing chronic hemodialysis. Rev Infect Dis 1981; 3:269–272.

16. Cunha BA. Vancomycin serum levels: unnecessary, unhelpful, and costly. Antibiot Clin 2004; 8:273–277.

17. Ristuccia AM, Cunha BA, eds. Antimicrobial Therapy. New York: Raven Press, 1984.

18. Gorbach SL, Bartlett JG, Blacklow NR, eds. Infectious Diseases. 4th ed. Philadelphia: Lippincott Williams Wilkins, 2004.

19. Mandell GL, Bennett JE, Dolin R, eds. Mandell, Douglas and Bennett's Principles and Practice of Infectious Diseases. 6th ed. Philadelphia: Elsevier, 2005.

20. Brook I. Management of anaerobic infection. Expert Rev Anti Infect Ther 2004; 2: 153–158.

21. Clark NM, Patterson J, Lynch JP III. Antimicrobial resistance among gram-negative organisms in the intensive care unit. Curr Opin Crit Care 2003; 9:413–423.

22. Clark NM, Hershberger E, Zervosc MJ, et al. Antimicrobial resistance among gram-positive organisms in the intensive care unit. Curr Opin Crit Care 2003; 9:403–412.

23. Acar JF. Resistance mechanisms. Semin Respir Infect 2002; 17:184–188.

24. Leibovici L, Soares-Weiser K, Paul M, et al. Considering resistance in systemic reviews of antibiotic treatment. J Antimicrob Chemother 2003; 52:564–571.

25. Carlet J, Ben Ali A, Chalfine A. Epidemiology and control of antibiotic resistance in the intensive care unit. Curr Opin Infect Dis 2004; 17:309–316.

26. Sasaki M, Hiyama E, Takesue Y, et al. Clinical surveillance of surgical imipenem-resistant *Pseudomonas aeruginosa* infection in a Japanese hospital. J Hosp Infect 2004; 56: 111–118.

27. Lee SO, Kim NJ, Choi SH, et al. Risk factors for acquisition of imipenem-resistant *Acinetobacter baumannii*: a case-control study. Antimicrob Agents Chemother 2004; 48:1070.

28. Ferraro MJ. The rise of fluoroquinolone resistance: fact or fiction. J Chemother 2002; 14(suppl 3):31–41.

29. Defez C, Fabbro-Peray P, Bouziges N, et al. Risk factors for multidrug-resistant *Pseudomonas aeruginosa* nosocomial infection. J Hosp Infect 2004; 57:209–216.

30. Cunha BA. *Pseudomonas aeruginosa*: Antibiotic resistance and antimicrobial therapy. Semin Respir Ther 2002; 17:231–239.

31. Cunha BA. Ciprofloxacin resistant *Streptococcus pneumoniae* not fluoroquinolone-resistant *Streptococcus pneumoniae*. Infect Dis Pract 2000; 24:30–31.

32. Cunha BA. Clinical manifestations and antimicrobial therapy of methicillin-resistant *Staphylococcus aureus* (MRSA). Clin Microbiol Infect 2005 11:33–42.

33. Cunha BA. Antibiotic side effects. Med Clin North Am 2001; 85:149–185.

34. Cunha BA, Klein NC. The selection and use of cephalosporins: a review. Adv Ther 1995; 12:83–101.

35. Cunha BA. Antimicrobial selection in the penicillin allergic patients. Drugs Today 2001; 37:337–383.

36. Cunha BA, Wu P, Qadri SMH. Meropenem inhibition of endotoxin release from *E. coli*. Adv Ther 1997; 14:168–171.

37. Bartlett JG. Clinical practice. Antibiotic-associated diarrhea. N Engl J Med 2002; 346:334–339.
38. Raymond DP, Pelletier SJ, Crabtree TD, et al. Impact of antibiotic-resistant gram-negative bacilli infections on outcome in hospitalized patients. Crit Care Med 2003; 31: 1035–1041.
39. Masterton R, Drusano G, Paterson DL, et al. Appropriate antimicrobial treatment in nosocomial infections—the clinical challenges. J Hosp Infect 2003; 55(suppl 1):1–12.
40. Hessen MT, Kaye D. Principles of use of antibacterial agents. Infect Dis Clin North Am 2004; 18:435–450.
41. Cunha BA. Antimicrobial resistance: myths, truths, and a rational formulary approach. Formulary 1999; 34:664–682.
42. Cunha BA. Antimicrobial resistance: strategies for control. Med Clin North Am 2000; 84:1407–1427.
43. Brown EM, Nathwani D. Antibiotic cycling or rotation: a systematic review of the evidence of efficacy. J Antimicrob Chemother 2005; 55:6–9.
44. Masterton RG. Antibiotic cycling: more than it might seem? J Antimicrob Chemother 2005; 55:1–5.
45. Gerding DN, Larson TA, Hughes RA, et al. Aminoglycoside resistance and aminoglycoside usage: ten years of experience in one hospital. Antimicrob Agents Chemother 1991; 35:1284–1290.
46. Cunha BA. Prevention of aminoglycoside resistance by the use of amikacin. Adv Ther 1987; 4:33–39.
47. Cunha BA. Formulary restrictions of streptogrammins/oxolinidones. J Crit Ill 2001; 16:522–523.
48. Cunha BA. Antibiotic resistance: control strategies. Crit Care Clin 1998; 8:309–328.
49. Cunha BA. Strategies to control antibiotic resistance. Semin Respir Crit Care Med 2000; 21:3–8.
50. Cunha BA. Effective antibiotic resistance and control strategies. Lancet 2001; 357: 1307–1308.

32

Antimicrobial Therapy in the Penicillin-Allergic Patient in the Critical Care Unit

Burke A. Cunha

Infectious Disease Division, Winthrop-University Hospital, Mineola, and State University of New York School of Medicine, Stony Brook, New York, U.S.A.

INTRODUCTION

Empiric antimicrobial therapy is a necessity in the critically ill patient with a life-threatening infectious disease. There are several factors that go into antibiotic selection including spectrum of activity against the presumed pathogens, which is related to the source of infection or organ system involved; second, pharmacokinetic and pharmacodynamic considerations which affect dosing and concentration in the source organ for the sepsis; third, the resistance potential of the antibiotic. Although cure of the patient is the immediate priority, drug selection has a subsequent effect on the flora of the critical care unit (CCU) and eventually may impact on the flora of the hospital. The fourth consideration is the safety profile of the drug, which has to do with adverse side effects and interactions, as well as the patient's allergic drug history. One of the most common problems encountered in treating critically ill patients is the question of penicillin allergy.

DETERMINING THE TYPE OF PENICILLIN ALLERGY

There are no good data on the incidence of penicillin allergy. Some studies are done using skin testing to derive their data. Other studies are based on clinical information, i.e., questioning the patient or relatives regarding the nature of the penicillin allergy. Many times, penicillin allergy is mentioned, and is not truly allergic reaction at all upon further or detailed questioning. Patients, if they are able to respond, are either vague or very clear about the nature of their penicillin allergy. In the critical care setting, there is often no way to get a drug allergy history. Relatives are usually uncertain as to the nature of the allergic reaction of the patient. There is a poor correlation between the patient reporting penicillin allergy and subsequent penicillin skin testing. In critical care medicine, the patient's history is the only piece of information that the clinician has to work with to make a decision regarding the nature of possible penicillin allergy (1–5). Because β-lactam antibiotics are one of the most common classes of antibiotics used, the question of using these agents in patients with penicillin allergy is a daily consideration. The clinical approach to the patient with a potential skin allergy involves determining the nature of the penicillin allergy as well as selecting an agent with a spectrum appropriate to the organ source of the sepsis. Penicillin allergies may be considered as those that result in anaphylactic reactions, i.e., anaphylaxis, laryngospasm, bronchospasm, hypotension, or total body hives, and those that result in nonanaphylactic reactions, i.e., drug fever or skin rash. Patients with nonanaphylactoid skin reactions may safely be given β-lactam antibiotics with a spectrum appropriate to the site of infection. Patients with a history of anaphylactic reaction to penicillin should be treated with an antibiotic of another class that has a spectrum appropriate to the focus of infection (6–11).

PENICILLIN ALLERGIC REACTIONS

In the critical care setting, when urgent antimicrobial therapy is necessary, there is no time for skin testing to rule out or confirm penicillin allergy. Patients who are communicative can indicate, on direct questioning, the nature of their penicillin reaction. Often times, what is considered a penicillin reaction by the patient is in fact an unrelated drug side effect. Patients often report a vague history of penicillin allergy during childhood, which has not recurred subsequently, while others report penicillin allergy occurred in close relatives but not themselves. Some patients were told they had a drug fever due to penicillin, but did not develop a rash; yet others report the reaction to a penicillin antibiotic was limited to a maculopapular rash. Responses to any of these indicate that if the patient had a reaction to penicillin, it was of the nonanaphylactoid variety. Patients with drug fever or rash due to penicillins may be safely given penicillins again (12,13). Reactions to β-lactams are stereotyped such that if the patient had a fever as the manifestation of penicillin allergy, on rechallenge, the patient will develop fever again as opposed to another clinical manifestation of penicillin allergy. Patients with drug fevers or drug rashes due to penicillins, at worst, will only have a similar nonanaphylactic reaction upon rechallenge with penicillin. Alternately, they may have no reaction at all if the β-lactam chosen is sufficiently different antigenetically than the one initially causing the reaction. It is not uncommon in clinical practice with third-generation cephalosporin allergies to have patients not react to cefoperazone, which is the most antigenemic member of third-generations cephalosporins. Among the second-generation cephalosporins, cefoxitin is the least likely to cross-react with other second-generation cephalosporins (12–14).

CROSS REACTIONS BETWEEN PENICILLINS AND β-LACTAMS

When cephalosporins were first introduced, the reported cross-reactivity rate with penicillins is was high as 30%. Subsequently, actual cross-allergic reactions were less than 3%. Many of the cross-reactions initially reported between penicillins and cephalosporins were nonspecific allergic reactions not based on penicillin/cephalosporin cross-reactivity. Patients with a penicillin allergy who have had a nonanaphylactic reaction may safely be given a β-lactam antibiotic. In the unlikely event the patient has a reaction, the patient would develop a drug fever or rash, but not anaphylaxis. The β-lactam class of drugs includes the penicillins, the semisynthetic penicillins, the modified penicillins, the amino-penicillins, and the ureido-penicillins (15–22).

CARBAPENEMS AND MONOBACTAMS

From an allergic perspective, β-lactams may be divided into carbapenems and noncarbapenems. Among the noncarbapenems are first-, second-, third-, and fourth-generation cephalosporins. Allergy to one is likely to result in cross-reactivity with another with the exceptions of cefoxitin among the second-generation cephalosporins, and cefoperazone among the third-generation cephalosporins. Although carbapenems are structurally related to β-lactam antibiotics from an allergic perspective, they should not be regarded as β-lactam antibiotics. Carbapenems, e.g., meropenem, do not react with other β-lactams or penicillin-derivatives. Therefore, carbapenems are frequently used as an alternative class of antibiotics to β-lactams and do not cross-react with any penicillin or β-lactam to such an extent that the reaction would be reportable in the literature. Carbapenems in general, and meropenem in particular, are completely safe to give patients with known/suspected history of penicillin anaphylaxis. The more likely the history of anaphylaxis to penicillin, the more confidently the clinician can use meropenem (23–25).

NON–β-LACTAM ANTIBIOTICS IN PATIENTS WITH PENICILLIN ANAPHYLACTIC REACTIONS

In patients giving a history of an anaphylactic reaction, i.e., anaphylaxis, laryngospasm, bronchospasm, hypotension, or total body hives, it is important to select a non–β-lactam antibiotic to avoid complicating the already serious situation in the critical care setting. As with nonanaphylactoid penicillin reactions, anaphylactic reactions tend to be stereotyped with repeated exposures. Patients who develop laryngospasm as the manifestation of their penicillin allergy do not develop total body hives on subsequent reexposure but will repeatedly develop laryngospasm as the main manifestation of their anaphylactic reaction. As with other manifestations of anaphylaxis, the reactions are stereotyped and will be repetitive and not change to another anaphylactoid manifestation. Fortunately, there are many highly effective non–β-lactam antibiotics available at the present time, therefore, invariably there are many appropriate non–β-lactam antibiotics to choose from to treat the life-threatening infections encountered in the CCU (Table 1) (22–25).

Antibiotic classes that have no allergic cross-reactivity with β-lactams include the macrolides, tetracyclines, clindamycin, chloramphenicol, trimethoprim-sulfamethoxazole (TMP-SMX), aminoglycosides, metronidazole, polymyxin B, vancomycin, quinupristin/dalfopristin, linezolid, daptomycin, quinolones, tigacycline, monobactams, and as previously mentioned, carbapenems. In 30 years of clinical experience in infectious disease, I have never had to resort to penicillin desensitization in order to treat a patient. There is always an alternative, non–β-lactam antibiotic, which is suitable for virtually every conceivable clinical situation. Although penicillin sensitivity testing/desensitization is a potential consideration in the noncritical ambulatory patient, in the critical care setting there is no time or need for penicillin testing/desensitization. If there is any question about a penicillin allergy in a noncommunicative patient in the CCU, then monotherapy or combination therapy with one of the non–β-lactam antibiotics mentioned above is appropriate and safe. The non–β-lactam antibiotics most useful in the critical care setting for the most common infectious disease syndromes encountered are presented here in tabular form (Table 2) (22,26).

Table 1 Antimicrobials Safe to Use in Penicillin-Allergic Patients in the Critical Care Unit

Antibacterials	*Antivirals*
Carbapenems	Amantadine
Imipenem	Rimantadine
Ertapenem	Acyclovir
Meropenem	Gancyclovir
Monobactams	Valganciclovir
Aztreonam	*Aminoglycosides*
Quinolones	Gentamicin
Ciprofloxacin	Tobramycin
Levofloxacin	Amikacin
Gatifloxacin	*Tetracyclines*
Moxifloxacin	Doxycycline
Antifungals	Minocycline
Amphotericin B	
Amphotericin B	*Other*
Lipid Preparations	Clindamycin
Flucytosine	Chloramphenicol
Fluconazole	TMP-SMX
Itraconazole	Rifampin
Posaconazole	Polymyxin B
Caspofungin	Vancomycin
Voriconazole	Quinupristin/
Anidulafungin	Dalfopristin
	Linezolid
	Daptomycin
	Tigacycline

Abbreviation: TMP-SMX, trimethoprim-sulfamethoxazole.

CONCLUSION

The incidence of penicillin allergy in the general population has been estimated to range between 1% to 10%, but no good reliable data exist on the actual incidence of penicillin allergy. Penicillin data derived from penicillin skin testing does not correlate with penicillin reactions in the clinical setting. Many patients reporting penicillin allergy have in fact had reactions to penicillin which are not on an allergic basis. Penicillin reactions are of the nonanaphylactic or anaphylactic variety if they are indeed penicillin reactions. Penicillin reactions may occur on a single exposure to a penicillin or β-lactam antibiotic. From questioning or previous history, patients' bona fide penicillin reactions may be classified as anaphylactic or nonanaphylactic. Because the cross-reactivity between β-lactams and penicillin is so low, β-lactam antibiotics may be used in patients who have had drug fever or a drug rash as the primary manifestation of their penicillin allergy. Should the patient develop an allergic cross-reaction between the β-lactam and the penicillin, the allergic manifestation will be of the same type as encountered previously.

In patients with a history of anaphylactic reactions to penicillin, it is essential to use a non–β-lactam antibiotic, i.e., a carbapenem, monobactam, quinolone, clindamycin, TMP-SMX, quinupristin/dalfopristin, linezolid, vancomycin, daptomycin, clindamycin, metronidazole, polymyxin B, or an aminoglycoside. As with nonanaphylactic

Table 2 Antibiotics Safe in Penicillin-Allergic Adult Patients in the Critical Care Unit

Clinical Syndrome	Penicillin Allergic	Non-Penicillin Allergic
Bacterial meningitis (pathogen unknown) S. pneumoniae, MSSA)	Meropenem (meningeal dose) TMP-SMX Vancomycin (plus I.T. dose) Chloramphenicol	Penicillin Ampicillin Ceftriaxone Cefepime (meningeal dose)
Brain abscess	Meropenem (meningeal dose) TMP-SMX Chloramphenicol TMP-SMX plus Metronidazole	Penicillin Ceftizoxime
Severe CAP	Respiratory quinolone Doxycycline	Ceftizoxime Cefepime
NP	Meropenem ± either Aztreonam or Amikacin	Cefepime Piperacillin/tazobactam
ABE (MSSA/MRSA)	Daptomycin Linezolid Quinupristin/dalfopristin Vancomycin	Nafcilllin Cefazolin
Pseudomonas aeruginosa	Polymyxin B Meropenem ± either Aztreonam or Amikacin	Piperacillin/tazobactam Cefepime
Cholangitis	Meropenem Tigacycline	Cefoxitin Cefoperazone Ceftizoxime Piperacillin/tazobactam Ampicillin plus 1st generation cephalosporin
Bacterial liver abscess	Meropenem Tigacycline	Cefoxitin Cefoperazone Ceftizoxime Piperacillin/tazobactam Ampicillin + 1st generation cephalosporin
Intra-abdominal source (colitis, peritonitis, obstruction, or abscess)	Meropenem Ertapenem Moxifloxacin Tigacycline Aztreonam plus either Metronidazole or Clindamycin	Piperacillin/tazobactam Cefoxitin Cefoperazone Ceftizoxime
Pelvic source (peritonitis, intraovarian abscess, septic pelvic thrombophlebitis)	Meropenem Ertapenem Moxifloxacin Tigacycline Aztreonam plus eith Metronidazole or Clindamycin	Piperacillin/tazobactam Cefoxitin Cefoperazone Ceftizoxime
Urosepsis (gram-negative aerobic bacilli)	Aztreonam Aminoglycoside TMP-SMX	

(Continued)

Table 2 Antibiotics Safe in Penicillin-Allergic Adult Patients in the Critical Care Unit (*Continued*)

Clinical Syndrome	Penicillin Allergic	Non-Penicillin Allergic
(Enterococci)	Linezolid	Ampicillin
E. faecalis (non-VRE)	Daptomycin	Piperacillin
	Vancomycin	
E. faecium (VRE)	Daptomycin	None
	Linezolid	
	Quinupristin/Dalfopristin	
Serious wound	Meropenem	
Infections	Ertapenem	Piperacillin/tazobactam
(Diabetic "fetid foot")	Moxifloxacin	
	Tigacycline	
Gas Gangrene	Clindamycin	Penicillin
	Meropenem	Piperacillin/tazobactam
Necrotizing fasciitis	Meropenem	Piperacillin/tazobactam
	Imipenem	Cefoxitin
	Ertapenem	
Sepsis (unknown source)	Meropenem	Piperacillin/tazobactam

Abbreviations: TMP-SMX, trimethoprim-sulfamethoxazole; I.T., intrathecal; MSSA, methicillin-sensitive *Staphylococcus aureus*; MRSA, methicillin-resistant *Staphylococcus aureus*; ABE, acute bacterial endocarditis; CAP, community-acquired pneumonia; NP, nosocomial pneumonia; VRE, vancomycin resistant enterococci.
Source: Adapted from Ref. 23, 25.

penicillin cross-reactions, anaphylactic reactions to penicillin also tend to be stereotyped, and upon repeated exposure have the same clinical expression as initially manifested in their allergic response. If there is any doubt about the exact nature of the penicillin allergy, it is not unreasonable to use a non–β-lactam antibiotic to eliminate the concern for potential penicillin allergy in such patients. Because the therapeutic armamentarium at the present time is so extensive, it is virtually never necessary to desensitize a patient in the critical care setting to receive a β-lactam when so many non–β-lactam antibiotics are available and effective.

REFERENCES

1. Salkind AR, Cuddy PG, Foxworth JW. Is this patient allergic to penicillin? JAMA 2001; 285:2498–2505
2. Surtees SJ, Stockton MG, Gietzen TW. Allergy to penicillin: fable or fact? Br J Med 1991; 302:1051–1052.
3. Lazarou J, Pomeranz BH, Corey PN. Incidence of adverse drug reactions in hospitalized patients: a meta-analysis of prospective studies. JAMA 1998; 279:1200–1205.
4. Kerr JR. Penicillin allergy: a study of incidence as reported by patients. Br J Clin Practr 1994; 48:5–7.
5. Solensky R, Earl HS, Gruchalla RS. Penicillin allergy: prevalence of vague history in skin test-positive patients. Ann Allergy Asthma Immunol 2000; 85:195–199.
6. Lin RY. A perspective on penicillin allergy. Arch Intern Med 1992; 152:930–937.
7. Green GR, Rosenblum AH, Sweet LC. Evaluation of penicillin hypersensitivity: value of clinical history and skin testing with penicilloyl-polylysine and penicillin G: a cooperative

prospective study of the penicillin study group of the American Academy of Allergy. J Allergy Clin Immunol 1977; 60:339–345.

 8. Idsoe O, Guthe T, Willcox RR, et al. Nature and extent of penicillin side-reactions, with particular reference to fatalities from anaphylactic shock. Bull World Health Organ 1968; 38:159–188.

 9. Sogn DD, Evans R III, Shepherd GM, et al. Results of the national institute of allergy and infectious disease collaborative clinical trial to test the predictive value of skin testing with major and minor penicillin derivatives in hospitalized adults. Arch Intern Med 1992; 152:1025–1032.

10. Fonacier L, Davis-Lorton M. Antibiotic adverse effects: penicillin allergy and desensitization. Antibiotics for Clin 1989; 2:109–113.

11. Levine BB, Zolov DM. Prediction of penicillin allergy by immunological tests. J Allergy 1969; 43:231–244.

12. Shapiro S, Slone D, Siskind V, et al. Drug rash with ampicillin and other penicillins. Lancet 1969; 2:969–972.

13. Shepherd GM. Allergy to β-lactam antibiotics. Immunol Allergy Clin North Am 1991; 11:611–633.

14. Cunha BA, Ristuccia A. The third-generation cephalosporins. Med Clin North Am 1982; 66:283–291.

15. Anne S, Reisman RE. Risk of administering cephalosporin antibiotics to patients with histories of penicillin allergy. Ann Allergy Asthma Immunol 1995; 74:167–170.

16. Blanca M, Fernandez J, Miranda A, et al. Cross-reactivity between penicillins and cephalosporins: clinical and immunological studies. J Allergy Clin Immunol 1989; 83:381–385.

17. Saxon A, Beall GN, Rohr AS, et al. Immediate hypersensitivity reactions to β-lactam antibiotics. Ann Intern Med 1987; 107:204–214.

18. Thethi AK, Van Dellen RG. Dilemmas and controversies in penicillin allergy. Immunol Allergy Clin North Am 2004; 24:445–461.

19. Weiss ME, Adkinson NF. Immediate hypersensitivity reactions to penicillin and related antibiotics. Clin Allergy 1988; 18:515–540.

20. Kelkar PS, Li JT. Cephalosporin allergy. N Engl J Med 2001; 345:804–809.

21. Daulat S, Solensky R, Earl HS, et al. Safety of cephalosporin administration to patients with histories of penicillin allergy. J Allergy Clin Immunol 2004; 113:1220–1222.

22. Novalbos A, Sastre J, Cuesta J, et al. Lack of allergic cross-reactivity to cephalosporins among patients allergic to penicillins. Clin Exp Allergy 2001; 31:438-443.

23. Cunha BA. Cross allergenicity of penicillin with carbapenems and monobactams. J Crit Illness 1998; 13:344.

24. Cunha BA. The safety of meropenem in elderly and renally-impaired patients. Int J Antimicrob Ther 1998; 10:109–117.

25. Cunha BA. Antimicrobial selection in the penicillin-allergic patient. Drugs of Today 2001; 37:377–383.

26. Cunha BA. Antibiotic side effects. Med Clin North Am 2001; 85:149–185.

Index

633

About the Editor

Burke A. Cunha is Chief, Infectious Disease Division, Winthrop-University Hospital, Mineola, New York, and Professor of Medicine, State University of New York School of Medicine, Stony Brook, New York. Dr. Cunha is the author or coauthor of more than 120 abstracts, 100 electronic publications, 950 articles, and 150 book chapters. He has edited 15 books on various infectious disease topics and is editor-in-chief of the journals *Infectious Disease Practice* and *Antibiotics for Clinicians*. Dr. Cunha is a fellow of the Infectious Diseases Society of America, the American Academy of Microbiology, the American College of Clinical Pharmacology, and the American College of Chest Physicians. Dr. Cunha's major clinical and research interests are fever, pneumonias, nosocomial infections, sepsis, infections in compromised hosts, antimicrobial therapy, antibiotic resistance, and surgical infections. Dr. Cunha received the M.D. degree from the Pennsylvania State University College of Medicine, Hershey, Pennsylvania.